T0076413

SAUNDERS

EDITION

Q&A REVIEW FOR THE NCLEX-PN® EXAMINATION

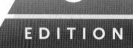

Linda Anne Silvestri, PhD, RN, FAAN

Nursing Instructor
University of Nevada, Las Vegas
Las Vegas, Nevada

President
Nursing Reviews, Inc. and Professional Nursing Seminars, Inc.
Henderson, Nevada

Elsevier
Next Generation NCLEX® (NGN) Thought Leader

Angela E. Silvestri, PhD, APRN, FNP-BC, CNE

Assistant Professor and *BSN Program Director*
University of Nevada, Las Vegas
Las Vegas, Nevada

President
Nurse Prep, LLC
Henderson, Nevada

Associate Editors

Eileen H. Gray, DNP, RN, CPNP

Nursing Instructor
University of Nevada, Las Vegas
Las Vegas, Nevada

Consultant and *Editor*
Nursing Reviews, Inc.
Henderson, Nevada

Allison E. Bowser, MEd, BS

Consultant and *Editor*
Nursing Reviews, Inc.
Henderson, Nevada

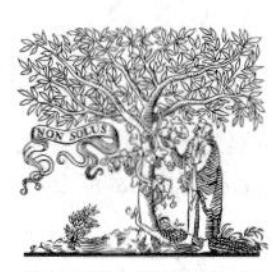

ELSEVIER

Elsevier
3251 Riverport Lane
St. Louis, Missouri 63043

SAUNDERS Q & A REVIEW FOR THE NCLEX-PN® EXAMINATION,
SIXTH EDITION
ISBN: 978-0-323-79534-0
Copyright © 2023 by Elsevier, Inc. All rights reserved.

No part of this publication may be reproduced or transmitted in any form or by any means, electronic or mechanical, including photocopying, recording, or any information storage and retrieval system, without permission in writing from the publisher. Details on how to seek permission, further information about the Publisher's permissions policies and our arrangements with organizations such as the Copyright Clearance Center and the Copyright Licensing Agency, can be found at our website: www.elsevier.com/permissions.

This book and the individual contributions contained in it are protected under copyright by the Publisher (other than as may be noted herein).

Notice

Practitioners and researchers must always rely on their own experience and knowledge in evaluating and using any information, methods, compounds or experiments described herein. Because of rapid advances in the medical sciences, in particular, independent verification of diagnoses and drug dosages should be made. To the fullest extent of the law, no responsibility is assumed by Elsevier, authors, editors or contributors for any injury and/or damage to persons or property as a matter of products liability, negligence or otherwise, or from any use or operation of any methods, products, instructions, or ideas contained in the material herein.

Previous editions copyrighted 2020, 2010, 2007, 2004, and 2000.
NCLEX®, NCLEX-RN®, and NCLEX-PN® are registered trademarks of the National Council of State Boards of Nursing, Inc.

Library of Congress Control Number: 2021943489

Content Strategist: Heather Bays-Petrovic
Senior Content Development Specialist: Laura Klein
Publishing Services Manager: Julie Eddy
Senior Project Manager: Cindy Thoms
Design Direction: Maggie Reid

Printed in India

Last digit is the print number: 9 8 7 6 5 4 3 2

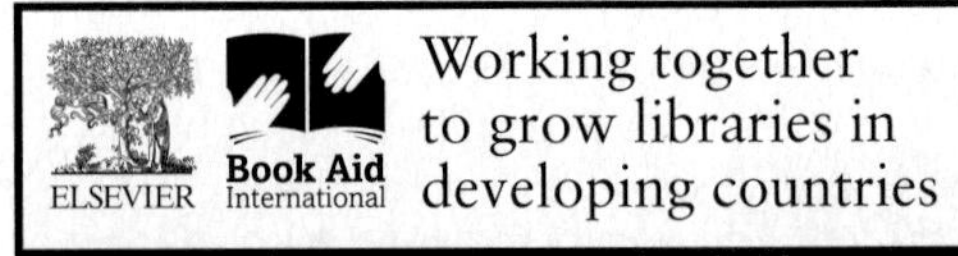

To my father and my mother and Angela's grandfather and grandmother,
Arnold Lawrence and Frances Mary
Our memories of their love, support, and words of encouragement will remain
in our hearts forever!
and
To our many nursing students, past, present, and future: their inspiration has brought many
personal and professional rewards to our lives!

To All Future Nurses,

Congratulations to you!

You should be very proud and pleased with yourself on your accomplishments in nursing, as well as your well-deserved success in completing your nursing program to become a licensed practical/vocational nurse. We know that you have worked very hard to be successful and that you have proven to yourself that indeed you can achieve your goals.

In our opinion, you are about to enter the most wonderful and rewarding profession that exists. Your willingness, desire, and ability to assist those who need nursing care will bring great satisfaction to your life. In the profession of nursing, learning is a lifelong process, which makes the profession stimulating and dynamic and ensures that your learning will continue to expand and grow as the profession continues to evolve. Your next very important endeavor will be the learning process needed to achieve success in your examination to become a licensed practical/vocational nurse.

We are excited and pleased to be able to provide you with the *Saunders Pyramid to Success* products, which will help you prepare for your next important professional goal: becoming a licensed practical/vocational nurse. We want to thank all our former nursing students whom we have assisted in their studies for the NCLEX-PN® examination for their willingness to offer ideas regarding their needs in preparing for licensure. Student ideas have certainly added a special uniqueness to all the products available in the *Saunders Pyramid to Success.*

Saunders Pyramid to Success products provide you with everything that you need to ready yourself for the NCLEX-PN® examination. These products include material that is required for the NCLEX-PN® examination for all nursing students regardless of educational background, specific strengths, areas in need of improvement, or clinical experience during the nursing program.

So, let's get started and begin our journey through the *Saunders Pyramid to Success,* and welcome to the wonderful profession of nursing!

Sincerely,

Linda Anne Silvestri, PhD, RN, FAAN

Angela E. Silvestri, PhD, APRN, FNP-BC, CNE

About the Authors

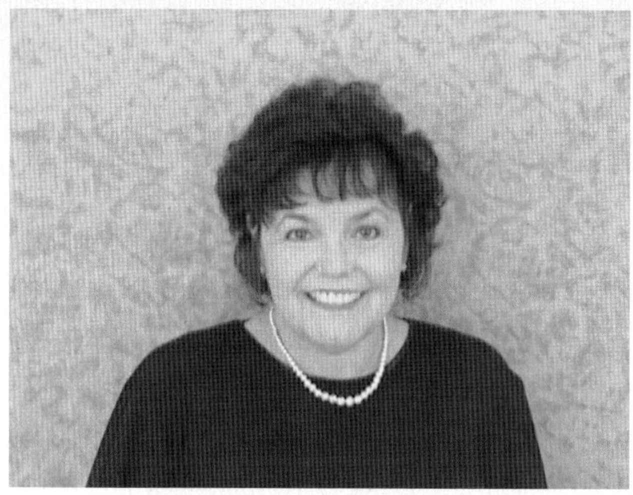

Linda Anne Silvestri (Photo by Laurent W. Valliere)

As a child, I always dreamed of becoming either a nurse or a teacher. Initially I chose to become a nurse because I really wanted to help others, especially those who were ill. Then I realized that both of my dreams could come true; I could be both a nurse and a teacher. So I pursued my dreams.

I received my diploma in nursing at Cooley Dickinson Hospital School of Nursing in Northampton, Massachusetts. Afterward, I worked at Baystate Medical Center in Springfield, Massachusetts, where I cared for clients in acute medical-surgical units, the intensive care unit, the emergency department, pediatric units, and other acute care units. Later, I received an associate degree from Holyoke Community College in Holyoke, Massachusetts, my BSN from American International College in Springfield, Massachusetts, and my MSN from Anna Maria College in Paxton, Massachusetts, with a dual major in nursing management and patient education. I received my PhD in nursing from the University of Nevada, Las Vegas (UNLV), and conducted research on self-efficacy and the predictors of NCLEX success. In 2012, I received the UNLV School of Nursing Alumna of the Year Award. In October 2019, I was inducted as a Fellow in the American Academy of Nursing. I am also a member of the Honor Society of Nursing, Sigma Theta Tau International, Phi Kappa Phi, the Western Institute of Nursing, the Golden Key International Honour Society, the National League for Nursing, and the American Nurses Association.

As a native of Springfield, Massachusetts, I began my teaching career as an instructor of medical-surgical nursing and leadership-management nursing in 1981 at Baystate Medical Center School of Nursing. In 1989, I relocated to Rhode Island and began teaching advanced medical-surgical nursing and psychiatric nursing to RN and LPN students at the Community College of Rhode Island. While I was teaching there, a group of students approached me for assistance in preparing for the NCLEX examination. I have always had a very special interest in test success for nursing students because of my own personal experiences with testing. Taking tests was never easy for me, and as a student I needed to find methods and strategies that would bring success. My own difficult experiences, desire, and dedication to assist nursing students to overcome the obstacles associated with testing inspired me to develop and write the many products that would foster success with testing. My experiences as a student, nursing educator, and item writer for the NCLEX examinations aided me as I developed a comprehensive review course to prepare nursing graduates for the NCLEX examination.

Later, in 1994, I began teaching medical-surgical nursing at Salve Regina University in Newport, Rhode Island. Currently, I am a part-time nursing instructor at the University of Nevada, Las Vegas, in Las Vegas, Nevada.

I am the president of Nursing Reviews, Inc. and Professional Nursing Seminars, Inc., located in Henderson, Nevada. Both companies are dedicated to helping nursing graduates achieve their goals of becoming licensed nurses.

Today, I am the successful author of numerous NCLEX review products published by Elsevier. Also, I am an Elsevier Next Generation NCLEX® (NGN) Thought Leader and focus on strategies to prepare students for the Next Generation NCLEX®. I am so pleased that you have decided to join us on your journey to success in testing for nursing examinations and for the NCLEX-PN® examination!

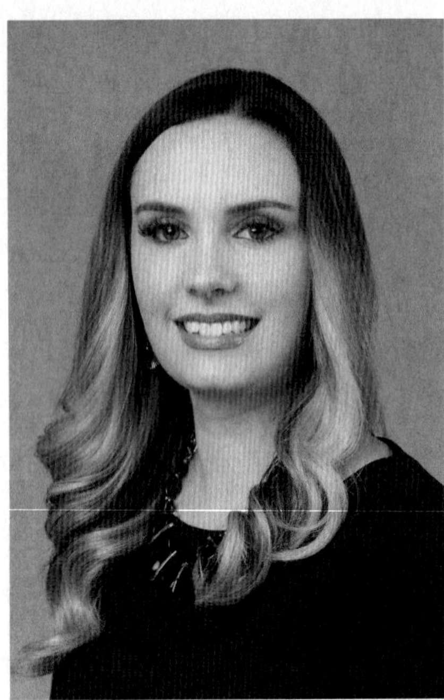

Angela E. Silvestri

Being a nurse is one of the most enriching aspects of my life. It is a career that is multifaceted and complex, and allows me to be challenged scientifically, technically, and spiritually. As a nurse educator, I feel honored to impart my knowledge and experience to others who are hoping to serve in this selfless, caring profession. As a nurse scientist, I aim to make an impact on health care delivery methods, quality of care provided, and overall health care outcomes.

I earned my baccalaureate of science in nursing at Salve Regina University in Newport, Rhode Island. Upon graduation, I worked in long-term care, subacute care, rehabilitation, and acute care settings. I had the opportunity to serve as a preceptor for new graduate RNs while working in these areas. With the desire to become an educator, I pursued my Master of Science in nursing with a focus in education from the University of Nevada, Las Vegas, and began my teaching career. I continued my studies in the Doctor of Philosophy program at the University of Nevada, Las Vegas, focusing on beginning my research program as a nurse scientist. I completed my postgraduate certificate in advanced practice and currently work as a board-certified family-nurse practitioner.

Throughout the years, I have worked extensively in the development of NCLEX review products, as well as with students in live review courses for the NCLEX. I am very excited at the prospect of helping graduates take the final step in becoming a licensed nurse. Thank you for your dedication to the profession of nursing, and I hope you find this resource useful as you move forward in your journey in becoming a licensed nurse. If you don't already know, Nursing is an amazing profession!

Contributors

ASSOCIATE EDITORS

Allison E. Bowser, M.Ed, BS
Consultant and Editor
Nursing Reviews, Inc.
Henderson, Nevada

Eileen H. Gray, DNP, RN, CPNP
Nursing Instructor
University of Nevada, Las Vegas
Las Vegas, Nevada
Former Nursing Chair/Dean
Salve Regina University
Newport, Rhode Island
Consultant and Editor
Nursing Reviews, Inc.
Henderson, Nevada

CONTRIBUTORS

Anthony Machnacz, LPN
The Atrium at Cardinal Drive
Senior Living
Agawam, Massachusetts

Laurent W. Valliere, BS, DD
Vice-President, Professional Nursing Seminars, Inc.
Henderson, Nevada
Alumni, Eastern New Mexico University
Portales, New Mexico

Reviewers

Julie Traynor, MS, RN, CNE
Consortium Director
Dakota Nursing Program
Devils Lake, North Dakota

Karen Petersen, MSN-L, RN
Nursing Faculty
Nursing Department
Paradise Valley Community College
Phoenix, Arizona

Kim Amos, PhD, MS(N), RN, CNE
ADN Director
Isothermal Community College
Spindale, North Carolina

Lisa Nicholas, RN, MSN
Lecturer
Nursing
University of Nevada, Las Vegas (UNLV)
Las Vegas, Nevada

Brianna Machnacz, BSN RN
Registered Nurse
Urgent Care
Medexpress
Springfield, Massachusetts

Preface

"Success is climbing a mountain, facing the challenge of obstacles, and reaching the top of the mountain."

—Linda Anne Silvestri PhD, RN, FAAN

"Success is never an accident. To be successful is to have been perseverant, to have sacrificed, and to have loved what you are cultivating to become successful."

—Angela Elizabeth Silvestri PhD, APRN, FNP-BC, CNE

Welcome to *Saunders Pyramid to Success!*
An Essential Resource for Test Success

Saunders Q&A Review for the NCLEX-PN® Examination is one in a series of products designed to assist you in achieving your goal of becoming a licensed practical/vocational nurse. This text and Evolve site package provide you with more than 5600 practice NCLEX-PN test questions based on the current NCLEX-PN test plan.

The current test plan for the NCLEX-PN identifies a framework based on *Client Needs.* The Client Needs categories include Physiological Integrity, Safe and Effective Care Environment, Health Promotion and Maintenance, and Psychosocial Integrity. *Integrated Processes* are also identified as a component of the test plan. These include Caring, Communication and Documentation, Culture and Spirituality, Nursing Process, and Teaching and Learning. This book has been uniquely designed and includes chapters that describe each specific component of the NCLEX-PN test plan framework and five practice tests with NCLEX-style questions specific to each component.

NCLEX-PN® TEST PREPARATION

This book begins with information regarding NCLEX-PN preparation. **Chapter 1** addresses information related to the NCLEX-PN test plan and testing procedures related to the examination. This chapter answers some of the questions that you may have regarding the testing procedures. Also included is important information about clinical judgment, the National Council of State Boards of Nursing (NCSBN) Clinical Judgment Measurement Model (NCJMM), and the cognitive skills of the model. The Next Generation NCLEX® (NGN) item types are introduced.

Chapter 2 discusses the NCLEX-PN from a nonacademic viewpoint and emphasizes a holistic approach for your individual test preparation. This chapter identifies the components of a structured study plan, anxiety-reducing techniques, and personal focus issues including self-efficacy.

Chapter 3 is a story of success written by a nursing graduate who took the NCLEX-PN and addresses the issue of what the examination is all about. Nursing students want to hear what other students have to say about their experiences with the NCLEX-PN and what it is really like to take this examination. Be sure to read what this graduate has to say.

Chapter 4 includes all of the important strategies that will assist in teaching you how to read a question, how not to read into a question, and how to use the process of elimination and various other strategies to select the correct response from the options presented. Cognitive skills of the NCJMM are introduced.

Client Needs

Chapters 5 through 9 address the NCLEX-PN test plan component, *Client Needs.* **Chapter 5** describes each category of Client Needs as identified by the test plan and lists any subcategories, the percentage of test questions for each category, and some of the content included on the NCLEX-PN. **Chapters 6 through 9** contain practice test questions related specifically to each category of Client Needs. Chapter 6 comprises questions related to Safe and Effective Care Environment, Chapter 7 contains questions dealing with Health Promotion and Maintenance, Chapter 8 is made up of questions concerned with Psychosocial Integrity, and Chapter 9 contains Physiological Integrity questions.

Integrated Processes

Chapter 10 and 11 address the *Integrated Processes* as identified in the NCLEX-PN test plan. **Chapter 10** describes each Integrated Process. **Chapter 11** contains practice test questions related specifically to each Integrated Process, including Caring, Communication and Documentation, Culture and Spirituality, Clinical Problem-Solving Process, and Teaching and Learning.

Book Design

The book is designed with a unique two-column format. The left column presents the practice questions and answer options, while the right column provides the corresponding answers, rationales, priority nursing tips, and test-taking strategies. The two-column format makes the review easier because you do not have to flip through pages in search of answers and rationales.

SPECIAL FEATURES FOUND ON EVOLVE

Pretest and Study Calendar

The accompanying Evolve site contains a 75-question pre-assessment test and a 75-question post-assessment test that provides you with feedback on your strengths and weaknesses. The results of your pretest will generate an individualized study calendar to guide you in your preparation for the NCLEX examination. Once you have completed your review of the practice questions in this resource, you can take the post-assessment test to evaluate your improvement and need for any additional review in preparation for the NCLEX. After completion of each test you are provided with the opportunity to review the answers, rationales, and strategies and we highly encourage you to do this.

Audio Questions

The accompanying Evolve site contains *Audio Questions* representative of content addressed in the current test plan for the NCLEX-PN examination. These questions are in NCLEX-style format, and each question presents an audio sound, such as lung sounds, as a component of the question.

Audio Review Summaries

The companion Evolve site includes three Audio Review Summaries that cover challenging subject areas under the 2020 NCLEX-PN test plan, including Pharmacology, Acid-Base Balance, and Fluids and Electrolytes.

NEXT GENERATION NCLEX® (NGN) CASE STUDIES AND NGN TEST QUESTIONS

The accompanying Evolve site contains stand-alone NGN test items and unfolding case studies. These case studies are accompanied by NGN test items representative of the NGN testing format. The stand-alone client situations are accompanied by one NGN test question that measures more than one or all of the cognitive skills of the NCSBN Clinical Judgment Measurement Model (NCJMM). The unfolding case studies are accompanied by 6 NGN test items and the questions measure all six cognitive skills of the NCJMM. These cognitive skills include Recognize Cues, Analyze Cues, Prioritize Hypotheses, Generate Solutions, Take Action, and Evaluate Outcomes.

PRACTICE QUESTIONS

While preparing for the NCLEX-PN examination, it is crucial for students to practice answering test questions. This book contains multiple-choice and alternate item format questions. The accompanying software includes all the questions from the book, plus additional new Evolve questions for a total of more than 5600 questions. The alternate item format questions in the book and on the accompanying Evolve site may be presented as one of the following:

- Fill-in-the-blank question
- Multiple response question
- Prioritizing (ordered response) question
- Figure/illustration question
- Graphic options question, in which each option contains a figure or illustration
- Chart/exhibit question
- Audio question

In addition, each practice question provides a review button that links you to common laboratory values for your reference while studying on the Evolve site.

The NGN® Case Studies and NGN test items are located on Evolve and provide you with practice in prioritizing, decision-making and critical thinking, and strengthen your clinical judgment skills.

ANSWER SECTIONS FOR PRACTICE QUESTIONS

- Each practice question is accompanied by the correct answer, rationale, priority nursing tip, test-taking strategy, and question categories. The structure of the answer section is unique and provides the following information for every question:
- **Rationale:** The rationale provides you with significant information regarding both correct and incorrect options.
- **Priority Nursing Tip:** The priority nursing tip provides you with an important piece of information that will be helpful to you when answering practice questions and questions on the NCLEX.
- **Test-Taking Strategy:** The test-taking strategy provides a logical path for selecting the correct option and helps you select an answer to a question on which you might have to guess. In each practice question, the specific strategy that will assist in answering the question correctly is in bold type.
- **Question Categories:** Each question on the accompanying Evolve site is identified based on

the categories used by the NCLEX-PN test plan. The question categories identified with each practice question include Level of Cognitive Ability, Client Needs, Integrated Process, Clinical Judgment/Cognitive Skill, the specific nursing Content Area, and Health Problem. Every question on the accompanying Evolve site is organized by these question codes, so you can customize your study session to be as specific or as generic as you need. All categories are identified by their full names so that you do not need to memorize codes or abbreviations. The codes will provide you with guidance on what topics to review for further remediation in the other resources in the Pyramid to Success. These resources are: *Saunders 2022-2023 Clinical Judgment and Test-Taking Strategies: Passing Nursing School and the NCLEX® Exam, Saunders Comprehensive Review for the NCLEX-PN® Exam,* and *the Saunders/HESI Online Review for the NCLEX®-PN Exam.*

HOW TO USE THIS BOOK

Saunders Q&A Review for the NCLEX-PN® Examination is specially designed to help you with your successful journey to the peak of the Pyramid to Success: becoming a licensed practical/vocational nurse. You should begin your journey through the Saunders Pyramid to Success by reading Chapter 1. Chapter 1 is titled "Clinical Judgment and the NCLEX-PN® Examination". It addresses information about clinical judgment and the related cognitive skills as defined by the National Council of State Boards of Nursing (NCSBN) and all of the information related to the NCLEX-PN test plan and the examination testing procedures. This chapter answers questions that you may have regarding this information. Continue on your journey through this book by reading Chapter 2 that describes the unique and special tips regarding how to prepare yourself both academically and nonacademically for this important examination. Read the chapter from the nursing graduate who passed the NCLEX-PN, and consider what the graduate had to say about the examination. Chapter 4, "Clinical Judgment and Test-Taking Strategies", includes information about using clinical judgment and the six cognitive skills to answer questions and all of the strategies that will assist in teaching you how to read a question, how not to read into a question, and how to use the process of elimination and various other strategies to select the correct response from the options presented. Read this chapter and practice these strategies as you proceed through your journey with this book.

Once you have read the introductory components of this book, it is time to begin the practice questions. As you read through each question and select an answer, be sure to read the rationale, the priority nursing tip, and the test-taking strategy. The rationale provides you with significant information regarding both the correct and incorrect options. The priority nursing tip provides you with a piece of important information to remember that will help answer questions on the NCLEX, and the test-taking strategy provides you with the logic for selecting the correct option.

CLIMBING THE PYRAMID TO SUCCESS

This step on the *Pyramid to Success* is to get additional practice with a **Q&A review** product. *Saunders Q&A Review for the NCLEX-PN® Examination* offers more than 5600 unique practice questions in the book and on the companion Evolve site. The questions are focused on the Client Needs and Integrated Processes of the NCLEX test plan, making it easy to access your study area of choice. For on-the-go Q&A review, you can pick up *Saunders Q&A Review Cards for the NCLEX-PN® Examination.*

As you work your way through *Saunders Q&A Review for the NCLEX-PN® Examination* and identify your areas of strength and weakness, you can return to the companion book, *Saunders Comprehensive Review for the NCLEX-PN® Examination,* to focus your study on these areas. The purpose of the *Saunders Comprehensive Review for the NCLEX-PN® Examination* is to provide a **comprehensive review** of the nursing content you will be tested on during the NCLEX-PN examination. However, *Saunders Comprehensive Review for the NCLEX-PN® Examination* is intended to do more than simply prepare you for the rigors of the NCLEX; this book is also meant to serve as a valuable study tool that you can refer to throughout your nursing program, with customizable Evolve site selections to help identify and reinforce key content areas. Your final step on the Pyramid to Success is to master the **online review.** *HESI/Saunders Online Review for the NCLEX-PN® Examination* provides an interactive and individualized platform to get you ready for your final licensure examination. This online course provides 10 high-level content modules, supplemented with instructional videos, audio, illustrations, testlets, and several subject matter examinations. End-of-module practice tests are provided along with several Crossing the Finish Line: Practice Tests and quizzes. In addition, you can assess your progress with a pretest and comprehensive examination in a computerized environment that prepares you for the actual NCLEX-PN examination.

At the base of the *Pyramid to Success* are our **test-taking strategies**, which provide a foundation for understanding and unpacking the complexities of NCLEX examination questions, including alternate item formats. *Saunders 2022-2023 Clinical Judgment and Test-Taking Strategies: Passing Nursing School and the NCLEX® Exam* takes a detailed look at all the test-taking strategies you will need to know in order to pass any nursing examination, including the NCLEX. Special tips are integrated for beginning nursing students, and there are 1200 practice questions included so that you can apply the testing strategies.

To obtain any of these resources that will prepare you for your nursing examinations and the NCLEX-PN examination, visit the Elsevier Health Sciences Web site at elsevierhealth.com.

Good luck with your journey through the *Saunders Pyramid to Success*. We wish you continued success throughout your new career as a licensed practical/vocational nurse!

Linda Anne Silvestri, PhD, RN, FAAN
Angela E. Silvestri, PhD, APRN, FNP-BC, CNE

Acknowledgments

A Few Words from Linda

There are many individuals who in their own ways have contributed to my success in making my professional dreams become a reality. My sincere appreciation and warmest thanks are extended to all of them.

First, I want to acknowledge my parents, who opened my door of opportunity in education. I thank my mother, Frances Mary, for all of her love, support, and assistance as I continuously worked to achieve my professional goals. I thank my father, Arnold Lawrence, who always provided insightful words of encouragement. My memories of their love and support will always remain in my heart. I also thank my best friend and love of my life, my husband, Larry; my sister, Dianne Elodia, and her husband, Lawrence; my brother, Lawrence Peter, and my sister-in-law, Mary Elizabeth; and my nieces and nephews, Gina, Karen, Angela, Katie, Gabrielle, Brianna, Nicholas, Anthony, and Nathan, who were continuously supportive, giving, and helpful during my research and preparation of this publication. They were always there and by my side whenever I needed them.

I want to thank my nursing students at the Community College of Rhode Island who approached me in 1991 and persuaded me to assist them in preparing to take the NCLEX examination. Their enthusiasm and inspiration led to the commencement of my professional endeavors in conducting review courses for the NCLEX examination for nursing students. I also thank the numerous nursing students who have attended my review courses for their willingness to share their needs and ideas. Their input has certainly added a special uniqueness to this publication.

I wish to acknowledge all of the nursing faculty who taught in my review courses for the NCLEX examination. Their commitment, dedication, and expertise have certainly assisted nursing students in achieving success with the NCLEX examination. Additionally, I want to especially acknowledge my husband, Laurent W. Valliere, for his contribution to this publication, for teaching in my review courses for the NCLEX examination, and for his commitment and dedication in assisting my nursing students to prepare for the examination from a nonacademic point of view. I also want to extend a VERY SPECIAL thank you to my niece, Angela, for joining me in preparing and authoring these NCLEX resources. Angela is wonderful to work with. We are an awesome team!!! Her ideas and expertise have certainly added to the content of this publication. She is very dedicated to promoting and ensuring student success. Thank you, Angela! And again, I thank my husband, Larry, for all of his continuous support as I moved through my personal challenges and professional endeavors; he has been my rock of support!

A Few Words from Angela

There are many people who contributed to my success in my work on this product. I am very grateful for their continued support in all of my endeavors.

First and foremost, I would like to thank my husband for his light-hearted and positive attitude. He always knows how to make me laugh, especially when I'm stressed. All of this would not be possible without him! I would also like to thank my kids, Scarlett, Addison, Maxwell, and Harlow for being such an inspiration to work hard, and to be a role model for them.

I would also like to thank my parents, Mary and Larry, for their continued support throughout the years. Their words of encouragement and wisdom have been tremendously important to my success. I also don't know what I would do without their support in caring for my kids!

I would like to thank my sister, Katie, who is a wonderful nurse herself and aspiring nurse practitioner. Her ambitions as a recent nursing graduate inspired me and reminded me every day why I'm so passionate about being an educator. Thank you to my brother, Nick, who always is positive and encouraging about my work. His wit and sarcasm are always a great way to lift your mood at the end of the day.

I want to extend a special thank you to Linda for her collaboration, guidance, and expertise. Without her I would not be where I am today. Thank you, Linda!

A Few Words from Linda and Angela

First and foremost, we want to thank our fabulous associate editors, Eileen Gray and Allison Bowser, for all of their dedication and hard work in editing and preparing the entire manuscript for this edition. Their expertise and close attention to details have certainly added to the quality of this resource. Eileen and Allison, thank you so much! You both are the best and we could not do this without you!

We also want to acknowledge and thank Laurent W. Valliere for writing a chapter addressing those important nonacademic test preparation issues.

In addition, we also sincerely thank Anthony Machnacz, LPN, for writing a chapter for this book about his experiences with preparing for and taking the NCLEX-PN examination.

A special thank you and acknowledgment goes to Katie Silvestri who updated and provided new practice questions for this edition. Thank you, Katie, for your expert work and dedication to the quality of this product. And we also want to thank all of the previous contributors. A very special thank you to all of you! We thank Dianne E. Fiorentino and Karen Machnacz for their continuous support and complete dedication to our work and in their reference support and other administrative responsibilities for the edition of this book. We also thank Jimmy Guibault, our pharmacist, for providing medication research support. Thank you, Jimmy! And a thank you to all of the other individuals on our beta review team: Mary and Larry Silvestri, Eileen Gray, Allison Bowser, Karen Machnacz, Gabby Machnacz, Brianna Machnacz, and Dianne Fiorentino.

We want to acknowledge all of the staff at Elsevier for their tremendous help throughout the preparation and production of this publication. A special thanks to all of them.

We want to especially acknowledge and thank some very important and special people from Elsevier. We thank Heather Bays-Petrovic, Content Strategist, for her continuous support, enthusiasm, and expert professional guidance throughout the preparation of this edition. We also want to thank Laura Klein, our Senior Content Development Specialist, for maintaining order for all of our manuscript submissions.

We also extend a very special thank you to Cindy Thoms, Senior Project Manager, who is always so supportive and so awesome to work with. Her attention to the many details to ensure and maintain the quality of all of our NCLEX® titles is so greatly appreciated. Thank you, Cindy! We could not have completed this publication without you!

We both want to thank and acknowledge our fantastic copyeditor, Babette Morgan, an Elsevier freelancer, and our fantastic proofreader, Melanie Benson Marshall, from Aptara. Their work and close attention to details was incredible and so appreciated. Thank you Babette and Melanie!

We thank Julie Eddy, Publishing Services Manager, and Maggie Reid, Senior Book Designer. You have all played such significant roles in finalizing this publication.

Lastly, a very special thank you to all our nursing students, past, present, and future. All of you light up our life! Your love and dedication to the profession of nursing and your commitment to provide health care will bring never-ending rewards!

Contents

UNIT

I

NCLEX-PN® Preparation

CHAPTER

1

Clinical Judgment and the NCLEX-PN® Examination

THE PYRAMID TO SUCCESS

Saunders Q&A Review for the NCLEX-PN® Examination

Welcome to the Pyramid to Success and *Saunders Q&A Review for the NCLEX-PN® Examination.*

At this time, you have completed the first step in your path toward the peak of the Pyramid with *Saunders Comprehensive Review for the NCLEX-PN® Examination.* Now it is time to continue the journey to becoming a licensed practical or vocational nurse with *Saunders Q&A Review for the NCLEX-PN® Examination!*

Clinical Judgment and Next Generation NCLEX® Items

Clinical judgment is the observed outcome of critical thinking and decision-making (Dickison, Haerling, & Lasater, 2019). In recent years, heightened attention has been paid to clinical judgment as a means of teaching, learning, and assessment and testing. The NCLEX-PN® examination requires candidates to demonstrate the ability to use clinical judgment in the delivery of client care. Clinical judgment should also be used as a test-taking strategy to answer test questions (see Chapter 4). The National Council of State Boards of Nursing (NCSBN) has created a Clinical Judgment Measurement Model (NCJMM) that consists of applying 6 cognitive skills or processes. These include: (1) recognizing cues; (2) analyzing cues; (3) prioritizing hypotheses; (4) generating solutions; (5) taking action; and (6) evaluating outcomes (Dickison et al., 2019). Table 1.1 provides a description of these six cognitive skills/processes identified in the NCJMM. The NCJMM also serves as a guide for the NCSBN to create NGN® questions. The NCJMM continues to evolve, as may the NGN® item types that will be presented in the exam. Stand-alone test items and unfolding case studies will be presented in the NGN. It is expected that the NGN® test items will be scored items in the new test plan implemented in 2023. Some of these NGN® item types can be found on the Evolve site accompanying this book. We highly encourage you to frequently access the NCSBN website at www.ncsbn.org for updates.

About This Resource and the NCLEX-PN® Examination

As you begin your journey through this book, you will be introduced to all of the important points regarding the NCLEX-PN examination, the process of testing, self-efficacy and the unique and special tips for preparing yourself for this very important examination. You will read what a nursing graduate who recently passed the NCLEX-PN has to say about the examination. All of the important test-taking strategies are detailed, which will guide you in selecting the correct option or in making a logical guess when you are unsure about an answer.

Saunders Q&A Review for the NCLEX-PN® Examination contains NCLEX-PN–style practice questions. The Evolve site accompanying this book contains all of the questions from the book plus additional Evolve questions for a total of more than 4700 practice questions. The types of practice questions include multiple choice; fill-in-the-blank; multiple-response; ordered-response; questions that contain a figure, chart/exhibit, or graphic option item; and audio item formats. Examples of question types can be located throughout this chapter. In addition, the Next Generation NCLEX® (NGN) item types are provided on the accompanying Evolve site.

The chapters have been developed to provide a description of the components of the NCLEX-PN test plan, including the Client Needs and the Integrated Processes. In addition, the included practice tests contain practice questions specific to each category of the Client Needs and the Integrated Processes. Each practice test contains practice questions. A rationale, a priority nursing tip, and a test-taking strategy are provided with each question. Each question is coded on the basis of the Level of Cognitive Ability, the Client Needs category, the Integrated Process, the Clinical Judgment/Cognitive Skill, the Health Problem if applicable, and the content area being tested. The rationale provides you with significant information regarding both the correct and incorrect options. The priority nursing tip provides you

Table 1.1 ▲ COGNITIVE SKILLS AND DESCRIPTIONS

COGNITIVE SKILL	DESCRIPTION
Recognize cues	Identifying significant data; data can be from many sources (assessment/data collection)
Analyze cues	Connecting data to the client's clinical presentation—determining whether the data is expected? Unexpected? (analysis)
Prioritize hypotheses	Ranking hypotheses; what are the concerns or client needs/problems and their priority? (analysis)
Generate solutions	Using hypotheses to determine interventions for an expected outcome (planning)
Take action	Implementing the generated solutions addressing the highest priorities or hypotheses (implementation)
Evaluate outcomes	Comparing observed outcomes with expected ones (evaluation)

From Dickison, P., Haerling, K. A., & Lasater, K. (2019). Integrating the National Council of State Boards of Nursing Clinical Judgment Model into nursing educational frameworks. *Journal of Nursing Education, 58*(2), 72-78.

with key information about a nursing point to remember. The test-taking strategy maps out a logical path for selecting the correct option, and the health problem code identifies the disorder to review, if necessary. On Evolve, the health problem code allows you to filter and select questions based on a disease process. For example, if heart failure is the area of interest, you can select "Adult Health, Cardiovascular, Heart Failure" on the Evolve site.

Other Resources in the Saunders Pyramid to Success

Additional products in Saunders Pyramid to Success include *Saunders Comprehensive Review for the NCLEX-PN® Examination, Saunders Clinical Judgment and Test-Taking Strategies: Passing Nursing School and the NCLEX® Exam, Saunders Q&A Review Cards for the NCLEX-PN® Exam,* and *HESI/Saunders Online Review for the NCLEX-PN® Examination*. Specific information about these ideal NCLEX preparation tools can be found in the preface of this book. Additionally, all products in the Saunders Pyramid to Success can be obtained online by visiting https://www.us.elsevierhealth.com or by calling 800-545-2522.

Let us continue with our journey up the Pyramid to Success!

EXAMINATION PROCESS

An important step in the Pyramid to Success is to become as familiar as possible with the examination process. Candidates facing the challenge of this examination can experience significant anxiety. Knowing what the examination is all about and knowing what you will encounter during the process of testing will assist in alleviating fear and anxiety. The information contained in this chapter was obtained from the NCSBN website (www.ncsbn.org) and from the NCSBN 2020 test plan for the NCLEX-PN and includes guidance related to registering for the exam, testing procedures, and answers to the questions most commonly asked by nursing students and graduates preparing to take the NCLEX. You can obtain additional information regarding the test and its development by accessing the NCSBN website and clicking on the NCLEX Examination tab or by writing to the National Council of State Boards of Nursing, 111 East Wacker Drive, Suite 2900, Chicago, IL 60601. You are encouraged to access the NCSBN website, because this site provides you with the most up-to-date and valuable information about the NCLEX and other resources available to an NCLEX candidate. You are also encouraged to access the most up-to-date *Candidate Bulletin.* This document provides you with everything you need to know about registration procedures and scheduling a test date.

COMPUTER ADAPTIVE TESTING

The acronym *CAT* stands for *computer adaptive test,* which means that the examination is created as the test-taker answers each question. All the test questions are categorized on the basis of the test plan structure and the level of difficulty of the question. As you answer a question, the computer determines your competency based on the answer you selected. If you selected a correct answer, the computer scans the question bank and selects a more difficult question. If you selected an incorrect answer, the computer scans the question bank and selects an easier question. This process continues until all test plan requirements are met and a reliable pass-or-fail decision is made.

When taking a CAT, once an answer is recorded, all subsequent questions administered depend, to an extent, on the answer selected for that question. Skipping questions or returning to earlier questions is incompatible with the logical methodology of a CAT. The inability to skip questions or go back to change previous answers will not be a disadvantage to you; you will not fall into that "trap" of changing a correct answer to an incorrect one with the CAT system.

If you are faced with a question that contains unfamiliar content, you may need to guess at the answer. There is no penalty for guessing, but you need to make an educated guess. With most of the questions, the answer will be right there in front of you. If you need to guess, use your nursing knowledge and clinical experiences and clinical judgment skills to their fullest extent and all of the test-taking strategies you have practiced in this review program.

Table 1.2 ▲ LEVELS OF COGNITIVE ABILITY: LEVEL AND DESCRIPTIONS AND EXAMPLES

LEVEL	DESCRIPTION AND EXAMPLE
Remembering	Recalling, recognizing, retrieving information from memorization, previous learning, or long-term memory. Example: A normal blood glucose level is 70 to 99 mg/dL.
Understanding	Interpreting the meaning of information. Example: A blood glucose level of 60 mg/dL is lower than the normal reference range.
Applying	Carrying out an appropriate action based on information. Example: Administering 10 g to 15 g of carbohydrate, such as a half-glass of fruit juice, to treat mild hypoglycemia.
Analyzing	Examining a broad concept, breaking it down into smaller parts, and determining how the parts relate to one another. Example: The broad concept is mild hypoglycemia and the smaller concepts are the signs and symptoms of mild hypoglycemia, such as hunger, irritability, weakness, headache, and blood glucose level lower than 60 mg/dL.
Evaluating	Making judgments, conclusions, or validations based on evidence. Example: Determining that treatment for mild hypoglycemia was effective if the blood glucose level returned to a normal level of 70 to 99 mg/dL.
Creating	Generating or producing a new outcome or plan by putting parts of information together. Example: Designing a safe and individualized plan of care with the interprofessional health care team for a client with diabetes mellitus that meets the client's physiological, psychosocial, and health maintenance needs.

Adapted from *Understanding Bloom's (and Anderson and Krathwohl's) Taxonomy,* 2015, ProEdit, Inc. http://www.proedit.com/understanding-blooms-and-anderson-and-krathwohls-taxonomy/.

You do not need any computer experience to take this examination. A keyboard tutorial is provided on the NCSBN website, and you are encouraged to view the tutorial when you are preparing for the NCLEX examination. The tutorial will instruct you on the use of the on-screen optional calculator, the use of the mouse, and how to record an answer. The tutorial also provides instructions on how to respond to the different question types on this examination. In addition, at the testing site, a test administrator is present to assist in explaining the use of the computer to ensure your full understanding of how to proceed.

DEVELOPMENT OF THE TEST PLAN

The test plan for the NCLEX-PN examination is developed by the NCSBN. The examination is a national examination; the NCSBN considers the legal scope of nursing practice as governed by state laws and regulations, including the nurse practice act, and uses these laws to define the areas on the examination that will assess the competence of the test-taker for licensure.

The NCSBN also conducts an important study every 3 years, known as a *practice analysis study,* to link the examination to nursing practice. The results of this study determine the framework for the test plan for the examination. The participants in this study include newly licensed practical/vocational nurses. From a list of nursing care activities (activity statements) provided, the participants are asked about the applicability, frequency, and importance of performing these activities in relation to client safety. A panel of content experts at the NCSBN analyzes the results of the study and makes decisions regarding the test plan framework. The results of this recently conducted study provided the structure for the test plan implemented in April 2020.

TEST PLAN

The content of the NCLEX-PN examination reflects the activities identified in the practice analysis study conducted by the NCSBN. The questions are written to address Level of Cognitive Ability, Client Needs, and Integrated Processes as identified in the test plan developed by the NCSBN.

Level of Cognitive Ability

Levels of cognitive ability include remembering, understanding, applying, analyzing, evaluating, and creating. The practice of nursing requires complex thought processing and critical thinking in decision making and in making clinical judgments. Therefore, you will not encounter any remembering or understanding questions on the NCLEX. Questions on this examination are written at the applying level or at higher levels of cognitive ability. Table 1.2 provides descriptions and examples of each level of cognitive ability. Box 1.1 presents an example of a question that requires you to apply data.

Box 1.1 ▲ LEVEL OF COGNITIVE ABILITY: APPLYING

The nurse notes blanching, coolness, and edema at the peripheral intravenous (IV) site. On the basis of these findings, the nurse would plan to implement which action?

1. Remove the IV.
2. Apply a warm compress.
3. Check for a blood return.
4. Measure the area of infiltration.

ANSWER: 1

This question requires you to determine that the client is experiencing an infiltration. Next, you need to consider the harmful effects of infiltration and determine the action that needs to be implemented. Because infiltration can be damaging to the surrounding tissue, the appropriate action is to remove the IV to prevent further damage. Once the IV is removed, further action would be taken depending on the medication infusing at the time of infiltration based on agency protocol, but may include aspiration of the fluid from the site, injection of an antidote, application of warm or cool compresses for specified time intervals, and elevation of the extremity. The licensed practical nurse would consult with the registered nurse (RN) about the necessary actions to take.

Client Needs

The NCSBN identifies a test plan framework based on Client Needs, which includes four major categories. Some of these categories are divided further into subcategories. The Client Needs categories are Safe and Effective Care Environment, Health Promotion and Maintenance, Psychosocial Integrity, and Physiological Integrity. Refer to Chapter 5 for a detailed description of the categories of Client Needs and the NCLEX-PN examination, and refer to Table 1.3 for the percentages of questions from each Client Needs category.

Integrated Processes

The NCSBN identifies five processes in the test plan that are fundamental to the practice of nursing. These processes are incorporated throughout the major categories of Client Needs. The Integrated Process subcategories are Caring, Communication and Documentation, Culture and Spirituality, Clinical Problem-Solving Process (Nursing Process; Data Collection, Planning, Implementation, and Evaluation), and Teaching and Learning. Refer to Chapter 10 for a detailed description of the Integrated Processes and the NCLEX-PN examination.

Table 1.3 ▲ THE FOUR CLIENT NEEDS CATEGORIES AND PERCENTAGE OF QUESTIONS ON THE NCLEX-PN EXAMINATION

CLIENT NEEDS CATEGORY AND SUBCATEGORY	PERCENTAGE OF QUESTIONS
SAFE AND EFFECTIVE CARE ENVIRONMENT	
Coordinated Care	18-24
Safety and Infection Control	10-16
HEALTH PROMOTION AND MAINTENANCE	6-12
PSYCHOSOCIAL INTEGRITY	9-15
PHYSIOLOGICAL INTEGRITY	
Basic Care and Comfort	7-13
Pharmacological Therapies	10-16
Reduction of Risk Potential	9-15
Physiological Adaptation	7-13

From National Council of State Boards of Nursing: *2020 NCLEX-PN® examination: Test plan for the National Council Licensure Examination for Practical Nurses*, Chicago, 2019, National Council of State Boards of Nursing.

TYPES OF QUESTIONS ON THE EXAMINATION

The types of questions that may be administered on the examination include multiple-choice; fill-in-the-blank; multiple-response; ordered-response (prioritizing); image (hot spot) questions; figure, chart/exhibit, or graphic option items; and audio formats. Additionally, the new Next Generation NCLEX® (NGN) items will be on the examination starting in 2023, according to the NCSBN. The NCSBN provides specific directions for you to follow with all question types to guide you through the testing process. Be sure to read these directions as they appear on the computer screen. Examples of some of these types of questions are noted in this chapter. Most question types are placed in this book, and all types, including the NGN items, are on the accompanying Evolve site.

Multiple-Choice Questions

Some of the questions that you will be asked to answer will be in the multiple-choice format. These questions provide you with data about a client situation and four answers, or options.

Fill-in-the-Blank Questions

Fill-in-the-blank questions may ask you to perform a medication calculation, determine an intravenous flow rate, or calculate an intake or output record on a client. You will need to type only a number (your answer) in the answer box. If the question requires rounding the answer, this needs to be performed at the end of the calculation. The rules for rounding an answer are described in the tutorial provided by the NCSBN and are also provided in the specific question on the computer screen. In addition, you must type in a decimal point if necessary. See Box 1.2 for an example.

Box 1.2 ▲ FILL-IN-THE-BLANK QUESTION

A physician's prescription reads digoxin 0.125 mg orally daily. The medication label reads digoxin 0.25 mg/tablet. The nurse prepares how many tablets to administer the dose? **Fill in the blank. Record the answer using one decimal place.**

ANSWER: 0.5 TABLET

For this fill-in-the-blank question, you need to focus on the prescription and the medication dosage that is available. Next, you will use the formula for calculating a medication dose. When you are taking the NCLEX examination, remember to use the on-screen calculator to verify your answer.

FORMULA:

$$\frac{\textit{Desired}}{\textit{Available}} \times \textit{Quantity} = \textit{Tablet}$$

$$\frac{0.125\text{ mg}}{0.25\text{ mg}} \times 1\text{ tablet} = 0.5\text{ tablet}$$

Multiple-Response Questions

For a multiple-response question, you will be asked to select or check all of the options, such as nursing interventions, that relate to the information in the question. In these question types, there may be one correct answer, there may be more than one correct answer, or all answers could be correct. See Box 1.3 for an example.

Ordered-Response Questions

In this type of question, you will be asked to place nursing actions in order of priority. Information will be presented in a question and, based on the data, you need to determine what you will do first, second, third, and so forth. Specific directions for answering are provided with the question. See Box 1.4 for an example. More practice questions of this type are located on the accompanying Evolve site.

Figure or Hot Spot Questions

A question with a picture or graphic will ask you to answer the question based on the picture or graphic. The question could contain a chart, a table, or a figure or illustration. You also may be asked to use the computer mouse to point and click on a specific area (hot spot) in the visual. A chart, table, figure, or illustration may appear in any type of question, including a multiple-choice question. See Box 1.5 for an example.

Box 1.3 ▲ MULTIPLE-RESPONSE QUESTION

The nurse is preparing to assist in the removal of a nasogastric tube from a client. Which actions would the nurse prepare to take to perform this procedure? **Select all that apply.**

- ❒ 1. Place the client in a supine position.
- ❒ 2. Assess for the presence of bowel sounds.
- ❒ 3. Untape the nasogastric tube from the client's nose.
- ❒ 4. Ask the client to hold his or her breath during the removal of the tube.
- ❒ 5. Keep the tube attached to the prescribed amount of suction during removal.
- ❒ 6. Instill 20 mL of air into the nasogastric tube to displace secretions back into the client's stomach.

ANSWER: 2, 3, 4, 6

With a multiple-response question, you will be asked to select or check all of the options (e.g., nursing actions) that relate to the information in the question. To answer this question, visualize the procedure and think about airway patency, prevention of aspiration, and prevention of mucosal irritation to identify the correct interventions. After explaining the procedure for tube removal to the client, the nurse checks for the presence of bowel sounds. The tube is not removed if bowel sounds are absent, and if bowel sounds are absent, the nurse would report this finding. The nurse dons clean gloves, places the client in an upright position, and places a towel across the client's chest. The suction is turned off, and the nasogastric tube is disconnected from the suction tube. The nurse instills 20 mL of air into the nasogastric tube to displace secretions back into the client's stomach and to decrease the client's risk of aspiration. The nasogastric tube is then untaped from the client's nose. Finally, the client is instructed to hold the breath during the removal of the tube, and the tube is pulled out in one quick but smooth and steady motion.

Chart/Exhibit Questions

In this type of question, you will be presented with a problem and a chart or exhibit. You will be provided with tabs or buttons that you need to click to obtain the information needed to answer the question. A prompt or message will appear that will indicate the need to click on a tab or button. See Box 1.6 for an example.

Graphic Item Option Questions

In this type of question, the option selections will be pictures rather than text. You will need to use the computer mouse to click on the option that represents your answer choice. See Box 1.7 for an example.

Box 1.4 ▲ ORDERED-RESPONSE QUESTION

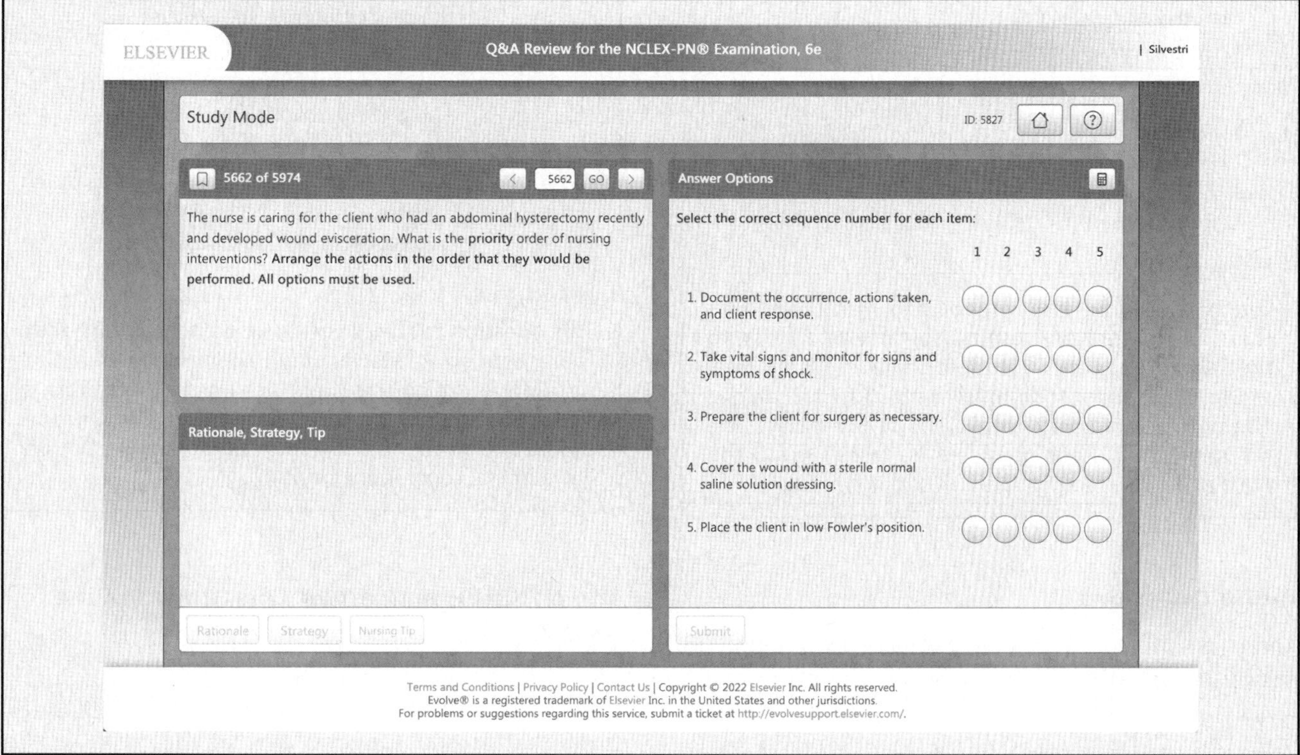

Box 1.5 ▲ FIGURE QUESTION

The nurse notes that this rhythm is being displayed on a client's cardiac monitor. Based on this rhythm, the nurse would take which action? **Refer to the figure.**

1. Contact the registered nurse.
2. Prepare to assist to administer atropine sulfate.
3. Ask the client to perform Valsalva's maneuver.
4. Document the rhythm in the client's medical record.

ANSWER: 4

For this question, you are provided with a figure of a rhythm strip and asked about it. Focus on the characteristics of the rhythm. Noting that the rhythm is a normal sinus rhythm will direct you to the correct option. In addition, note that all of the incorrect options identify nursing actions that are performed if the rhythm is abnormal.

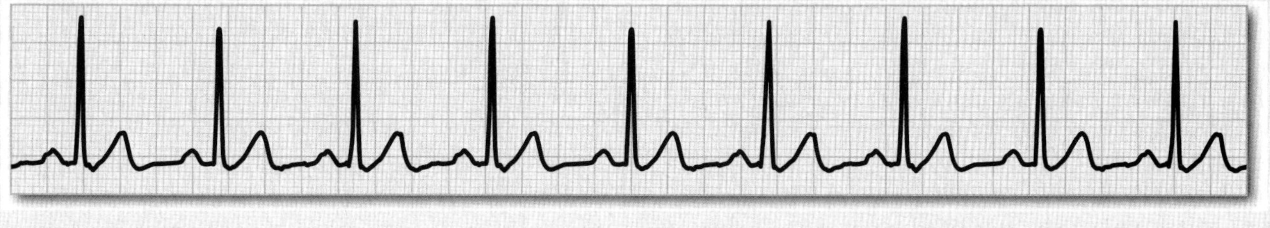

Box 1.6 ▲ CHART/EXHIBIT QUESTION

The nurse reviews the laboratory results form in a client's chart and reports which abnormal result to the primary health care provider? **Refer to the chart.**

CLIENT'S MEDICAL RECORD

Laboratory	Medications	Progress Reports
Sodium 150 mEq/L		
Potassium 4 mEq/L		
Fasting glucose 99 mg/dL		
Blood urea nitrogen 10 mg/dL		

1. Sodium
2. Potassium
3. Fasting glucose
4. Blood urea nitrogen

ANSWER: 1

For this question, you are provided with the client's chart and laboratory results. You need to refer to the laboratory results to determine the abnormal result. The normal sodium level is 135 to 145 mEq/L. The normal potassium level is 3.5 to 5.0 mEq/L. The normal fasting blood glucose is 70 to 99 mg/dL. The normal blood urea nitrogen is 10 to 20 mg/dL.

Box 1.7 ▲ GRAPHIC OPTIONS QUESTION

The primary health care provider writes a prescription for a client to be placed in a supine position. The nurse places the client in which position? **Refer to Figures 1-4.**

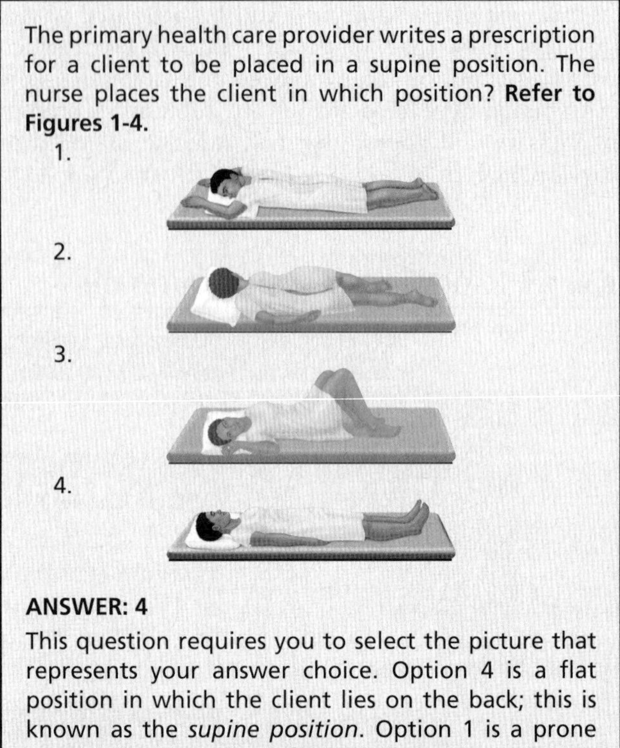

ANSWER: 4

This question requires you to select the picture that represents your answer choice. Option 4 is a flat position in which the client lies on the back; this is known as the *supine position*. Option 1 is a prone position. Option 2 is a left side-lying position. Option 3 is a dorsal recumbent position.

Audio Questions

Audio questions will require listening to a sound to answer the question. These questions will prompt you to use the headset provided and to click on the sound icon. You will be able to click on the volume button to adjust the volume to your comfort level, and you will be able to listen to the sound as many times as necessary. Content examples include, but are not limited to, various lung sounds, heart sounds, or bowel sounds. Box 1.8 illustrates an example of an audio question. Practice audio questions are located on the accompanying Evolve site.

NEXT GENERATION NCLEX® (NGN) ITEM TYPES

The NGN question item types will be presented as a stand-alone case accompanied by one question or as an unfolding case study accompanied by six questions. Stand-alone questions will measure one or more than one of the cognitive skills. The unfolding case studies will be accompanied by six questions; all six cognitive skills will be measured (see Table 1.1). The Evolve site accompanying this book provides you with practice with all NGN item types. You are encouraged to access www.ncsbn.org for the most current information on these test items, their description, and how they will be presented.

The NCSBN Practice Test Questions for the NCLEX

The NCSBN provides a practice test for candidates that is composed of previously used NCLEX questions that are no longer a part of the NCLEX. This exam simulates the look of the real exam and provides the candidate with practice for the NCLEX. This practice test can be purchased through the NCSBN at www.ncsbn.org.

REGISTERING TO TAKE THE EXAMINATION

It is important to obtain an NCLEX Examination Candidate Bulletin from the NCSBN website at www.ncsbn.org, because this bulletin provides all of the information you need to register for and schedule your examination. It also provides you with website and telephone information for NCLEX examination contacts. The initial step in the registration process is to submit an application to the state board of nursing in the state in which you intend to obtain licensure. You need to obtain information from the board of nursing regarding the specific registration process, because the process may vary from state to state. Then, use the NCLEX Examination Candidate Bulletin as your guide to complete the registration process.

Box 1.8 ▲ AUDIO QUESTION

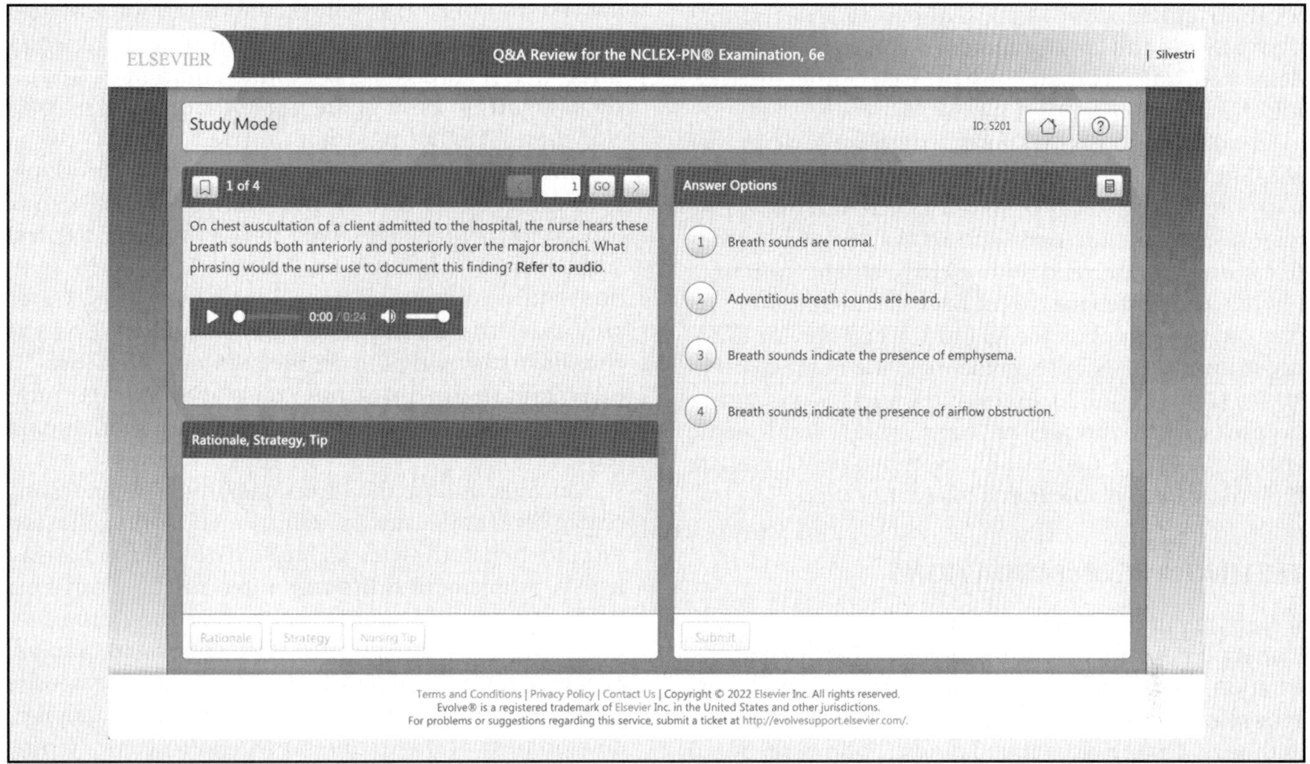

Following the registration instructions and completing the registration forms precisely and accurately are important. Registration forms not properly completed or not accompanied by the proper fees in the required method of payment will be returned to you and will delay testing. You must pay a fee for taking the examination; you also may have to pay additional fees to the board of nursing in the state in which you are applying.

AUTHORIZATION TO TEST FORM AND SCHEDULING AN APPOINTMENT

Once you are eligible to test, you will receive an Authorization to Test (ATT) form. You cannot make an appointment until you receive an ATT form. Note the validity dates on the ATT form, and schedule a testing date and time before the expiration date on the ATT form. The NCLEX Examination Candidate Bulletin provides you with the directions for scheduling an appointment; you do not have to take the examination in the same state in which you are seeking licensure.

The ATT form contains important information, including your test authorization number, candidate identification number, and validity date. You need to take your ATT form to the testing center on the day of your examination. You will not be admitted to the examination if you do not have it.

CHANGING YOUR SCHEDULED APPOINTMENT

If for any reason you need to change your appointment to test, you can make the change on the candidate website or by calling candidate services. Refer to the NCLEX Examination Candidate Bulletin for this contact information and other important procedures for canceling and changing an appointment. If you fail to arrive for the examination or fail to cancel your appointment to test without providing appropriate notice, you will forfeit your examination fee and your ATT form will be invalidated. This information will be reported to the board of nursing in the state in which you have applied for licensure, and you will be required to register and pay the testing fees again.

DAY OF THE EXAMINATION

It is important that you arrive at the testing center at least 30 minutes before the test is scheduled. If you arrive late for the scheduled testing appointment, you may be required to forfeit your examination appointment. If it is necessary to forfeit your appointment, you will need to reregister for the examination and pay an additional fee. The board of nursing will be notified that you did not take the test. A few days before your scheduled date of testing, take the time to drive to the testing center to determine its exact location, the length of time required to arrive at that destination, and any potential obstacles that might delay you, such as road construction, traffic, or parking sites.

In addition to the ATT form, you must have proper identification (ID), such as a U.S. driver's license, a passport, a U.S. state ID, or a U.S. military ID, to be admitted to take the examination. All acceptable identification must be valid and not expired and contain a photograph and signature (in English). In addition, the first and last names on the ID must match the ATT form. According to the NCSBN guidelines, any name discrepancies require legal documentation, such as a marriage license, divorce decree, or court action legal name change. Refer to the NCLEX Examination Candidate Bulletin for acceptable forms of identification.

TESTING ACCOMMODATIONS

If you require testing accommodations, you should contact the board of nursing before submitting a registration form. The board of nursing will provide the procedures for the request. The board of nursing must authorize testing accommodations. Following board of nursing approval, the NCSBN reviews the requested accommodations and must approve the request. If the request is approved, the candidate will be notified and provided the procedure for registering for and scheduling the examination.

TESTING CENTER

The testing center is designed to ensure complete security of the testing process. Strict candidate identification requirements have been established. You will be asked to read the rules related to testing. A digital fingerprint and palm vein print will be taken. A digital signature and photograph will also be taken at the testing center. These identity confirmations will accompany the NCLEX exam results. In addition, if you leave the testing room for any reason, you may be required to perform these identity confirmation procedures again to be readmitted to the room.

Personal belongings are not allowed in the testing room; all electronic devices must be placed in a sealable bag provided by the test administrator and kept in a locker. Any evidence of tampering with the bag could result in the need to report the incident and test cancellation. A locker and locker key will be provided for you; however, storage space is limited, so you must plan accordingly. In addition, the testing center will not assume responsibility for your personal belongings. The testing waiting areas are generally small; friends or family members who accompany you are not permitted to wait in the testing center while you are taking the examination.

Once you have completed the admission process, the test administrator will escort you to the assigned computer. You will be seated at an individual workspace area that includes computer equipment, appropriate lighting, an erasable note board, and a marker. No items, including unauthorized scratch paper, are allowed into the testing room. Eating, drinking, or the use of tobacco is not allowed in the testing room. You will be observed at all times by the test administrator while taking the examination. In addition, video and audio recordings of all test sessions are made. The testing center has no control over the sounds made by typing on the computer by others. If these sounds are distracting, raise your hand to summon the test administrator. Earplugs are available on request.

You must follow the directions given by the testing center staff and must remain seated during the test except when authorized to leave. If you think that you have a problem with the computer, need a clean note board, need to take a break, or need the test administrator for any reason, you must raise your hand. You are also encouraged to access the NCSBN candidate website to obtain additional information about the physical environment of the testing center and to view a virtual tour of the testing center.

TESTING TIME AND LENGTH OF THE EXAMINATION

The maximum testing time is 5 hours; this period includes all breaks and the examination. All breaks are optional. If you take a break, you must leave the testing room; when you return, you may be required to perform identity confirmation procedures to be readmitted.

Currently, the number of scored items ranges from 60 (minimum number) to 130 (maximum). It is also important to know that the NCLEX will include 15 pretest questions. The pretest questions are questions that may be presented as scored questions on future examinations. These pretest questions are not identified as such. In other words, you do not know which questions are the pretest (unscored) questions.

The NCSBN proposed NGN test design, to be implemented in 2023, will be made up of scored items ranging from 70 (minimum) to 135 (maximum). In addition to the current NCLEX item types, the NGN will include case studies with accompanying test questions. Refer to Chapter 4 for information on these NGN case studies and item types. Additionally, go to the Evolve site accompanying this book for practice with these case studies and NGN items. Refer to the NCSBN website at www.ncsbn.org. It is important that you access this site frequently for the latest updates regarding testing.

COMPLETING THE EXAMINATION

When the examination has ended, you may be asked to complete a brief computer-delivered questionnaire about your testing experience. After you complete this questionnaire, you need to raise your hand to summon the test administrator. The test administrator will collect and inventory all note boards and then permit you to leave.

PROCESSING RESULTS

Every computerized examination is scored twice, once by the computer at the testing center and again after the examination is transmitted to the test scoring center. No results are released at the testing center; testing center staff do not have access to examination results. The board of nursing receives your result, and your result will be mailed to you approximately 6 weeks after you take the examination. In some states, an unofficial result can be obtained via the Quick Results Service 2 business days after taking the examination. There is a fee for this service, and information about obtaining your NCLEX result by this method can be obtained on the NCSBN website under candidate services.

PASS-OR-FAIL DECISIONS AND THE CANDIDATE PERFORMANCE REPORT

All examination questions are categorized by test plan area and level of difficulty. This is an important point to keep in mind when you consider how the computer makes a pass-or-fail decision, because a pass-or-fail decision is not based on a percentage of correctly answered questions.

A candidate performance report is provided to a test-taker who fails the examination. This report provides the test-taker with information about personal strengths and weaknesses in relation to the test plan framework and provides a guide for studying and retaking the examination. If a retake is necessary, the candidate must wait 45 days before retaking the examination, depending on state procedures. Test-takers should refer to the state board of nursing in the state in which licensure is sought for procedures regarding when the examination can be taken again.

Additional information about pass-or-fail decisions and the candidate performance report can be found in the NCLEX Examination Candidate Bulletin located at www.ncsbn.org.

INTERSTATE ENDORSEMENT AND NURSE LICENSURE COMPACT

Because the NCLEX-PN examination is a national examination, you can apply to take the examination in any state. When licensure is received, you can apply for interstate endorsement, which is obtaining another license in another state to practice nursing in that state. The procedures and requirements for interstate endorsement may vary from state to state, and these procedures can be obtained from the state board of nursing in the state in which endorsement is sought. It may be possible to practice nursing in another state under the mutual recognition model of nursing licensure if the state has enacted a Nurse Licensure Compact. To obtain information about the Nurse Licensure Compact and the states that are part of this interstate compact, access the NCSBN website at www.ncsbn.org.

THE INTERNATIONALLY EDUCATED NURSE

An important first step in the process of obtaining information about becoming a licensed nurse in the United States is to access the NCSBN website at www.ncsbn.org and obtain information provided for international nurses in the NCLEX website link. The NCSBN provides information about some of the documents you need to obtain as an international nurse seeking licensure in the United States and about credentialing agencies. Refer to Box 1.9 for a listing of some of these documents. The NCSBN also provides information regarding the requirements for education and English proficiency, and immigration requirements such as visas and VisaScreen.

An important factor to consider as you pursue this process is that requirements may vary from state to

Box 1.9 ▲ INTERNATIONALLY EDUCATED NURSE: SOME DOCUMENTS NEEDED TO OBTAIN LICENSURE

1. Proof of citizenship or lawful alien status
2. Work visa
3. VisaScreen certificate
4. Commission on Graduates of Foreign Nursing Schools (CGFNS) certificate
5. Criminal background check documents
6. Official transcripts of educational credentials sent directly to credentialing agency or board of nursing from home country school of nursing
7. Validation of a comparable nursing education as that provided in U.S. nursing programs; this may include theoretical instruction and clinical practice in a variety of nursing areas, including, but not limited to, medical nursing, surgical nursing, pediatric nursing, maternity and newborn nursing, community and public health nursing, and mental health nursing
8. Validation of safe professional nursing practice in home country
9. Copy of nursing license or diploma or both
10. Proof of proficiency in the English language
11. Photograph(s)
12. Social Security number
13. Application and fees

state. You need to contact the board of nursing in the state in which you are planning to obtain licensure to determine the specific requirements and documents that you need to submit.

Boards of nursing can decide either to use a credentialing agency to evaluate your documents or to review your documents at the specific state board, known as in-house evaluation. When you contact the board of nursing in the state in which you intend to work as a nurse, inform the board that you were educated outside the United States and ask it to send you an application to apply for licensure by examination. Be sure to specify that you are applying for a licensed practical/vocational nurse licensure. You should also ask about the specific documents needed to become eligible to take the NCLEX exam. You can obtain contact information for each state board of nursing through the NCSBN website at www.ncsbn.org. In addition, you can write to the NCSBN regarding the NCLEX exam. The address is 111 East Wacker Drive, Suite 2900, Chicago, IL 60601. The telephone number for the NCSBN is 1-866-293-9600; international telephone is 1 011 312 525 3600; the fax number is 1-312-279-1032.

CHAPTER 2

Self-Efficacy and Profiles to Success

LAURENT W. VALLIERE, BS, DD, LINDA ANNE SILVESTRI, PhD, RN, FAAN, AND
ANGELA SILVESTRI, PhD, APRN, FNP-BC, CNE

THE PYRAMID TO SUCCESS

Preparing to take the NCLEX-PN® examination can produce a great deal of anxiety. You may be thinking that this exam is the most important test you will ever have to take and that it reflects the culmination of everything you have worked so hard for. This is an important examination because passing the exam means that you can begin your career as a licensed nurse. A vital ingredient to your success on the NCLEX is to avoid the negative thoughts that allow this examination to seem overwhelming and intimidating. Such thoughts will take control over your destiny. A strong positive attitude, self-efficacy, a structured plan for preparation, and the development of control through discipline and perseverance ensure reaching the peak of the Pyramid to Success, becoming a licensed nurse (Box 2.1). For additional information about testing, study habits, and test anxiety, we refer you to *Saunders 2022-2023 Clinical Judgment and Test-Taking Strategies: Passing Nursing School and the NCLEX® Exam.*

Self-Efficacy

The concept of self-efficacy was originally proposed in social science research by Albert Bandura (1977) in developing social cognitive theory. This theory has been used extensively in the field of psychology. Central to Bandura's work are the concepts of self-efficacy and self-efficacy (outcome) expectations. The concept of self-efficacy is described as a type of self-reflection that affects one's behavior (Bandura, 1977). Self-reflection enables an individual to assess his or her own experiences, develop perceptions about his or her own capabilities that guide behavior, and determine how much effort will ensue for performance. Thus, self-reflection leads to an individual's self-efficacy expectations and confidence in the ability to succeed.

⚠ *A study by Silvestri, Clark, & Moonie (2013) showed that self-efficacy expectations were an important predictor for NCLEX success.*

Self-Efficacy Expectations

Self-efficacy expectations are focused on the belief in one's own capacity to carry out particular behaviors. These expectations determine the behaviors a person chooses to perform, the degree of perseverance, and the quality of the performance. Bandura (1977) describes self-efficacy as an individual's belief regarding his or her abilities to successfully perform activities or tasks and indicates that the stronger the sense of self-efficacy, the more confident one is to succeed. In applying Bandura's (1977) theory to NCLEX success, if you have high self-efficacy expectations, you will work hard and persevere and believe that you will achieve NCLEX success. Conversely, if your self-efficacy expectations are low, this could lead to self-doubt about your ability to achieve success on NCLEX.

YOUR PROFILE TO SUCCESS

Increasing Self-Efficacy

Self-Reflection

Self-reflection enables individuals to assess their own experiences, develop perceptions about their capabilities that guide behavior, and determine how much effort will ensue for performance. Thus, self-reflection leads to an individual's self-efficacy expectations and confidence in the ability to succeed. According to Bandura (1977), individuals possess a self-regulatory function that provides the capability to influence their own cognitive processes and actions and thus alter their environments. Therefore, whatever self-efficacy beliefs an individual holds will help to determine what activities the individual will pursue, the effort that he or she will expend in pursuing these activities, and how long he or she will persist in the face of obstacles and hardships.

To start, take time to self-reflect. Think about your accomplishments and how you achieved them. Journal these accomplishments and keep them in mind. Review them whenever you begin to feel self-doubt about your

Box 2.1 ▲ PROFILES TO SUCCESS

Avoid negative thoughts that allow the examination to seem overwhelming and intimidating.
Maintain a strong positive attitude and self-efficacy expectations.
Develop a comprehensive plan to prepare for the examination.
Examine the study methods and strategies that you used to prepare for exams during nursing school.
Develop realistic time goals.
Select a study time period and place that will be most conducive to your success.
Commit to your own special study methods and strategies.
Incorporate a balance of exercise, rest, and relaxation into your preparation schedule.
Maintain healthy eating habits.
Learn to control anxiety.
Remember that discipline and perseverance will automatically bring control.
Remember that this examination is all about you.
Remember that your self-confidence and your belief in yourself will lead you to success!

ability to succeed on the NCLEX. Some self-reflection questions to ask yourself include:

1. Am I a goal-setter?
2. Do I develop a plan and determine what activities I need to pursue to achieve my goals?
3. Do I set goals that are unrealistic to achieve in a specific time frame?
4. Do I accomplish the goals that I set?
5. How much time and effort do I put in to accomplish my goals?
6. Do I find ways to achieve my goals when I am faced with life challenges and obstacles?
7. How do I feel when I accomplish a goal?

Developing Your Preparation Plan

Nursing graduates preparing for the NCLEX must develop a comprehensive plan. The most important component of this plan is to identify the study patterns that helped you obtain your nursing degree. Begin your planning by reflecting on the personal and academic challenges that you experienced during your nursing education. Take time to focus on the thoughts, feelings, and emotions that you experienced before taking an examination while in your nursing program. Examine the methods that you used to prepare for those exams, both academically and psychologically.

These factors are important considerations when preparing for the NCLEX, because they identify the patterns that proved successful for you. Think about this for a moment. Your own methods of study must have worked, or you would not be at this point of preparing for the NCLEX-PN.

Each individual has developed his or her own methods of successfully preparing for an examination. Graduates who have taken the NCLEX-PN will probably share their experiences and methods of preparing for this challenge with you, and they will provide you with important strategies that they have used. Listen closely to what they have to say, but remember that this examination is all about you. Your identity and what you require in terms of preparation are most important.

Reflect on the methods and strategies that worked for you throughout your nursing program. Do not think that you need to develop new methods and strategies when preparing for the NCLEX. Use what has worked for you. Take some time to reflect on these strategies, write them down on a large blank card, sign your name, and write "LPN" or "LVN" after your name. Post this card in a place where you will see it every morning. Commit to your own special strategies. These strategies reflect your profile and identity and will lead you to success!

A frequent concern of graduates preparing for the NCLEX relates to deciding whether to study alone or join a study group. Examining your profile will help you make this decision. Again, reflect on what has worked for you throughout your nursing program as you prepared for your exams. Remember that *your* needs are most important. Address your own needs, and do not become pressured by peers who are encouraging you to join a study group if this is not your normal pattern of study. Additional pressure is not what you need at this important time in your life.

Graduates who are preparing for NCLEX frequently inquire about the best method of preparing. First, remember that you are already prepared. In fact, you began preparing for this examination on the first day of your nursing program. The task that you are faced with is to review, in a comprehensive manner, the nursing content that you learned as part of your nursing program. It can be overwhelming to look at your bookshelf overflowing with the nursing books that you used during nursing school, and your challenge becomes monumental when you look at the boxes of nursing lecture notes that you have accumulated. It is unrealistic to even think that you could read all of those nursing books and lecture notes in preparation for the NCLEX. These books and notes should be used as reference sources, if needed, during your preparation for the NCLEX.

Saunders Comprehensive Review for the NCLEX-PN® Examination has identified for you all of the important nursing content areas relevant to the examination. While you are undertaking this comprehensive review, you should note the areas that were unfamiliar or unclear. Be sure that you have taken the necessary time to become familiar with the necessary areas. Now, progress through the Pyramid to Success, and test your knowledge with this book, *Saunders Q&A Review for the NCLEX-PN® Examination*. You may identify nursing content areas that still require further review. Take the time to review these areas as you are guided to do by this book.

Identifying Your Goals for Success

⚠ *Create a list of your goals related to NCLEX preparation. Open your calendar and start with listing your daily goals and what you want to accomplish each day. Your daily goal could be to practice a specific number of questions, review a specific content area, or even to take a day of rest and relaxation!*

Your profile to success requires that you develop realistic time goals for preparing for the NCLEX. It is necessary to take the time to examine your life and all of the commitments that you may have, including family, work, and friends. As you develop your goals, remember to plan time for fun and exercise. To achieve success, you require a balance of both work and enjoyment. If you do not plan for some leisure time, you will become frustrated and perhaps even angry. These sorts of feelings will block your ability to focus and concentrate. Remember that you need time for yourself.

Goal development may be a relatively easy process, because you have probably been juggling your life commitments ever since you entered nursing school. Remember that your goal is to identify a daily time frame and period for you to use when reviewing and preparing for the NCLEX. Open your calendar, and identify the days on which life commitments will not allow you to spend this time preparing. Block those days off, and do not consider them as a part of your review time. Identify the time that is best for you in terms of your ability to concentrate and focus so that you can accomplish the most in your identified time frame. Consider a time that is quiet and free of distractions. Many individuals find morning hours to be the most productive, whereas others find that afternoon and evening hours are the most useful. Remember that the NCLEX is all about you; select the time period that will be most conducive to your success.

Selecting Your Study Place

The place of study is also very important. Select a place that is quiet and comfortable and where you normally do your studying and preparing. Some individuals prefer to study at home in their own environment; if this is your normal pattern, be sure that you are able to free yourself of distractions during your scheduled preparation time. If this is not an option, you may consider spending your preparation time in a library. When selecting your place of study, reflect on what worked best for you during your nursing program.

Deciding on Your Amount of Daily Study Time

Selecting the amount of daily preparation time has frequently been a dilemma for many graduates who are preparing for the NCLEX. It is very important to determine a realistic time period that can be adhered to on a daily basis. Set a time frame that will provide you with quality time and that can be realistically achieved. If you do not follow these guidelines, you will become frustrated. This frustration will block your journey toward the peak of the Pyramid to Success.

It is a good idea for you to spend at least 2 hours each day preparing for the NCLEX. This is a realistic time period in terms of both quality and achievability. You may find that, after 2 hours, your ability to focus will diminish. However, you may find on some days that you are able to spend more than the scheduled 2 hours and that your concentration is still present; when these days occur, use them to your advantage.

DEVELOPING CONTROL

Discipline and perseverance will automatically bring control. Control will provide you with the momentum that will sweep you to the peak of the Pyramid to Success.

Discipline yourself to spend time preparing for the NCLEX every day. Daily preparation is very important because it maintains a consistent pattern and keeps you in synchrony with the mind flow required for the day that you are scheduled to take the NCLEX. Some days you may think about skipping your scheduled preparation time because you are not in the mood for study or because you just do not feel like studying. On these days, practice your discipline and persevere. Stand yourself up, shake off the thoughts of skipping a day, take a deep breath, and get the oxygen flowing throughout your body. Look in the mirror, smile, and say to yourself, "This time is for me, and I will do this!" Look at your card that displays your name with "LPN" or "LVN" after it, and get yourself to that special study place. Remember that discipline and perseverance will bring control.

Dealing With Anxiety

In the profile to success, academic preparation directs the path to the peak of the Pyramid to Success. However, additional factors will influence your successful achievement, including your control of anxiety, physical stamina, rest, relaxation, self-confidence, and your complete belief that you will achieve success on the NCLEX. You need to take time to think about these important factors and to incorporate them into your daily preparation schedule.

Anxiety is a common concern among students who are preparing to take the NCLEX. A low level of anxiety is normal and will keep your senses sharp and alert. However, a great deal of anxiety can block your process of thinking and hamper your ability to focus and concentrate. You have already practiced the task of controlling anxiety when you took exams in nursing school. Now you need to continue with this practice and incorporate this control on a daily basis. Each day, before beginning your scheduled preparation time, sit in your quiet special study place, close your eyes, and take a slow, deep breath through your nose. Fill your body with oxygen, hold your breath to a count of 4, and then exhale slowly through your mouth. Continue with this exercise, and repeat it four to six times. This exercise will help you relieve your mind of any unnecessary chatter, and it will deliver oxygen to all of your body tissues and to your brain. On the day that you take the NCLEX, after the necessary pretesting procedures, you will be escorted to your test computer. Practice this breathing exercise before beginning the exam, and use it during the examination if you feel yourself becoming anxious or distracted. Remember that breathing will move oxygen to your brain!

Ensuring Physical Readiness

Physical stamina is a necessary component of your readiness for the NCLEX. Plan to incorporate a balance of exercise, rest, and relaxation into your preparation schedule. It is also important that you maintain healthy eating habits. Begin to practice these healthy habits now, if you have not already done so. There are a few points to keep in mind each day as you plan your daily meals. Three balanced meals are important, with snacks such as fruit included between meals. Remember that food items that contain fat will slow you down and that food items that contain caffeine will cause nervousness and sometimes shakiness. These items should be limited in the diet. Healthy foods that are high in complex carbohydrates work best to supply you with your energy needs. Remember that your brain can work like a muscle, so it requires those carbohydrates. In addition, be sure that you include necessary fruits and vegetables in your diet and drink plenty of water (Box 2.2).

If you are the type of individual who does not eat breakfast, work on changing that habit as you are preparing for the NCLEX. Provide your brain with energy in the morning with some form of complex carbohydrate food; it will make a difference. On the day of the NCLEX, feed your brain, and eat a healthy breakfast. In addition, on this very important day, bring a snack such as fruit or a bagel for break time, and feed your brain again so that you will have the energy to concentrate, focus, and successfully complete your examination.

Box 2.2 ▲ HEALTHY EATING HABITS

Eat three balanced meals each day.
Include snacks, such as fruits and vegetables, between meals.
Drink ample amounts of water.
Avoid food items that contain fat.
Avoid food items that contain caffeine.
Consume healthy foods that contain complex and healthy carbohydrates.

▲ *Take time for you! Holistic preparation is important, so be sure to include self-care and positive pampering in your preparation plan.*

Adequate rest, relaxation, and exercise are important to your preparation process. Many graduates who are preparing for NCLEX have difficulty sleeping, particularly the night before the examination. Begin now to develop methods that will assist you with relaxing your body and mind and that will help you obtain restful sleep. You may already have a particular method that you use to help you sleep. If not, it may be helpful to try the breathing exercise while you lie in bed to help you eliminate any mind chatter that is present.

It is also helpful to visualize a special place and time that is a totally relaxing memory while you do these breathing exercises. Graduates have also stated that listening to quiet music or relaxation tapes has assisted them with relaxing and sleeping. Begin to practice some of these helpful methods now, while you are preparing for the NCLEX, and identify those that work best for you. The night before your scheduled examination is an important one. Spend some time having fun, get to bed early, and incorporate the relaxation methods that you have been using to help you sleep (Box 2.3).

CONFIDENCE AND BELIEF IN YOURSELF

Your self-confidence and the belief that you have the ability to achieve success will bring your goals to fruition (Box 2.4). Reflect on the profile to success that you

Box 2.3 ▲ RELAXATION METHODS

Inhale through your nose and fill your body with oxygen.
Hold your breath to a count of 4.
Exhale slowly through your mouth.
Visualize a special place and time that is a totally relaxing memory.

Box 2.4 ▲ YOUR PYRAMID TO SUCCESS WORDS!

Believe: Believe in your success every day.
Plan: Plan the study strategies that work for you.
Control: Always maintain command of your emotions, and breathe.
Practice: Review, review, review: practice questions, practice questions, and more practice questions!
Succeed: Believe, plan, control, and practice: "Yes, I can!"

maintained during your nursing education. Your confidence and belief in yourself, along with your academic achievements, have brought you to the status of a graduate. Now you are facing one more important challenge.

Can you meet this challenge successfully? Yes, you can! There is no reason to think otherwise if you have taken all of the necessary steps to ensure that profile to success. Each morning, place your feet on the floor, stand tall, take a deep breath, and smile. With both hands, imagine yourself brushing off any negative feelings. Look at the card that bears your name with the letters "LPN" or "LVN" after it, and tell yourself, "Yes, I can!"

Believe in yourself, and you will reach the peak of the Pyramid to Success!

Congratulations, and we wish you continued success in your career as a licensed practical or vocational nurse!

CHAPTER

3

The NCLEX-PN® Examination: From a Graduate's Perspective

ANTHONY MACHNACZ, LPN

The day I graduated from nursing school, all I could think was "I did it! What an accomplishment!" I worked through many obstacles to achieve my nursing degree. On my path, I faced many challenges, from juggling family and study commitments while in nursing school all the way to landing a job. I needed to find a balance to make it come together while enjoying my family life and having some relaxation and fun in my life. This is a learning process, which is challenging, but with the support of my family and other nursing students, it all worked out. It is really important that you accept the support from family and, just as important, accept support from your fellow nursing students. If you support each other, then you will all work together to achieve your desire and goal to become a nurse.

When my fellow nursing students and I graduated from nursing school, we all knew we had to pass the NCLEX®. So many things were going through our minds. It was overwhelming. We thought: How are we going to pass this major exam, and how are we going to study? We were all nervous and anxious and welcomed all of the suggestions for preparing that our instructors and former graduates provided. All the information and suggestions they provided were overwhelming for me. I needed to take some time to think about what I had been doing to prepare for nursing exams while in school and about what learning style was going to work for me to prepare for the NCLEX. I needed to fight my feelings of lacking confidence and being unsure of myself. I wanted to be successful, so I put together all the suggestions I was given and focused on what would work for my learning style. This really helped me stay on track.

I want to tell you that it is important to listen to your instructors and former students about how to prepare for this exam, but always remember that this test is about *you*, so do what is going to work for you to be successful. I prepared for the NCLEX using *Saunders Comprehensive Review for the NCLEX-PN® Examination* and *Saunders Q&A Review for the NCLEX-PN® Examination*. I also carried around the *Saunders Review Cards for the NCLEX-PN®* and practiced these questions whenever I could. In fact, I brought them to work and studied when I could. These cards are so easy to carry around. When deciding what resources you want to use to prepare for NCLEX, I recommend these two books because they are packed with all the information and practice questions that you need to be ready for the exam. This is all you need, so don't think that you need to go out and buy all the NCLEX products that are on the market.

When planning your preparation time and goals, remember to be realistic so that you do not become overwhelmed. You are already anxious and nervous, so don't make things worse for yourself. Develop a self-focused plan that will work for you, but be sure that it is a structured plan. Knowing what I needed to do to plan my time around work and other commitments, I made sure that my plan was structured and realistic so that I could stick to it. I suggest doing practice questions as the primary way to prepare for the NCLEX. Just keep doing practice question after practice question after practice question. This is the best study strategy. Always read the rationales and strategies. Reading those rationales will really help you understand why the answer is correct and why the incorrect options are incorrect. Also during your study session, make a list of the content areas that you are having difficulty with. These are the areas that you will want to review in *Saunders Comprehensive Review for the NCLEX-PN® Examination* or your nursing textbooks if necessary.

My goal was to do 250 practice questions a day, and I did achieve my daily goal. In fact, I practiced 6000 questions before taking the NCLEX. I would start my practice questions in the morning for a couple of hours and then take a break to clear my mind. I have a passion for hiking. It calms and relaxes me—plus I am getting some exercise. I highly recommend that you take the time to do something that relaxes you and clears your mind. Of course, all I could think about was passing the NCLEX, but seriously, after a couple of hours of studying, your mind becomes distracted and you lose focus, so you need to take a break and clear your mind. This really helped me stay focused and on track with my study plan. Make sure to take time to have some fun, and be sure to eat healthy to keep your body and mind fueled for success.

The day before my exam I studied and took breaks in between. I went for a hike later in the day and had a good dinner with family. I slept well but felt as if I had knots in my stomach. The morning of the exam I woke up early, feeling nervous and anxious. I did a few practice questions just to get my mind in question mode. Then I had something light but healthy to eat. I went for a walk to clear my mind and prepare myself mentally and physically for the exam. Then I was ready to head to the testing center. The center was 50 minutes away, and my mom drove with me. She is an LPN and took the NCLEX not so long ago, so she gave me support during the entire drive. She said, "Keep taking those deep breaths to get the oxygen into your body and brain, relax because you have prepared yourself, and be confident because you have used all the tools to pass and be successful." She was so right. So I entered the testing center thinking of what she had said and confident that I could do this!

When I entered the testing center, I needed to go through all of the COVID-19 requirements and was asked several related questions. I needed to wait in a separate room until my name was called. I needed to stay 6 feet apart from others and maintain social distancing, and of course I had to wear a mask. I needed to show identification, and I provided my driver's license. I also needed my ATT form. Then they asked me to scan the palm of my hand on a reader. They provide you with a locker to store your belongings. I recommend that you don't bring your phone because they ask you to place it in a plastic bag; then they seal it, and when you want it, they need to open the sealed bag for you. They have strict policies, and you already may feel overwhelmed, so the less that you have to deal with, the better. Once all of the preadmission requirements were done, I was brought to my testing area. Here I was—ready to go! Just remember that, yes, you can do this. Know that for just about every question presented to you, the answers are there in front of you in the options. Read the question, reread the question again, and answer the question the way you answered your practice questions.

When I finished the exam, I felt overwhelmed and I felt a sigh of relief. But I did keep thinking and wondering if I passed. Waiting the two days to receive the quick results felt like weeks. While waiting, at times I thought I did great. But then, going over the exam in my mind, I became nervous and anxious that I had failed. I am told that this is a normal and natural feeling. The day came when I could check to see my results. Anxiously typing and accessing the website, I came to being one click away from seeing whether my results would say "pass" or "fail." I clicked the results and saw the word "PASS." I could not believe it! I took a double look and actually started crying tears of joy. I am a nurse! All the hard work, dedication, and family support from my mom, aunt, and sisters led me to fulfill my dream of becoming a nurse.

Just remember, you prepared for this exam all the way through nursing school. You can do this and have the confidence that you will pass. My final thoughts for you are to put together a study plan that works for you and your schedule and to practice, practice, and practice those questions. Plan to practice about 200 to 250 questions a day. Take breaks, regroup, and practice questions again. Always believe and be confident in yourself. Have a positive outlook, and you will be successful. I wish you much success on your journey, and I congratulate you on becoming an LPN.

CHAPTER

4

Clinical Judgment and Test-Taking Strategies

INTRODUCTION

Throughout this book, *strategic words* presented in the question, such as those that indicate the need to prioritize, are **bolded**. In addition, the specific test-taking strategy to use to answer correctly is **bolded** in that section for each question. For example, if the test-taking strategy is to focus on *strategic words*, then *strategic words* is **bolded.** The specific content area to review is noted in the ***Health Problem*** code. So, for example, if heart failure is the content to review, the ***Health Problem*** code will read: ***Health Problem***: Heart Failure.

The highlighting of the strategy and the Health Problem code provides you with guidance on what strategies and topics to review for further remediation in *Saunders Comprehensive Review for the NCLEX-PN® Examination* and *Saunders Clinical Judgment and Test-Taking Strategies: Passing Nursing School and the NCLEX® Exam*.

If you would like to read more about test-taking strategies after completing this chapter, *Saunders Clinical Judgment and Test-Taking Strategies: Passing Nursing School and the NCLEX® Exam* focuses on the test-taking strategies that will help you pass your nursing examinations while in nursing school and will prepare you for the NCLEX-PN examination.

I. CLINICAL JUDGMENT

Clinical judgment is the observed outcome of critical thinking and decision-making (Dickison, Haerling, & Lasater, 2019). The NCLEX-PN examination requires candidates to demonstrate the ability to use clinical judgment in client care. Thus, clinical judgment skills along with other traditional test-taking strategies should be used to answer test questions. The National Council of State Boards of Nursing (NCSBN) has created a Clinical Judgment Measurement Model (NCJMM) that consists of applying six cognitive skills or processes: (1) recognize cues; (2) analyze cues; (3) prioritize hypotheses; (4) generate solutions; (5) take action; and (6) evaluate outcomes. See Chapter 1, Table 1.1 for a description of these six cognitive skills/processes.

II. KEY TEST-TAKING STRATEGIES (BOX 4.1)

III. HOW TO AVOID READING INTO THE QUESTION (BOX 4.2)

A. Pyramid Points
   1. For traditional NCLEX items, such as multiple choice or multiple response, avoid asking yourself the forbidden words, "Well, what if …?" because this will lead you to the "forbidden" area: reading into the question.

⚠ *For NGN® items, you will have to ask yourself "What if…?" because you need to think about and consider all existing and potential concerns, such as complications, that can occur in the client. For NGN items, be sure to focus on what the question is asking to assist you in determining what you need to consider in answering.*

   2. Focus only on the data in the question, read every word, and make a decision about what the question is asking. Reread the question more than one time. Ask yourself, "What is this question asking?" and "What content is this question testing?" (see Box 4.2).
   3. Determine whether an abnormality exists. Look at data in the question and in the responses and decide what is abnormal. Pay close attention to this information as you answer the question.
   4. Focus on the client in the question. At times, there are other people discussed in the question who also impact how the question should be answered. Remember the concepts of client-centered and family-centered care.
   5. Consider available resources as you answer the question. Remember that you will have all the resources you need at the client's bedside to provide quality client care.
   6. Look for strategic words in the question, such as *immediate, initial, first, priority, initial, best, need for follow-up,* and *need for further teaching;* strategic

Box 4.1 ▲ KEY TEST-TAKING STRATEGIES

THE QUESTION

- Focus on the data in the case study or question. Read every word, and make a decision about what the question is asking.
- Note the subject and determine what content is being tested.
- Visualize the event and recognize cues; note whether an abnormality exists in the data, and analyze or interpret the data provided.
- Determine who "the client of the question" is.
- Look for the strategic words; strategic words make a difference regarding what the question is asking about.
- Determine whether the question presents a positive or negative event query.
- For traditional NCLEX items, such as multiple choice or multiple response, avoid asking yourself the forbidden words "Well, what if ...?" because this will lead you to the "forbidden" area: reading into the question.
- Remember, for NGN items, you will have to ask yourself "What if...?" because you need to think about and consider all existing and potential concerns, such as complications, that can occur in the client. For NGN items, be sure to focus on what the question is asking to assist you in determining what you need to consider in answering.
- Apply the NCSBN Clinical Judgment Measurement Model (NCJMM) and the six cognitive skills/processes alongside other test-taking strategies.

THE OPTIONS

- Always use the process of elimination when choices or options are presented, and always read each option carefully; once you have eliminated options, reread the question before selecting your final choice or choices.
- In multiple-choice questions, look for comparable or alike options, and eliminate these.
- Determine whether there is an umbrella option; if so, this could be the correct option.
- Identify any closed-ended words; if present, the option is likely incorrect.
- Use the ABCs (airway, breathing, and circulation), Maslow's Hierarchy of Needs, the steps of the nursing process, and the NCJMM to answer questions that require prioritizing; use CAB (compressions, airway, breathing) for cardiopulmonary resuscitation (CPR).
- Use therapeutic communication techniques to answer communication questions, and remember to focus on the client's thoughts, feelings, concerns, anxiety, and fears.
- Use delegating and assignment-making guidelines to match the client's needs with the scope of practice of the health care provider.
- Use pharmacology guidelines to select the correct option if the question addresses a medication.

Box 4.2 ▲ PRACTICE QUESTION: AVOIDING THE "WHAT IF ...?" SYNDROME AND READING INTO THE QUESTION

The nurse is caring for a hospitalized client with a diagnosis of heart failure who suddenly complains of shortness of breath and dyspnea during activity. After assisting the client to bed and placing the client in high Fowler's position, the nurse would take which **immediate** action?

1. Administer high-flow oxygen to the client.
2. Call the consulting cardiologist to report the findings.
3. Prepare to administer an additional dose of furosemide.
4. Obtain a set of vital signs and perform focused respiratory and cardiovascular assessments.

ANSWER: 4

Test-Taking Strategy. You may immediately think that the client has developed pulmonary edema, a complication of heart failure, and needs additional diuresis. Pulmonary edema is an emergency, and you might think an action needs to be taken before further assessment, which may lead you to choose option 3. Although pulmonary edema is a complication of heart failure, the question does not specifically state that pulmonary edema has developed; the client could be experiencing shortness of breath or dyspnea as a symptom of heart failure exacerbation, which may be expected, particularly on exertion or during activity. This is why it is important to base your answer only on the information presented, without assuming something else could be occurring. Read the question carefully. Note the **strategic word,** ***immediate,*** and focus on the **data in the question**, the client's complaints. Use the **nursing process,** and note that vital signs and assessment data would be needed before administering oxygen, administering medications, or contacting the cardiologist. Although the cardiologist may need to be notified, this is not the immediate action. Because there are no data in the question that indicate the presence of pulmonary edema, option 4 is correct. Additionally, focus on what the question is asking. The question is asking you for a nursing action, so that is what you need to look for as you eliminate the incorrect options. Use nursing knowledge, clinical experiences, clinical judgment abilities, and test-taking strategies to assist in answering the question. Remember to focus on the **data in the question** and what the question is asking and to avoid the "What if ...?" syndrome and reading into the question.

words make a difference regarding what the question is asking (Box 4.3).

7. In multiple-choice questions, multiple-response questions, or questions that require you to arrange nursing interventions or other data in order of priority, read every choice or option presented before answering.
8. *Always* use the process of elimination when choices or options are presented; after you have eliminated options, reread the question before selecting your final choice or choices. Focus on the data in both the question and the options to assist in the process of elimination and to direct you to the correct answer (see Box 4.2).
9. With questions that require you to fill in the blank, focus on the data in the question and determine what the question is asking. If the question requires you to calculate a medication dose, an intravenous flow rate, or intake and output amounts, recheck your work in calculating, and always use the on-screen calculator to verify the answer.

B. Ingredients of a question (Box 4.4)

1. The *ingredients of a question* include the event, which is a client or clinical situation; the event query or the stem of the question; and the options or answers.
2. The *event* provides you with the content about the client or clinical situation that you need to think about when answering the question.
3. The *event query* asks something specific about the content of the event.
4. The *options* are all of the answers provided with the question.
5. In a multiple-choice question, there will be four options and you must select one; read every option carefully and think about the event and the event query as you use the process of elimination.
6. In a multiple-response question, there will be several options and you must select all options that apply to the event in the question; one option, more than one option, or all options can be correct in these question types. Each option provided is a true or false statement; choose the true statements. Also, visualize the event and use your nursing knowledge, clinical experiences, and clinical judgment strategies to answer the question.
7. In an ordered-response (prioritizing) question, you will be required to arrange in order of priority nursing interventions or other data; visualize the event and use your nursing knowledge, clinical experiences, and clinical judgment strategies to answer the question.
8. A fill-in-the-blank question does not contain options, and some figure/illustration questions and audio item formats may or may not contain options. A graphic option item will contain options in the form of a picture or graphic.
9. A chart/exhibit question will most likely contain options; read the question carefully and all of the data in the chart or exhibit before selecting an answer. In this question type, there will be information in the chart/exhibit that is pertinent to how the question is answered, and there may also be information that is not pertinent. It is necessary to discern what information is important and what the "distractors" are.
10. The NGN item types will use a case study approach. The stand-alone cases will be accompanied by a question that tests one or more cognitive skills. The unfolding case studies will be accompanied by six NGN item type questions, and each cognitive skill will be tested. Examples of both standalone and unfolding case studies and NGN items can be located on the Evolve site accompanying this book. Additionally, the unique test-taking strategies used to answer NGN items are illustrated with each NGN item.

Box 4.3 ▲ COMMON STRATEGIC WORDS

WORDS THAT INDICATE THE NEED TO PRIORITIZE

Best
Early or late
Essential
First
Highest priority
Immediate
Initial
Most
Most appropriate
Most important
Most likely
Next
Priority
Primary

WORDS THAT REFLECT ASSESSMENT

Ascertain
Assess
Check
Collect data
Determine
Find out
Gather
Identify
Monitor
Observe
Obtain information
Recognize cues

ADDITIONAL STRATEGIC WORDS

Need for further teaching
Need for further education
Need for follow-up

Box 4.4 ▲ INGREDIENTS OF A QUESTION: EVENT, EVENT QUERY, AND OPTIONS

EVENT. The nurse caring for a client with myocardial infarction is helping the client fill out the diet menu request form.

EVENT QUERY. The nurse recommends that the client select which beverage from the menu?

OPTIONS

1. Tea
2. Cola
3. Coffee
4. Fruit juice

ANSWER: 4
Test-Taking Strategy. Focus on the client's diagnosis and recall that caffeine needs to be eliminated from the diet because of its stimulating effects. Also, note that options 1, 2, and 3 are **comparable or alike**, in that they are products that contain caffeine; this will direct you to the correct option.

As you read a question, remember to note its ingredients: the event, event query, and options!

Remember to focus on the **subject,** what the question is asking, and look at each part of the question to answer correctly.

IV. STRATEGIC WORDS (Box 4.5)

A. *Strategic words* focus your attention on a critical point to consider when answering the question and will assist you in eliminating the incorrect options. These words can be located in either the event or the query of the question.

B. Some strategic words may indicate that all options are correct and that it will be necessary to prioritize to select the correct option; words that reflect the process of assessment/data collection are also important to note (see Box 4.3). Words that reflect assessment/data collection usually indicate the need to look for an option that is a first step, because data collection is the first step in the nursing process.

C. As you read the question, look for the strategic words; strategic words make a difference regarding the focus of the question.

V. SUBJECT OF THE QUESTION (BOX 4.6)

A. The *subject of the question* is the specific topic that the question is asking about.

B. Identifying the subject of the question will assist you in eliminating the incorrect options and direct you in selecting the correct option. Throughout this book, if the *subject* of the question is a specific strategy to use in answering the question correctly, it is bolded in the test-taking strategy.

Box 4.5 ▲ PRACTICE QUESTION: STRATEGIC WORDS

The nurse is caring for a client receiving digoxin. The nurse monitors the client for which **early** manifestation of digoxin toxicity?

1. Anorexia
2. Facial pain
3. Photophobia
4. Yellow color perception

ANSWER: 1
Test-Taking Strategy. Focus on the **strategic word,** *early.* The most common early manifestations of toxicity include gastrointestinal disturbances such as anorexia, nausea, and vomiting. Facial pain, personality changes, and ocular disturbances (photophobia, light flashes, halos around bright objects, yellow or green color perception) are also signs of toxicity, but they are not early signs. Remember to look for **strategic words** and recognize cues!

Box 4.6 ▲ PRACTICE QUESTION: SUBJECT OF THE QUESTION

A client who underwent a bronchoscopy was returned to the nursing unit 1 hour ago. The nurse determines that the client is experiencing a complication of the procedure if the nurse notes which finding on data collection?

1. An oxygen saturation of 95%
2. A weak gag and cough reflex
3. A respiratory rate of 20 breaths per minute
4. Breath sounds that are greater on the right than on the left

ANSWER: 4
Test-Taking Strategy. Focus on the **subject,** a complication of bronchoscopy. Therefore, look for the abnormal piece of data in the options. Begin to answer this question by eliminating options 1 and 3, which are acceptable data. From the remaining options, recall that the client is medicated before this procedure, which would cause a weak gag and cough reflex. Unequal breath sounds are always abnormal. Remember to focus on the **subject**!

▲ *The test-taking strategy for every practice question in this book is bolded. Bolding the strategy will point out and provide you with guidance on what strategies you need to review in* Saunders Clinical Judgment and Test-Taking Strategies: Passing Nursing School and the NCLEX® Exam. *The Health Problem code that accompanies each practice question will provide insight into the content areas in need of further remediation in* Saunders Comprehensive Review for the NCLEX-PN® Examination.

VI. POSITIVE AND NEGATIVE EVENT QUERIES (BOXES 4.7 AND 4.8)

A. A *positive event query* uses strategic words that ask you to select an option that is correct; for example, the event query may read, "Which statement by a client *indicates an understanding* of the side effects of the prescribed medication?"

B. A *negative event query* uses strategic words that ask you to select an option that is an incorrect item or statement; for example, the event query may read, "Which statement by a client *indicates a need for further teaching* about the side effects of the prescribed medication?"

VII. QUESTIONS THAT REQUIRE PRIORITIZING

A. Many questions in the examination will require you to use the skill of prioritizing nursing actions.

B. Look for the strategic words in the question that indicate the need to prioritize (see Box 4.3).

C. Remember that when a question requires prioritization, all options may be correct, and you will need to determine the correct order of action.

Box 4.7 ▲ PRACTICE QUESTION: POSITIVE EVENT QUERY

A client admitted to the hospital with coronary artery disease complains of dyspnea when at rest. The nurse determines that which item would be of the **most** help to the client?

1. Providing a walker to aid in ambulation
2. Elevating the head of the bed to at least 45 degrees
3. Performing continuous monitoring of oxygen saturation
4. Placing an oxygen cannula at the bedside for use if needed

ANSWER: 2

Test-Taking Strategy. This question is an example of a **positive event query.** Note the **strategic word,** *most,* and focus on the **data in the question** and the **subject,** the item that is *most* helpful to the client. The management of dyspnea is generally directed toward alleviating the cause. Symptom relief may be achieved, or at least aided, by placing the client with the head of the bed elevated. In severe cases, supplemental oxygen is used. Monitoring the oxygen saturation level detects early complications, but it does not help the client. Likewise, placing an oxygen cannula at the bedside for use would not help the client. Remember that **positive event queries** ask you to select an option that is a correct item or statement. Remember to read the event query and note whether it is a positive event type.

Box 4.8 ▲ PRACTICE QUESTION: NEGATIVE EVENT QUERY

The nurse has reinforced discharge instructions to a client who underwent a right mastectomy with axillary lymph node dissection. Which statement by the client indicates the **need for further teaching** regarding home care measures?

1. "It is all right to use a straight razor to shave under my arms."
2. "I should inform all of my other doctors that I have had this surgical procedure."
3. "I need to be sure that I do not have blood pressures taken or blood drawn from my right arm."
4. "I need to be sure to wear thick mitt hand covers or to use thick pot holders when I am cooking and touching hot pans."

ANSWER: 1

Test-Taking Strategy. This question identifies an example of a **negative event query**. Note the **strategic words,** *need for further teaching;* these words indicate that you need to select an option that identifies an incorrect client statement. Recalling that edema and infection are of concern with this client and that the client needs to be instructed regarding the measures that will avoid trauma to the affected arm will direct you to the correct option. Remember that **negative event queries** frequently ask you to evaluate outcomes and select an option that is an incorrect item or client statement!

D. Strategies to use to prioritize include the ABCs (airway, breathing, and circulation), Maslow's Hierarchy of Needs theory, the steps of the nursing process, and the cognitive skills in the NCJMM (recognize cues, analyze cues, prioritize hypotheses, generate solutions, take action, and evaluate outcomes).

E. The ABCs (Box 4.9)
   1. Use the ABCs—airway, breathing, and circulation—when selecting an answer or determining the order of priority.
   2. Remember the order of priority: airway, breathing, and circulation.
   3. Airway is always the first priority. Note that an exception occurs when cardiopulmonary resuscitation (CPR) is performed; in this situation, the nurse follows the CAB (compressions, airway, breathing) guidelines.

F. Maslow's Hierarchy of Needs theory (Box 4.10 and Fig. 4.1)
   1. According to Maslow's Hierarchy of Needs theory, physiological needs are the priority, followed by safety and security needs, love and belonging needs, self-esteem needs, and finally, self-actualization needs; select the option or determine the order of priority by addressing physiological needs first.

Box 4.9 ▲ PRACTICE QUESTION: USE OF THE ABCS

The nurse is caring for a client with Buerger's disease. Which finding would the nurse determine to be a potential complication associated with this disease?

1. Pain with diaphoresis
2. Discomfort in one digit
3. Numbness and tingling in the legs
4. Cramping in the foot while resting

ANSWER: 3

Test-Taking Strategy. Use the **ABCs—airway, breathing, and circulation**—to answer this question. Buerger's disease (thromboangiitis obliterans) is a recurring inflammation of the small- and medium-sized arteries and veins of the upper and lower extremities that results in thrombus formation and the occlusion of blood vessels. Numbness and tingling in the legs indicate cardiovascular and neurovascular impairment. Remember to use the **ABCs—airway, breathing, and circulation**—to analyze cues and prioritize.

Box 4.10 ▲ PRACTICE QUESTION: MASLOW'S HIERARCHY OF NEEDS THEORY

The nurse working in a long-term care facility is assigned to care for four clients on the hospice unit. When planning client rounds, which client would the nurse collect data from **first**?

1. The client who was complaining of severe back pain during the previous shift
2. The client who is being discharged home today and will need assistance packing
3. The client who is bed bound and needs to be turned and repositioned every 2 hours
4. The client who needs assistance applying antiembolic stockings before ambulating to the dining room for breakfast

ANSWER: 1

Test-Taking Strategy. Note the **strategic word,** *first;* this word tells you that you need to prioritize. Use **Maslow's Hierarchy of Needs theory.** The nurse is working on a hospice unit, which means that the nurse is caring for terminally ill clients. These clients need to be comforted, and the nurse needs to maintain a satisfactory lifestyle for these clients throughout the phases of dying. Although all of these clients need the nurse's attention, the client who needs to be seen first would be the client who was in severe pain during the previous shift. The nurse would evaluate this client to see whether further pain medication is needed or if the pain indicates a potential complication. Alleviating suffering is a priority nursing responsibility. Because pain is often an element of suffering, promoting optimal pain relief is a primary goal. Also, noting the word *severe* in option 1 will direct you to the correct option. Remember to use **Maslow's Hierarchy of Needs theory** to help prioritize and generate solutions!

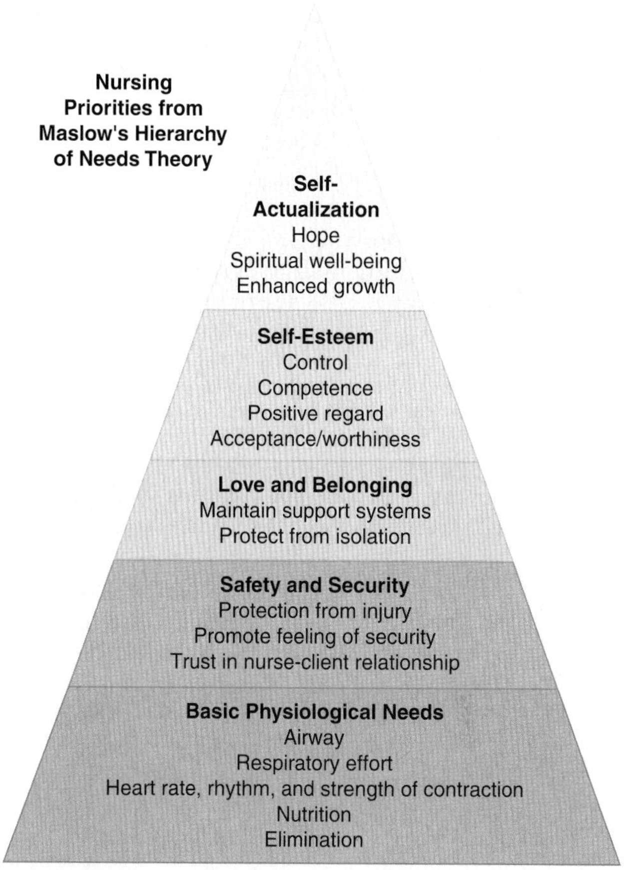

Nursing Priorities from Maslow's Hierarchy of Needs Theory

Self-Actualization
Hope
Spiritual well-being
Enhanced growth

Self-Esteem
Control
Competence
Positive regard
Acceptance/worthiness

Love and Belonging
Maintain support systems
Protect from isolation

Safety and Security
Protection from injury
Promote feeling of security
Trust in nurse-client relationship

Basic Physiological Needs
Airway
Respiratory effort
Heart rate, rhythm, and strength of contraction
Nutrition
Elimination

Figure 4.1 Use Maslow's Hierarchy of Needs theory to establish priorities.

2. When a physiological need is not addressed in the question or noted in one of the options, continue to use Maslow's Hierarchy of Needs theory sequentially as a guide, and look for the option that addresses safety.

▲ *The steps of the nursing process are data collection, planning, implementation, and evaluation. Cognitive skills identified in the NCJMM include recognize cues, analyze cues, prioritize hypotheses, generate solutions, take action, and evaluate outcomes.*

G. Steps of the nursing process and NCJMM cognitive skills
   1. Data Collection (Focused Assessment)/Recognize Cues
      a. The nurse recognizes cues by identifying significant data from many sources.
      b. These questions address the process of gathering subjective and objective data relative to the client, confirming the data, and communicating and documenting the data.
      c. Remember that data collection/recognizing cues is the first step.
      d. When you are asked to select your first, immediate, or initial nursing action, collect data/recognize cues first to prioritize when selecting the correct option.

e. Look for strategic words in the options that reflect data collection/recognizing cues (see Box 4.3).
f. If an option contains the concept of collection of client data, the best choice is to select that option (Box 4.11).
g. Possible exception to the guideline: If the question presents an emergency situation, read carefully; in an emergency situation, an action may be the priority rather than taking the time to collect further data.

2. Analyze Cues and Prioritize Hypotheses (Box 4.12)
   a. *Analyze Cues* and *Prioritize Hypotheses* are not specific steps of the Clinical Problem-Solving Process, but they are cognitive skills identified in the NCJMM. The nurse analyzes cues by connecting significant data to the client's clinical presentation and then determining the answers to these questions: Are the data expected? Unexpected? What are the concerns?
   b. After analyzing cues, the nurse identifies concerns and client needs (hypotheses) and prioritizes by ranking the hypotheses from highest to lowest priority.
   c. These questions are the most difficult questions because they require an understanding of the principles of physiological responses and interpretation of the data collected.

Box 4.11 ▲ PRACTICE QUESTION: DATA COLLECTION/RECOGNIZE CUES

The nurse enters a client's room and finds the client slumped down in a chair. The client's breathing is shallow, and a pulse is present. Based on these data, the nurse determines that which action is the **priority**?

1. Have the secretary call a code blue.
2. Call the primary health care provider (PHCP).
3. Check the vital signs and level of consciousness.
4. Ask the unit clerk to call the family immediately.

ANSWER: 3

Test-Taking Strategy. Focus on the **data in the question** and note the **strategic word,** *priority.* Use the **steps of the nursing process.** Option 3 is the only option that addresses data collection. In addition, the use of the **ABCs—airway, breathing, and circulation**—will direct you to the correct option. The client is breathing and has a pulse; therefore, additional data are needed before any other action is performed. The vital signs and level of consciousness need to be checked. After these data are obtained, the registered nurse is notified, further assessment is done, and then the PHCP is notified, who will then contact the family if deemed necessary. A code blue is not indicated at the present time. Remember to recognize cues and that data collection is the first **step of the nursing process.**

Box 4.12 ▲ PRACTICE QUESTION: ANALYZE CUES/PRIORITIZE HYPOTHESES

The nurse reviews the arterial blood gas results of a client and notes the following: pH 7.45, Pco_2 30 mm Hg, and HCO_3 22 mEq/L (22 mmol/L). The nurse analyzes these results as indicating which condition?

1. Metabolic acidosis, compensated
2. Respiratory alkalosis, compensated
3. Metabolic alkalosis, uncompensated
4. Respiratory acidosis, uncompensated

ANSWER: 2

Test-Taking Strategy. This question requires you to analyze cues. Focus on the **data in the question** and the **subject,** interpreting arterial blood gas results. The nurse needs to analyze the cues provided in the question and have knowledge of normal arterial blood gas results and acid-base disorders to determine the condition the client is experiencing. The normal pH is 7.35 to 7.45. In a respiratory condition, an opposite effect will be seen between the pH and the Pco_2. In this situation, the pH is at the high end of the normal value and the Pco_2 is low. So, you can eliminate options 1 and 3. In an alkalotic condition, the pH is elevated. The values identified indicate a respiratory alkalosis. Compensation occurs when the pH returns to a normal value. Because the pH is in the normal range at the high end, compensation has occurred. Although analysis is not a step in the Clinical Problem-Solving Process, remember that *Analyze Cues* and *Prioritize Hypotheses* are cognitive skills identified in the NCJMM, and the nurse needs to analyze cues and connect data to the presentation in the question.

   d. They require critical thinking, decision-making, and determining priority concerns and client needs.
   e. These questions may also include the communication and documentation of the results from the process of analyzing cues and identifying priority hypotheses.
   f. Often, these types of questions require examining a broad concept and breaking it down into smaller parts, assimilation of the information, and application to a client scenario.
   g. The licensed practical/vocational nurse may need to collaborate with the registered nurse when analyzing cues and prioritizing hypotheses.

3. Planning/Generate Solutions (Box 4.13)
   a. The nurse generates solutions by using hypotheses to determine interventions for an expected outcome.
   b. These questions require prioritizing client problems, determining goals and outcome criteria for goals of care, developing the plan of care, and communicating and documenting the plan of care.

Box 4.13 ▲ PRACTICE QUESTION: PLANNING/ GENERATING SOLUTIONS

A client is admitted to the hospital with a diagnosis of acute pancreatitis. The nurse plans care, knowing that which problem occurs with this disorder?

1. Hyperkalemia
2. Hypoglycemia
3. Abdominal pain
4. Sodium retention

ANSWER: 3

Test-Taking Strategy. Focus on the **subject,** planning nursing care for a problem that occurs with acute pancreatitis. The question specifically addresses the planning **step of the nursing process**. Note the word *acute,* and use your medical terminology skills. Remember that *-itis* indicates inflammation; this will direct you to the correct option. Additionally, the remaining options are unrelated to the client's diagnosis. Remember that planning is the second **step of the nursing process** and that the nurse needs to plan and generate solutions to determine interventions for an expected outcome.

c. Remember that actual client problems rather than potential client problems will be the priority in most client situations.

4. Implementation/Take Action (Box 4.14)
   a. The nurse implements the generated solutions, addressing the highest priorities or hypotheses.
   b. These questions address further data collection or analyzing, organizing and managing care, counseling and teaching, providing care to achieve established goals, supervising and coordinating care, and communicating and documenting nursing interventions.
   c. Focus on a nursing action rather than on a medical action when you are answering a question, unless the question is asking you to determine what prescribed medical action is anticipated and necessary.
   d. On the NCLEX-PN examination, the only client whom you need to be concerned about is the client in the case study or question that you are answering; avoid the "What if …?" syndrome, and remember that the client in the question on the computer screen is your *only* assigned client.
   e. Answer the question from a textbook and ideal point of view. Think about and visualize the data in the question as if the problem were in real time or represented a real clinical situation; however, remember that this is your *only* assigned client and that you have all of the time and all of the equipment needed to care for the client readily available at the bedside; remember that you do not need to run to the supply room to obtain, for example, sterile gloves because the sterile gloves will be at the client's bedside (see section XII).

Box 4.14 ▲ PRACTICE QUESTION: IMPLEMENTATION/TAKE ACTION

A visitor brings a client who is on suicide precautions a brightly packaged gift. The nurse caring for the client takes which action?

1. Suggests that the client open the gift
2. Reinforces the safety policies with the client
3. Tells the client what a beautiful package this is
4. Lets the visitor spend time alone with the client

ANSWER: 1

Test-Taking Strategy. This question specifically addresses the take action or implementation **step of the nursing process**. Note the **data in the question** and the **subject,** the action that the nurse takes. Implementation questions address the process of organizing and managing care. The nurse must be concerned with the safety of the client. The visitor may or may not be aware of the client's suicidal thoughts or of the hospital's safety policies. The client should open the gift in the presence of the nurse so that sharp or unsafe objects can be locked in the client's safety box. Leaving the package unattended in the room with the client is hazardous. Options 2, 3, and 4 are incorrect and unsafe. Remember that implementation is the third **step of the nursing process.** The nurse needs to consider generated solutions and then take action.

5. Evaluation/Evaluate Outcomes (Box 4.15)
   a. The nurse compares observed outcomes with expected ones.
   b. These questions focus on comparing the actual outcomes of care with the generated solutions and expected outcomes and on communicating and documenting findings.
   c. They also focus on assisting in determining the client's response to care and on identifying factors that may interfere with achieving expected outcomes.
   d. In these question types, watch for negative event queries because they are frequently used.

H. Determine whether an abnormality exists (Box 4.16)

1. In the question, the client scenario will be described. Use your nursing knowledge and recognize cues to determine whether any of the information presented indicates an abnormality.
2. If an abnormality exists, either further data collection and analysis or further nursing action will be required. Therefore, options that focus on documenting care or continuing to monitor the client are unlikely to be correct answers; do not select these options if they are presented!

Box 4.15 ▲ PRACTICE QUESTION: EVALUATION/ EVALUATE OUTCOMES

The nurse provides instructions to a pregnant woman about food items to consume that contain folic acid. Which statement made by the client indicates an adequate understanding of these food items?

1. "I will eat yogurt every day."
2. "I will eat a banana every day."
3. "A glass of milk each day will be sufficient."
4. "Green leafy vegetables, whole grains, and fruits are important to eat."

ANSWER: 4

Test-Taking Strategy. Evaluation is the fourth **step of the nursing process**. Note the words *indicates an adequate understanding.* These words indicate that this is an evaluation-type question. Options 1 and 3 can be eliminated first because they are **comparable or alike** in that both yogurt and milk are dairy products and are high in calcium. To select from the remaining options, remember that bananas are high in potassium. Remember that evaluation is the fourth **step of the nursing process.** The nurse needs to evaluate outcomes by comparing observed outcomes with expected ones.

Box 4.16 ▲ PRACTICE QUESTION: DETERMINE WHETHER AN ABNORMALITY EXISTS

The nurse is caring for a client who is taking digoxin and is complaining of nausea. The nurse gathers additional assessment data and checks the most recent laboratory results. Which laboratory value requires the **need for follow-up** by the nurse?

1. Sodium 138 mEq/L
2. Potassium 3.3 mEq/L
3. Phosphorus 3.1 mg/dL
4. Magnesium 1.8 mg/dL

ANSWER: 2

Test-Taking Strategy. Note the **strategic words,** *need for follow-up.* The first step in approaching the answer to this question is to **determine whether an abnormality exists**. Recognize cues in the question that are significant, and analyze the cues by connecting the data to a possible hypothesis. Because the client is taking digoxin and is complaining of nausea, the nurse would suspect toxicity. The normal reference range for sodium is 135 to 145 mEq/L; potassium, 3.5 to 5.0 mEq/L; phosphorus, 3.0 to 4.5 mg/dL; and magnesium, 1.8 to 2.6 mEq/L. The laboratory values noted in the options are all within normal range except for the potassium level. Recall that the potassium level must stay consistent while the client is taking digoxin to prevent adverse effects such as toxicity from occurring. Remember to recognize cues, analyze them, and **determine whether an abnormality exists** in the event before choosing the correct option.

I. Focus on the data in the question and recognize cues (Box 4.17)
   1. With this strategy, data are provided in either the question or the options (or both) that are important in answering the question correctly.
   2. Data needed to answer the question will be abnormal and will not be borderline. In other words, using nursing knowledge, clinical experiences, and clinical judgment abilities will assist you in recognizing the abnormal data. If it is borderline, there will be another event in the question that could cause the data to become abnormal.

J. Choose options that ensure client safety (see Box 4.17)
   1. When choosing an option, think about whether the option could cause a compromise in client safety.
   2. If an option could potentially result in an adverse effect or increase the client's risk for injury, eliminate that option.
   3. Address client concerns using therapeutic communication techniques (Box 4.18).

Box 4.17 ▲ PRACTICE QUESTION: FOCUS ON THE DATA IN THE QUESTION AND ENSURE CLIENT SAFETY

The nurse is providing discharge instructions to a client with diabetes mellitus. The client's glycosylated hemoglobin (HbA1c) level is 10%. How would the nurse inform the client?

1. "Increase the amount of vegetables and water intake in your diet regimen."
2. "Change the time of day you exercise because it may cause hypoglycemia."
3. "Continue with the same diet and exercise regimen you are currently using."
4. "Utilize a high-intensity exercise regimen and decrease carbohydrate consumption."

ANSWER: 1

Test-Taking Strategy. Focus on the **data in the question,** an HbA1c level of 10%. The nurse needs to recognize cues and analyze those cues to determine that the HbA1c level is above the recommended range for a client with diabetes mellitus and indicates poor glycemic control. Therefore, an **abnormality exists.** Choose the option that addresses this abnormality and ensures client safety. Option 1 is a safe recommendation to make to a diabetic client, and will help to reduce the HbA1c level. Changing the time of day for exercise and continuing with the same diet and exercise regimen will not address the client's problem. Note the words *high-intensity* in option 4. Utilizing a high-intensity exercise regimen and decreasing carbohydrate consumption could potentially result in a hypoglycemic reaction and does not ensure client safety. Remember to ensure client safety. Focus on the **data in the question;** recognize cues and analyze them to determine whether an abnormality is present.

Box 4.18 ▲ PRACTICE QUESTION: COMMUNICATION AND THE CLIENT OF THE QUESTION

A client who is scheduled for surgery for placement of skeletal traction says to the nurse, "I'm not sure if I want to have this skeletal traction or if the skin traction would be best to fix my fracture." Based on the client's statement, the nurse would make which response?

1. "There is no reason to be concerned. I have seen lots of these procedures."
2. "Skeletal traction is much more effective than skin traction in your situation."
3. "You have concerns about skeletal versus skin traction for your type of fracture?"
4. "Your fracture is very unstable. You will die if you do not have this surgery performed."

ANSWER: 3

Test-Taking Strategy. Use **therapeutic communication techniques**. Select the option that enhances communication and addresses the client's feelings and concerns; this will direct you to the correct option. The incorrect responses are nontherapeutic. Remember to recognize and analyze cues, use **therapeutic communication techniques,** and focus on the client.

VIII. ELIMINATE COMPARABLE OR ALIKE OPTIONS (BOX 4.19)

A. When reading the options in multiple-choice questions, look for options that are comparable or alike.

B. Comparable or alike options can be eliminated as possible answers because it is unlikely that both options will be correct.

Box 4.19 ▲ PRACTICE QUESTION: ELIMINATE COMPARABLE OR ALIKE OPTIONS

The nurse is caring for a group of clients. On review of the clients' medical records, the nurse determines that which client is at risk for excess fluid volume?

1. The client taking diuretics
2. The client with an ileostomy
3. The client with kidney disease
4. The client undergoing gastrointestinal suctioning

ANSWER: 3

Test-Taking Strategy. Focus on the **subject**, the client at risk for excess fluid volume. Think about the pathophysiology associated with each condition identified in the options. The only client who retains fluid is the client with kidney disease. The client taking diuretics, the client with an ileostomy, and the client undergoing gastrointestinal suctioning all lose fluid; these are **comparable or alike** options. Remember to think about the pathophysiology of each condition and to eliminate **comparable or alike** options.

IX. ELIMINATE OPTIONS CONTAINING CLOSED-ENDED WORDS (BOX 4.20)

A. Some closed-ended words are *all, always, every, must, none, never,* and *only.*

B. Eliminate options that contain closed-ended words because these words imply a fixed or extreme meaning; these types of options are usually incorrect.

C. Options that contain open-ended words such as *may, usually, normally, commonly,* or *generally* should be considered as possibly correct.

Box 4.20 ▲ PRACTICE QUESTION: ELIMINATE OPTIONS THAT CONTAIN CLOSED-ENDED WORDS

A client is to undergo a computed tomography (CT) scan of the abdomen with oral contrast, and the nurse provides preprocedure instructions. The nurse instructs the client to take which action in the preprocedure period?

1. Avoid eating or drinking for at least 3 hours before the test.
2. Limit self to only two cigarettes on the morning of the test.
3. Have a clear liquid breakfast only on the morning of the test.
4. Take all routine medications with a glass of water on the morning of the test.

ANSWER: 1

Test-Taking Strategy. The nurse needs to use knowledge about the preparation for a CT scan of the abdomen to take action with regard to preprocedure instructions. Note the **closed-ended words** "only" in options 2 and 3 and "all" in option 4. Eliminate options that contain **closed-ended words,** because these options are usually incorrect. Also, note that options 2, 3, and 4 are **comparable or alike** options in that they all involve taking in something on the morning of the test. Remember to eliminate options that contain **closed-ended words.**

X. LOOK FOR THE UMBRELLA OPTION (BOX 4.21)

A. When answering a question, look for the umbrella option.

B. The umbrella option is a broad, comprehensive, or universal statement that usually contains the concepts of the other options within it.

C. The umbrella option will be the correct answer.

XI. USE THE GUIDELINES FOR DELEGATING AND ASSIGNMENT-MAKING (BOX 4.22)

A. You may be asked a question that will require you to decide how you will delegate a task or assign clients to other health care providers (HCPs).

Box 4.21 ▲ PRACTICE QUESTION: LOOK FOR THE UMBRELLA OPTION

A client admitted to the hospital is diagnosed with a pressure injury on the coccyx and has a wound dressing and a wound vac. The wound culture results indicate methicillin-resistant *Staphylococcus aureus* is present. The wound dressing and wound vac foam are due to be changed. The nurse would employ which protective precautions to prevent contraction of the infection during care?

1. Gloves and a mask
2. Contact precautions
3. Airborne precautions
4. Face shield and gloves

ANSWER: 2

Test-Taking Strategy. Focus on the client's diagnosis, and recall that this infection is through direct contact. Recall that contact precautions involve the use of gown and gloves for routine care and the use of gown, gloves, and face shield if splashing is anticipated during care. Note that the correct option is the **umbrella option.** Remember to look for the **umbrella option,** a broad or universal option that includes the concepts of the other options in it.

B. Focus on the data in the question and what task or assignment is to be delegated and the available HCPs.
C. When you have determined what task or assignment is to be delegated and the available HCPs, consider the client's needs and match the client's needs with the scope of practice of the HCPs identified.
D. The Nurse Practice Act and any practice limitations define which aspects of care can be delegated and which must be performed by a registered nurse. Use nursing scope of practice as a guide to assist in answering questions. Remember that the NCLEX is a national examination and that national standards rather than agency-specific standards must be followed when delegating.
E. In general, noninvasive interventions, such as skin care, range-of-motion exercises, ambulation, grooming, and hygiene measures, can be assigned to an assistive personnel (AP), also known as a nursing assistant or certified nursing assistant.
F. A licensed practical/vocational nurse (LPN/LVN) can perform focused assessments and the tasks that an AP can perform and can usually perform certain invasive tasks, such as dressings, suctioning, urinary catheterization, and administering medications orally or by the subcutaneous or intramuscular route; some selected piggyback intravenous medications may also be administered. The LPN/LVN can also reinforce teaching initiated by the RN.
G. A registered nurse can perform the tasks that an LPN can perform and is responsible for performing comprehensive assessments, supervising care, initiating teaching, and administering medications intravenously.

Box 4.22 ▲ PRACTICE QUESTION: USE GUIDELINES FOR DELEGATING AND ASSIGNMENT MAKING

The nurse in charge of a long-term care facility is planning the client assignments for the day. Which client would be assigned to the assistive personnel (AP)?

1. A client on strict bed rest
2. A client with dyspnea who is receiving oxygen therapy
3. A client scheduled for transfer to the hospital for surgery
4. A client with a gastrostomy tube who requires tube feedings every 4 hours

ANSWER: 1

Test-Taking Strategy. Note the **subject** of the question, the assignment to be delegated to the AP. When asked questions about delegation, think about the role description and scope of practice of the employee and the needs of the client. A client with dyspnea who is receiving oxygen therapy, a client scheduled for transfer to the hospital for surgery, or a client with a gastrostomy tube who requires tube feedings every 4 hours has both physiological and psychosocial needs that require care by a licensed nurse. The AP has been trained to care for a client on bed rest. Remember the nurse needs to match the client's needs with the scope of practice of the health care provider in order to plan and generate solutions for a safe client assignment!

XII. AVAILABLE RESOURCES AND IDEAL SITUATIONS (BOX 4.23)

A. When providing care to a client, particularly in emergency situations, keep in mind that all of the resources needed to provide client care (e.g., blood pressure cuff, dressing supplies) will be readily available. Remember, you have everything you need wherever and whenever you need it!
B. Answer the question as if it were an ideal situation. Remember that NCLEX requires you to answer questions based on textbook information, and you also will need to use knowledge and clinical judgment when making decisions about the client's health problem and condition and apply the cognitive skills identified in the NCJMM.

XIII. ANSWERING PHARMACOLOGY QUESTIONS (BOX 4.24)

A. If you are familiar with the medication, use nursing knowledge to answer the question.
B. Remember that the question will identify the generic name of the medication only.
C. If the question identifies a medical diagnosis, try to form a relationship between the medication and the diagnosis; for example, you can determine that

Box 4.23 ▲ AVAILABLE RESOURCES

The nurse is called to the room of a client with a chest tube. The client states that it feels as if the tube has pulled out of the chest. The nurse assesses the client and finds that the tube has dislodged and is lying on the floor. What action would the nurse take **next**?

1. Obtain a pair of sterile gloves.
2. Contact the charge nurse for help.
3. Cover the insertion site with a sterile dressing.
4. Submerge the dislodged tube into sterile water.

ANSWER: 3

Test-Taking Strategy. Note the **strategic word,** *next.* Recognize cues in the question, and analyze the cues for their significance to identify the action that needs to be taken. When providing care to a client, particularly in emergency situations, keep in mind that all of the resources needed to provide client care will be readily available at the client's bedside. Most students would eliminate option 4 first, knowing that this action is unnecessary in this scenario. From the remaining options, you may think, "I don't have sterile gloves or a sterile dressing with me, so let me call for help first." Remember, you have everything you need wherever and whenever you need it!

cyclophosphamide is an antineoplastic medication if the question refers to a client with breast cancer who is taking this medication. Remember though that on the NCLEX a diagnosis may or may not be presented in a question.

D. Try to determine the classification of the medication being addressed to assist in answering the question. Identifying the classification will assist in determining a medication's action or its side effects and adverse effects or both.

▲ *Recognize the common side effects and adverse effects associated with each medication classification and relate the appropriate nursing interventions to each effect; for example, if a side effect is hypertension, the associated nursing intervention would be to monitor the blood pressure.*

E. Focus on what the question is asking or the subject of the question—for example, intended effect, side effect, adverse effect, or toxic effect.

F. Learn medications that belong to a classification by commonalities in their medication names; for example, medications that act as beta blockers end with "*-lol*" (e.g., aten*olol*).

G. If the question requires a medication calculation, remember that a calculator is available on the computer; talk yourself through each step to be sure that the answer makes sense, and recheck the calculation before answering the question, particularly if the answer seems like an unusual dosage.

Box 4.24 ▲ PRACTICE QUESTION: ANSWERING PHARMACOLOGY QUESTIONS

Lisinopril is prescribed as adjunctive therapy in the treatment of heart failure. After administering the first dose, the nurse would monitor which item as the **priority?**

1. Weight
2. Urine output
3. Lung sounds
4. Blood pressure

ANSWER: 4

Test-Taking Strategy. Focus on the name of the medication and note the **strategic word,** *priority.* Recall that the medication names of most angiotensin-converting enzyme (ACE) inhibitors end with "-*pril,*" and one of the indications for use of these medications is hypertension. Excessive hypotension ("first-dose syncope") can occur in clients with heart failure or in clients who are severely sodium-depleted or volume-depleted. Although weight, urine output, and lung sounds would be monitored, monitoring the blood pressure is the priority. Remember to use pharmacology guidelines to assist in answering questions about medications and to note the **strategic words.**

H. Pharmacology: Pyramid Points to remember
   1. In general, the client should not take an antacid with medication because the antacid will affect the absorption of the medication.
   2. Enteric-coated and sustained-release tablets should not be crushed; also, capsules should not be opened.
   3. The client should never adjust or change a medication dose or abruptly stop taking a medication.
   4. The nurse never adjusts or changes the client's medication dosage and never discontinues a medication.
   5. The client needs to avoid taking any over-the-counter medications or any other medications, such as herbal preparations, unless they are approved for use by the primary health care provider.
   6. The client needs to avoid consuming alcohol.
   7. Medications are never administered if the prescription is difficult to read, is unclear, or identifies a medication dose that is not a normal one.
   8. Additional strategies for answering pharmacology questions are presented in *Saunders Clinical Judgment and Test-Taking Strategies: Passing Nursing School and the NCLEX® Exam.*

UNIT

II

Client Needs

CHAPTER

5

Client Needs and the NCLEX-PN® Test Plan

CLIENT NEEDS

In the new test plan implemented in April 2020, the National Council of State Boards of Nursing (NCSBN) identified a framework based on Client Needs. This framework was selected on the basis of the findings of a practice analysis study of newly licensed practical and vocational nurses in the United States. The study identified the nursing activities performed by these entry-level nurses. In addition, according to the NCSBN, the Client Needs categories provide a structure for defining nursing actions and competencies across all settings for all clients. The NCSBN identifies four major categories of Client Needs. Some categories are further divided into subcategories, and the percentage of test questions in each subcategory is identified (Table 5.1). Refer to the NCSBN website at www.ncsbn.org for additional information about the NCLEX test plan.

Safe and Effective Care Environment

According to the NCSBN, these questions test the concepts that the nurse (1) provides nursing care; (2) collaborates with interprofessional team members to facilitate effective client care; and (3) protects clients, significant others, and health care personnel from environmental hazards.

Table 5.1 ▲ CLIENT NEEDS CATEGORIES AND PERCENTAGE OF QUESTIONS ON THE NCLEX-PN EXAMINATION

CLIENT NEEDS CATEGORY	PERCENTAGE OF QUESTIONS
SAFE AND EFFECTIVE CARE ENVIRONMENT	
Coordinated Care	18–24
Safety and Infection Control	10–16
HEALTH PROMOTION AND MAINTENANCE	6–12
PSYCHOSOCIAL INTEGRITY	9–15
PHYSIOLOGICAL INTEGRITY	
Basic Care and Comfort	7–13
Pharmacological Therapies	10–16
Reduction of Risk Potential	9–15
Physiological Adaptation	7–13

From: National Council of State Boards of Nursing: *NCLEX-PN® detailed test plan*. Chicago, 2019, National Council of State Boards of Nursing.

The Safe and Effective Care Environment category includes two subcategories: Coordinated Care and Safety and Infection Control. The NCSBN identifies nursing content related to the subcategories of this Client Needs category (Box 5.1). The Coordinated Care subcategory addresses content related to facilitating effective client

Box 5.1 ▲ NCLEX-PN CONTENT: SAFE AND EFFECTIVE CARE ENVIRONMENT

COORDINATED CARE

Advance directives
Advocacy
Client-care assignments
Client rights
Collaboration with the health care team
Concepts of management and supervision
Confidentiality and information security
Continuity of care
Establishing priorities
Ethical practice
Information technology
Informed consent
Legal responsibilities
Performance improvement (quality improvement)
Referral processes
Resource management

SAFETY AND INFECTION CONTROL

Accident, error, and injury prevention
Emergency response plan
Ergonomic principles
Handling hazardous and infectious materials
Home safety
Least restrictive restraints and safety devices
Reporting of incidents, events, irregular occurrences, and variances
Safe use of equipment
Security plan
Standard precautions, transmission-based precautions, and surgical asepsis

From the National Council of State Boards of Nursing, eds: *NCLEX-PN® Examination: Detailed test plan for the National Council Licensure Examination for Practical Nurses.* Chicago, 2019: National Council of State Boards of Nursing. Portions copyrighted by the National Council of State Boards of Nursing, Inc. All rights reserved. Refer to the National Council of State Boards of Nursing website for more information about the test plan: www.ncsbn.org.

Box 5.2 ▲ SAFE AND EFFECTIVE CARE ENVIRONMENT QUESTIONS

COORDINATED CARE

The nurse is planning the client assignments for the day. Which is the **most appropriate** assignment for the assistive personnel (AP)?

1. The client who requires colostomy irrigation
2. The client receiving continuous tube feedings
3. The client who requires stool specimen collections
4. The client who has difficulty swallowing food and fluids

ANSWER: 3

This question addresses the subcategory Coordinated Care in the Client Needs category of Safe and Effective Care Environment, and it specifically addresses content related to client care assignments. Delegation of tasks must be consistent with the individual's level of expertise and licensure or lack of licensure. Note the **strategic words,** *most appropriate.* In this situation, the most appropriate assignment for the AP would be to care for the client who requires stool specimen collections, which is a noninvasive task. The client with difficulty swallowing food and fluids is at risk for aspiration, and colostomy irrigations and tube feedings are not performed by AP. Remember that the health care provider needs to be competent and skilled at performing the task or activity that has been assigned.

SAFETY AND INFECTION CONTROL

A client with tuberculosis (TB) is scheduled to go to the radiology department for a chest x-ray. Which nursing intervention would be appropriate when preparing to transport the client?

1. Apply a mask to the client.
2. Apply a mask and gown to the client.
3. Apply a mask, gown, and gloves to the client.
4. Notify the x-ray department so that personnel can be sure to wear masks when the client arrives.

ANSWER: 1

This question addresses the subcategory Safety and Infection Control in the Client Needs category of Safe and Effective Care Environment, and it specifically addresses content that is related to airborne precautions. Clients who have or are suspected of having TB should wear a mask when out of the hospital room to prevent the spread of the infection to others. A gown and gloves are not necessary.

care through collaboration with other health care team members. The Safety and Infection Control subcategory addresses content that tests the knowledge, skills, and abilities required to protect clients and health care personnel from health and environmental hazards. Focus on safety with these types of questions, and remember the importance of hand washing, call bells, bed positioning, appropriate use of side rails, asepsis, use of standard and other precautions, prioritizing, triage principles, and emergency response planning.

Box 5.2 presents examples of questions that address these two subcategories. Refer to Chapter 6, "Safe and Effective Care Environment Practice Questions," for practice with questions that reflect this Client Needs category.

Health Promotion and Maintenance

According to the NCSBN, the Health Promotion and Maintenance category tests the concepts that the nurse provides and assists in directing nursing care to promote and maintain health. Content addressed in these questions relates to assisting the client and significant others during the normal expected stages of growth and development, and providing client care related to the prevention and early detection of health problems.

The NCSBN identifies nursing content that is related to this Client Needs category (Boxes 5.3 and 5.4). Use the Teaching and Learning theory if the question addresses client teaching, remembering that the client's willingness, desire, and readiness to learn are the first priorities. With questions in this Client Needs category, watch for negative event queries because they are frequently used in questions that address Health Promotion and Maintenance and client education. Also, refer to Chapter 7, "Health Promotion and Maintenance Practice Questions," for practice with questions that reflect this Client Needs category.

Box 5.3 ▲ NCLEX-PN CONTENT: HEALTH PROMOTION AND MAINTENANCE

- Aging process
- Antepartum, intrapartum, and postpartum periods and newborn care
- Community resources
- Data collection techniques
- Developmental stages and transitions
- Health promotion and disease prevention
- High-risk behaviors
- Lifestyle choices
- Self-care

From the National Council of State Boards of Nursing, eds: *NCLEX-PN® Examination: Detailed test plan for the National Council Licensure Examination for Practical Nurses.* Chicago, 2019, National Council of State Boards of Nursing. Portions copyrighted by the National Council of State Boards of Nursing, Inc. All rights reserved. Refer to the National Council of State Boards of Nursing website for more information about the test plan: www.ncsbn.org.

Box 5.4 ▲ HEALTH PROMOTION AND MAINTENANCE QUESTIONS

A postpartum nurse has instructed a new parent regarding how to bathe their newborn infant. The nurse demonstrates the procedure to the parent and asks the parent to perform the procedure on the following day. Which observation by the nurse indicates that the parent is performing the procedure correctly?

1. The parent cleans the ears and then moves to the eyes and the face.
2. The parent begins to wash the newborn infant by starting with the eyes and face.
3. The parent washes the arms, chest, and back, followed by the neck, arms, and face.
4. The parent washes the newborn infant's entire body and then washes the eyes, face, and scalp.

ANSWER: 2

This question addresses the Client Needs category of Health Promotion and Maintenance, and it specifically addresses the postpartum period and newborn care. The bathing of a newborn should start with the eyes and face and with the cleanest area first. Next, the external ears and behind the ears are cleaned. The newborn infant's neck should be washed, because formula, lint, and breast milk will often accumulate in the folds of the neck. The hands and arms are then washed. The infant's legs are washed next, with the diaper area washed last. Remember to always start with the cleanest area of the body and to proceed to the dirtiest area.

A client with atherosclerosis asks the nurse about dietary modifications to lower the risk of heart disease. The nurse encourages the client to eat which food to lower this risk?

1. Fresh cantaloupe
2. Broiled cheeseburger
3. Baked chicken with skin
4. Mashed potato with gravy

ANSWER: 1

This question addresses the Client Needs category of Health Promotion and Maintenance, and it specifically addresses health and wellness. To lower the risk of heart disease, the diet should be low in saturated fat, with the appropriate number of total calories. The diet should be low in red meat and include more white meat with the skin removed. Dairy products should be low in fat, and foods with high amounts of empty calories should be avoided. Fresh fruits and vegetables are naturally low in fat.

Box 5.5 ▲ NCLEX-PN CONTENT: PSYCHOSOCIAL INTEGRITY

Abuse or neglect
Behavioral management
Chemical and other dependencies
Coping mechanisms
Crisis intervention
Cultural awareness
End-of-life concepts
Grief and loss
Mental health concepts
Religious and spiritual influences on health
Sensory and perceptual alterations
Stress management
Support systems
Therapeutic communication
Therapeutic environment

From the National Council of State Boards of Nursing, eds: *NCLEX-PN® Examination: Detailed test plan for the National Council Licensure Examination for Practical Nurses.* Chicago, 2019, National Council of State Boards of Nursing. Portions copyrighted by the National Council of State Boards of Nursing, Inc. All rights reserved. Refer to the National Council of State Boards of Nursing website for more information about the test plan: www.ncsbn.org.

Psychosocial Integrity

The NCSBN notes that these questions test the concepts that the nurse provides nursing care that promotes and supports the emotional, mental, and social well-being of the client and significant others. Content addressed in these questions relates to supporting and promoting the client's or significant others' ability to cope, adapt, or problem-solve in situations such as illnesses; disabilities; or stressful events, including abuse, neglect, or violence.

In this Client Needs category, you may be asked communication-type questions that relate to how you would respond to a client, a client's family member or significant other, or other health care team members. To answer communication questions focus on the client in the question and use therapeutic communication techniques because of their effectiveness in the communication process. Remember to select the option that focuses on the thoughts, feelings, concerns, anxieties, or fears of the client, client's family member, or significant other.

The NCSBN identifies nursing content related to this Client Needs category (Boxes 5.5 and 5.6). Refer to Chapter 8, "Psychosocial Integrity Practice Questions," for practice with questions that reflect this Client Needs category.

Physiological Integrity

The Physiological Integrity category includes four subcategories: Basic Care and Comfort, Pharmacological Therapies, Reduction of Risk Potential, and Physiological Adaptation.

The NCSBN indicates that questions in this Client Needs category test the concepts that the nurse provides

Box 5.6 ▲ PSYCHOSOCIAL INTEGRITY QUESTIONS

The nurse is planning care for a client who is experiencing anxiety after a myocardial infarction. Which **priority** nursing intervention should be included in the plan of care?

1. Answer questions with factual information.
2. Provide detailed explanations of all procedures.
3. Limit family involvement during the acute phase.
4. Administer an antianxiety medication to promote relaxation.

ANSWER: 1

This question addresses the Client Needs category of Psychosocial Integrity, and it specifically addresses content related to fear and anxiety. Note the **strategic word,** *priority.* Accurate information reduces fear, strengthens the nurse–client relationship, and assists the client with dealing realistically with the situation. Providing detailed information may increase the client's anxiety, so information should be provided simply and clearly. Limiting family involvement may or may not be helpful, because the client's family may be a source of support for the client. Medication should not be used unless necessary.

The nurse in the mental health clinic is assisting with collecting data from a family with a diagnosis of domestic violence. Which factor would the nurse **initially** want to include during data collection?

1. The coping style of each family member
2. The family's anger toward the intrusiveness of the nurse
3. The family's current ability to use community resources
4. The family's denial of the violent nature of their behavior

ANSWER: 1

This question addresses the Client Needs category of Psychosocial Integrity, and it specifically addresses domestic violence and crisis intervention. Note the **strategic word,** *initially.* At the beginning, data collection includes a careful history of each family member. The correct option addresses each family member. The incorrect options address the family as a whole.

Box 5.7 ▲ NCLEX-PN CONTENT: PHYSIOLOGICAL INTEGRITY

BASIC CARE AND COMFORT

Assistive devices
Elimination
Mobility and immobility
Nonpharmacological comfort interventions
Nutrition and oral hydration
Personal hygiene
Postmortem care
Rest and sleep

PHARMACOLOGICAL THERAPIES

Side effects/adverse effects/contraindications/interactions
Dosage calculations
Expected actions and outcomes
Medication administration
Pharmacological pain management

REDUCTION OF RISK POTENTIAL

Changes/abnormalities in vital signs
Diagnostic tests
Laboratory values
Potential for alterations in body systems
Potential for complications of diagnostic tests, treatments, and procedures
Potential for complications from surgical procedures and health alterations
Therapeutic procedures

PHYSIOLOGICAL ADAPTATION

Alterations in body systems
Basic pathophysiology
Fluid and electrolyte imbalances
Medical emergencies
Unexpected responses to therapies

From the National Council of State Boards of Nursing, eds: *NCLEX-PN® Examination: Detailed test plan for the National Council Licensure Examination for Practical Nurses.* Chicago, 2019, National Council of State Boards of Nursing. Portions copyrighted by the National Council of State Boards of Nursing, Inc. All rights reserved. Refer to the National Council of State Boards of Nursing website for more information about the test plan: www.ncsbn.org.

comfort and assistance in the performance of activities of daily living and provides care related to the administration of medications and selected intravenous therapies.

These questions also address the nurse's ability to reduce the client's potential for developing complications or health problems related to treatments, procedures, or existing conditions and to provide care to clients with acute, chronic, or life-threatening physical health conditions. Focus on the Maslow's Hierarchy of Needs theory in these types of questions, and remember that physiological needs are a priority and are addressed first. Also, use the ABCs—airway, breathing, and circulation—and the steps of the nursing process when selecting an option addressing Physiological Integrity.

The NCSBN identifies nursing content related to the subcategories of this Client Needs category (Box 5.7). Box 5.8 provides practice questions that address these subcategories. Also, refer to Chapter 9, "Physiological Integrity Practice Questions," for practice with questions that reflect this Client Needs category.

Box 5.8 ▲ PHYSIOLOGICAL INTEGRITY QUESTIONS

BASIC CARE AND COMFORT

A client with right-sided weakness needs to learn how to use a cane for home maintenance of mobility. The nurse plans to teach the client to position the cane by holding it in which way?

1. With the left hand and 6 inches lateral to the left foot
2. With the right hand and 6 inches lateral to the right foot
3. With the left hand, with the cane placed in front of the left foot
4. With the right hand, with the cane placed in front of the right foot

ANSWER: 1

This question addresses the subcategory Basic Care and Comfort in the Client Needs category of Physiological Integrity, and it specifically addresses content related to the use of an assistive device. The client is taught to hold the cane on the opposite side of the weakness because, with normal walking, the opposite arm and leg move together (called *reciprocal motion*). The cane is placed 6 inches lateral to the fifth toe.

PHARMACOLOGICAL THERAPIES

The nurse is caring for a client with hypertension who is receiving furosemide orally daily. Which laboratory result would indicate to the nurse that the client may be experiencing an adverse effect related to the medication?

1. A chloride level of 98 mEq/L
2. A sodium level of 135 mEq/L
3. A potassium level of 3.1 mEq/L
4. A blood urea nitrogen (BUN) level of 15 mg/dL

ANSWER: 3

This question addresses the subcategory Pharmacological Therapies in the Client Needs category of Physiological Integrity, and it specifically addresses content related to the adverse effect of a medication. Furosemide is a loop diuretic that can produce acute, profound water loss; volume and electrolyte depletion; dehydration; decreased blood volume; and circulatory collapse. Option 3 is the only option that indicates an electrolyte depletion, because the normal potassium level is 3.5 to 5.0 mEq/L. The normal chloride level is 98 to 106 mEq/L, the normal sodium level is 135 to 145 mEq/L, and the normal BUN level is 10 to 20 mg/dL.

REDUCTION OF RISK POTENTIAL

The nurse is caring for a client scheduled to undergo a renal biopsy. To minimize the risk of postprocedure complications, the nurse would report which laboratory result to the primary health care provider before the procedure?

1. Potassium: 3.8 mEq/L
2. Serum creatinine: 1.2 mg/dL
3. Prothrombin time: 15 seconds
4. Blood urea nitrogen (BUN): 18 mg/dL

ANSWER: 3

This question addresses the subcategory Reduction of Risk Potential in the Client Needs category of Physiological Integrity, and it specifically addresses a potential postprocedure complication of a diagnostic test. Postprocedure hemorrhage is a complication after renal biopsy. Because of this, the prothrombin time is checked before the procedure. The normal prothrombin time range is 11 to 12.5 seconds. The nurse ensures that these results are available and reports abnormalities promptly. The normal potassium level is 3.5 to 5.0 mEq/L, the normal serum creatinine level is 0.6 to 1.2 mg/dL, and the normal BUN level is approximately 10 to 20 mg/dL.

PHYSIOLOGICAL ADAPTATION

A pregnant client tells the nurse that she felt wetness on her peripad and that she found some clear fluid. The nurse quickly inspects the perineum and notes the presence of the umbilical cord. Which action should the nurse take **first**?

1. Notify the registered nurse.
2. Monitor the fetal heart rate.
3. Transfer the client to the delivery room.
4. Place the client in Trendelenburg's position.

ANSWER: 4

This question addresses the subcategory Physiological Adaptation in the Client Needs category of Physiological Integrity, and it specifically addresses an acute and life-threatening physical health condition. Note the **strategic word,** *first.* On inspection of the perineum, if the umbilical cord is noted, the nurse immediately places the client into Trendelenburg's position to relieve cord compression. The registered nurse is notified, who then contacts the obstetrician. The nurse monitors the fetal heart rate, and the client is transferred to the delivery room as prescribed by the obstetrician.

CHAPTER

6

Safe and Effective Care Environment Practice Questions

1. The nurse is preparing to transfer an average-sized client from the bed to the wheelchair. The client recently suffered a stroke and is experiencing right-sided hemiplegia. The client can support weight on the unaffected side, and the nurse plans to use the hemiplegic transfer technique. The client is sitting upright in bed with the legs dangling over the side. For the safest transfer, where would the wheelchair be positioned?
   1 Next to either leg
   2 Near the client's left leg
   3 Near the client's right leg
   4 As space in the room permits

Level of Cognitive Ability: Applying
Client Needs: Safe and Effective Care Environment
Clinical Judgment/Cognitive Skills: Generate Solutions
Integrated Process: Nursing Process/Planning
Content Area: Foundations of Care: Safety
Health Problem: Adult Health: Neurological: Stroke

Answer: 2
Rationale: Although the space in the room is an important consideration for the placement of a wheelchair for a transfer, when the client has an affected lower extremity, movement would always occur toward the client's unaffected (strong) side. For example, if the client's right leg is affected and the client is sitting on the edge of the bed, then the wheelchair is positioned next to the client's left side; this wheelchair position allows the client to use the unaffected leg effectively and safely.
Priority Nursing Tip: When transferring clients experiencing hemiplegia, support needs to be provided by the unaffected side.

Test-Taking Strategy: Focus on the **subject,** the safest transfer for the client. The correct option will provide the safest transfer, because positioning the wheelchair next to the client's unaffected leg allows the client to use the stronger leg more effectively for a safe transfer. Therefore options 1 and 3 are incorrect. Although option 4 is a consideration for wheelchair positioning, it is not the safest answer.

---

2. The nurse, preparing to leave the room of a client with a tracheostomy, would ensure that the client has which means of communication readily available before leaving the room?
   1 Call bell
   2 Letter board
   3 Picture board
   4 Pen and paper

Level of Cognitive Ability: Applying
Client Needs: Safe and Effective Care Environment
Clinical Judgment/Cognitive Skills: Generate Solutions
Integrated Process: Nursing Process: Planning
Content Area: Foundations of Care: Safety
Health Problem: Adult Health: Respiratory: Upper Airway

Answer: 1
Rationale: Before leaving the room, the nurse would ensure that the call bell is readily available to the client. A client who cannot speak needs to have a means of contacting the nurse who is not in the room. The other options facilitate communication only when the nurse is already present in the client's room.
Priority Nursing Tip: Keep in mind that when a tracheostomy is present, air cannot pass over the vocal cords to create audible speech, so the client needs to be provided with alternate means of communication.

Test-Taking Strategy: Focus on the **subject,** communication needs of the client, and note the words, *tracheostomy* and *leaving the room.* Remember that options that are **comparable or alike** are often incorrect; in this case, all are forms of paper communication.

---

3. A licensed practical nurse (LPN) is asked to prepare a room for a child who will be admitted to the pediatric unit with a diagnosis of tonic-clonic seizures. The LPN prepares the room and plans to place which items at the bedside?

1 A tracheotomy set and oxygen
2 Suction apparatus and oxygen
3 An endotracheal tube and an oral airway
4 An emergency cart and padded side rails

Level of Cognitive Ability: Applying
Client Needs: Safe and Effective Care Environment
Clinical Judgment/Cognitive Skills: Generate Solutions
Integrated Process: Nursing Process/Planning
Content Area: Pediatrics: Neurological
Health Problem: Pediatric-Specific: Seizures

Answer: 2

Rationale: Tonic-clonic seizures cause a tightening of all the body's muscles followed by rhythmic jerking of all extremities. An obstructed airway and increased oral secretions are the major complications during and after a seizure, making availability to suctioning equipment and oxygen a priority. During the postictal phase, a suction apparatus, oxygen, and airway are helpful to prevent aspiration and treat cyanosis, which may have occurred during the seizure. Options 1, 3, and 4 present incorrect information. Inserting a tracheostomy or endotracheal tube is not done in this situation. It is not necessary to have an emergency cart at the bedside, but a cart would be available in the treatment room or on the nursing unit. The effectiveness of the use of padded side rails is now debatable and may embarrass the client.

Priority Nursing Tip: Although seizures seem to last a long time, they usually do not last more than 60 to 90 seconds.

Test-Taking Strategy: Focus on the **subject,** seizure precautions and the associated risks of a seizure. Recalling that tonic-clonic seizures produce excessive oral secretions and result in airway obstruction will assist you with selecting the correct option.

---

4. A child is admitted to the hospital with an undiagnosed exanthema (rash) that covers the trunk but is sparse on the extremities. During data collection, the nurse discovers that the child was exposed to varicella 2 weeks ago. Which is the appropriate, **immediate** nursing intervention?

1 Place the child in a private room and maintain strict isolation.
2 Place the child in any available bed as long as it is near the nursing station.
3 Encourage a parent to remain with the child until a diagnosis is confirmed.
4 Check the progression of the exanthema and report it to the primary health care provider.

Level of Cognitive Ability: Applying
Client Needs: Safe and Effective Care Environment
Clinical Judgment/Cognitive Skills: Take Action
Integrated Process: Nursing Process/Implementation
Content Area: Pediatrics: Infectious and Communicable Diseases
Health Problem: Pediatric-Specific: Skin Inflammation and Infection

Answer: 1

Rationale: A child with undiagnosed exanthema would be placed on strict isolation in a private room. Varicella causes a profuse rash on the trunk with a sparse rash on the extremities. It is important to prevent the spread of this communicable disease by placing the child in isolation until further diagnosis and treatment can be started. This information makes options 2, 3, and 4 incorrect because none address the spread of the disease.

Priority Nursing Tip: Remember that transmission of varicella can be airborne or by direct contact with contaminated objects.

Test-Taking Strategy: Note the **strategic word,** *immediate,* and the **data in the question**. The correct option prevents the child from exposing other children and keeps staff, visitors, and others at minimal risk. Admitting the child to "any" room is inappropriate. Checking the progression of the exanthema is correct, but it is not the immediate intervention. Option 3, although supportive of the child, does not address the immediate issue of disease containment.

5. A licensed practical nurse (LPN) is assisting the registered nurse (RN) in the planning of the client assignments for the day. Which client would be assigned to the assistive personnel (AP)?

1 A client who had a below-the-knee amputation
2 A client on strict bed rest undergoing a 24-hour urine collection
3 A client scheduled for transfer to the hospital for coronary artery bypass surgery
4 A client scheduled for transfer to the hospital for an invasive diagnostic procedure

Level of Cognitive Ability: Applying
Client Needs: Safe and Effective Care Environment
Clinical Judgment/Cognitive Skills: Generate Solutions
Integrated Process: Nursing Process/Planning
Content Area: Leadership/Management: Delegating/Supervising
Health Problem: N/A

Answer: 2

Rationale: The nurse is legally responsible for client assignments and needs to assign tasks based on the guidelines of nurse practice acts and the job description of the employing agency. Clients who have had below-the-knee amputations, who are scheduled for invasive diagnostic procedures, or who are scheduled to be transferred to a hospital for coronary artery bypass surgery have both physiological and psychosocial needs that require nursing assessment, planning, and interventions. The AP has been trained to care for clients who are on bed rest and require urine collections. The nurse will provide instructions, but the tasks required for these duties are within the role description of an AP.

Priority Nursing Tip: AP are paraprofessionals who assist individuals with physical disabilities, mental impairments, and other health care needs with their activities of daily living (ADLs) along with very basic nursing tasks.

Test-Taking Strategy: Note the **subject**, the assignment that can be delegated to the AP. When you are asked questions that relate to delegation, think about the role description of the employee and the needs of the client. This knowledge directs you to the correct option because that client has needs that the AP has been trained to address.

---

6. The nurse is preparing to administer a continuous tube feeding via a feeding pump and notes that the electrical cord for the pump has only two prongs. What is the appropriate action to ensure safety?

1 Use the pump if the plug fits snugly into the wall socket.
2 Use the pump but put it on the battery when long feedings are needed.
3 Contact the unit's nurse manager to report the problem and get a replacement.
4 Label the pump as being "out of service," and notify the biomedical department.

Level of Cognitive Ability: Applying
Client Needs: Safe and Effective Care Environment
Clinical Judgment/Cognitive Skills: Take Action
Integrated Process: Nursing Process/Implementation
Content Area: Foundations of Care: Safety
Health Problem: N/A

Answer: 4

Rationale: Electrical equipment needs to be maintained in good working order and would be grounded. (The third, longer prong in an electrical plug is the ground prong.) Theoretically, the ground prong carries any stray electrical current back to the ground, whereas the other two prongs carry the power to the piece of electrical equipment. Because this is a safety issue, the equipment would not be used and the biomedical department would be notified so that the problem can be properly handled. There is no reason to contact the nurse manager. Running the pump on the battery is not the most appropriate nursing action because the battery will run out, especially with the feeding being continuous.

Priority Nursing Tip: Focus on safe use of equipment ultimately with the client's safety in mind; this is a primary nursing responsibility.

Test-Taking Strategy: Focus on the **subject**, electrical safety. Eliminate options 1 and 2 first because they are **comparable or alike** and indicate using the pump. Understanding the principles of basic electrical safety and the role of the biomedical department would assist with directing you to the correct option from those remaining.

---

7. The nurse is assessing a client's home in preparation for hospital discharge. Which observation made by the nurse is an indication that the older adult client **needs further instruction** about home safety?
   1 Stairs are carpeted and carpets are secured with tacks.
   2 There is a clothes hamper at the end of the hallway.
   3 There are wet spots on the ceramic-tiled bathroom floor.
   4 Area rugs in the living room are skid-resistant.

Level of Cognitive Ability: Evaluating
Client Needs: Safe and Effective Care Environment
Clinical Judgment/Cognitive Skills: Evaluate Outcomes
Integrated Process: Teaching and Learning
Content Area: Foundations of Care: Safety
Health Problem: N/A

Answer: 3
Rationale: Injuries in the home frequently result from wet spots on the floor (regardless of the type of flooring); small rugs on the stairs and floor; and clutter on bedside tables, closet shelves, the top of the refrigerator, and bookshelves. Area rugs and runners would not be used on or near stairs. Any carpeting on the stairs would be secured with carpet tacks. Pathways would be kept clear. Nonessential items would be placed in drawers to eliminate clutter.
Priority Nursing Tip: Because falls are the leading cause of morbidity and mortality among older adults, nursing interventions would be focused on risk reduction interventions.

Test-Taking Strategy: Note the **strategic words,** *needs further instruction.* These words indicate a **negative event query** and ask you to select an option that is an unsafe situation. Recalling the principles related to home safety and evaluating the options for possible risk-related outcomes will assist with directing you to the correct option.

---

8. A hospitalized client with a history of alcohol abuse tells the licensed practical nurse (LPN), "I am leaving now. I don't want any more treatment." There are no discharge orders, and the client is scheduled for an important diagnostic test in 1 hour. After the nurse discusses the client's concerns with the client, the client dresses and begins to walk out of the hospital room. What is the **most appropriate** nursing action to address client risks?
   1 Call security to block all the exit areas.
   2 Insist that the client stay until the primary health care provider (PHCP) can be reached.
   3 Tell the client that he or she cannot return to the hospital if he or she leaves now.
   4 Notify the registered nurse (RN) for prompt assessment of the client and situation.

Level of Cognitive Ability: Applying
Client Needs: Safe and Effective Care Environment
Clinical Judgment/Cognitive Skills: Take Action
Integrated Process: Nursing Process/Implementation
Content Area: Leadership/Management: Ethical/Legal
Health Problem: Mental Health: Addictions

Answer: 4
Rationale: The LPN should notify the RN for assessment of the client to determine whether there is a physiological basis for the behavior. In addition, most health care facilities have documents that the client is asked to sign that relate to the client's responsibilities when the client leaves against medical advice. The RN will ask the client to sign these documents before he or she leaves. The RN should request that the client wait to speak to the PHCP before leaving, but if the client refuses to do so, the nurse cannot hold the client against his or her will. Calling security to block the exits constitutes false imprisonment. All clients have a right to health care at any time and cannot be told otherwise.
Priority Nursing Tip: A client experiencing alcohol withdrawal can demonstrate poor decision-making skills and so require appropriate monitoring for safety risks.

Test-Taking Strategy: Note the **strategic words,** *most appropriate.* Focus on the **subject**, a client leaving against medical advice (AMA). Keeping the concept of false imprisonment in mind, eliminate options 1 and 2, because they are **comparable or alike** in that they resort to restricting the client. Eliminate option 3, because all clients have a right to health care.

---

9. While in the cafeteria, two nurses and a physical therapist discuss a client who has been physically abused. While later providing therapy to the client, the physical therapist asks the client questions about the physical abuse. The client is upset that the information has been shared and reports the incident to the hospital's administration. The outcome associated with the nurses' discussion about the client is associated with which consequence for the nurses?

❒ 1 The nurses can be charged with libel.
❒ 2 The nurses can be charged with slander.
❒ 3 There are no consequences, because the discussion took place within a health care facility.
❒ 4 There are no consequences, because the physical therapist is involved in the client's care.

Level of Cognitive Ability: Analyzing
Client Needs: Safe and Effective Care Environment
Clinical Judgment/Cognitive Skills: Analyze Cues
Integrated Process: Nursing Process/Implementation
Content Area: Leadership/Management: Ethical/Legal
Health Problem: N/A

Answer: 2
Rationale: Defamation is false communication or careless disregard for the truth that causes damage to someone's reputation, either in writing (libel) or verbally (slander). The most common examples are giving out inaccurate or inappropriate information from the medical record; discussing clients, families, or visitors in public areas (cafeteria); or speaking negatively about coworkers. The event described could cause emotional harm to the client, and the nurses could be charged with slander. This event also violates the client's right to confidentiality. Based on this understanding of the situation, options 1, 3, and 4 are incorrect.
Priority Nursing Tip: Clients have the right to confidentiality, and it is a nursing responsibility to respect this right at all times.

Test-Taking Strategy: Focus on the **subject,** confidentiality. Use your knowledge about the law and the legal responsibilities of the nurse to protect the client. Eliminate options 3 and 4 first because there are consequences to the nurses' actions. From the remaining options, it is necessary to know that slander involves a verbal discussion about a client.

---

10. The nurse, having administered a dose of diazepam to the client with a muscle injury, would implement which interventions before leaving the client's room to ensure safety? **Select all that apply.**

❒ 1 Close the shades to minimize sun exposure.
❒ 2 Turn off the overhead light to decrease unnecessary stimuli.
❒ 3 Turn down the volume of the television to encourage restful sleep.
❒ 4 Educate the client to the possible risk for medication-related dizziness.
❒ 5 Provide the client with access to the call bell to facilitate communication with staff.

Level of Cognitive Ability: Applying
Client Needs: Safe and Effective Care Environment
Clinical Judgment/Cognitive Skills: Take Action
Integrated Process: Nursing Process/Implementation
Content Area: Pharmacology: Psychotherapeutic: Barbiturate and Sedative-Hypnotics
Health Problem: Adult Health: Musculoskeletal: Tissue or Ligament Injury

Answer: 4, 5
Rationale: Diazepam is a sedative/hypnotic medication with anticonvulsant and skeletal muscle relaxant properties. The nurse would institute safety measures before leaving the client's room to ensure that the client does not injure himself or herself. The most frequent side effects of this medication are dizziness, drowsiness, and lethargy. Therefore, the nurse would educate the client to the possibility of experiencing dizziness and provide the client with easy access to the call bell. Options 1, 2, and 3 may be helpful measures that provide a comfortable, restful environment; however, options 4 and 5 are the ones that provide for the client's safety.
Priority Nursing Tip: The administration of any medication that affects a client's level of consciousness requires that the nurse do frequent monitoring of the client.

Test-Taking Strategy: Focus on the **subject,** client safety after medication administration. Recalling that this medication has a sedative/hypnotic effect directs you to options that are safety related, especially for falls.

11. A client demonstrates difficulty with fine motor coordination due to a stroke. The nurse would review the progress notes from which health care team member to obtain suggestions for addressing the resulting client needs?

1 Social worker
2 Speech pathologist
3 Recreational therapist
4 Occupational therapist

Level of Cognitive Ability: Applying
Client Needs: Safe and Effective Care Environment
Clinical Judgment/Cognitive Skills: Take Action
Integrated Process: Nursing Process/Implementation
Content Area: Leadership/Management: Management of Care
Health Problem: Adult Health: Neurological: Stroke

Answer: 4

Rationale: The occupational therapist focuses on the development or relearning of fine motor skills. Social workers, speech pathologists, and recreational therapists do not address this type of client problem. Social workers focus on social problems such as securing community services, speech pathology addresses communication and swallowing issues, whereas recreational therapists provide activities that increase socialization and interpersonal skills.

Priority Nursing Tip: Fine motor coordination is needed for activities such as eating, maintaining hygiene, and dressing.

Test-Taking Strategy: Focus on the **subject,** fine motor coordination, and the health care team member whose practice would focus on such issues. Understanding the roles of the other health care team members will help in selecting the correct option.

---

12. A postpartum client has been diagnosed with endometritis. The nurse would encourage the parent to implement what intervention to prevent the spread of infection to the newborn while in the hospital?

1 Keeping the newborn in the isolette
2 Asking visitors to not hold the newborn
3 Wearing a mask to prevent the spread of airborne droplets
4 Washing the hands carefully before picking up the newborn

Level of Cognitive Ability: Applying
Client Needs: Safe and Effective Care Environment
Clinical Judgment/Cognitive Skills: Take Action
Integrated Process: Teaching and Learning
Content Area: Foundations of Care: Infection Control
Health Problem: Maternity: Infections/Inflammations

Answer: 4

Rationale: Infections like endometritis can be transmitted through contaminated items (e.g., hands, bed linens) of clients with endometritis. Hand washing is one of the most effective methods for preventing the transmission of this infectious disease because it breaks the chain of infection. Options 2 and 3 are unrelated to the route of transmission of this infection because the infection is present only in the parent, and option 1 is unnecessary when considering the route of transmission.

Priority Nursing Tip: Endometritis is an inflammatory condition of the lining of the uterus and is usually due to an infection.

Test-Taking Strategy: Focus on the **subject,** infection prevention. Eliminate options 2 and 3 first because they are unrelated to the route of transmission for this type of infection—direct contact between source of infection (the parent or objects infected by the parent) and the child. Choose correctly from the remaining options by using concepts related to the spread of infectious disease while supporting maternal-infant bonding.

---

13. A 2-month-old infant is admitted to the hospital. The nurse would perform which action to maintain the infant's safety and reduce the risk of sudden infant death syndrome (SIDS)?

1 Avoid placing plastic items in contact with the infant's skin.
2 Place the infant in a supine position in preparation for sleep.
3 Take the pacifier out of the infant's mouth before the infant falls asleep.
4 Cover the crib with netting when the child is not being directly observed.

Answer: 2

Rationale: The American Academy of Pediatrics recommends the supine position for sleep to reduce the risk of SIDS. None of the other options are known to be related to SIDS. The situation presents no evidence that the infant is allergic to plastic, so that intervention is not needed. Pacifiers are considered safe and appropriate at this age. Safety netting is unnecessary at this age, because the infant cannot roll over or stand alone.

Priority Nursing Tip: Consider the age of the infant and the infant's associated physical abilities when choosing appropriate measures to best reduce the risk for injury,

Level of Cognitive Ability: Applying
Client Needs: Safe and Effective Care Environment
Clinical Judgment/Cognitive Skills: Take Action
Integrated Process: Nursing Process/Implementation
Content Area: Foundations of Care: Safety
Health Problem: Pediatric-Specific: Sudden Infant Death Syndrome (SIDS)

Test-Taking Strategy: Focus on the **subject,** infant safety related to SIDS. Your knowledge of age-appropriate care and techniques to reduce the risk of SIDS will assist you with selecting the correct option from those unrelated to SIDS. Remember that the supine position for sleep is recommended to reduce the risk of SIDS.

---

14. The primary health care provider prescribes sertraline to the client with depression. The nurse reviewing the client's record would question the prescription if which notation is documented?

1 A history of diabetes mellitus
2 A history of myocardial infarction
3 Currently prescribed phenelzine sulfate
4 Currently being treated for irritable bowel syndrome

Level of Cognitive Ability: Analyzing
Client Needs: Safe and Effective Care Environment
Clinical Judgment/Cognitive Skills: Recognize Cues
Integrated Process: Nursing Process/Data Collection
Content Area: Pharmacology: Psychotherapeutic: Selective Serotonin Reuptake Inhibitors (SSRIs)
Health Problem: Mental Health: Mood Disorders

Answer: 3
Rationale: Sertraline is a serotonin reuptake inhibitor and an antidepressant medication. Potentially fatal reactions may occur if sertraline is administered concurrently with a monoamine oxidase inhibitor (MAOI), such as phenelzine sulfate. MAOIs would be stopped at least 14 days before sertraline therapy is started to prevent the risk of neuroleptic malignant syndrome. Conversely, sertraline would be stopped at least 14 days before MAOI therapy begins. None of the other options present situations that would result in a risk for injury.
Priority Nursing Tip: Neuroleptic malignant syndrome is characterized by a high fever, irregular pulse, tachycardia, tachypnea, muscle rigidity, and altered mental state.

Test-Taking Strategy: Focus on the **subject,** interactions and contraindications associated with the use of sertraline. It is necessary to know that potentially fatal reactions may occur if sertraline is administered concurrently with an MAOI; this will help direct you to the correct option.

---

15. The nurse performing which action after the administration of medication via intermuscular injection demonstrates appropriate knowledge concerning standard precautions?

1 Recaps the needle and discards the syringe in the disposal unit
2 Breaks the needle and discards it in a regulated disposal container
3 Discards the uncapped needle and syringe in a labeled cardboard box
4 Discards the uncapped needle and syringe in a labeled, rigid plastic container

Level of Cognitive Ability: Evaluating
Client Needs: Safe and Effective Care Environment
Clinical Judgment/Cognitive Skills: Take Action
Integrated Process: Nursing Process/Implementation
Content Area: Foundations of Care: Safety
Health Problem: N/A

Answer: 4
Rationale: Standard precautions include specific guidelines for the handling of sharps and needles. Needles would not be recapped, bent, broken, or cut after use; rather, they would be disposed of in a labeled, impermeable container specifically used for this purpose. Needles would not be discarded in cardboard boxes because they could puncture the cardboard and cause a needlestick injury.
Priority Nursing Tip: Standard precautions are a set of infection control practices used to prevent the transmission of diseases that can be acquired by contact with blood, body fluids, nonintact skin (including rashes), and mucous membranes.

Test-Taking Strategy: Focus on the **subject,** needle safety and standard precautions. Recalling that needles would never be broken or recapped assists with eliminating options 1 and 2. Noting that option 3 identifies a container that could be punctured assists with its elimination.

---

16. A licensed practical nurse (LPN) is assisting a registered nurse (RN) with developing a plan of care for a client who will be hospitalized for the insertion of an internal cervical radiation implant to treat cervical cancer. What action would the nurse take to provide for safety related to the procedure?

1 Limiting visitors' time to 60-minute visits
2 Placing the client in a private room close to the nurses' station
3 Placing a lead container and long-handled forceps in the client's room
4 Reinserting the implant into the vagina immediately if it becomes dislodged

Level of Cognitive Ability: Applying
Client Needs: Safe and Effective Care Environment
Clinical Judgment/Cognitive Skills: Take Action
Integrated Process: Nursing Process/Planning
Content Area: Adult Health: Oncology
Health Problem: Adult Health: Cancer: Cervical/Uterine/Ovarian

Answer: 3
Rationale: A lead container and long-handled forceps need to be kept in the client's room at all times during internal radiation therapy. If the implant becomes dislodged, the nurse would pick it up with long-handled forceps and place it in the lead container; it would not be reinserted by the nurse. The client's room would be marked with appropriate signs that state the presence of radiation. Visitors are limited to 30-minute visits to help manage environmental exposure risks. Additionally, pregnant women and children are not allowed to visit. The client would be placed in a private room at the end of the hall, because this location provides less of a chance of exposing others to radiation.
Priority Nursing Tip: A radiation implant is a type of radiation therapy in which radioactive material sealed in needles, seeds, wires, or catheters is placed directly into or near a tumor. It is also called brachytherapy, internal radiation therapy, or radiation brachytherapy.

Test-Taking Strategy: Focus on the **subject,** internal cervical radiation implant. Use your knowledge about the precautions and care for a client with a radiation implant to answer the question. Eliminate option 1 because of the lengthy time frame for visits, increasing the risk for exposure. Eliminate option 2 because of the words *close to the nurses' station;* this would increase the risk of exposure to both staff and visitors. Knowing that it is not within the scope of nursing practice to reinsert the implant assists with the elimination of option 4.

---

17. The nurse is assigned to care for a 4-week-old infant with pyloric stenosis scheduled for a pyloromyotomy. What intervention would the nurse plan to implement when caring for this infant?

1 Elevating the head of the infant's bed
2 Feeding the infant in an upright position
3 Feeding the infant 1 oz of formula every hour
4 Placing the infant in a side-lying position for sleeping

Level of Cognitive Ability: Applying
Client Needs: Safe and Effective Care Environment
Clinical Judgment/Cognitive Skills: Generate Solutions
Integrated Process: Nursing Process/Planning
Content Area: Pediatrics: Gastrointestinal
Health Problem: Pediatric-Specific: GI and Rectal Problems

Answer: 1
Rationale: Pyloric stenosis is the most common surgical disorder causing vomiting in infancy and is addressed with a pyloromyotomy. The head of the bed is elevated to reduce the risk of aspiration, making that option correct. Options 2 and 3 are unnecessary during the preoperative period, because the infant is kept nothing by mouth (NPO). Preoperatively, the infant's status is NPO, and the infant is stabilized with intravenous fluids and electrolytes. The side-lying position would not be required for sleeping as long as the head of the bed was appropriately elevated.
Priority Nursing Tip: Although the true cause of pyloric stenosis is unknown, it is believed to begin as the muscle at the bottom of the stomach thickens.

Test-Taking Strategy: Focus on the **subject,** an infant with pyloric stenosis. Use your knowledge about the condition and its common symptoms and signs as well as preoperative routine to eliminate incorrect options.

---

18. What action on the part of the nurse would constitute an invasion of privacy?

1 Inserting a urinary catheter into a client against his or her expressed wishes
2 Threatening to restrain a client if she or he does not cooperate with a prescribed treatment
3 Using a vest restraint to keep a client with a history of falling from getting out of bed
4 Releasing a photograph of a client to the local newspaper without his or her written consent

Level of Cognitive Ability: Applying
Client Needs: Safe and Effective Care Environment
Clinical Judgment/Cognitive Skills: Analyze Cues
Integrated Process: Nursing Process/Implementation
Content Area: Leadership/Management: Ethical/Legal
Health Problem: N/A

Answer: 4
Rationale: Invasion of privacy takes place when an individual's private affairs are unreasonably invaded. Taking photographs of a client and submitting for publication without the client's written permission is an example of such a violation. The described restraining of a client constitutes an example of false imprisonment. Threatening to place a client in restraints is an example of an assault. Performing a procedure without consent is an example of battery.
Priority Nursing Tip: The legal term for a harmful or offensive touching without permission is battery.

Test-Taking Strategy: Note the **subject**, invasion of privacy. Understanding of the various legal concerns related to nursing care and an analysis of the provided options related to what is considered privacy will assist with directing you to the correct option.

---

19. The nurse overhears the physician telling a client that the results of a biopsy have not been returned when in fact the results clearly indicated the presence of malignancy. Which resulting action would place the nurse in jeopardy of committing slander?

1 Sending an anonymous letter to the unit's nurse manager
2 Sharing the details of the incident with another nurse
3 Telling another nurse, "That physician always lies to clients."
4 Immediately telling the client the result of the biopsy

Level of Cognitive Ability: Applying
Client Needs: Safe and Effective Care Environment
Clinical Judgment/Cognitive Skills: Analyze Cues
Integrated Process: Nursing Process/Implementation
Content Area: Leadership/Management: Ethical/Legal
Health Problem: N/A

Answer: 3
Rationale: Defamation is false communication or careless disregard for the truth that causes damage to someone's reputation, either in writing (libel) or verbally (slander). The nurse is committing slander when making the statement in option 3. A breach of confidentiality occurs when the information is shared inappropriately, as in options 1 and 2. It is not the nurse's responsibility to share the information with the client. Although the physician may be aware of the client's biopsy results, the physician decides when it is best to share such a diagnosis with the client.
Priority Nursing Tip: According to the law, negligence is the failure to use reasonable care, resulting in damage or injury to another.

Test-Taking Strategy: Focus on the **subject**, identifying a slanderous act. You can eliminate options 1 and 2, which are **comparable or alike** in that they involve sharing the information with others. An understanding that slander constitutes verbal defamation will direct you to the correct option from those remaining.

---

20. The nurse notes that the prescription for furosemide is higher than the recommended dosage. When the nurse calls the prescribing physician to clarify the prescription, the request to change the dosage is denied and the nurse is told to administer the medication as prescribed. What action would the nurse take **immediately**?

1 Document that the medication dose was missed and why that occurred.
2 Administer the dose as prescribed and document the refusal to change the dose.
3 Contact the nursing supervisor to explain the situation while delaying administration.
4 Call the state medical board and report the physician for malpractice.

Level of Cognitive Ability: Applying
Client Needs: Safe and Effective Care Environment
Clinical Judgment/Cognitive Skills: Take Action
Integrated Process: Nursing Process/Implementation
Content Area: Leadership/Management: Ethical/Legal
Health Problem: N/A

Answer: 3

Rationale: If the physician writes a prescription that requires clarification, it is the nurse's responsibility to contact the physician for clarification. If there is no resolution regarding the prescription after speaking with the physician, the nurse would contact the nurse manager or supervisor for further clarification regarding what the next step would be. Under no circumstances would the nurse proceed to carry out the prescription until clarification is obtained. Option 1 is not an ethical solution and fails to resolve the problem, and option 4 is a premature action and does nothing to resolve the immediate issue at hand.

Priority Nursing Tip: The nurse acts as client advocate when questioning a prescribed treatment.

Test-Taking Strategy: Note the **strategic word,** *immediately*. Focus on the **subject,** questioning a medication prescription. Consider client safety when determining the correct option. Eliminate options that fail to resolve or at least attempt to resolve the issue or that place the client at risk for injury.

---

21. The nurse administers a 50-mg oral dose of metoprolol instead of the prescribed 25-mg dose to a client with hypertension. Once the error is discovered, what actions would the nurse take to ensure client safety and act responsibly? **Select all that apply.**

❒ 1 Complete an irregular occurrence report.
❒ 2 Elevate all side rails of the bed.
❒ 3 Monitor the client's heart rate.
❒ 4 Monitor the client's blood pressure.
❒ 5 Make a copy of the irregular occurrence report for the physician.

Level of Cognitive Ability: Applying
Client Needs: Safe and Effective Care Environment
Clinical Judgment/Cognitive Skills: Take Action
Integrated Process: Nursing Process/Implementation
Content Area: Leadership/Management: Ethical/Legal
Health Problem: Adult Health: Cardiovascular: Hypertension

Answer: 1, 3, 4

Rationale: An irregular occurrence report needs to be completed whenever an unusual incident occurs. The report is confidential and privileged information; it would not be copied, placed in the chart, or have any reference made to it in the client's record. Even though the client is at higher risk for fall due to possible bradycardia, elevating all side rails of the bed is considered a restraint and would not be done. The client's blood pressure and heart rate would be monitored because this medication can cause the side effect of hypotension and bradycardia.

Priority Nursing Tip: Metoprolol, a beta blocker that affects the heart and circulation (blood flow through arteries and veins), is used to treat angina (chest pain), dysrhythmias, and hypertension (high blood pressure).

Test-Taking Strategy: Focus on the **subject,** medication error. Knowing that metoprolol is a beta blocker with potential side effects of bradycardia and hypotension will assist you with selecting options related to cardiac function. Knowing the purpose and management of irregular occurrence reports will help you answer correctly.

22. A newly licensed practical nurse (LPN) asks about the need to obtain professional liability insurance. What is the appropriate response to the LPN?

1 "The hospital insurance covers your actions."
2 "It is very expensive, and you really don't need it."
3 "All nurses should have their own malpractice insurance."
4 "Lawsuits are filed against the hospital, so you are safe without it."

Level of Cognitive Ability: Applying
Client Needs: Safe and Effective Care Environment
Clinical Judgment/Cognitive Skills: Generate Solutions
Integrated Process: Nursing Process/Implementation
Content Area: Leadership/Management: Ethical/Legal
Health Problem: N/A

Answer: 3
Rationale: Nurses need their own professional liability insurance for protection against malpractice lawsuits. Nurses erroneously assume that they are protected by an agency's professional liability policies. Usually, when the nurse is sued, the employer is also sued for the nurse's actions or inactions. Regardless of the perceived expense, nurses are encouraged to have their own malpractice insurance.
Priority Nursing Tip: Professional liability insurance protects you against covered claims arising from real or alleged errors or omissions, including negligence, in the course of your professional duties.

Test-Taking Strategy: Note the **subject** of the question, the need to obtain professional liability insurance. Note that options 1, 2, and 4 are **comparable or alike** in that they all refer to not obtaining the malpractice insurance.

---

23. A licensed practical nurse (LPN) stops at the scene of an accident and administers safe care to the victim, who sustained a compound fracture of the femur. The victim is hospitalized and later develops sepsis because of the fractured femur. The victim files suit against the nurse who provided care at the scene of the accident. What statement **best** describes the immunity the *Good Samaritan law* provides the nurse?

1 It is not applicable in this situation and will not provide protection.
2 It protects laypersons and not professional health care providers.
3 It provides protection if the care given at the scene was not negligent.
4 It provides immunity, even if the nurse accepted compensation for the care provided.

Level of Cognitive Ability: Analyzing
Client Needs: Safe and Effective Care Environment
Clinical Judgment/Cognitive Skills: Analyze Cues
Integrated Process: Nursing Process/Implementation
Content Area: Leadership/Management: Ethical/Legal
Health Problem: N/A

Answer: 3
Rationale: Good Samaritan laws have been enacted by state legislatures to encourage nurses and other health care providers to provide care to a person when an accident, emergency, or injury occurs without fear of being sued for the care provided. Called *immunity from suit,* this protection usually applies only if all the conditions of the law are met, such as the health care provider receives no compensation for the care provided and the care given is not willfully and wantonly negligent.
Priority Nursing Tip: Good Samaritan laws protect the health care provider as long as training and scope of practice during provision of emergency care have not been exceeded.

Test-Taking Strategy: Note the **strategic word,** *best.* Focus on the **data in the question** and the **subject,** the Good Samaritan law. An understanding of the law, who is protected, and under what circumstances that protection occurs will help direct you to the correct option.

---

24. Upon entering the room, the nurse finds an older client attempting to use a pillow to put out the flames on a bedspread. Which action would the nurse take **first** to safely manage this situation?

1 Pull the nearest fire alarm.
2 Close the door of the room.
3 Remove the client from the room.
4 Run to get the nearest fire extinguisher.

Level of Cognitive Ability: Applying
Client Needs: Safe and Effective Care Environment
Clinical Judgment/Cognitive Skills: Take Action
Integrated Process: Nursing Process/Implementation
Content Area: Foundations of Care: Safety
Health Problem: N/A

Answer: 3
Rationale: During a fire emergency, the steps to follow are summed up with the acronym *RACE:* **R**emove the victim; **A**ctivate the alarm; **C**ontain the fire; and **E**xtinguish as needed. This is a universal standard that may be applied to any type of fire emergency. Option 3 is correct, because the client is removed from the area. Option 1 would be the next step (activate the alarm), followed by option 2 (contain the fire), and then option 4 (extinguish as needed).
Priority Nursing Tip: There are four classes of fire extinguishers—A, B, C, and D—and each class can put out a different type of fire. Multipurpose extinguishers can be used on different types of fires and will be labeled with more than one class, such as A-B, B-C, or A-B-C.

Test-Taking Strategy: Note the **strategic word,** *first.* With client safety in mind, sequence the activities with the use of the RACE acronym; this will direct you to the correct option.

---

25. An unconscious, unaccompanied adult client is suspected of having a perforated spleen, and emergency surgery is required immediately. When considering informed consent for the surgical procedure, what is the **best** nursing action?

1 Ask the hospital chaplain to sign the consent form.
2 Consider that the concept of implied consent applies.
3 Call the nursing supervisor to initiate a court order for the surgical procedure.
4 Call a family member to obtain telephone consent before the surgical procedure.

Level of Cognitive Ability: Applying
Client Needs: Safe and Effective Care Environment
Clinical Judgment/Cognitive Skills: Generate Solutions
Integrated Process: Nursing Process/Implementation
Content Area: Leadership/Management: Ethical/Legal
Health Problem: N/A

Answer: 2
Rationale: Generally, there are only two instances in which the informed consent of an adult client is not needed. One instance is when an emergency is present and delaying treatment for obtaining informed consent would result in injury or death. The concept of implied consent is then considered. The second instance is when the client waives the right to give informed consent. It is inappropriate to ask the hospital chaplain to sign the consent form because he/she has no legal right to do that. Requesting that the nursing supervisor initiate a court order for the surgical procedure delays necessary lifesaving interventions. Although the client's family needs to be notified, calling a family member to obtain telephone consent before the surgical procedure also delays necessary lifesaving interventions.
Priority Nursing Tip: For informed consent, you need to have the capacity (or ability) to make the decision. The medical provider needs to disclose information on the treatment, test, or procedure in question, including the expected benefits and risks, and the likelihood (or probability) that the benefits and risks will occur.

Test-Taking Strategy: Note the **strategic word,** *best.* Focus on the **data in the question** and note the phrase *surgery is required immediately.* An understanding of the requirements for both informed and implied consent is necessary to answer this item correctly. Options 3 and 4 are **comparable or alike** in that they require delaying treatment and would then be eliminated.

---

26. The nurse is asked to assess the corneal reflex of an unconscious client. What would the nurse use as the safest stimulus when touching the client's cornea?

1 Sterile glove
2 Wisp of cotton
3 Sterile drop of saline
4 Tip of a 1-mL syringe

Level of Cognitive Ability: Applying
Client Needs: Safe and Effective Care Environment
Clinical Judgment/Cognitive Skills: Generate Solutions
Integrated Process: Nursing Process/Implementation
Content Area: Health Assessment/Physical Exam: Neurological
Health Problem: N/A

Answer: 3
Rationale: The client who is unconscious is at great risk for corneal abrasion. The safest way to test the corneal reflex is by using a drop of sterile saline to stimulate a blink. Options 1, 2, and 4 can cause injury to the cornea.
Priority Nursing Tip: The corneal reflex, also known as the blink reflex, is an involuntary blinking of the eyelids elicited by stimulation of the cornea.

Test-Taking Strategy: Focus on the **subject**, safely assessing for corneal reflex. Eliminate options that are **comparable or alike** because they are unlikely to be correct. In this case, each of the incorrect options is a solid object, and the correct option is a liquid.

---

27. What statement by the nurse demonstrates an understanding of case management?

1 "It represents an interdisciplinary health care delivery system."
2 "One nurse takes care of one client and is responsible for that client."
3 "One nurse supervises all of the other employees when they care for clients."
4 "A single case manager plans the care for all of the clients in the nursing unit."

Level of Cognitive Ability: Applying
Client Needs: Safe and Effective Care Environment
Clinical Judgment/Cognitive Skills: Evaluate Outcomes
Integrated Process: Nursing Process/Implementation
Content Area: Leadership/Management: Management of Care
Health Problem: N/A

Answer: 1
Rationale: Case management represents an interdisciplinary health care delivery system to promote the appropriate use of hospital personnel and material resources to maximize hospital revenues while providing for optimal outcomes of care. Case management involves managing client care by managing the client care environment. Options 2, 3, and 4 are incorrect descriptions because the nurse case manager may be responsible for more than one client, is not responsible for non-nursing–related care or personnel, and may not be the only case manager assigned to a particular nursing unit.
Priority Nursing Tip: The case manager accomplishes clients' care by assessing treatment needs; developing, monitoring, and evaluating treatment plans and progress; facilitating interdisciplinary approaches; and monitoring staff performance.

Test-Taking Strategy: Focus on the **subject**, case management. Note that options 2, 3, and 4 are **comparable or alike** in that they all address a single individual managing the client care environment.

---

28. A client is scheduled for a bone marrow aspiration. When collecting needed supplies, the nurse will provide which skin-cleansing agent for the purpose of decontaminating the skin at the insertion site?

1 Alcohol swabs
2 Soap and water
3 Povidone-iodine
4 Hydrogen peroxide

Level of Cognitive Ability: Applying
Client Needs: Safe and Effective Care Environment
Clinical Judgment/Cognitive Skills: Generate Solutions
Integrated Process: Nursing Process/Planning
Content Area: Foundations of Care: Infection Control
Health Problem: N/A

Answer: 3

Rationale: Bone marrow aspiration involves the removal of a small amount of liquid bone marrow through a needle. Before a bone marrow aspiration procedure, the needle insertion site is cleansed with an antiseptic solution such as povidone-iodine or chlorhexidine-alcohol to minimize the risk of infection related to breeching the skin. The other options are incorrect because they would not produce the necessary antibacterial effect.

Priority Nursing Tip: During a bone marrow aspiration, the needle is placed through the top layer of bone, and a liquid sample containing bone marrow cells is obtained through the needle by sucking (aspirating) it into a syringe.

Test-Taking Strategy: Focus on the **subject,** bone marrow aspiration. Use your knowledge of general asepsis and topical cleansing agents to answer this question. Recalling that a bone marrow aspiration procedure is invasive will assist with directing you to the correct option.

---

29. A client reports, "I'm so glad you're here. The medicine didn't work when the nurse who cared for me last night gave it to me." The nurse has previously observed this same occurrence with both this client and other clients and suspects that the night nurse is substance impaired. Which action would the nurse take to appropriately respond to this potential risk to client care?

1 Report the information to the police.
2 Report the information to a supervisor.
3 Call the impaired nurse's organization, and report the nurse.
4 Call the involved nurse and discuss the event with him/her.

Level of Cognitive Ability: Applying
Client Needs: Safe and Effective Care Environment
Clinical Judgment/Cognitive Skills: Take Action
Integrated Process: Nursing Process/Implementation
Content Area: Leadership/Management: Ethical/Legal
Health Problem: N/A

Answer: 2

Rationale: Nurse practice acts require reporting any suspicion of substance-impaired nurses to the immediate nursing supervisor. The situation described would be reported to the nursing supervisor, who will then report it to the board of nursing and police as is appropriate. The board of nursing has jurisdiction over the practice of nursing and then may develop plans for treatment and supervision. Discussing the suspicion with the involved nurse is an inappropriate action if done by someone without the authority of the nursing supervisor.

Priority Nursing Tip: Follow the chain of command to report issues requiring further investigation and follow-up.

Test-Taking Strategy: Focus on the **subject,** reporting responsibilities. Remember to follow the channel of organizational structure to report events such as this one. By reporting the information, the nurse alerts the institution about the potential problem and sets the stage for further investigation and appropriate action.

---

30. While assisting with providing emergency treatment for a client experiencing ventricular tachycardia, the licensed practical nurse (LPN) identifies what intervention as adhering to the safe principles of defibrillation?

1 Wiping the paddles free of any lubricant
2 Performing a visual and verbal check of "all clear"
3 Holding the client's upper torso stable while the defibrillation is performed
4 Handing the charged paddles to the person performing the defibrillation

Level of Cognitive Ability: Applying
Client Needs: Safe and Effective Care Environment
Clinical Judgment/Cognitive Skills: Recognize Cues
Integrated Process: Nursing Process/Implementation
Content Area: Foundations of Care: Safety
Health Problem: Adult Health: Cardiovascular: Dysrhythmias

Answer: 2

Rationale: Safety during defibrillation is essential for preventing injury to the client and to the personnel assisting with the procedure. The person performing the defibrillation ensures that all personnel are standing clear of the bed with a verbal and visual check of "all clear." Charged paddles would never be handed to other personnel. For the shock to be effective, some type of conductive medium (e.g., lubricant, gel) needs to be placed between the paddles and the skin. The client is not touched during the defibrillation procedure to best minimize the risk of a transfer of electrical current to staff.

Priority Nursing Tip: In ventricular tachycardia (V-tach or VT), abnormal electrical signals in the ventricles cause the heart to beat faster than normal, usually 100 or more beats a minute, out of sync with the upper chambers.

Test-Taking Strategy: Focus on the **subject,** safe principles of defibrillation. An understanding of the role electricity plays in the defibrillation process is required to identify safe practice during the treatment. Option 2 involves a verbal and visual check of "all clear," which provides for the safety of all involved. All the remaining options describe a process that interferes with the safe performance of the defibrillation by not effectively managing the related risks.

---

31. While giving a client a bed bath, the nurse is asked to answer an emergency telephone call. What is the appropriate nursing action to address the safety issues created by this situation?

1 Complete the bath before answering the call.
2 Leave the room to maintain confidentiality while answering the call.
3 Place the call light within the client's reach, and answer the call.
4 Leave the door open so that the client can be monitored, and answer the call.

Level of Cognitive Ability: Applying
Client Needs: Safe and Effective Care Environment
Clinical Judgment/Cognitive Skills: Take Action
Integrated Process: Nursing Process/Implementation
Content Area: Leadership/Management: Prioritizing
Health Problem: N/A

Answer: 3

Rationale: If it is necessary for the nurse to answer the call and to leave the room temporarily, the door would be closed or the room curtains pulled around the bathing area to provide privacy. The client would be covered with a blanket, and, to maintain safety, the call light would be placed within the client's reach.

Priority Nursing Tip: When an emergency phone call needs to be answered, one appropriate action is to ask another nurse to accept the call.

Test-Taking Strategy: Note the **data in the question**, especially the phrase *an emergency telephone call.* When considering safety, the only option that addresses client safety and comfort is the correct option.

---

32. What information would the nurse provide to the client interested in providing consent for organ donation?

1 Written consent is not necessary to become a donor.
2 A donor needs to be 18 years old or older to provide consent.
3 A guardian's request for organ donation is invalid if unconfirmed prior to the donor's death.
4 Only the family can give consent at the time of the donor's death.

Level of Cognitive Ability: Applying
Client Needs: Safe and Effective Care Environment
Clinical Judgment/Cognitive Skills: Generate Solutions
Integrated Process: Nursing Process/Implementation
Content Area: Leadership/Management: Ethical/Legal
Health Problem: N/A

Answer: 2

Rationale: Any person 18 years old or older may become an organ donor by indicating his or her consent in writing. In the absence of appropriate documentation, a family member or legal guardian may authorize the donation of the decedent's organs at the time of death.

Priority Nursing Tip: Potential donors under the age of 18 require parental consent.

Test-Taking Strategy: Focus on the **subject,** organ donation. An understanding of the age requirements and other circumstances surrounding consent will help in directing you to the correct options.

---

33. The nurse employed in the medical unit of a local hospital arrives at work and is told to report (float) to the pediatric unit for the day. The nurse assigned as temporary staff (float) has never worked in the pediatric unit and is anxious about floating to this area. What **initial** action would the nurse take to ensure safe nursing care?

1 Calling the nursing supervisor to report being concerned
2 Refusing to float to the pediatric unit until being cross-trained
3 Asking another nurse with more years of experience to float to the pediatric unit
4 Reporting to the pediatric unit and helping identify tasks that can be safely performed

Level of Cognitive Ability: Applying
Client Needs: Safe and Effective Care Environment
Clinical Judgment/Cognitive Skills: Take Action
Integrated Process: Nursing Process/Implementation
Content Area: Leadership/Management: Ethical/Legal
Health Problem: N/A

Answer: 4

Rationale: Floating is an acceptable legal practice used by hospitals to solve their understaffing problems. Legally, the nurse cannot refuse to float unless a union contract guarantees that nurses can work only in specified areas or the nurse can prove a lack of knowledge for the performance of assigned tasks. When this situation occurs, the nurse and the pediatric nurse manager would set priorities, identify such potential areas, and then make an assignment that maximizes the nurse's ability to provide safe nursing care. The nurse would not ask another nurse to accept the assignment; staffing is a complicated process that needs to be directed by a supervisor with knowledge of the existing needs. The supervisor would be called if the nurse is asked to perform a task that could not be safely performed.

Priority Nursing Tip: In some cases, nurses who are permanently assigned to a specific unit may be asked to float to another unit because of staffing needs. However, some facilities establish a float pool.

Test-Taking Strategy: Note the **strategic word,** *initial.* Note that options 2 and 3 are **comparable or alike** in that the nurse does not fulfill the assignment. Option 1 does not attempt to address the issue or to provide for safe nursing care. Understanding the nurse's rights concerning the practice of "floating" will help direct you to the correct option.

---

34. The nurse determines that if the assistive personnel (AP) performs which action during a routine hand-washing procedure, **additional instruction is needed** in performing appropriate hand hygiene?

1 Keeps the hands lower than the elbows
2 Uses 3 to 5 mL of soap from the dispenser
3 Washes continuously for at least 15 seconds
4 Dries the hands from the forearm down to the fingers

Level of Cognitive Ability: Evaluating
Client Needs: Safe and Effective Care Environment
Clinical Judgment/Cognitive Skills: Evaluate Outcomes
Integrated Process: Nursing Process/Implementation
Content Area: Skills: Infection Control
Health Problem: N/A

Answer: 4
Rationale: Proper hand-washing procedure involves wetting the hands and wrists and keeping the hands lower than the forearms so that water flows toward the fingertips. The nurse uses 3 to 5 mL of soap and scrubs for at least 15 seconds using a rubbing and circular motion. The hands are rinsed and then dried from the fingers to the forearms. The paper towel is discarded, and a second paper towel is used to turn off the faucet to avoid hand contamination.
Priority Nursing Tip: Hand hygiene is a general term applying to the use of soap/solution (non-antimicrobial or antimicrobial) and water or the use of a waterless antimicrobial agent on the surface of the hands.

Test-Taking Strategy: Focus on the **subject**, effective hand hygiene. Note the **strategic words,** *additional instruction is needed.* These words indicate a **negative event query** and ask you to select an option that is an incorrect action performed by the AP. Visualize each option, and use basic principles of asepsis to answer this question.

---

35. In anticipation that a recently deceased client's eyes will be donated, what would the nurse do **initially** to support the condition of the corneas and a successful transplantation? **Select all that apply.**

❒ 1 Close the client's eyes.
❒ 2 Confirm the client is a donor with the National Eye Bank Center.
❒ 3 Place the client in the supine position.
❒ 4 Elevate the head of the client's bed.
❒ 5 Place dry sterile dressings over the eyes.

Level of Cognitive Ability: Applying
Client Needs: Safe and Effective Care Environment
Clinical Judgment/Cognitive Skills: Take Action
Integrated Process: Nursing Process/Implementation
Content Area: Developmental Stages/End-of-Life Care
Health Problem: N/A

Answer: 1, 4
Rationale: When a corneal donation is anticipated, the head of the bed is elevated, the deceased client's eyes are closed, and a small ice pack is placed on the client's eyes. Options 3 and 5 are incorrect actions that would impair the integrity of the corneas. Although appropriate, option 2 is not an initial action because it does not support the condition of the corneas.
Priority Nursing Tip: Human tissues—such as bone, skin, heart valves, and cornea—can be donated within the first 24 hours of death.

Test-Taking Strategy: Note the **strategic word**, *initially,* while focusing on the **subject,** organ donation of the eyes. Knowing how to care for the eyes to preserve the corneal tissue will help in correctly answering this question.

---

36. During data collection, the client tells the nurse that a living will was prepared 2 years ago and asks whether the will needs to be updated. Which nursing response demonstrates the nurse has an understanding of living wills?

1 "Living wills are valid for 6 months and then should be renewed or revised."
2 "The will deals with very basic issues and doesn't need to be changed very often."
3 "You will need to update the document with your lawyer's help as soon as possible."
4 "A living will should be reviewed yearly with your physician."

Level of Cognitive Ability: Applying
Client Needs: Safe and Effective Care Environment
Clinical Judgment/Cognitive Skills: Evaluate Outcomes
Integrated Process: Nursing Process/Implementation
Content Area: Leadership/Management: Ethical/Legal
Health Problem: N/A

Answer: 4
Rationale: The client should discuss the living will with the physician, and it should be reviewed annually to ensure that it contains the client's current wishes and desires. Options 1 and 2 include inaccurate information. Option 3 is not an appropriate response because a lawyer is not needed for the implementation or revision of a living will.
Priority Nursing Tip: Living wills are legal documents that instruct physicians and family members on what to do regarding life-sustaining treatments clients may or may not want. Changes in a client's health status may prompt a reevaluation of the initial decisions made.

Test-Taking Strategy: Focus on the **subject,** revising a living will. An understanding of the purpose of a living will and the possible needs for revision will direct you to the correct option.

---

37. The licensed practical nurse (LPN) is preparing to suction a client diagnosed with acquired immunodeficiency syndrome. The LPN would gather which supplies to perform this procedure safely?

1 Gloves and gown
2 Gown and protective eyewear
3 Gloves, mask, and protective eyewear
4 Gloves, gown, and protective eyewear

Level of Cognitive Ability: Applying
Client Needs: Safe and Effective Care Environment
Clinical Judgment/Cognitive Skills: Generate Solutions
Integrated Process: Nursing Process/Implementation
Content Area: Skills: Infection Control
Health Problem: Adult Health: Immune: Immunodeficiency Syndrome

Answer: 3
Rationale: Standard precautions include the use of gloves whenever there is actual or potential contact with blood or body fluids. During suctioning, the nurse wears gloves, a mask, and protective eyewear or a face shield. Impervious gowns are worn in those instances when it is anticipated that there will be contact with a large amount of body fluids or blood.
Priority Nursing Tip: Acquired immunodeficiency syndrome (AIDS) is a disease due to infection with the human immunodeficiency virus (HIV). It is also referred to as acquired immunodeficiency disease.

Test-Taking Strategy: Note that the **subject** of the question is suctioning, so expect airborne secretions with this procedure. Basic knowledge of standard precautions would direct you to an option that includes a mask, protective eyewear, and gloves; the only option that contains these three items is option 3.

---

38. The licensed practical nurse (LPN) determines that an assistive personnel (AP) ambulating a client with right-sided weakness is performing the procedure safely when the AP's position is where?

1 Behind the client
2 In front of the client
3 On the left side of the client
4 To the right side of the client

Level of Cognitive Ability: Evaluating
Client Needs: Safe and Effective Care Environment
Clinical Judgment/Cognitive Skills: Evaluate Outcomes
Integrated Process: Nursing Process/Evaluation
Content Area: Skills: Activity/Mobility
Health Problem: N/A

Answer: 4
Rationale: When walking with a client, the AP would stand on the client's affected side to provide support. The AP would position the free hand on the client's shoulder so that the client can be pulled toward the nurse if the client falls forward. Options 1, 2, and 3 are incorrect because they would not provide sufficient support.
Priority Nursing Tip: The client would be instructed to look up and outward rather than at his or her feet when ambulating.

Test-Taking Strategy: Focus on the **subject,** ambulating a client with right-sided weakness. This information will assist you with placing the nurse in a strategic position should the client lose balance and begin to fall forward or backward. Recalling that support is needed on a client's affected side will direct you to the correct option.

---

39. A licensed practical nurse (LPN) has a client who is refusing the administration of an intramuscular medication. What response would the registered nurse (RN) provide about consequences when the LPN suggests, "I'll just give it anyway"?

1 "You are talking about assaulting your client."
2 "If the client doesn't consent, what you are suggesting is battery."
3 "If the client is refusing, you can't give it unless the primary health care provider insists."
4 "That's a difficult question; I'd suggest talking to the nurse manager to be really sure."

Level of Cognitive Ability: Analyzing
Client Needs: Safe and Effective Care Environment
Clinical Judgment/Cognitive Skills: Take Action
Integrated Process: Nursing Process/Implementation
Content Area: Leadership/Management: Ethical/Legal
Health Problem: N/A

Answer: 2
Rationale: An assault occurs when a person puts another person in fear of a harmful or offensive contact. Battery is actual contact with one's body. In the event described, the nurse can be charged with battery because the nurse administers a medication that the client has refused. Neither of the remaining options clearly provides accurate information about consequence of the nurse's proposed action.
Priority Nursing Tip: For assault to be accountable, the victim needs to be aware of the threat of harmful or offensive contact.

Test-Taking Strategy: Focus on the **subject,** a client's right to refuse treatment. An understanding of the legal consequences for the nurse of such actions would direct you to the correct option.

---

40. A licensed practical nurse (LPN) is reinforcing teaching given by a registered nurse (RN) to the parents of a child diagnosed with celiac disease. What would the LPN remind the parents to do to ensure that the diet is based on the child's physical needs?

1 Restrict corn and rice in the diet.
2 Serve pasta dishes instead of cereals with grain.
3 Keep the intake of fresh starchy vegetables to a minimum.
4 Read food labels carefully to avoid hidden sources of gluten.

Level of Cognitive Ability: Applying
Client Needs: Safe and Effective Care Environment
Clinical Judgment/Cognitive Skills: Generate Solutions
Integrated Process: Teaching and Learning
Content Area: Skills: Client Teaching
Health Problem: Pediatric-Specific: Gastrointestinal and Rectal Problems

Answer: 4
Rationale: Celiac disease is a disease in which the small intestine is hypersensitive to gluten, leading to difficulty in digesting food. Gluten is added to many foods, such as hydrolyzed vegetable protein derived from cereal grains. Grains are also frequently added to processed foods as thickening or fillers. Because of this, it is important to read food labels. Gluten is found primarily in the grains of wheat and rye. Rice, corn, and other vegetables are acceptable in a gluten-free diet. Many pasta products contain gluten and would be avoided.
Priority Nursing Tip: A primary responsibility of the nurse is to teach the parents of a child with celiac disease about foods that need to be eliminated from the child's diet.

Test-Taking Strategy: Focus on the **subject,** client teaching about celiac disease. Begin to answer this question by recalling that a gluten-free diet is indicated for the management of celiac disease, and remember which foods are high in gluten.

---

41. The nurse notes that a child who has been diagnosed with intussusception has a formed brown bowel movement. The nurse would take which **initial** action to ensure that a safe plan of care is implemented for the child?

1 Prepare the child for hydrostatic reduction.
2 Ask the child about any increase in abdominal pain.
3 Warn the child and the parents that surgery is imminent.
4 Report the passage of the normal stool to the registered nurse (RN).

Level of Cognitive Ability: Applying
Client Needs: Safe and Effective Care Environment
Clinical Judgment/Cognitive Skills: Take Action
Integrated Process: Nursing Process/Implementation
Content Area: Pediatrics: Gastrointestinal
Health Problem: Pediatric-Specific: Gastrointestinal and Rectal Problems

Answer: 4
Rationale: Intussusception is a medical condition in which a part of the intestine folds into the section next to it. The passage of a formed brown bowel movement usually indicates that an intussusception has reduced itself. The nurse immediately reports this data to the RN, who will in turn report it to the primary health care provider. This finding may change the course of the plan of care. Hydrostatic reduction is prescribed to help decrease, improve, or reduce the affected intestinal area. Increased abdominal pain is not expected, because the child's gastrointestinal tract is likely to be more functional. The finding does not indicate the need for immediate surgery.
Priority Nursing Tip: The child diagnosed with intussusception will pass currant jelly–like stools.

Test-Taking Strategy: Focus on the **subject,** care for a client with intussusception. Note the **strategic word,** *initial.* Understanding of this pathology is necessary to answer this question correctly. Recognizing the characteristics of normal stool and that the passage of a normal stool may indicate that an intussusception is resolving or has resolved will direct you to the correct option.

---

42. A client with schizophrenia is demonstrating psychotic behavior. The client is belligerent and agitated, making aggressive gestures, and pacing in the hallway. To ensure a therapeutic environment, what is the nurse's **highest priority**?

1 Assisting other staff with restraining the client
2 Providing safety for the client and for other clients on the unit
3 Offering comfort and consolation to the other clients on the unit
4 Politely asking the client to calm down and regain control over his or her behavior

Level of Cognitive Ability: Applying
Client Needs: Safe and Effective Care Environment
Clinical Judgment/Cognitive Skills: Prioritize Hypotheses
Integrated Process: Nursing Process/ Implementation
Content Area: Foundations of Care: Safety
Health Problem: Mental Health: Schizophrenia

Answer: 2
Rationale: Psychosis is characterized as disruptions to a person's thoughts and perceptions that make it difficult for them to recognize what is real and what is not real. A psychotic client who is out of control may require seclusion to ensure the safety of the client and of the other clients on the unit. The correct option is the only one that addresses the safety needs of both the client and others. Options 1 and 3 do not provide for the client's safety needs or rights. In addition, specific policies and guidelines on restraining a client need to be followed. Option 4 may be ineffective, and it does not address the safety needs of others in the unit.
Priority Nursing Tip: Two of the main symptoms of psychosis are delusions and hallucinations.

Test-Taking Strategy: Focus on the **subject**, therapeutic environment related to the client demonstrating psychotic behaviors. Note the **strategic words,** *highest priority.* Use **Maslow's Hierarchy of Needs theory** to prioritize the nursing actions. The correct option addresses safety, which is the nurse's priority.

---

43. A client diagnosed with Bell's palsy is scheduled for magnetic resonance imaging (MRI). The nurse would implement which intervention to ensure a safe environment in preparation for this test?

1 Apply metal-tipped electrodes to the client's chest.
2 Remove all objects that contain metal from the client.
3 Shave the client's groin for the insertion of a femoral catheter.
4 Ensure that the client maintains nothing-by-mouth (NPO) status for 24 hours.

Level of Cognitive Ability: Applying
Client Needs: Safe and Effective Care Environment
Clinical Judgment/Cognitive Skills: Take Action
Integrated Process: Nursing Process/ Implementation
Content Area: Foundations of Care: Safety
Health Problem: Adult Health: Neurological: Bell's Palsy

Answer: 2
Rationale: Bell's palsy is a form of temporary facial paralysis resulting from damage or trauma to the facial nerves. An MRI uses magnetic fields to produce a diagnostic image. All metal objects (e.g., rings, bracelets, hairpins, watches) would be removed from the client. The client's history would also be reviewed to determine whether the client has any internal metallic devices (e.g., orthopedic hardware, pacemakers, shrapnel). A femoral catheter is not inserted for this procedure. For an abdominal MRI, the client is usually NPO; however, this is unnecessary for an MRI of the head. In addition, maintaining NPO status for 24 hours is unnecessary and may be harmful to the client. Metal-tipped electrodes are not used for this test.
Priority Nursing Tip: Movement of external metal objects (such as a watch, jewelry, clothing with fasteners, and metal hair fasteners) during MRI testing can be injurious to anyone in the field.

Test-Taking Strategy: Focus on the **subject,** care for a client with Bell's palsy. Note the physiological location as it relates to the client's diagnosis. Recalling that metallic objects cannot be in place during an MRI and focusing on the client's diagnosis will direct you to the correct option.

---

44. The nurse caring for a client who has been in a coma for more than 1 year is told by the primary health care provider to stop the tube feeding providing sustenance to the client. The nurse, acting as the client's advocate, **first** determines whether which requirement has been met?

1 Institutional ethics committee approval
2 A court order to discontinue the treatment
3 Authorization by the family to discontinue the treatment
4 A written order by the primary health care provider to remove the tube

Level of Cognitive Ability: Applying
Client Needs: Safe and Effective Care Environment
Clinical Judgment/Cognitive Skills: Take Action
Integrated Process: Nursing Process/Implementation
Content Area: Leadership/Management: Ethical/Legal
Health Problem: N/A

Answer: 3
Rationale: The client's family or legal guardian can make treatment decisions, generally in collaboration with primary health care providers, other health care workers, and other trusted advisers. The nurse first checks for family authorization before discontinuing the treatment. After doing this, option 4 would be appropriate. Although options 1 and 2 may be necessary in some events, these options are not the first actions to take in this situation.
Priority Nursing Tip: A legal guardian is a person who has the legal authority (and the corresponding duty) to care for the personal and property interests of another person, called a ward.

Test-Taking Strategy: Focus on the **subject,** decision making for the unconscious client, and note the **strategic word,** *first;* this tells you that the correct option is determined according to a proper sequence of action. Recalling that the family or legal guardian can make decisions about discontinuing treatment will direct you to the correct option.

---

45. The nurse assisting a physician with the insertion of a Miller-Abbott tube in a client with a bowel obstruction would implement what intervention to ensure a safe environment and to decrease the client's risk of aspiration?

1 Place the client in a high-Fowler's position.
2 Assist with inserting the tube with the balloon inflated.
3 Instruct the client to bear down if there is an urge to gag.
4 Ask the client to cough when the tube reaches the nasopharynx.

Level of Cognitive Ability: Applying
Client Needs: Safe and Effective Care Environment
Clinical Judgment/Cognitive Skills: Take Action
Integrated Process: Nursing Process/Implementation
Content Area: Foundations of Care: Safety
Health Problem: Adult Health: Gastrointestinal: Lower GI Disorders

Answer: 1
Rationale: A Miller-Abbott tube is a nasoenteric tube used to correct a bowel obstruction and to decompress the intestine. A high-Fowler's position decreases the risk of aspiration if vomiting occurs. The primary health care provider inserts the tube with the balloon deflated in a manner like that used with a nasogastric tube. Option 3 would not help manage the gag reflex. Option 4 would not be helpful.
Priority Nursing Tip: Bowel obstruction, also known as intestinal obstruction, is a mechanical or functional obstruction of the intestines that prevents the normal movement of the products of digestion. Either the small bowel or large bowel may be affected.

Test-Taking Strategy: Focus on the **subject,** decreasing the risk of aspiration during the insertion of a Miller-Abbott tube. An understanding of the process implemented for the insertion of any tube into the gastrointestinal tract is helpful in arriving at the correct object. Eliminate option 2 first, because the tube could not be inserted with the balloon inflated. Next, eliminate options 3 and 4, because coughing and bearing down will not facilitate the passage of the tube.

46. The nurse is administering medication prescriptions to manage the client's cancer pain. Which strategy would the nurse follow to ensure adequate and safe pain control?

1 Try multiple simultaneous medications for maximum pain relief, paying attention to any existing medication interactions.
2 Rely entirely on prescription and over-the-counter medications for pain relief to ensure client adherence to the treatment.
3 Ensure that the client is kept at a low baseline pain level to avoid sedation or addiction and to allow for interaction with family and friends.
4 Start with low medication doses and gradually increase to a dose that relieves the pain without exceeding the maximal daily dose.

Level of Cognitive Ability: Applying
Client Needs: Safe and Effective Care Environment
Clinical Judgment/Cognitive Skills: Take Action
Integrated Process: Nursing Process/Implementation
Content Area: Foundations of Care: Safety
Health Problem: N/A

Answer: 4
Rationale: The most appropriate approach to pain management is to begin with low doses and to increase the dose as needed to maintain a dose that relieves the pain while not increasing the risk for toxicity. Option 2 ignores the benefits of other options that may relieve pain, such as massage, therapeutic touch, and music. Keeping the client at a baseline level of pain is an inappropriate practice. Multiple medication interventions do not guarantee effectiveness and can also be unsafe.
Priority Nursing Tip: Cancer pain is a complex, temporally changing symptom that is the end result of mixed-mechanism pain. It involves inflammatory, neuropathic, ischemic, and compression mechanisms at multiple sites.

Test-Taking Strategy: Focus on the **subject,** managing a client's pain. Begin to answer this question by eliminating options 1 and 2 because of the words *multiple* and *entirely.* Choose correctly between the remaining options by remembering the basic principles of pain management and the need for pain relief in order to function and interact effectively.

---

47. A licensed practical nurse (LPN) is reinforcing instructions given to a client regarding medication administration after discharge. The LPN would use what approach to **best** ensure the safe administration of medication in the home?

1 Show the client the proper way to take the prescribed medications.
2 Tell the client to double up on the medications if a dose has been missed.
3 Count the number of pills remaining in the prescription bottle once a week.
4 Allow the client to verbalize and demonstrate the correct administration procedure.

Level of Cognitive Ability: Applying
Client Needs: Safe and Effective Care Environment
Clinical Judgment/Cognitive Skills: Generate Solutions
Integrated Process: Teaching and Learning
Content Area: Skills: Client Teaching
Health Problem: N/A

Answer: 4
Rationale: The most effective method of teaching to ensure the safe self-administration of medications in any setting is to have the client verbalize and demonstrate how to take medications. This ensures that the client has both the knowledge and the physical ability to adhere to medication therapy. Option 1 is useful early in the teaching or learning process, but it does not allow the nurse to evaluate the client's own knowledge and abilities. Option 2 is incorrect because it is a dangerous practice. Option 3 is unrealistic and does not enhance self-care.
Priority Nursing Tip: Focus on the cognitive, affective, and psychomotor behaviors that the client would be able to achieve after reinforcement of teaching.

Test-Taking Strategy: Focus on the **subject,** client teaching about home medications. Note the **strategic word,** *best.* Eliminate options 2 and 3 first by remembering the general guidelines for safe medication administration as well as teaching and learning principles. From the remaining options, select the one that most universally addresses the full abilities needed by the client after discharge.

---

48. A client diagnosed with thrombophlebitis is being treated with heparin sodium therapy. The registered nurse (RN) asks the licensed practical nurse (LPN) to check the medication supply to ensure that the antidote for this therapy is available. The nurse checks the medication supply for which medication?

1 Streptokinase
2 Phytonadione
3 Protamine sulfate
4 Aminocaproic acid

Level of Cognitive Ability: Applying
Client Needs: Safe and Effective Care Environment
Clinical Judgment/Cognitive Skills: Take Action
Integrated Process: Nursing Process/Implementation
Content Area: Pharmacology: Cardiovascular: Anticoagulants
Health Problem: Adult Health: Cardiovascular: Vascular Disorders

Answer: 3

Rationale: Protamine sulfate is the antidote for heparin sodium. Streptokinase is a thrombolytic agent used to dissolve blood clots. Phytonadione (vitamin K) is the antidote for warfarin. Aminocaproic acid is an antifibrinolytic used to prevent the breakdown of clots that have already been formed.

Priority Nursing Tip: Thrombophlebitis is an inflammatory process that causes a blood clot to form and block one or more veins, usually in the lower extremities.

Test-Taking Strategy: Focus on the **subject**, heparin sodium antidote. Specific knowledge of the antidote to heparin sodium is needed to answer this question correctly. A knowledge of the function of the medications offered as options will assist in eliminating inappropriate medications.

---

49. The nurse assisting with the care of a client diagnosed with cardiomyopathy would place **priority** on what intervention to ensure client safety?

1 Administering vasodilator medications
2 Conducting a thorough pain assessment
3 Taking measures to prevent orthostatic changes when the client stands
4 Telling the client about the importance of avoiding over-the-counter medications

Level of Cognitive Ability: Applying
Client Needs: Safe and Effective Care Environment
Clinical Judgment/Cognitive Skills: Prioritize Hypotheses
Integrated Process: Nursing Process/Implementation
Content Area: Adult Health: Cardiovascular
Health Problem: Adult Health: Cardiovascular: Inflammatory and Structural Heart Disorders

Answer: 3

Rationale: Orthostatic changes can occur in the client with cardiomyopathy because of impaired venous return; these changes could lead to dizziness and falls. Vasodilators would not be administered because they would exacerbate the potential risk for hypotension. There is no mention of pain in the question, and pain may not directly affect safety in this event. Option 4 is an accurate statement, but it is not directly related to the subject of the question.

Priority Nursing Tip: Orthostatic hypotension is defined as a decrease in systolic blood pressure of 20 mm Hg or a decrease in diastolic blood pressure of 10 mm Hg within 3 minutes of standing when compared with blood pressure from the sitting or supine position.

Test-Taking Strategy: Note the **strategic word,** *priority.* Focus on the **subject,** the safety of a client diagnosed with cardiomyopathy. The correct option is the one that deals with the prevention of a condition that can be related to cardiomyopathy. Knowledge of the pathological and physiological outcomes of cardiomyopathy will help you arrive at the correct option.

50. A licensed practical nurse (LPN) is reinforcing teaching given to a client who has been diagnosed with infective endocarditis. What intervention does the LPN stress as being important for this client to perform regarding oral hygiene?

1 Floss the teeth twice a day.
2 Use an oral irrigation device daily.
3 Brush the teeth twice a day using a soft toothbrush.
4 Use an organic toothpaste to avoid unnecessary additives.

Level of Cognitive Ability: Applying
Client Needs: Safe and Effective Care Environment
Clinical Judgment/Cognitive Skills: Take Action
Integrated Process: Teaching and Learning
Content Area: Skills: Client Teaching
Health Problem: Adult Health: Cardiovascular: Inflammatory and structural heart disorders

Answer: 3

Rationale: The oral cavity is a possible portal of entry for infecting organisms in endocarditis. The LPN would reinforce the importance of good oral hygiene, using a soft toothbrush to brush the teeth at least twice a day and rinsing the mouth with water after brushing. Oral irrigation devices and flossing can be traumatizing to the gums and would be avoided, as bacteremia may result. Organic toothpaste is an unnecessary intervention because the issue is bacteria, not additives.

Priority Nursing Tip: Infective endocarditis (IE) is defined as an infection of the endocardial surface of the heart that may include one or more heart valves, the mural endocardium, or a septal defect.

Test-Taking Strategy: Focus on the **subject,** oral hygiene and endocarditis. The risk involves the introduction of bacteria via the mouth. Avoid options that might damage the mucous membrane in the oral cavity. Eliminate any option that is not focused on the introduction of bacteria.

---

51. A licensed practical nurse (LPN) is assisting a registered nurse (RN) with caring for a client who just underwent cardiac catheterization via the femoral approach. What action by the LPN would **require additional instructions** if performed immediately after the client returns from the procedure?

1 Having the client logroll side-to-side to remove the soiled linen
2 Having the client sit upright for a meal consisting of clear liquids
3 Encouraging the client to drink extra fluids to encourage kidney function
4 Asking the client to wiggle the toes when collecting data about the neurovascular status

Level of Cognitive Ability: Evaluating
Client Needs: Safe and Effective Care Environment
Clinical Judgment/Cognitive Skills: Evaluate Outcomes
Integrated Process: Teaching and Learning
Content Area: Adult Health: Cardiovascular
Health Problem: N/A

Answer: 2

Rationale: For 6 hours after cardiac catheterization via the femoral approach (or per primary health care provider's prescriptions), the client would not bend or hyperextend the affected leg to avoid blood vessel occlusion or hemorrhage. This means that having the client sit upright would be contraindicated. Logrolling is acceptable because flexion of the lower affected extremity is not required. Asking the client to wiggle the toes to determine neurovascular status is acceptable and would be done, because vascular status could be impaired if a hematoma or thrombus were developing. Fluids would be increased to help with replacing losses from the osmotic effects of the dye and eliminating the contrast medium through the kidneys.

Priority Nursing Tip: Focus on ensuring adequate circulation to the affected extremity when helping to determine an unsafe practice.

Test-Taking Strategy: Focus on the **subject,** care postcardiac catheterization via femoral approach. Note the **strategic words,** *require additional instructions.* This phrase indicates a **negative event query** and asks you to select an option that is an incorrect action. To identify the incorrect action, use your knowledge of nursing care after cardiac catheterization, and keep in mind that the femoral access site was used and the possible adverse reactions that may occur.

---

52. The nurse is delivering a meal tray to a client diagnosed with heart failure. Which item would the nurse remove from the tray before bringing it to the client's bedside?

1 Sherbet
2 Green beans
3 Baked chicken
4 Saltine crackers

Answer: 4

Rationale: Clients with heart failure would monitor and restrict their sodium intake. Saltine crackers are high in sodium and would be avoided. Green beans and sherbet are low in sodium. Baked chicken would contain only physiological saline because it is an animal product and thus would not have to be avoided by the client.

Priority Nursing Tip: The restriction of dietary sodium will help prevent fluid retention.

Test-Taking Strategy: Focus on the **subject,** diet for a client experiencing heart failure. First, you need to be able to identify the type of diet that a client with heart failure would eat: a low-sodium diet. Use the process of elimination to select the food highest in sodium.

Level of Cognitive Ability: Applying
Client Needs: Safe and Effective Care Environment
Clinical Judgment/Cognitive Skills: Take Action
Integrated Process: Nursing Process/ Implementation
Content Area: Adult Health: Cardiovascular
Health Problem: Adult Health: Cardiovascular: Heart Failure

---

53. An older adult client with a history of diabetes mellitus is vomiting as a result of gastroenteritis. The nurse would implement which intervention to maintain oral intake and safely minimize the risk of dehydration?

1 Give only sips of water until the client is able to tolerate solid foods.
2 Withhold all food and fluids until vomiting has ceased for at least 8 hours.
3 Encourage the client to drink up to 8 to 12 ounces of enriched fluid every hour while awake.
4 Provide the client with 50 mL of clear liquids hourly for at least 3 days to allow for bowel rest.

Answer: 3

Rationale: Dehydration is a harmful reduction in the amount of water in the body. Small amounts of fluid may be tolerated even when vomiting is present. The client would be offered up to 8 to 12 ounces of liquid that contains both glucose and electrolytes hourly. The diet would be advanced to a regular diet as soon as it is tolerated and would include a minimum of 100 to 150 grams of carbohydrates daily. Options 1, 2, and 4 are incorrect actions because they will not maintain adequate oral intake.

Priority Nursing Tip: The dehydrated client with diabetes will need adequate glucose and electrolytes as replacements from losses due to vomiting.

Test-Taking Strategy: Focus on the **subject,** interventions for a dehydrated client diagnosed with diabetes. Begin to answer this question by eliminating options 1 and 2 because of the **closed-ended words** "only" and "all." Choose correctly from the remaining options, knowing that a 3-day time frame is excessive.

Level of Cognitive Ability: Applying
Client Needs: Safe and Effective Care Environment
Clinical Judgment/Cognitive Skills: Take Action
Integrated Process: Nursing Process/ Implementation
Content Area: Foundations of Care: Fluids & Electrolytes
Health Problem: Adult Health: Endocrine: Diabetes Mellitus

---

54. A client is asked to produce a sputum culture. The nurse demonstrates a **need for further education** on this diagnostic test when observed encouraging what action?

1 Obtaining the specimen early in the morning
2 Having the client take deep breaths before coughing
3 Giving the client a clean cup to expectorate in
4 Asking the client to rinse the mouth with water before expectoration

Level of Cognitive Ability: Applying
Client Needs: Safe and Effective Care Environment
Clinical Judgment/Cognitive Skills: Evaluate Outcomes
Integrated Process: Nursing Process/Implementation
Content Area: Skills: Specimen Collection
Health Problem: N/A

Answer: 3

Rationale: A sterile sputum container, not a clean cup, is necessary to avoid contamination. The client would rinse the mouth with water before specimen collection to avoid contaminating the specimen with particles from the oropharynx. The client would take deep breaths before expectoration for best sputum production. The specimen is optimally obtained early in the morning, because sputum has a longer amount of time to collect in the airways during sleep.

Priority Nursing Tip: A sputum culture is a test to detect and identify bacteria or fungi that infect the lungs or breathing passages.

Test-Taking Strategy: Note the **strategic words,** *need for further education.* This phrase indicates a **negative event query** and asks you to select an option that is an incorrect nursing action. Use your knowledge of the principles of aseptic technique to choose correctly.

---

55. The nurse suggesting measures to prevent the spread of infection to other clients will encourage staff to implement what practice as the **best** method?

1 Use proper hand-washing techniques.
2 Use sterile technique with all procedures.
3 Never stop in the middle of performing a procedure.
4 Read the policy and procedure manual before performing treatments.

Level of Cognitive Ability: Applying
Client Needs: Safe and Effective Care Environment
Clinical Judgment/Cognitive Skills: Generate Solutions
Integrated Process: Nursing Process/Implementation
Content Area: Foundations of Care: Infection Control
Health Problem: N/A

Answer: 1

Rationale: Proper hand washing is the best way to prevent the spread of infection. Not all procedures require sterile technique. Reading the policy and procedure manual does not guarantee that infection will not spread. It may be necessary in some situations to stop in the middle of a procedure, but option 3 is not the best way to prevent the spread of infection.

Priority Nursing Tip: Hand hygiene is effective in preventing and controlling spread of infection.

Test-Taking Strategy: Focus on the **subject,** the best way to prevent the spread of infection. Note the **strategic word,** *best.* Recalling the basic principles of infection prevention will direct you to the correct option.

---

56. The nurse is carrying out an order to obtain a sputum sample, which needs to be obtained via the saline inhalation method. What would the nurse do to help the client use the nebulizer safely and correctly?

1 Hold the nebulizer under the nose.
2 Keep the lips closed lightly over the seal.
3 Keep the lips closed tightly over the seal.
4 Alternate one vapor breath with one breath from room air.

Answer: 2

Rationale: A nebulizer is a medication delivery device used to administer medication in the form of a mist inhaled into the lungs. Inhaling vaporized saline is an effective means of helping a client cough productively. The vapor condenses on the respiratory mucosa, thus stimulating the cough reflex and the expectoration of secretions. The nurse tells the client to close the mouth lightly over the mouthpiece; it is not necessary to form a tight seal. The client inhales vaporized saline with each breath until coughing results. The nebulizer is not held under the nose.

Level of Cognitive Ability: Applying
Client Needs: Safe and Effective Care Environment
Clinical Judgment/Cognitive Skills: Take Action
Integrated Process: Nursing Process/Implementation
Content Area: Skills: Specimen Collection
Health Problem: N/A

Priority Nursing Tip: Nebulizers are commonly used for the treatment of cystic fibrosis, asthma, chronic obstructive pulmonary disease, and other respiratory diseases or disorders.

Test-Taking Strategy: Focus on the **subject**, using the saline inhalation method to obtain a sputum specimen. Being familiar with and visualizing this procedure will direct you to the correct option.

---

57. The nurse has completed tracheostomy care on a client with a nondisposable inner cannula. What would the nurse do **immediately** before reinserting the inner cannula into the tracheostomy?

1 Rinse the cannula in sterile water.
2 Suction the airway with a sterile catheter.
3 Dry the cannula with a sterile cotton ball.
4 Lightly tap the cannula dry against a sterile surface.

Answer: 4
Rationale: The nurse reinserts the inner cannula after tapping it dry against a sterile surface. It would not be dried with a cotton ball, which could leave cotton particles on the cannula. The client's airway is suctioned before tracheostomy care is performed. The cannula is rinsed in sterile water before it is tapped dry.
Priority Nursing Tip: Make sure the inner cannula is as dry as possible to avoid client aspiration.

Test-Taking Strategy: Note the **strategic word,** *immediately.* Focus on the **subject,** tracheostomy care. The wording of the question tells you that there is a sequence that needs to be followed to complete the steps of the procedure. Determining which step would be performed immediately before reinsertion will direct you to the correct option.

Level of Cognitive Ability: Applying
Client Needs: Safe and Effective Care Environment
Clinical Judgment/Cognitive Skills: Take Action
Integrated Process: Nursing Process/Implementation
Content Area: Adult Health: Respiratory
Health Problem: N/A

---

58. A licensed practical nurse (LPN) is assisting with the care of a client with a nasogastric (NG) tube. The registered nurse (RN) determines that the LPN **needs additional education** regarding confirmation of NG tube placement if he/she is observed doing what?

1 Measuring the pH of the gastric aspirate
2 Reviewing the report of the abdominal flat plate x-ray
3 Aspirating the NG tube with a 50-mL syringe to retrieve gastric contents
4 Instilling 20 mL of air into the NG tube while auscultating over the stomach

Answer: 4
Rationale: The auscultatory method is no longer considered reliable and would indicate that the LPN requires additional education on best practices. The best method of determining tube placement is to verify it by x-ray. Once confirmed by initial x-ray, measuring gastric pH and assessing for gastric contents are acceptable.
Priority Nursing Tip: An NG tube is used to treat gastric immobility and bowel obstruction.

Test-Taking Strategy: Focus on the **subject,** verifying the placement of an NG tube, and note the **strategic words,** *needs additional education.* These words indicate a **negative event query** and the need to select the incorrect action. This tells you that the correct answer is an option that puts the client at risk for possible injury because it is an unreliable method.

Level of Cognitive Ability: Evaluating
Client Needs: Safe and Effective Care Environment
Clinical Judgment/Cognitive Skills: Evaluate Outcomes
Integrated Process: Teaching and Learning
Content Area: Skills: Tube Care
Health Problem: N/A

59. What intervention would the nurse implement to provide a safe environment for an older adult client to minimize the stress and resulting anxiety caused by hospitalization?

1 Restrict visitors to the minimum number possible.
2 Keep the door open and the room lights on at all times.
3 Admit the client to a room far away from the noisy nurses' station.
4 Allow the client to have as many choices related to care as possible.

Level of Cognitive Ability: Applying
Client Needs: Safe and Effective Care Environment
Clinical Judgment/Cognitive Skills: Take Action
Integrated Process: Nursing Process/Implementation
Content Area: Mental Health
Health Problem: Mental Health: Coping

Answer: 4
Rationale: Several general interventions will reduce the hospitalized client's level of stress. These include acknowledging the client's feelings, offering information, providing social support, and letting the client have control over choices related to care. Options 1 and 3 could increase anxiety, whereas option 2 could add to the disruption created by the hospitalization and interfere with the client's sleep pattern.
Priority Nursing Tip: The hospital setting may exert negative psychological consequences, causing older clients to feel worthless, fearful, or not in control of what is happening to them.

Test-Taking Strategy: Focus on the **subject,** effects of hospitalization on an older adult client. Consider the words *safe, stress,* and *anxiety;* this tells you that the correct option is one that calms the client's feelings of fear and anxiety after being placed in a foreign environment. Use general principles related to safety and stress reduction to answer the question.

---

60. The nurse reinforces teaching provided to a client recently diagnosed with pulmonary tuberculosis (TB). The nurse determines that the teaching was **effective** when the client makes what statement about spreading the disease?

1 "I have to be very careful about not sneezing around people."
2 "Once I start treatment, I can't spread the TB bacteria to other people."
3 "Wearing disposable gloves will make it difficult for the TB germs to spread."
4 "Hand washing, especially after using the bathroom, is very important to staying healthy."

Level of Cognitive Ability: Evaluating
Client Needs: Safe and Effective Care Environment
Clinical Judgment/Cognitive Skills: Evaluate Outcomes
Integrated Process: Teaching and Learning
Content Area: Adult Health: Respiratory
Health Problem: Adult Health: Pulmonary: Tuberculosis

Answer: 1
Rationale: TB is spread by droplet nuclei, which become airborne when the infected client laughs, sings, sneezes, or coughs. An individual needs to inhale the droplet nuclei for the chain of infection to continue. TB is not spread by hand contact, although effective hand washing is a good practice. The client is still contagious when treatment first begins.
Priority Nursing Tip: TB is an infectious disease that may affect almost any tissue of the body, especially the lungs, which is caused by the organism *Mycobacterium tuberculosis* and characterized by tubercles.

Test-Taking Strategy: Focus on the **subject,** the method of TB transmission. Note the **strategic word,** *effective.* Recalling that TB is a respiratory disorder and spread by droplet nuclei will direct you to the correct option.

---

61. The nurse is collecting data about a client's risk of attempting suicide. What is the **best** question for the nurse to ask the client?

1 "Do you have a death wish?"
2 "Do you wish your life was over?"
3 "Do you ever think about ending it all?"
4 "Have you ever thought of killing yourself?"

Level of Cognitive Ability: Applying
Client Needs: Safe and Effective Care Environment
Clinical Judgment/Cognitive Skills: Generate Solutions
Integrated Process: Nursing Process/Data Collection
Content Area: Mental Health
Health Problem: Mental Health: Suicide

Answer: 4
Rationale: A suicide risk assessment requires direct communication between the client and the nurse. It is important to provide a question directly related to the risk for suicide. Options 1, 2, and 3 do not directly address the subject of the question. The correct option is the most direct because it clearly asks the client about suicide.
Priority Nursing Tip: Suicidal ideation, also known as suicidal thoughts, is thinking about or an unusual preoccupation with suicide.

Test-Taking Strategy: Focus on the **subject,** assessing for suicidal thoughts, and note the **strategic word,** *best.* Also, note that the correct option contains the word *killing.* Option 4 directly addresses the subject of suicide.

---

62. The registered nurse (RN) determines that the licensed practical nurse (LPN) understands the importance of the admission process for a suicidal client when he/she identifies what as its **primary** function?

1 Collecting baseline data
2 Identifying abnormalities
3 Confirming existing medical problems
4 Noting evidence of physical self-harm

Level of Cognitive Ability: Evaluating
Client Needs: Safe and Effective Care Environment
Clinical Judgment/Cognitive Skills: Evaluating Outcomes
Integrated Process: Nursing Process/Data Collection
Content Area: Mental Health
Health Problem: Mental Health: Suicide

Answer: 4
Rationale: The physical assessment of a suicidal client would be thorough and would focus on the evidence of self-harm and the formulation of a plan for the suicide attempt. Observed cuts, bruises, and other injuries would be inquired about during the assessment. Although all the options are correct, option 4 is most appropriate for the suicidal client. Clients with a history or evidence of self-harm are greater suicide risks.
Priority Nursing Tip: Psychological evaluation is defined as a way of assessing an individual's behavior, personality, cognitive abilities, and several other domains.

Test-Taking Strategy: Focus on the **subject,** assessment of the suicidal client. Note the **strategic word,** *primary.* Remember that physical evidence of self-harm is an important component of the assessment process of suicidal clients because it presents objective evidence that such clients have possibly engaged in behaviors intended to hurt or kill themselves.

---

63. The nurse assisting with the care of suicidal clients in a psychiatric nursing unit would plan to implement special precautions at what time generally considered a period of increased risk?

1 Day shift
2 Weekdays
3 Shift change
4 8 AM to 2 PM

Level of Cognitive Ability: Applying
Client Needs: Safe and Effective Care Environment
Clinical Judgment/Cognitive Skills: Generate Solutions
Integrated Process: Nursing Process/Planning
Content Area: Mental Health
Health Problem: Mental Health: Suicide

Answer: 3
Rationale: During shift changes, fewer staff members may be available to observe clients. The staff in a psychiatric nursing unit would increase precautions during shift changes for clients identified as suicidal. Other times of increased risk for suicides are weekends (not weekdays) and night shifts (not day shifts).
Priority Nursing Tip: Client safety is a priority.

Test-Taking Strategy: Focus on the **subject,** times of increased suicide risk. Remember that options that are **comparable or alike** are unlikely to be correct, so eliminate options 1 and 4 first because both are related to similar time periods. Consider factors that influence suicidal attempt planning. Choose between the remaining options by selecting the time when fewer staff members would be available to observe clients.

---

64. The nurse is assisting with the admission of a client from the postanesthesia care unit to the surgical nursing unit. What intervention would be implemented to **best** ensure the safety of this client?

1 Assist the client with moving from the transport stretcher to the bed.
2 Show concern for client's comfort when transferring to the bed.
3 Put the top side rails up after positioning the client in the bed.
4 Keep the client covered when transferring to the bed.

Level of Cognitive Ability: Applying
Client Needs: Safe and Effective Care Environment
Clinical Judgment/Cognitive Skills: Generate Solutions
Integrated Process: Nursing Process/Implementation
Content Area: Skills: Perioperative Care
Health Problem: N/A

Answer: 3
Rationale: Because the client may still be experiencing residual effects of anesthesia, per agency policy, the nurse would raise the side rails after transferring the client from the stretcher to the bed to address issues of dizziness. Although all the options are appropriate, client safety is best addressed by minimizing the risk of falling.
Priority Nursing Tip: General anesthesia suppresses many of your body's normal automatic functions, such as those that control breathing, heartbeat, circulation of the blood (such as blood pressure), movements of the digestive system, and throat reflexes such as swallowing, coughing, or gagging.

Test-Taking Strategy: Focus on the **subject,** safety of the postsurgical client, and note the **strategic word,** *best.* Considering the effects of anesthesia would help you in identifying the correct option.

---

65. The nurse caring for a child with a fever would implement which intervention to enhance safety when giving the child a prescribed tepid tub bath?

1 Add isopropyl alcohol to the bathwater.
2 Let the child soak in the tub for 10 minutes.
3 Slowly add cool water to the warmer bath water.
4 Warm the water to the same body temperature of the child.

Level of Cognitive Ability: Applying
Client Needs: Safe and Effective Care Environment
Clinical Judgment/Cognitive Skills: Take Action
Integrated Process: Nursing Process/Implementation
Content Area: Foundations of Care: Safety
Health Problem: Pediatric-Specific: Fever

Answer: 3
Rationale: Cool water would be added to an already warm bath, because this will cause the water temperature to slowly drop. The child will be able to gradually adjust to the changing water temperature and will not experience chilling. The child would be kept in a tepid tub bath for 20 to 30 minutes to achieve maximum results. Alcohol is toxic and contraindicated for tepid sponge or tub baths. To achieve the best cooling results for the child with a fever, the water temperature would be at least 2 degrees lower than the child's body temperature.
Priority Nursing Tip: The child with fever would be monitored for signs and symptoms of dehydration and electrolyte imbalance.

Test-Taking Strategy: Focus on the **subject,** care for client with fever. Begin to answer this question by eliminating option 4 because this would not lower the child's temperature. Eliminate option 1 next, knowing that isopropyl alcohol would not be used. To choose correctly between the remaining options, you need to be familiar with either the time frames indicated to lower a temperature with a tepid bath or the proper methods for cooling the bathwater.

---

66. The nurse assisting with the care of a child who underwent the surgical repair of a cleft lip the previous day would implement which safety-focused nursing intervention when caring for the surgical incision?

1 Clean the incision only if serous exudate forms.
2 Remove the Logan bar carefully to clean the incision.
3 Rub the incision gently with a sterile cotton-tipped swab.
4 Rinse the incision with sterile water after using diluted hydrogen peroxide, if prescribed.

Level of Cognitive Ability: Applying
Client Needs: Safe and Effective Care Environment
Clinical Judgment/Cognitive Skills: Take Action
Integrated Process: Nursing Process/Implementation
Content Area: Skills: Wound Care/Dressings
Health Problem: Pediatric-Specific: Disorders of Prenatal Development

Answer: 4

Rationale: The incision would be rinsed with sterile water when it is cleaned with a solution other than water or saline. The Logan bar is intended to maintain the integrity of the suture line; removing the Logan bar on the first postoperative day is incorrect because removal would increase tension on the surgical incision. The incision is cleaned after every feeding and when serous exudate forms. The incision would be dabbed and not rubbed to maintain its integrity.

Priority Nursing Tip: All surgical incisions need to be monitored for signs and symptoms of infection.

Test-Taking Strategy: Focus on the **subject,** care of incisions. Knowledge of basic incision care and infection control is needed for answering this item correctly. Eliminate option 2 first, recalling that the Logan bar maintains the integrity of the suture line. Eliminate option 1 because of the word *only* and option 3 because of the word *rub.*

---

67. The nurse is assigned to care for an older adult client who has been identified as a victim of physical abuse. When assisting with the planning of care for this client, the nurse's **priority** is focused toward what client need?

1 Adhering to the mandatory abuse reporting laws
2 Removing the client from any immediate danger
3 Referring the abusing family member for treatment
4 Encouraging the client to file charges against the abuser

Level of Cognitive Ability: Applying
Client Needs: Safe and Effective Care Environment
Clinical Judgment/Cognitive Skills: Prioritize Hypotheses
Integrated Process: Nursing Process/Planning
Content Area: Mental Health
Health Problem: Mental Health: Abusive Behaviors

Answer: 2

Rationale: Whenever the abused client remains in the abusive environment, priority needs to be placed on determining whether the person is in any immediate danger. If so, emergency action needs to be taken to remove the client from the abusive situation. Options 1 and 3 may be appropriate interventions but are not the priority. Option 4 is not an appropriate intervention at this time and may produce increased fear and anxiety in the client.

Priority Nursing Tip: The safety of the client is the number one priority.

Test-Taking Strategy: Focus on the **subject,** the needs of an abused adult, and note the **strategic word,** *priority.* Use **Maslow's Hierarchy of Needs theory** to select the correct option. Remember that if a physiological need is not present, then safety is the priority.

---

68. What intervention would the nurse implement when considering activities for the depressed client during the **early** stages of hospitalization?

1 Avoid planned activities until the client asks to participate in milieu activities.
2 Offer the client a menu of daily activities, and insist that the client participate in all of them.
3 Provide a structured daily program of activities, and encourage the client to participate in them.
4 Provide an activity that is quiet and solitary in nature, such as working on a puzzle or reading a book, to avoid increased fatigue.

Level of Cognitive Ability: Applying
Client Needs: Safe and Effective Care Environment
Clinical Judgment/Cognitive Skills: Take Action
Integrated Process: Nursing Process/Implementation
Content Area: Mental Health
Health Problem: Mental Health: Mood Disorders

Answer: 3
Rationale: A depressed person is often withdrawn. In addition, the person may have difficulty concentrating, a loss of interest or pleasure, low energy, fatigue, feelings of worthlessness, and poor self-esteem. The plan of care needs to provide successful experiences in a stimulating yet structured environment. Options 1 and 4 are restrictive, and option 2 is demanding.
Priority Nursing Tip: Depression can cause physical symptoms of pain, appetite changes, and sleep problems.

Test-Taking Strategy: Focus on the **subject,** care for a client with depression. Note the **strategic word,** *early*. Remember that the depressed client requires a structured and stimulating program that gradually encourages interaction with others. Options 1 and 4 are too restrictive and offer little or no structure or stimulation. Option 2 is eliminated because of the high demands placed on the client.

---

69. The nurse caring for a client who requires contact isolation demonstrates an understanding of infection control when making what statement about the order of removing items of protective equipment when leaving the room?

1 "I untie the gown just before I take off my gloves."
2 "The goggles are removed right before removing the mask."
3 "The mask comes off last to avoid any contact with contaminates."
4 "The gloves are removed first because they are the most contaminated."

Level of Cognitive Ability: Applying
Client Needs: Safe and Effective Care Environment
Clinical Judgment/Cognitive Skills: Evaluate Outcomes
Integrated Process: Nursing Process/Implementation
Content Area: Foundations of Care: Infection Control
Health Problem: N/A

Answer: 4
Rationale: The nurse would remove gloves first because these are the items that are the most contaminated. The nurse then carefully removes the mask by touching only the elastic or mask strings; ungloved hands will not become contaminated by touching only these areas. The nurse then unties the neck strings and the back strings of the gown and allows the gown to fall from his or her shoulders. The nurse removes his or her hands from the sleeves without touching the outside of the gown, holds the gown inside at the shoulder seams, folds it inside out, and discards it in the appropriate trash receptacle or laundry bag. The nurse removes eyewear or goggles and then washes his or her hands.
Priority Nursing Tip: Contact precautions are used to prevent the spread of germs, infections, or diseases that can be contracted and spread from touching the client or items in the room.

Test-Taking Strategy: Focus on the **subject,** taking off personal protective equipment. Use your knowledge of standard precautions and of the methods used to prevent contamination. Visualize the correct process of removing contaminated clothing and items. Remember that the gloves are the items that are the most contaminated.

---

70. Ultraviolet light (UVL) therapy is prescribed in the treatment plan of a client diagnosed with psoriasis. Which statement made by the client indicates the **need for further instruction** regarding safety measures related to the therapy?

1 "Each treatment will last 30 minutes."
2 "I will wear eye goggles during the treatment."
3 "I will expose only the area that requires treatment."
4 "I will cover my face with a loosely applied covering."

Level of Cognitive Ability: Evaluating
Client Needs: Safe and Effective Care Environment
Clinical Judgment/Cognitive Skills: Evaluate Outcomes
Integrated Process: Teaching and Learning
Content Area: Adult Health: Integumentary
Health Problem: Adult Health: Integumentary: Inflammation/Infection

Answer: 1
Rationale: Safety precautions are required during UVL therapy. Most UVL treatments require the person to stand in a light-treatment chamber for up to 15 minutes. It is best to expose only those areas that require treatment to the UVL. Wearing protective wraparound goggles prevents the exposure of the eyes to UVL. If it does not require treatment, the face would be shielded with a loosely applied cloth.
Priority Nursing Tip: Direct contact with the UVL bulbs of the treatment unit would be avoided to prevent the burning of the skin.

Test-Taking Strategy: Focus on the **subject,** UVL therapy, and note the **strategic words,** *need for further instruction.* These words indicate a **negative event query** and ask you to select an option that is an incorrect client statement. Knowledge related to this therapy will help you determine an appropriate length of time for exposure to UVL, whereas the other options describe appropriate interventions.

---

71. The nurse is assigned to care for a client during the acute phase of a burn injury. The nurse reviews the physician's prescriptions and would question the registered nurse (RN) about which prescription?

1 Monitor the weight daily.
2 Monitor the urine output hourly.
3 Maintain the nasogastric tube with intermittent suction.
4 Administer morphine sulfate intramuscularly every 3 hours as needed for pain.

Level of Cognitive Ability: Applying
Client Needs: Safe and Effective Care Environment
Clinical Judgment/Cognitive Skills: Take Action
Integrated Process: Nursing Process/Implementation
Content Area: Adult Health: Integumentary
Health Problem: Adult Health: Integumentary: Burns

Answer: 4
Rationale: During the acute phase of a burn, oral, subcutaneous, and intramuscular routes for administering medications are contraindicated because of the poor absorption from the client's stomach, subcutaneous tissue, and muscle. Consequently, as fluid shifts back into the vasculature, doses that have remained in the tissue spaces can move rapidly to the vascular space and lead to lethal dosages. When the fluid balance is stabilized and the gut is functioning, oral opioid agents can be used. Options 1, 2, and 3 are all appropriate interventions for a client with a burn.
Priority Nursing Tip: The fluid shifts begin into the interstitial spaces after the burn injury and can continue for 36 hours before fluids begin to remobilize back to the vasculature.

Test-Taking Strategy: Note the **subject,** the prescription that would be questioned. Read each option carefully, and think about the physiology that occurs in the client with a burn. Recalling that poor absorption will occur with medications administered by the oral, subcutaneous, or intramuscular routes will direct you to the correct option.

72. The nurse caring for an older adult client who has begun ambulating after having a surgical fixation of a fractured hip would plan to implement what intervention to minimize the chance of further injury? **Select all that apply.**

❒ 1 Keeping all the side rails up
❒ 2 Answering the call bell promptly
❒ 3 Keeping the call bell within reach
❒ 4 Ensuring that the night-light is working
❒ 5 Checking in on the client every 6 hours

Level of Cognitive Ability: Applying
Client Needs: Safe and Effective Care Environment
Clinical Judgment/Cognitive Skills: Generate Solutions
Integrated Process: Nursing Process/Planning
Content Area: Adult Health/Musculoskeletal
Health Problem: Adult Health: Musculoskeletal: Skeletal Injury

Answer: 2, 3, 4

Rationale: Falls are a major risk for postsurgical clients, especially those with ambulation issues. Safe nursing actions for preventing injury to the client include providing a call bell within the client's reach. Responding promptly to the client's use of the call light minimizes the chance that the client will try to get up alone, which could result in a fall. Night-lights are built into the lighting systems of most facilities, and the bulbs in these lights need to be routinely checked to ensure that they are working. Checking the client hourly needs to be completed to assess for pain, surgical incision, vital signs, safety, and need for elimination. Keeping all side rails up acts as a restraint and could lead to client injury.

Priority Nursing Tip: Hip repair involves stabilizing broken bones with surgical screws, nails, rods, or plates. This may also be called "hip pinning."

Test-Taking Strategy: Focus on the **subject,** client safety related to ambulation. Your knowledge of safety issues will help you to identify that it is inappropriate to have all side rails up for a client who is ambulatory and to recognize the need for frequent assessment of such clients.

---

73. The nurse has reinforced instructions to a parent regarding methods of preventing Lyme disease. Which statement made by the parent would indicate the **need for further teaching**?

1 "We will wear hats when we go on our hiking trip."
2 "Wearing long-sleeved tops and long pants is important."
3 "We will wear closed shoes and socks that can be pulled up over our pants."
4 "We will avoid the use of insect repellents because they will attract the ticks."

Level of Cognitive Ability: Evaluating
Client Needs: Safe and Effective Care Environment
Clinical Judgment/Cognitive Skills: Evaluate Outcomes
Integrated Process: Teaching and Learning
Content Area: Adult Health: Immune
Health Problem: Adult Health: Immune: Lyme Disease

Answer: 4

Rationale: Lyme disease, also known as Lyme borreliosis, is an infectious disease caused by bacteria of the Borrelia type, which is spread by ticks. To prevent Lyme disease, individuals would be instructed to use an insect repellent on the skin and clothes when the individuals are in areas in which ticks are likely to be found. Long-sleeved tops, long pants, closed shoes, and a hat or cap would be worn. If possible, heavily wooded areas or areas with thick underbrush would be avoided. Socks can be pulled up and over pant legs to prevent ticks from entering under the clothing.

Priority Nursing Tip: Lyme disease can cause a rash, often in a bull's-eye pattern, and flulike symptoms. Joint pain and weakness in the limbs also can occur.

Test-Taking Strategy: Focus on the **subject,** Lyme disease, and note the **strategic words,** *need for further teaching.* These words indicate a **negative event query** and ask you to select an option that is an incorrect client statement. Using your knowledge that the disease results from a tick bite will help direct you to the correct option.

---

74. The registered nurse (RN) is discussing the care of a client with a spinal cord injury with paraplegia and spasticity of the leg muscles with the licensed practical nurse (LPN). What actions by the LPN indicate a **need for further teaching? Select all that apply.**

- ❒ 1 Using restraints to minimize the painful spasms
- ❒ 2 Administering an as-needed prescription for a muscle relaxant
- ❒ 3 Massaging reddened areas on the heels to prevent skin breakdown
- ❒ 4 Performing range-of-motion exercises to stretch leg muscles
- ❒ 5 Avoiding the frequent repositioning of lower limbs to improve comfort

Level of Cognitive Ability: Evaluating
Client Needs: Safe and Effective Care Environment
Clinical Judgment/Cognitive Skills: Evaluate Outcomes
Integrated Process: Teaching and Learning
Content Area: Adult Health: Neurological
Health Problem: Adult Health: Neurological: Spinal Cord Injury

Answer: 1, 3, 5

Rationale: Paraplegia and spasticity create issues related to immobility, pressure ulcers, extremity pain, and joint contractures. Using limb restraints will not alleviate spasticity and could harm the client, and so would be avoided. The use of muscle relaxants may be helpful if the spasms cause discomfort to the client or pose a risk to the client's safety. Massaging reddened areas is to be avoided because doing so may further injure the skin. Range-of-motion exercises are beneficial for stretching muscles and exercising joints, which may diminish spasticity. Leaving the affected limb in one position can predispose the client to pressure ulcers and cause worsening spasticity.

Priority Nursing Tip: Spasticity is a feature of altered skeletal muscle performance with a combination of paralysis, increased tendon reflex activity, and hypertonia.

Test-Taking Strategy: Focus on the **subject,** care related to paraplegia and spasticity, and note the **strategic words,** *need for further teaching;* these words indicate a **negative event query** and ask you to select an option that is an incorrect action and one that is potentially harmful to the client. Understanding the care needed to address the issues created by paraplegia and muscle spasticity will help direct you to the correct options.

---

75. What intervention would the nurse implement to promote client safety regarding a client admitted with a diagnosis of hypoparathyroidism?

1 Keep the room slightly cool.
2 Institute seizure precautions.
3 Keep the head of the bed lowered.
4 Close the window blinds to minimize sunlight.

Level of Cognitive Ability: Applying
Client Needs: Safe and Effective Care Environment
Clinical Judgment/Cognitive Skills: Take Action
Integrated Process: Nursing Process/Implementation
Content Area: Adult Health: Endocrine
Health Problem: Adult Health: Endocrine: Parathyroid Disorders

Answer: 2

Rationale: Hypoparathyroidism results from insufficient parathyroid hormone, which leads to low serum calcium levels. Hypocalcemia can cause tetany, which, if untreated, can lead to seizures. The nurse would institute seizure precautions to maintain a safe environment. The other options do nothing to help this health problem or to promote a safe environment for this client.

Priority Nursing Tip: Insufficient parathyroid hormone levels can result in tingling or burning (paresthesia) in fingertips, toes, and lips.

Test-Taking Strategy: Note the **subject,** hypoparathyroidism and client safety. A knowledge of the complications associated with deficiency will help you identify the effects of low calcium levels. With these in mind and a focus on safety, eliminate each of the incorrect options.

76. The nurse assisting with preparing a plan of care for a client being admitted to the hospital for the insertion of a cervical radiation implant will implement what intervention to ensure client safety?

1 Sit in a chair when out of bed.
2 Maintain a side-lying position.
3 Elevate the head of the bed 60 degrees.
4 Maintain bed rest in the supine position.

Level of Cognitive Ability: Applying
Client Needs: Safe and Effective Care Environment
Clinical Judgment/Cognitive Skills: Take Action
Integrated Process: Nursing Process/Planning
Content Area: Adult Health: Oncology
Health Problem: Adult Health: Cancer: Cervical/Uterine/Ovarian

Answer: 4

Rationale: The client with a cervical radiation implant would be maintained on bed rest in the supine position to prevent the movement of the radiation source. The head of the bed is elevated to a maximum of 10 to 15 degrees for comfort. Turning the client on the side is avoided.

Priority Nursing Tip: Radiation therapy can be administered by a machine that aims x-rays at the body (external beam radiation) or by placing small capsules of radioactive material directly into the cervix (internal or implant radiation or brachytherapy).

Test-Taking Strategy: Focus on the **subject,** care for a client with a radiation implant. Consider the anatomical location of the implant and the risk of dislodgment. Options 1, 2, and 3 can cause dislodgment of the implant.

---

77. The nurse is assigned to a client who has just returned after an oral cholecystogram. At this time, which physician's prescription **requires follow-up**?

1 Maintain the client's mobility.
2 Monitor the client's hydration status.
3 Maintain a clear liquid status for 72 hours.
4 Monitor the client for abdominal discomfort.

Level of Cognitive Ability: Analyzing
Client Needs: Safe and Effective Care Environment
Clinical Judgment/Cognitive Skills: Take Action
Integrated Process: Nursing Process/Implementation
Content Area: Foundations of Care: Diagnostic Tests
Health Problem: Adult Health: Gastrointestinal: GI Accessory Organs

Answer: 3

Rationale: An oral cholecystogram is an x-ray procedure for diagnosing gallstones. The client would be able to resume a normal diet after the nurse has ensured that the client's gastrointestinal (GI) function is normal. It is unnecessary to keep the client on clear liquids for 72 hours after the procedure. The nurse would help the client maintain mobility as the client's ability allows. The nurse would also assess the hydration status as part of routine care for the client undergoing a GI diagnostic test. Monitoring for pain is an appropriate intervention.

Priority Nursing Tip: A cholecystogram requires the client to take contrast agent tablets in the evening of the day before the test.

Test-Taking Strategy: Focus on the **subject,** postcholecystogram care, and note the **strategic words,** *requires follow-up.* This tells you that the correct option is not necessary. A knowledge of the procedure and needed care will help you in determining which interventions are appropriate after this procedure; option 3 is an intervention that is unnecessary at this time.

---

78. The nurse is checking a client for the results of a purified protein derivative (PPD) test implanted 72 hours previously. The nurse determines that the PPD induration has a diameter of 11 mm. What action would the nurse take **next**?

1 Ask the client for permission to repeat the test.
2 Notify the primary health care provider (PHCP).
3 Document the normal finding in the client's record.
4 Tell the client to make an appointment with a pulmonologist.

Level of Cognitive Ability: Applying
Client Needs: Safe and Effective Care Environment
Clinical Judgment/Cognitive Skills: Take Action
Integrated Process: Nursing Process/ Implementation
Content Area: Adult Health: Respiratory
Health Problem: Adult Health: Respiratory: Tuberculosis

Answer: 2

Rationale: A PPD skin test is a screening test for tuberculosis (TB). An area of induration that measures 10 mm or more is considered a positive reading and indicates exposure to TB. The nurse who observes a positive PPD reading notifies the PHCP immediately. The PHCP would then order a chest x-ray to determine whether the client has clinically active TB or old, healed TB lesions. A sputum culture would then be performed to confirm a diagnosis of active TB. Option 3 is incorrect because the reading is not a normal finding. Option 1 is incorrect because the test results are positive. The PHCP rather than the nurse would request a consultation with a pulmonologist.

Priority Nursing Tip: A negative test PPD does not always mean that a person is free of tuberculosis.

Test-Taking Strategy: Note the **abnormal data,** *the diameter of the induration,* as well as the **strategic word,** *next.* Begin to answer this question by eliminating options 1 and 4 because it is not a nursing responsibility to prescribe another test or to provide consultations. Knowing that the results indicate a positive test will direct you to the correct option.

---

79. The nurse reinforcing information about tuberculosis (TB) disease and recuperation determines that the client understands the information presented when identifying what criteria for a return to work?

1 The client is no longer febrile.
2 Three consecutive sputum cultures are negative.
3 The purified protein derivative test and chest x-ray are negative.
4 The sputum culture and purified protein derivative test are negative.

Level of Cognitive Ability: Evaluating
Client Needs: Safe and Effective Care Environment
Clinical Judgment/Cognitive Skills: Evaluate Outcomes
Integrated Process: Teaching and Learning
Content Area: Adult Health: Respiratory
Health Problem: Adult Health: Respiratory: Tuberculosis

Answer: 2

Rationale: The client needs to have sputum cultures performed every 2 to 4 weeks after the initiation of anti-TB medication therapy. The client may return to work when the results of three sputum cultures are negative, because the client is considered noninfectious at that point. A positive purified protein derivative test never reverts to negative, while TB does not always result in a positive chest x-ray.

Priority Nursing Tip: Tuberculosis is spread via airborne particles.

Test-Taking Strategy: Focus on the **subject,** tuberculosis teaching. Use your knowledge on TB testing and transmission to answer correctly.

---

80. What room feature would the nurse determine is necessary for a client being admitted to the hospital with possible tuberculosis (TB)? **Select all that apply.**

❒ 1 Private room
❒ 2 Ultraviolet lighting
❒ 3 Two air exchanges per hour
❒ 4 Venting to the outside
❒ 5 Located near the nursing station

Level of Cognitive Ability: Applying
Client Needs: Safe and Effective Care Environment
Clinical Judgment/Cognitive Skills: Generate Solutions
Integrated Process: Nursing Process/Planning
Content Area: Adult Health: Respiratory
Health Problem: Adult Health: Respiratory: Tuberculosis

Answer: 1, 2, 4

Rationale: The client with TB needs to be admitted to a private room that provides at least six air exchanges per hour. The room would provide venting to the outside and have ultraviolet lights installed. The room need not be close to the nursing station.

Priority Nursing Tip: A person with latent TB infection, but not disease, cannot spread the infection to others, because there are no TB germs in the sputum.

Test-Taking Strategy: Focus on the **subject,** environmental needs for the care of a client diagnosed with tuberculosis. Begin to answer this question by recalling the method of transmission and then think about the specific requirements of physical facilities that are used when caring for clients with TB.

---

81. Which nursing intervention is appropriate for the nurse to implement when transporting a client diagnosed with active tuberculosis (TB) to the x-ray department?

1 Applying a mask to the client
2 Applying both a mask and gown to the client
3 Applying a mask, gown, and gloves to the client
4 Applying a particulate air respirator, gown, and gloves to the client

Level of Cognitive Ability: Applying
Client Needs: Safe and Effective Care Environment
Clinical Judgment/Cognitive Skills: Take Action
Integrated Process: Nursing Process/Implementation
Content Area: Foundations of Care: Infection control
Health Problem: Adult Health: Respiratory: Tuberculosis

Answer: 1

Rationale: TB requires airborne precautions. Clients who have or who are suspected of having TB would wear a mask when they are out of their rooms. A high-efficiency particulate air respirator (mask) is worn by the nurse when caring for the client with TB. Neither a gown nor gloves are needed for the client because the transmission mode for this disease is airborne.

Priority Nursing Tip: Tuberculosis is an infectious disease usually caused by *Mycobacterium tuberculosis* bacteria. TB can be spread by the infected person during coughing and sneezing.

Test-Taking Strategy: Focus on the **subject,** measures for airborne-transmitted diseases. An understanding of airborne precautions is necessary for answering this item correctly. Understanding how contact and airborne precautions differ will help eliminate options 2, 3, and 4.

---

82. A client's aggressive behavior has required four-point restraints. When will the nurse consider the client is demonstrating the ability to be safely returned to the milieu?

1 The client is able to identify the reasons for the aggressive behavior.
2 The client has been medicated and is still experiencing sedative effects.
3 The client apologizes and tells the nurse that such behavior will not happen again.
4 The client initiates no aggressive acts for an hour after the release of two leg restraints.

Level of Cognitive Ability: Evaluating
Client Needs: Safe and Effective Care Environment
Clinical Judgment/Cognitive Skills: Evaluate Outcomes
Integrated Process: Nursing Process/Evaluation
Content Area: Mental Health
Health Problem: Mental Health: Violence

Answer: 4
Rationale: Restraints are used as a last resort to provide external control over a client's unsafe behaviors. The best indicator that the client's behavior is under control is when the client demonstrates the ability to internally control these unacceptable behaviors. Although understanding the triggers for the behaviors is necessary, understanding alone does not demonstrate self-control over the actions. None of the other options demonstrate sufficient behavior control on the part of the client.
Priority Nursing Tip: When a client in restraints demonstrates the ability to control aggressive behaviors, the ankle restraints are removed first, one at a time, at regular intervals. The wrist and waist restraints are removed together when the client continues to exhibit nonaggressive behavior.

Test-Taking Strategy: Focus on the **subject,** restraint use and indicators that restraints can be safely removed. To answer this question accurately, you need to be familiar with the clinical concerns that first made the restraints necessary. Review the options for the degree of client self-control needed to manage the aggressive behavior and eliminate those that involve external controls (medication) or verbal assurances only.

---

83. A client becomes enraged and has started to bite and kick a roommate for occupying the bathroom. Which action would the nurse take **first**?

1 Physically restrain the client.
2 Notify the risk-management department.
3 Provide a safe environment for both clients.
4 Administer a medication to provide chemical restraint.

Level of Cognitive Ability: Applying
Client Needs: Safe and Effective Care Environment
Clinical Judgment/Cognitive Skills: Take Action
Integrated Process: Nursing Process/Implementation
Content Area: Mental Health
Health Problem: Mental Health: Violence

Answer: 3
Rationale: This situation places both clients at a risk for physical injury. The first action of the nurse is to provide an environment that is safe for both clients. This may take a variety of forms, depending on individual circumstances, agency protocols, and written primary health care provider orders. Seclusion, chemical restraint, and physical restraint are used only when alternative and less restrictive measures are ineffective for controlling the client's behavior.
Priority Nursing Tip: A chemical restraint is a form of medical restraint in which a medication is used to restrict the freedom of movement of a client or in some cases to sedate a client.

Test-Taking Strategy: Note the **strategic word,** *first.* Use **Maslow's Hierarchy of Needs theory** to answer this question. Physiological and safety needs come first. In this situation, the correct answer is the option that is an **umbrella option** because it *meets the needs of both clients* identified in the question.

---

84. After a cardiologist prescribes a 12-lead electrocardiogram (ECG), the nurse reinforces teaching to the client about the procedure. What comment by the client indicates an understanding about the test?

1 "I should lie very still while the ECG is being done."
2 "When the ECG begins, I need to take a deep breath."
3 "I should try to hold my breath while the ECG is running."
4 "I need to be prepared for the loud noise the ECG will make."

Level of Cognitive Ability: Evaluating
Client Needs: Safe and Effective Care Environment
Clinical Judgment/Cognitive Skills: Evaluate Outcomes
Integrated Process: Nursing Process/Evaluation
Content Area: Foundations of Care: Diagnostic Tests
Health Problem: N/A

Answer: 1
Rationale: Electrocardiogram is a recording of the electrical activity of the heart and is abbreviated as ECG and EKG. Good contact between the skin and electrodes is necessary to obtain a clear 12-lead ECG printout. Movement may cause a disruption in that contact and artifact, which makes the ECG printout difficult to read. The client does not have to hold the breath or take a deep breath during the procedure. The client would be reassured that the procedure will not produce loud noises.
Priority Nursing Tip: An ECG provides information about heart rate and rhythm, and it can show evidence of a previous heart attack (myocardial infarction).

Test-Taking Strategy: Focus on the **subject,** client understanding of an ECG. First, eliminate options that are **comparable or alike,** such as those that refer to breathing. Next, think about what the test involves to eliminate option 4.

---

85. The nurse, assisting with planning the discharge of a client diagnosed with chronic anxiety, documents which statement that demonstrates the client's efforts to promote a safe, therapeutic environment at home?

1 Is identifying anxiety-producing events
2 Is initiating contact with a crisis counselor
3 Is making an effort to ignore feelings of anxiety
4 Is attempting to eliminate all anxiety from daily events

Level of Cognitive Ability: Evaluating
Client Needs: Safe and Effective Care Environment
Clinical Judgment/Cognitive Skills: Evaluate Outcomes
Integrated Process: Nursing Process/Evaluation
Content Area: Mental Health
Health Problem: Mental Health: Anxiety Disorder

Answer: 1
Rationale: Recognizing events that produce anxiety allows the client to prepare to cope with anxiety or to avoid a specific stimulus. Counselors will not be available for all anxiety-producing events, and this option does not encourage the development of internal strengths. Ignoring feelings will not resolve anxiety. It is impossible to eliminate all anxiety from daily events.
Priority Nursing Tip: Anxiety may arise preceding a new experience or when values are threatened, whereas fear is a reaction to current events. These feelings may cause physical symptoms, such as a fast heart rate and shakiness.

Test-Taking Strategy: Focus on the **subject,** managing anxiety. Eliminate option 4 first because of the **closed-ended word** "all." Eliminate option 3 next because feelings would not be ignored. From the remaining options, select option 1; it is more client-centered, and it provides preparation for the client to deal with anxiety when it occurs.

---

86. The nurse is planning to reinforce safety instructions to prevent injury to a client diagnosed with Ménière's disease with chronic vertigo. What safety instruction would the nurse provide to the client?

1 Remove all floor clutter in the home.
2 Turn the head slowly when spoken to.
3 Drive at times when you do not feel dizzy.
4 Go to the bedroom and lie down when vertigo occurs.

Level of Cognitive Ability: Applying
Client Needs: Safe and Effective Care Environment
Clinical Judgment/Cognitive Skills: Take Action
Integrated Process: Teaching and Learning
Content Area: Adult Health/Ear
Health Problem: Adult Health/Ear/Ménière's Disease

Answer: 1

Rationale: The client would maintain a clutter-free home with throw rugs removed, because the effort of regaining balance after slipping could trigger vertigo. This action also demonstrates a proactive one to promote safety. The client with chronic vertigo would avoid driving and using public transportation; the sudden movements involved in each could precipitate an attack. To further prevent vertigo attacks, the client would change position slowly and turn the entire body (not just the head) when spoken to. If vertigo does occur, the client would immediately sit down or grasp the nearest piece of stable furniture.

Priority Nursing Tip: A viral infection of the vestibular nerve, called vestibular neuritis, can cause intense, constant vertigo.

Test-Taking Strategy: Focus on the **subject**, safety instructions for the client with vertigo. Begin to answer this question by applying an understanding of vertigo to eliminate options 3 and 4 first because they put the client at greatest risk of injury. From the remaining options, note that the correct option demonstrates a proactive action to minimize vertigo.

---

87. What is the **most important** assessment for the nurse to make before ambulating a client with Parkinson's disease who is taking newly prescribed levodopa-carbidopa?

1 The client's current orthostatic vital signs
2 The client's history of falls within the last 2 months
3 The degree of intention tremors exhibited by the client
4 Effectiveness of the assistive devices used by the client

Level of Cognitive Ability: Analyzing
Client Needs: Safe and Effective Care Environment
Clinical Judgment/Cognitive Skills: Prioritize Hypotheses
Integrated Process: Nursing Process/Data Collection
Content Area: Pharmacology: Neurological: Antiparkinsonians
Health Problem: Adult Health: Neurological: Parkinson's Disease

Answer: 1

Rationale: Clients diagnosed with Parkinson's disease are at risk for postural (orthostatic) hypotension from the pathophysiology associated with the disease. This problem worsens when levodopa-carbidopa is introduced, because the medication can also cause postural hypotension, thus increasing the client's risk for falls. Although knowledge of the client's use of assistive devices and history of falls is helpful, it is not the most important piece of data based on the information in this question. Clients with Parkinson's disease generally have resting rather than intention tremors.

Priority Nursing Tip: Levodopa-carbidopa is a combination medication used to treat symptoms of Parkinson's disease or Parkinson-like symptoms (such as shakiness, stiffness, difficulty moving). Carbidopa can also reduce some of levodopa's side effects such as nausea and vomiting.

Test-Taking Strategy: Focus on the **subject** of the question, assessments and ambulating a client taking levodopa-carbidopa. Note the **strategic words,** *most important.* Knowledge of the disease and its effect on ambulation, as well as the adverse effects of the prescribed medication, will help direct you to the correct option.

---

88. While bathing a client on strict bed rest, how can the nurse safely increase venous return in the extremities?

1 Long, firm strokes from distal to proximal areas
2 Short, patting strokes from distal to proximal areas
3 Firm, circular strokes from proximal to distal areas
4 Smooth, light strokes back and forth from proximal to distal areas

Level of Cognitive Ability: Applying
Client Needs: Safe and Effective Care Environment
Clinical Judgment/Cognitive Skills: Take Action
Integrated Process: Nursing Process/Implementation
Content Area: Skills: Hygiene
Health Problem: N/A

Answer: 1
Rationale: Long, firm strokes in the direction of venous flow promote venous return when the extremities are bathed. Circular strokes are used on the face. Short, patting strokes and light strokes are not as comfortable for the client and do not promote venous return.
Priority Nursing Tip: Bed rest can mean resting in bed at home, resting in bed and being monitored while in the hospital, or partly restricting activity. The client's condition and the physician's prescriptions will determine the amount of restrictions.

Test-Taking Strategy: Focus on the **subject,** encouraging venous return. Understanding the physiology associated with venous return will help eliminate options 3 and 4 first because a stroke from proximal to distal will not promote venous return. Next, visualize the remaining options and the subject to answer correctly.

---

89. The nurse is preparing to give an intramuscular (IM) injection using the Z-track technique. The nurse demonstrates a **need for further teaching** regarding this technique when observed performing which action?

1 Massaging the site after injecting the medication
2 Retracting the skin to the side before piercing the skin with the needle
3 Preparing a 0.25-mL air lock in the syringe after drawing up the medication
4 Attaching a new sterile needle to the syringe after drawing up the medication

Level of Cognitive Ability: Evaluating
Client Needs: Safe and Effective Care Environment
Clinical Judgment/Cognitive Skills: Evaluate Outcomes
Integrated Process: Teaching and Learning
Content Area: Skills: Medication Administration
Health Problem: N/A

Answer: 1
Rationale: The Z-track variation of the standard IM technique is used to administer IM medications that are highly irritating to subcutaneous and skin tissues. The site would not be massaged because this can lead to tissue irritation. Attaching a new sterile needle is done after drawing up the medication so that the new needle will not have any medication adhering to the outside that could be irritating to the tissues. Preparing an air lock keeps the needle clean of medication on insertion, and, as the air is injected behind the medication, it will provide a seal at the point of insertion to prevent tracking of the medication. Retracting the skin provides a seal over the injected medication to prevent tracking through the subcutaneous tissues.
Priority Nursing Tip: The Z-track method of IM injection prevents leakage of medications such as iron dextran into the subcutaneous tissue.

Test-Taking Strategy: Focus on the **subject** of the question, Z-tracking of the medication, and note the **strategic words,** *need for further teaching.* Note that the item is presenting a **negative event query,** requiring you to select an inappropriate action. An understanding of the purpose and process of Z-tracking will help you identify options 2, 3, and 4 as appropriate.

---

90. In which position would the client be placed to safely promote deep breathing and coughing when their tracheostomy is being suctioned?

1 Supine
2 Lateral
3 High Fowler's
4 Semi-Fowler's

Level of Cognitive Ability: Applying
Client Needs: Safe and Effective Care Environment
Clinical Judgment/Cognitive Skills: Take Action
Integrated Process: Nursing Process/Implementation
Content Area: Skills: Oxygenation
Health Problem: N/A

Answer: 4

Rationale: Unless it is contraindicated, the client is placed in semi-Fowler's position to promote deep breathing, maximum lung expansion, and productive coughing. With the client in this position, gravity pulls downward on the diaphragm, which allows greater chest expansion and lung volume. Options 1 and 2 would impede lung expansion. The high Fowler's position would not allow for easy visualization of the tracheotomy or easy access of the suction catheter.

Priority Nursing Tip: Upright at 90 degrees is full or high Fowler's position. With semi-Fowler's position, the head and trunk would be raised to 15 to 45 degrees, with 30 degrees as most common.

Test-Taking Strategy: Focus on the **subject,** suctioning a client with a tracheostomy. An understanding of the positions and their impact on breathing will assist in answering the item correctly. Eliminate options 1 and 2 first because they are **comparable or alike** options in that *they impede chest expansion*. From the remaining options, eliminate option 3 because the high Fowler's position would not allow for easy visualization of the tracheostomy or easy access of the suction catheter.

---

91. Which finding by the nurse indicates a normal fetal heart rate (FHR) for a full-term pregnancy?

1 FHR of 80 beats per minute
2 FHR of 90 beats per minute
3 FHR of 140 beats per minute
4 FHR of 170 beats per minute

Level of Cognitive Ability: Analyzing
Client Needs: Safe and Effective Care Environment
Clinical Judgment/Cognitive Skills: Analyze Cues
Integrated Process: Nursing Process/Data Collection
Content Area: Maternity: Antepartum
Health Problem: N/A

Answer: 3

Rationale: The normal FHR at term is 140 beats per minute. The normal range is 110 to 160 beats per minute; therefore, option 3 is the only correct option.

Priority Nursing Tip: A baby is considered preterm if born before 37 weeks of pregnancy.

Test-Taking Strategy: Focus on the **subject,** a normal fetal heart rate at term. Knowledge of the normal FHR is required to answer this question. This knowledge will direct you to the correct option.

---

92. Which is a contraindication to heart organ donation at the time of the client's death?

1 Age of 38 years
2 Hepatitis B infection
3 Allergy to penicillin-type antibiotics
4 Negative rapid plasma reagin laboratory result

Answer: 2

Rationale: A potential organ donor needs to meet age eligibility requirements, which vary by organ; for example, donors need to be less than 65 years old for kidney donation, less than 55 years old for pancreas and liver donation, and less than 40 years old for heart donation. The donor needs to be free of communicable disease (e.g., human immunodeficiency virus, hepatitis, syphilis), and the involved organ cannot be diseased. A negative rapid plasma reagin laboratory result indicates an absence of syphilis. Allergies are not relevant for possible donors.

Level of Cognitive Ability: Analyzing
Client Needs: Safe and Effective Care Environment
Clinical Judgment/Cognitive Skills: Recognize Cues
Integrated Process: Nursing Process/Data Collection
Content Area: Developmental Stages: End-of-Life Care
Health Problem: N/A

Priority Nursing Tip: Organs that can be transplanted are the heart, kidneys, liver, lungs, pancreas, and intestines. Transplantable forms of tissue include the skin, bone tissue (including tendons and cartilage), eye tissue, heart valves, and blood vessels.

Test-Taking Strategy: Note the **subject,** contraindication to organ donation. Note that the correct option relates to an infectious and communicable disease. Your understanding of the criteria for donation will help you in eliminating options not directly associated with the presence of communicable diseases.

---

93. A client diagnosed with chronic kidney disease has an indwelling abdominal catheter used for peritoneal dialysis. While bathing, the client spills water on the dressing that covers the catheter. The licensed practical nurse (LPN) reports the occurrence to the registered nurse (RN) and plans to **immediately** assist with which intervention?

1 Changing the dressing
2 Removing the catheter
3 Flushing the peritoneal dialysis catheter
4 Scrubbing the catheter with povidone-iodine

Level of Cognitive Ability: Applying
Client Needs: Safe and Effective Care Environment
Clinical Judgment/Cognitive Skills: Generate Solutions
Integrated Process: Nursing Process/Planning
Content Area: Skills: Infection Control
Health Problem: Adult Health: Renal and Urinary: Acute Kidney Injury and Chronic Kidney Disease

Answer: 1
Rationale: Clients with peritoneal dialysis catheters are at high risk for infection. Because bacteria can reach the catheter insertion site more easily through a wet dressing, the nurse ensures that the dressing is kept dry at all times. The catheter is not removed; it is placed surgically by the primary health care provider, and it is needed for further dialysis treatments. Flushing the catheter is not indicated. Scrubbing the catheter with povidone-iodine is done at the time of connection or disconnection of peritoneal dialysis by the RN.
Priority Nursing Tip: Peritoneal dialysis (PD) is a type of dialysis that uses the peritoneum in a person's abdomen as the membrane through which fluid and dissolved substances are exchanged with the blood.

Test-Taking Strategy: Note the **data in the question** and focus on the **subject,** a wet dressing. Note the **strategic word,** *immediately.* Understanding that the risk of infection is a concern will help you focus on the dressing rather than the catheter.

---

94. Which intervention will maintain the viability of the kidneys of a terminally ill client in the death process after a head injury to support organ donation?

1 Regular monitoring of the client's respirations
2 Medicating the client to avoid an elevated temperature
3 Administering intravenous (IV) fluids to establish and maintain hydration
4 Performing frequent range-of-motion exercises on the legs to facilitate venous return

Answer: 3
Rationale: Perfusion to the kidney is affected by blood pressure, which is in turn affected by blood vessel tone and fluid volume. Therefore, the client who was previously dehydrated to control intracranial pressure is now in need of rehydration to maintain perfusion to the kidneys. The nurse prepares to infuse IV fluids as prescribed and to continue monitoring the urine output. Checking the respirations and temperature and performing frequent range-of-motion exercises with extremities will not maintain the viability of the kidneys.
Priority Nursing Tip: Kidney donor recovery time will vary, depending on the type of surgical procedure. Most donors resume normal activities about a month after surgery.

Level of Cognitive Ability: Applying
Client Needs: Safe and Effective Care Environment
Clinical Judgment/Cognitive Skills: Take Action
Integrated Process: Nursing Process/Implementation
Content Area: Developmental Stages: End-of-Life Care
Health Problem: N/A

Test-Taking Strategy: Note the **subject,** maintaining the viability of the kidneys. This implies an action orientation, which guides you to look for options that involve intervention rather than data collection. Knowledge of interventions to support kidney perfusion will assist in answering this question correctly.

---

95. Which action by the nurse demonstrates a **need for further teaching** regarding the proper handling of legal evidence?

1 Initiating a custody log
2 Releasing personal items to the family
3 Placing all evidence into labeled, sealed paper bags
4 Cutting the clothing along seams, avoiding sites of damage

Level of Cognitive Ability: Evaluating
Client Needs: Safe and Effective Care Environment
Clinical Judgment/Cognitive Skills: Evaluate Outcomes
Integrated Process: Teaching and Learning
Content Area: Leadership/Management: Ethical/Legal
Health Problem: N/A

Answer: 2
Rationale: Basic rules for handling evidence include limiting the number of people with access to the evidence, including family members; initiating a chain-of-custody log to track the handling and movement of evidence; and carefully removing clothing to avoid destroying evidence. This usually includes cutting clothes along seams and avoiding areas where there are obvious holes or tears. Potential evidence is never released to the family to take home.
Priority Nursing Tip: A Sexual Assault Evidence Collection Kit is used to collect evidence from a victim of assault.

Test-Taking Strategy: Focus on the **subject,** handling legal evidence, and note the **strategic words,** *need for further teaching;* this phrase indicates a **negative event query** and asks you to select the option that is an incorrect action. Review each option and use your knowledge of evidence handling to select the option that may jeopardize evidence.

---

96. Using principles of prioritization during a disaster, the nurse initiates care **first** for the client presenting with what injury?

1 Fractured tibia
2 Penetrating abdominal injury
3 Bright red bleeding from a neck wound
4 Open severe head injury and a deep coma

Level of Cognitive Ability: Applying
Client Needs: Safe and Effective Care Environment
Clinical Judgment/Cognitive Skills: Take Action
Integrated Process: Nursing Process/Implementation
Content Area: Leadership/Management: Prioritizing
Health Problem: N/A

Answer: 3
Rationale: The client with arterial bleeding from a neck wound is in immediate need of treatment to save the client's life because the wound is directly associated with circulation and potentially with airway and breathing. According to the triage process, the client in this classification would be issued a red tag. The client with a penetrating abdominal injury would be tagged yellow and classified as "delayed," requiring intervention within 30 to 60 minutes. A green or "minimal" designation would be given to the client with a fractured tibia; this client requires intervention but can provide self-care, if needed. A designation of "expectant" and a color code of black would be applied to the client with massive injuries and a minimal chance of survival; these clients are given supportive care and pain management but are given definitive treatment last.
Priority Nursing Tip: Bright red bleeding indicates active bleeding and can be life-threatening if not controlled.

Test-Taking Strategy: Note the **strategic word,** *first.* To answer this question accurately, you need to be able to apply principles of prioritizing and the concept of **ABCs—airway, breathing, and circulation**. Review the options and select the client with injuries associated with airway, breathing, and circulation who is considered treatable at the scene.

---

97. The nurse is collecting data about home safety from an older client who is at risk for falls. The nurse determines that which item commonly found in the home poses a potential risk for the client and needs to be removed?

1 Scatter rugs
2 Wood flooring
3 Baseboard lighting
4 Motion lighting in the bathroom

Level of Cognitive Ability: Applying
Client Needs: Safe and Effective Care Environment
Clinical Judgment/Cognitive Skills: Recognize Cues
Integrated Process: Nursing Process/Data Collection
Content Area: Foundations of Care: Safety
Health Problem: Adult Health: Musculoskeletal: Skeletal Injury

Answer: 1

Rationale: Scatter rugs could potentially cause the older client to fall and would be removed or at least secured with a nonskid backing. The incidence of falls by older clients can be reduced with the use of bathroom safety equipment such as automatic lighting. In addition, the home needs to have railings on all staircases and ample lighting to illuminate floors. Wood floors are less likely to trigger slips and associated falls.

Priority Nursing Tip: The side effects of some medications can upset balance and increase the risk for falls. Medications for depression, sleep problems, and high blood pressure often cause falls.

Test-Taking Strategy: Focus on the **subject,** home situations that poses a risk for falls. Answer correctly by identifying the option that is most likely to trigger a fall.

---

98. A client who received a dose of chemotherapy 12 hours ago is incontinent of urine while in bed. The nurse would wear what personal protective barriers to safely clean the client and change bedding?

1 Mask and gloves
2 Gown and gloves
3 Mask, gown, and gloves
4 Gown, gloves, and eyewear

Level of Cognitive Ability: Applying
Client Needs: Safe and Effective Care Environment
Clinical Judgment/Cognitive Skills: Take Action
Integrated Process: Nursing Process/Implementation
Content Area: Foundations of Care: Safety
Health Problem: N/A

Answer: 2

Rationale: The client who has received chemotherapy will have antineoplastic agents or their metabolites in body fluids and excreta for 48 hours. For this reason, the nurse needs to wear protection when dealing with likely sources of contamination. In this instance, the nurse would wear gloves and a gown to protect the hands and uniform from contamination.

Priority Nursing Tip: While receiving chemotherapy, it is safe for the client to touch other people (including hugging or kissing). However, special care is needed to protect those who come into direct contact with the medication.

Test-Taking Strategy: Focus on the **subject,** safety after chemotherapy administration. Begin to answer this question by reasoning that the potential source of contamination in this event is the client's urine. Because urine present on the hospital gown and bedclothes is unlikely to splash, you can eliminate the options that identify a mask or eyewear.

---

99. A clinic nurse is reinforcing instructions to the parent of a child who has been diagnosed with mumps. The parent is concerned about their other children and asks the nurse how the infection is transmitted. What statement made by the parent indicates that the education provided by the nurse has been **effective**?

1 "Everyone gets extra vitamin C until this is over."
2 "Hand washing frequently will be really stressed in our house."
3 "The children won't play together until everyone is well again."
4 "I'll be sure that my children don't sneeze without covering the mouth and nose."

Answer: 4

Rationale: Mumps is transmitted via airborne droplets, salivary secretions, and possibly the urine. Addressing sneezing would demonstrate understanding. Options 1, 2, and 3 are incorrect because none focuses on the appropriate mode of transmission of mumps.

Priority Nursing Tip: Mumps, a contagious disease caused by a virus, typically starts with a few days of fever, headache, muscle aches, tiredness, and loss of appetite, followed by swollen salivary glands.

Level of Cognitive Ability: Evaluating
Client Needs: Safe and Effective Care Environment
Clinical Judgment/Cognitive Skills: Evaluate Outcomes
Integrated Process: Teaching and Learning
Content Area: Skills: Infection Control
Health Problem: Pediatric-Specific: Communicable Diseases

Test-Taking Strategy: Note the **strategic word,** *effective*. Focus on the **subject,** the method of transmission of mumps. Remembering that mumps is transmitted via airborne droplets, salivary secretions, and possibly the urine will help direct you to the statement associated with airborne transmission interventions.

---

100. To provide the client with accurate education regarding a planned bone marrow aspiration, the nurse would provide the client with which information?

1 Most clients report no pain from the procedure.
2 The procedure is painful, but the client will be under anesthesia.
3 A local anesthetic is used, but there is some pain during aspiration.
4 The procedure is very painful, but the client will be heavily medicated beforehand.

Level of Cognitive Ability: Applying
Client Needs: Safe and Effective Care Environment
Clinical Judgment/Cognitive Skills: Take Action
Integrated Process: Nursing Process/Implementation
Content Area: Foundations of Care: Diagnostic Tests
Health Problem: N/A

Answer: 3
Rationale: A local anesthetic is used to anesthetize the skin and subcutaneous tissue to minimize tissue discomfort with needle insertion. The client will feel some pain briefly when the sample is aspirated out of the marrow. Options 1, 2, and 4 are not true statements regarding this procedure.
Priority Nursing Tip: Providing accurate and truthful information to the client will help reduce fear and anxiety.

Test-Taking Strategy: Focus on the **subject,** bone marrow aspiration. Recalling that the procedure may be performed at the bedside will assist you with eliminating options 2 and 4. Knowing that the procedure is invasive will help you eliminate option 1.

---

101. The nurse would perform what action when attempting to move the client safely from the bed to a chair using a hydraulic lift?

1 Positioning the client in the center of the sling
2 Arranging to have four staff members available to assist
3 Having the client grasp the chains that attach the sling to the lift
4 Lowering the client quickly after he or she is positioned over the chair

Level of Cognitive Ability: Applying
Client Needs: Safe and Effective Care Environment
Clinical Judgment/Cognitive Skills: Take Action
Integrated Process: Nursing Process/Implementation
Content Area: Skills: Activity/Mobility
Health Problem: N/A

Answer: 1
Rationale: One person may operate a hydraulic lift. The client is positioned in the center of the sling, which is then attached to chains or straps that connect the sling to the lift. The client's hands and arms are crossed over the chest, and the client is raised from the bed into a sitting position. The lift raises the client off the mattress and lowers the client slowly after the sling is positioned over the chair.
Priority Nursing Tip: Manual client lifts feature a hydraulic mechanism that allows the nurse to operate the lift via a minimal effort pump lever.

Test-Taking Strategy: Focus on the **subject,** safe transfer using a hydraulic lift. Having an understanding of the process while visualizing this procedure will assist with directing you to the correct option.

---

102. An older adult client in a long-term care facility is at risk for injury related to confusion. Because the client's gait is stable, which method of restraint, if prescribed, would be **best** to prevent injury to the client?

1 Vest restraint
2 Waist restraint
3 Alarm-activating bracelet
4 Chair with a locking lap tray

Answer: 3

Rationale: If the client is confused and has a stable gait, the least intrusive method of restraint is the use of an alarm-activating bracelet or "wandering bracelet." This allows the client to move about the residence freely while preventing him or her from leaving the premises. A vest or waist restraint or a chair with a locking lap tray is more intrusive than an alarm-activating bracelet.

Priority Nursing Tip: A physician's order is necessary for the use of a restraint. If restraints are prescribed, the least invasive type needs to be used.

Level of Cognitive Ability: Applying
Client Needs: Safe and Effective Care Environment
Clinical Judgment/Cognitive Skills: Generate Solutions
Integrated Process: Nursing Process/Planning
Content Area: Foundations of Care: Safety
Health Problem: N/A

Test-Taking Strategy: Note the **strategic word,** *best.* Your knowledge of the various restraint methods and your focus on each type of restraint will help you eliminate options. Also, focus on the **data in the question.** The words *gait is stable* will also guide your selection.

---

103. The nurse, suctioning the airway of a client with a tracheostomy, safely performs the procedure by implementing which action?

1 Turning on wall suction to 190 mm Hg
2 Withdrawing the catheter while continuously suctioning
3 Inserting the catheter until the client coughs or resistance is felt
4 Reentering the catheter into the tracheostomy after suctioning the client's mouth

Answer: 3

Rationale: The nurse inserts the catheter until resistance is felt or it triggers the cough reflex and then withdraws it 1 cm to move it away from the mucosa. The wall suction unit is maintained between 80 and 120 mm Hg of pressure; this allows for the adequate removal of secretions while protecting the airway from trauma. The nurse suctions intermittently and does not reenter the tracheostomy after suctioning the client's mouth; doing so would introduce cross-contamination.

Priority Nursing Tip: Suctioning of the tracheostomy tube is necessary to remove mucus, maintain a patent airway, and avoid tracheostomy tube blockages.

Level of Cognitive Ability: Applying
Client Needs: Safe and Effective Care Environment
Clinical Judgment/Cognitive Skills: Take Action
Integrated Process: Nursing Process/Implementation
Content Area: Skills: Oxygenation
Health Problem: N/A

Test-Taking Strategy: Focus on the **subject,** suctioning the client with tracheostomy. Remembering that mucosal trauma can occur during suctioning will assist you with eliminating options 1 and 2. From the remaining options, visualizing this procedure and recognizing cross-contamination–related actions will direct you to the correct option.

---

104. Furosemide 40 mg orally has been prescribed for a client. The nurse administers furosemide 80 mg to the client at 10:00 AM. After discovering the error, the nurse would document what statement on an irregular occurrence report?

1 "Furosemide 80 mg was administered at 10:00 AM."
2 "Furosemide 80 mg was given to the client accidentally."
3 "The wrong dose of medication was given to the client at 10:00 AM."
4 "I meant to give 40 mg of furosemide, but I was rushed and I gave the wrong dose."

Answer: 1

Rationale: When filing an irregular occurrence report, the nurse needs to state the facts clearly. The nurse would not record assumptions, opinions, judgments, or conclusions about what occurred. The correct option is the only statement that states the facts clearly and without unnecessary comments.

Priority Nursing Tip: Any preventable event that may cause or lead to inappropriate medication use or client harm needs to be considered a medication error.

Level of Cognitive Ability: Applying
Client Needs: Safe and Effective Care Environment
Clinical Judgment/Cognitive Skills: Take Action
Integrated Process: Communication and Documentation
Content Area: Leadership/Management: Ethical/Legal
Health Problem: N/A

Test-Taking Strategy: Focus on the **subject,** documentation after a medication error. Using the **data in the question,** select the option that clearly and most directly states what has occurred. Option 4 is eliminated first because it contains unnecessary information. Option 2 provides information that it was unintentional and is an attempt to rationalize. Option 3 is incorrect because it assigns blame to the nurse.

---

105. The registered nurse (RN) employed in a long-term care facility assists a licensed practical nurse (LPN) with completing an irregular occurrence report for a client who was found sitting on the floor. After completing the report, which action by the LPN demonstrates a **need for further education** on the reporting process?

1 Immediately notifying the nursing supervisor
2 Forwarding the report to the nursing director's office
3 Asking the unit secretary to call the primary health care provider
4 Documenting in the nurses' notes that an irregular occurrence report was filed

Answer: 4
Rationale: An irregular occurrence form is an administrative document, not part of the medical record, so nurses are advised not to document the filing of an irregular occurrence report in the nurses' notes. Options 1, 2, and 3 are accurate interventions to notify appropriate persons, as well to provide for client safety.
Priority Nursing Tip: Irregular occurrence reports contain confidential information.

Test-Taking Strategy: Focus on the **subject,** appropriate handling of an irregular occurrence report, and note the **strategic words,** *need for further education;* this indicates a **negative event query** and asks you to select an option that is an incorrect action. Apply your knowledge of the purpose and management of this document to determine appropriate handling as identified in options 1, 2, and 3.

Level of Cognitive Ability: Evaluating
Client Needs: Safe and Effective Care Environment
Clinical Judgment/Cognitive Skills: Evaluate Outcomes
Integrated Process: Nursing Process/Evaluation
Content Area: Leadership/Management: Ethical/Legal
Health Problem: N/A

---

106. The physician tells the nurse, "I'm in a hurry. Write a prescription to decrease the atenolol to 25 mg daily for my client." Which is the appropriate nursing action in response to the request?

1 Writing the prescription exactly as stated
2 Informing the client of the change of medication
3 Calling the nursing supervisor to write the prescription
4 Asking the physician to return to the nursing unit to write the prescription

Answer: 4
Rationale: Nurses are not to accept verbal orders from physicians because of the risk of errors. Although the client will be informed about the change in the treatment plan, this is not the most appropriate action now. The physician would be made aware that the new order needs to be written to be implemented.
Priority Nursing Tip: Verbal orders present the risk for miscommunication of what is really intended.

Level of Cognitive Ability: Applying
Client Needs: Safe and Effective Care Environment
Clinical Judgment/Cognitive Skills: Take Action
Integrated Process: Nursing Process/Implementation
Content Area: Leadership/Management: Ethical/Legal
Health Problem: N/A

Test-Taking Strategy: Focus on the **subject,** a verbal order. Recalling that verbal orders are not acceptable will assist you with selecting the correct option. Options 1 and 3 are **comparable or alike** because both suggest the prescription would be written by someone other than the physician, so both would be eliminated. Option 2 does not address the issue. Option 4 clearly identifies the nurse's responsibility in this event.

---

107. The nurse determines the teaching related to a prescribed intravenous pyelogram (IVP) was **effective** when the client states the need to report which related complication immediately?

1 Nausea
2 Itching
3 Salty taste in the mouth
4 Warm, flushed feeling in the body

Level of Cognitive Ability: Evaluating
Client Needs: Safe and Effective Care Environment
Clinical Judgment/Cognitive Skills: Evaluate Outcomes
Integrated Process: Nursing Process/Evaluation
Content Area: Foundations of Care: Diagnostic Testing
Health Problem: N/A

Answer: 2
Rationale: IVP is a contrast study of the kidneys that determines the presence of a variety of disorders of the kidneys, ureters, and bladder. Difficulty breathing, wheezing, hives, and itching signal an allergic response and would be reported immediately. Normal sensations during the injection of the iodine-based radiopaque dye include a warm, flushed feeling; a salty taste in the mouth; and transient nausea.
Priority Nursing Tip: When anaphylaxis occurs, histamine is released and leads to bronchoconstriction, mucosal edema, and excess mucous production.

Test-Taking Strategy: Note the **strategic word,** *effective.* Focus on the **subject,** adverse reactions to IVP. Applying your knowledge concerning this procedure's risk for adverse reactions will help in identifying the possible existence of an allergic reaction.

---

108. An infant diagnosed with respiratory syncytial virus is prescribed ribavirin. What observation indicates a **need for further teaching** regarding the management of the disease process?

1 The infant's pregnant aunt visits.
2 The infant's asthmatic grandfather is asked not to visit.
3 All visitors wash their hands just prior to leaving the infant's room.
4 All visitors don gowns, gloves, masks, and hair coverings while visiting.

Level of Cognitive Ability: Evaluating
Client Needs: Safe and Effective Care Environment
Clinical Judgment/Cognitive Skills: Evaluate Outcomes
Integrated Process: Teaching and Learning
Content Area: Foundations of Care: Safety
Health Problem: Pediatric-Specific: Bronchitis/Bronchiolitis/Respiratory Syncytial Virus

Answer: 1
Rationale: Ribavirin, also known as tribavirin, is an antiviral medication used to treat respiratory syncytial virus infection, hepatitis C, and viral hemorrhagic fever. Whenever anyone is receiving ribavirin, there are precautions taken to prevent exposure to the medication. Everyone who enters the room while the client is receiving ribavirin needs to wear gowns, masks, gloves, and hair coverings. Anyone who is pregnant or considering pregnancy and anyone with a history of respiratory problems or reactive airway disease would not care for or visit anyone receiving ribavirin. Good hand washing is necessary before leaving the room, because hand washing prevents the spread of germs.
Priority Nursing Tip: Ribavirin is aerosolized and administered via small-particle generator and can pose risk to others.

Test-Taking Strategy: Focus on the **subject,** ribavirin precautions, and note the **strategic words,** *need for further teaching;* these words indicate a **negative event query** and ask you to select an option that is an incorrect activity by a family member. Applying your knowledge about the disease and medication and its possible effects will assist with directing you to the correct option.

---

109. When the client is prescribed dextroamphetamine sulfate 25 mg orally daily, the nurse educates the client to limit the consumption of what?

1 Iron
2 Starch
3 Protein
4 Caffeine

Level of Cognitive Ability: Applying
Client Needs: Safe and Effective Care Environment
Clinical Judgment/Cognitive Skills: Take Action
Integrated Process: Nursing Process/ Implementation
Content Area: Pharmacology: Neurological: Central Nervous System Stimulants
Health Problem: N/A

Answer: 4

Rationale: Dextroamphetamine sulfate is a central nervous system (CNS) stimulant. Caffeine is also a stimulant and needs to be limited for the client taking this medication. In addition, the client would be taught to limit his or her own caffeine intake. Neither iron, starch, nor protein needs to be limited while taking this medication.

Priority Nursing Tip: Dextroamphetamine sulfate stimulates release of norepinephrine.

Test-Taking Strategy: Focus on the **subject,** administration of dextroamphetamine. Recall that this medication is a CNS stimulant. Next, evaluate each of the options to determine the additive stimulation that each provides. Knowing that caffeine is a stimulant will direct you to the correct option.

---

110. To ensure client safety, the nurse would encourage the client prescribed enalapril for hypertension to engage in what action to avoid its common adverse effect?

1 Avoid long-term sun exposure
2 Consume a variety of foods high in potassium
3 Change from a sitting to standing position slowly
4 Ensure that the diet contains sufficient amounts of high-fiber foods

Level of Cognitive Ability: Applying
Client Needs: Safe and Effective Care Environment
Clinical Judgment/Cognitive Skills: Take Action
Integrated Process: Teaching and Learning
Content Area: Pharmacology: Cardiovascular Angiotensin-Converting Enzyme (ACE) Inhibitor
Health Problem: Adult Health: Cardiovascular: Hypertension

Answer: 3

Rationale: Orthostatic hypotension is a concern for clients taking antihypertensive medications such as enalapril. Clients are advised to avoid standing in one position for significant amounts of time, to change positions slowly, and to avoid extreme warmth (e.g., showers, baths, hot tubs, weather). The use of this medication does not require any special consideration regarding foods high in potassium or fiber. Photosensitivity is not generally associated with enalapril.

Priority Nursing Tip: Enalapril is an ACE inhibitor, and the net effect of ACE inhibitors is systemic vasodilation.

Test-Taking Strategy: Focus on the **subject,** adverse effects of enalapril. Recalling that most medications that end with the letters *-pril* are ACE inhibitors and that ACE inhibitors are often prescribed for hypertension will assist in determining its effects and lead you to the correct option.

---

111. The nurse assisting with planning care of a client who is recovering after femoral–popliteal bypass grafting will support extremity circulation and minimize the risk for harm by implementing what interventions? **Select all that apply.**

❒ 1 Using a bed cradle to keep bed linen off the client's legs
❒ 2 Placing a sheepskin directly beneath the client's affected leg
❒ 3 Keeping a lightweight blanket on the bed to promote warmth
❒ 4 Applying elastic wraps to facilitate venous return in the affected leg
❒ 5 Placing a pneumatic boot on the affected leg when ambulating the client

Answer: 1, 2, 3

Rationale: The use of sheepskin, a bed cradle, and lightweight blankets can promote warmth to the extremity and protect it from harm. Elastic wraps would be used when the client is out of bed to reduce edema, but they could impair circulation and wound healing. Frequently, the limb that has been operated on is left unwrapped for monitoring and is not covered by elastic wraps or pneumatic boots. However, these devices may be placed on the alternate extremity.

Priority Nursing Tip: The section of vein used for grafting or the man-made blood vessel graft is sewn onto both the femoral and popliteal arteries so that blood can travel through the new graft vessel and around the narrowed or blocked area.

Level of Cognitive Ability: Applying
Client Needs: Safe and Effective Care Environment
Clinical Judgment/Cognitive Skills: Generate Solutions
Integrated Process: Nursing Process/Planning
Content Area: Skills: Perioperative Care
Health Problem: Adult Health: Cardiovascular: Vascular Disorders

Test-Taking Strategy: Focus on the **subject**, postoperative care for a femoral–popliteal bypass graft. Recall that the limb that has been operated on needs frequent monitoring, warmth, and protection; this will direct you to the correct options.

---

112. The nurse is changing a dressing on a venous stasis ulcer that is a clean wound and has a growing bed of granulation tissue. The nurse demonstrates a **need for further education** regarding wound integrity if the nurse intends to use which dressing material?

1 Hydrocolloid dressing
2 Vaseline gauze dressing
3 Wet-to-dry saline dressing
4 Wet-to-wet saline dressing

Level of Cognitive Ability: Evaluating
Client Needs: Safe and Effective Care Environment
Clinical Judgment/Cognitive Skills: Evaluate Outcomes
Integrated Process: Teaching and Learning
Content Area: Skills: Wound Care/Dressings
Health Problem: Adult Health: Integumentary: Wounds

Answer: 3
Rationale: The use of wet-to-dry saline dressings provides a mechanical debridement whereby both devitalized and viable tissue are removed; this method would not be used on a clean, granulating wound. Granulation tissue in a venous stasis ulcer is protected with the use of wet-to-wet saline dressings, Vaseline gauze, or moist occlusive dressings such as hydrocolloid dressings, which are used only if prescribed.
Priority Nursing Tip: Debridement is the removal of unhealthy tissue from a wound to promote healing. It can be done by surgical, chemical, mechanical, or autolytic (using the body's own processes) removal of the tissue.

Test-Taking Strategy: Note the **strategic words,** *need for further education;* these words indicate a **negative event query** and ask you to select an option that is an incorrect type of dressing. Note that the wound is clean with granulation tissue, which needs protection. Note that options 1, 2, and 4 all have one thing in common—continuous moisture; this will direct you to option 3 because it is the only dressing that could disrupt this healing tissue.

---

113. An older adult client is admitted to the nursing unit with severe digoxin toxicity from the accidental ingestion of a week's supply of the medication. The licensed practical nurse (LPN) checks to see whether what antidote is in the unit's medication supply?

1 Furosemide
2 Protamine sulfate
3 Potassium chloride
4 Digoxin immune Fab

Level of Cognitive Ability: Applying
Client Needs: Safe and Effective Care Environment
Clinical Judgment/Cognitive Skills: Take Action
Integrated Process: Nursing Process/Implementation
Content Area: Pharmacology: Cardiovascular: Antidysrhythmics
Health Problem: N/A

Answer: 4
Rationale: Digoxin immune Fab is an antidote for severe digoxin toxicity. It contains an antibody produced in sheep that antigenically binds any unbound digoxin in the serum and removes it. It also binds the digoxin reentering the bloodstream from the tissues, which is then excreted by the kidneys. Potassium chloride and furosemide are other medications commonly used in conjunction with digoxin for cardiac conditions. Protamine sulfate is the antidote for heparin.
Priority Nursing Tip: The early manifestations of digoxin toxicity are gastrointestinal and include nausea, vomiting, abdominal pain, and diarrhea. Another manifestation is visual disturbances (blurred or yellow vision).

Test-Taking Strategy: Focus on the **subject,** digoxin toxicity. Apply your knowledge of the medications noted in the options, especially their functions and use as antidotes, and note the relationship between the name of the medication in the question and the correct option.

---

114. A client prescribed lisinopril has a white blood cell (WBC) count of 3800 mm^3. The nurse would plan to implement what intervention to minimize the client's risk for infection?

1 Follow aseptic technique diligently.
2 Place the client on respiratory isolation.
3 Use antibacterial soap when bathing the client.
4 Request oral antibiotics from the primary health care provider.

Level of Cognitive Ability: Applying
Client Needs: Safe and Effective Care Environment
Clinical Judgment/Cognitive Skills: Generate Solutions
Integrated Process: Nursing Process/Planning
Content Area: Pharmacology: Cardiovascular: Angiotensin-Converting Enzyme (ACE) Inhibitors
Health Problem: N/A

Answer: 1
Rationale: Clients taking angiotensin-converting enzyme inhibitors such as lisinopril are at risk for the development of neutropenia. Recall that the normal range of white blood cells is 5000 to 10,000 mm^3. Clients with a low blood cell count require the use of strict aseptic technique to minimize their risk for infection. Options 2 and 4 are unrelated to the information in the question because the focus is on infection prevention, not treatment. Antibacterial soap is inappropriate because there is no indication that the skin barrier has been damaged.
Priority Nursing Tip: A client diagnosed with neutropenia needs to be taught to report signs and symptoms of infection (e.g., sore throat, fever) to the primary health care provider. The WBC count with differential may be monitored monthly for up to 6 months in clients deemed at risk.

Test-Taking Strategy: Focus on the **subject,** a client taking lisinopril, while noting the **data in the question,** a white blood cell (WBC) count of 3800 mm^3. Recalling the normal WBC count and noting that the count is low, which places the client at risk for infection, will direct you to the appropriate intervention.

---

115. A nursing student is providing care for a client diagnosed with obsessive-compulsive disorder (OCD). The nursing student observes that the client spends many hours during the day and night washing their hands. Which statement by the nursing student reflects an understanding regarding this client's repetitive behavior?

1 "It increases the client's self-esteem."
2 "It relieves the client's chronic anxiety."
3 "It decreases the chance of developing an infection."
4 "It provides the client with a feeling of self-control."

Level of Cognitive Ability: Evaluation
Client Needs: Safe and Effective Care Environment
Clinical Judgment/Cognitive Skills: Evaluate Outcomes
Integrated Process: Teaching and Learning
Content Area: Mental Health
Health Problem: Mental Health: OCD

Answer: 2
Rationale: The compulsive, repetitive act provides immediate relief from anxiety and is used to cope with stress, conflict, or pain. Although the client may feel the need to increase self-esteem and regain self-control, the action is not related to meeting those needs. Infection is a physiological issue; this behavior is directed toward managing a psychosocial issue.
Priority Nursing Tip: The term *coping* generally refers to adaptive (constructive) coping strategies, that is, strategies that reduce stress.

Test-Taking Strategy: Focus on the **subject,** a client with OCD exhibiting repetitive behavior. Applying knowledge related to behaviors associated with compulsive disorders and the relief of anxiety will direct you to option 2.

---

116. What information would the nurse plan to include when preparing to reinforce the preprocedure information for a client scheduled for a cardiac catheterization?

1 The procedure is performed in the operating room.
2 The initial catheter insertion is quite painful; after that, there is little or no pain.
3 The client may feel various sensations, such as palpitations when the dye is injected.
4 The client may feel fatigue and have various aches because it is necessary to lie quietly on a hard x-ray table for approximately 4 hours.

Level of Cognitive Ability: Applying
Client Needs: Safe and Effective Care Environment
Clinical Judgment/Cognitive Skills: Generate Solutions
Integrated Process: Nursing Process/Planning
Content Area: Skills: Client Teaching
Health Problem: Adult Health: Cardiovascular: Coronary Artery Disease

Answer: 3

Rationale: During the preprocedure teaching, the client would be told that the procedure is performed in a darkened cardiac catheterization room and that electrocardiogram leads are attached to the limbs. A local anesthetic is used, so there is little to no pain with catheter insertion. The x-ray table is hard and may be tilted periodically. The procedure may take up to 2 hours, and the client may feel various sensations with catheter passage and dye injection.

Priority Nursing Tip: The client scheduled for a diagnostic procedure needs to be provided with factual information to help decrease anxiety.

Test-Taking Strategy: Focus on the **subject,** preprocedure information about cardiac catheterization. Applying knowledge of the procedure and expected outcomes will help in eliminating options that are inaccurate regarding where and how long the procedure will last and the amount of discomfort that will occur.

---

117. What nursing action would the nurse take when a client reports pain during the inflation of an indwelling urinary catheter balloon?

1 Stop and contact the prescribing physician.
2 Ensure the client that the discomfort will pass.
3 Withdraw 1 mL of air from the balloon of the catheter.
4 Deflate the balloon and insert it farther into the bladder.

Level of Cognitive Ability: Applying
Client Needs: Safe and Effective Care Environment
Clinical Judgment/Cognitive Skills: Take Action
Integrated Process: Nursing Process/Implementation
Content Area: Skills: Elimination
Health Problem: N/A

Answer: 4

Rationale: The procedure may be expected to be uncomfortable but not painful. If the client reports pain after the balloon is inflated, it is necessary to deflate the balloon and insert it farther into the bladder because it is most likely positioned in the urethra. Options 2 and 3 are incorrect actions because they do not address the need to correctly position the balloon. It is unnecessary to call the physician.

Priority Nursing Tip: Sterile technique is required when inserting a urinary catheter.

Test-Taking Strategy: Focus on the **subject,** pain with inflation of a urinary catheter balloon. Apply your knowledge of the intervention and then visualize the procedure when selecting the correct option. A client's report of pain would never be dismissed by suggesting that "discomfort will pass."

---

118. The nurse is caring for a client scheduled for an arthrogram. What question has **priority** during the preprocedure assessment to minimize the risk for injury?

1 "Do you have any allergies?"
2 "Do you want to void before the procedure?"
3 "Are you confident you can lie still for the entire procedure?"
4 "Have you talked with your physician about this procedure?"

Level of Cognitive Ability: Applying
Client Needs: Safe and Effective Care Environment
Clinical Judgment/Cognitive Skills: Take Action
Integrated Process: Nursing Process/Data Collection
Content Area: Foundations of Care: Diagnostic Tests
Health Problem: N/A

Answer: 1

Rationale: Because of the risk of allergy to the contrast medium, the nurse places highest priority on determining whether the client has an allergy to contrast dye, iodine, or shellfish. The nurse also reinforces information about the test, tells the client about the need to remain still during the procedure, and encourages the client to void before the procedure for comfort. The question related to allergies has priority because this knowledge is directly related to avoiding an allergic reaction to the contrast dye.

Priority Nursing Tip: An arthrogram is a test using x-rays to obtain a series of pictures of a joint after a contrast material (such as a dye, water, air, or a combination of these) has been injected into the joint.

Test-Taking Strategy: Focus on the **subject,** preprocedure assessment for an arthrogram. Note the **strategic word,** *priority*. Although all the options are relevant, only option 1 is related to a potential risk. The consequence of a possible allergic reaction makes this the correct option.

---

119. The nurse, reinforcing discharge instructions for a client with a spinal cord injury, stresses what action as a **priority** in providing a safe home-care environment?

1 Being aware of community services
2 Working toward securing long-term care placement
3 Including the significant others in the teaching session
4 Keeping all follow-up laboratory and diagnostic test appointments

Level of Cognitive Ability: Applying
Client Needs: Safe and Effective Care Environment
Clinical Judgment/Cognitive Skills: Take Action
Integrated Process: Teaching and Learning
Content Area: Leadership/Management: Management of Care
Health Problem: Adult Health: Neurological: Spinal Cord Injury

Answer: 3

Rationale: Involving the client's significant others in discharge teaching is a priority for the client with a spinal cord injury, because the client will need the support of the significant others. Knowledge and understanding of what to expect will help both the client and the significant others deal with the limitations. While community services may be able to support the client, it is not the priority action in preparation for discharge. Laboratory and diagnostic testing are inappropriate discharge instructions for this client. Long-term placement is not the only option for clients with spinal cord injuries.

Priority Nursing Tip: Community service is work performed by a nurse, layperson, or a group of people that benefits and assists others in the community.

Test-Taking Strategy: Focus on the **subject,** home care for a client with spinal cord injury. Note the **strategic word,** *priority*. Apply your knowledge about the needs of a client who has mobility issues when considering needs related to the home environment and supporting autonomy. The support of family and caregivers is vital to providing a safe home-care environment. Eliminate option 2 first because long-term placement is not the only discharge option. The remaining options are related to health issues rather than environmental concerns.

---

120. The nurse is asked to assist with applying electrocardiogram (ECG) electrodes to a client. The nurse would implement what intervention to keep the electrodes in place during the procedure?

1 Securing the electrodes with adhesive tape
2 Placing clear, transparent dressings over the electrodes
3 Applying lanolin to the skin before applying the electrodes
4 Cleaning the skin with an alcohol pad just before applying the electrodes

Level of Cognitive Ability: Applying
Client Needs: Safe and Effective Care Environment
Clinical Judgment/Cognitive Skills: Take Action
Integrated Process: Nursing Process/Implementation
Content Area: Foundations of Care: Diagnostic Tests
Health Problem: N/A

Answer: 4
Rationale: A secure connection between the skin and the electrodes is necessary to achieve an accurate ECG. Alcohol pads are commonly used to prepare the skin to help the electrodes adhere. Placing adhesive tape or a clear dressing over the electrodes will not help the adhesive gel of the actual electrode make better contact with the skin. Lanolin or any other lotion makes the skin slippery and prevents good initial adherence.
Priority Nursing Tip: Improper electrode placement will negatively impact the quality of the electrocardiogram.

Test-Taking Strategy: Focus on the **subject**, ensuring adherence of ECG electrodes. Note that options 1 and 2 are **comparable or alike** in that they both provide an external form of providing security for the electrodes. Eliminate option 3 because of the moisturizing effect of lanolin. Only option 4 addresses direct contact with the skin.

---

121. The nurse observes a client who is wringing his hands, looking frightened, and reports "feeling out of control." Which approach by the nurse will help maintain a safe client environment?

1 Moving the client to a "time-out" room to provide privacy
2 Taking the client to a quiet room to talk about his feelings
3 Observing the client in an ongoing manner without intervening
4 Administering the prescribed as-needed anxiety medication immediately

Level of Cognitive Ability: Applying
Client Needs: Safe and Effective Care Environment
Clinical Judgment/Cognitive Skills: Take Action
Integrated Process: Nursing Process/Implementation
Content Area: Mental Health
Health Problem: Mental Health: Anxiety Disorder

Answer: 2
Rationale: The anxiety symptoms demonstrated by this client require some form of intervention. Moving the client decreases environmental stimulus, and talking gives the nurse an opportunity to identify the cause of the client's feelings and to identify appropriate interventions. Isolation is appropriate only if the client is a danger to self or others. There is no indication in the question that the client poses a threat to others. Medication is used only when other noninvasive approaches have been unsuccessful.
Priority Nursing Tip: Many individuals who suffer with panic attacks experience what they describe as a feeling of disconnect from reality that scares and confuses them.

Test-Taking Strategy: Focus on the **subject,** a client expressing feelings of anxiousness. The client is in distress, and intervention is necessary. Eliminate options 1 and 4, which are **comparable or alike** because both suggest forms of restraints. The option that addresses the client's feelings while providing safety is the correct option.

---

122. A client has Buck's extension traction applied to the right leg. The nurse would perform which intervention to prevent complications resulting from the use of the device?

1 Provide pin care once per shift.
2 Inspect the skin of the right leg frequently for breakdown.
3 Massage the skin of the right leg with lotion every 8 hours.
4 Release the weights on the right leg for range-of-motion exercises daily.

Level of Cognitive Ability: Applying
Client Needs: Safe and Effective Care Environment
Clinical Judgment/Cognitive Skills: Take Action
Integrated Process: Nursing Process/Implementation
Content Area: Foundations of Care: Safety
Health Problem: Adult Health: Musculoskeletal: Skeletal Injury

Answer: 2
Rationale: Buck's extension traction is a type of skin traction. The nurse inspects the skin of the limb in traction frequently for irritation or inflammation. Massaging the skin with lotion is not indicated. The nurse never releases the weights of traction unless specifically prescribed to do so by the physician. There are no pins to care for with skin traction.
Priority Nursing Tip: Skin traction usually does not reduce a fracture, but pain reduction can be achieved.

Test-Taking Strategy: Focus on the **subject,** Buck's extension traction. Knowledge of this form of traction will allow you to eliminate options 1 and 4 because there are no pins, and the nurse never removes weights without a specific prescription to do so. To select from the remaining options, visualize this type of traction to answer correctly.

---

123. The nurse, assisting during a code, can safely allow what item to remain in close contact with the client while being defibrillated?

1 Ventilator
2 Backboard
3 Oxygen canister
4 Nitroglycerin transdermal patch

Level of Cognitive Ability: Applying
Client Needs: Safe and Effective Care Environment
Clinical Judgment/Cognitive Skills: Take Action
Integrated Process: Nursing Process/Implementation
Content Area: Complex Care: Basic Life Support/Cardiopulmonary Resuscitation/Cardiac Arrest
Health Problem: N/A

Answer: 2
Rationale: Flammable materials such as oxygen, metal devices, and liquids that can carry or transfer/conduct electricity are removed from the client and bed before defibrillation. The nitroglycerin patch may have a metal backing and needs to be removed. A ventilator delivers oxygen to the client. The backboard is needed to immediately resume cardiopulmonary resuscitation (CPR) if defibrillation is unsuccessful and is made of a material that does not conduct electricity.
Priority Nursing Tip: Nitroglycerin belongs to a class of medications known as nitrates and works by relaxing and widening blood vessels so that blood can flow more easily through the heart.

Test-Taking Strategy: Focus on the **subject,** safety during defibrillation. Apply your understanding of the defibrillation process and the risks it creates. Options 1 and 3 are **comparable or alike** because both are flammable and so are eliminated first. From the remaining options, remember that the nitroglycerin patch may have a metallic backing that conducts electricity and would need to be removed.

---

124. A licensed practical nurse (LPN) is reinforcing the discharge instructions provided to an adult client who has experienced family violence. What information has the **priority** for this client regarding further risks of physical abuse?

1 Specific information about self-defense classes
2 Instructions to call the police the next time the abuse occurs

Answer: 4
Rationale: Discharge instruction for this client would include information regarding safety from further abuse. Assisting the victim of family violence with a specific plan for removing himself or herself from the abuser (e.g., safe havens, hotlines) is essential. An abused person is usually reluctant to call the police but needs to be educated on how to safely leave before the abuse begins. Although feeling the security of being able to defend oneself may be empowering, teaching the victim to fight back (e.g., self-defense classes) is inappropriate when dealing with a violent

3 Exploration of the pros and cons of remaining with the abusive family member
4 Specific information regarding safe havens and shelters in the client's neighborhood

Level of Cognitive Ability: Applying
Client Needs: Safe and Effective Care Environment
Clinical Judgment/Cognitive Skills: Prioritize Hypotheses
Integrated Process: Nursing Process/Planning
Content Area: Mental Health
Health Problem: Mental Health: Violence

person, because often the abuser is more powerful. An exploration of the pros and cons of remaining with the abusive family member is inappropriate and unhelpful. The focus is on safety so that abuse does not occur.
Priority Nursing Tip: Babies and children are particularly vulnerable to physical abuse. Physical abuse is more likely to lead to death in this age-group than in any other age-group.

Test-Taking Strategy: Focus on the **subject**, information regarding further risks of physical abuse, and note the **strategic word**, *priority*. Apply your knowledge regarding family violence, and select the option that has the greatest potential to minimize the risk of physical abuse. This will direct you to the correct option.

---

125. The nurse, caring for a client with a recently applied plaster leg cast, would take which action to prevent the development of compartment syndrome?
1 Elevate the limb and apply ice to it.
2 Elevate the limb and cover it with bath blankets.
3 Keep the affected leg horizontal and apply heat to it.
4 Place the leg in a slightly dependent position and apply ice to it.

Level of Cognitive Ability: Applying
Client Needs: Safe and Effective Care Environment
Clinical Judgment/Cognitive Skills: Take Action
Integrated Process: Nursing Process/Implementation
Content Area: Adult Health: Musculoskeletal
Health Problem: Adult Health: Musculoskeletal: Skeletal Injury

Answer: 1
Rationale: Compartment syndrome is a painful condition that occurs when pressure within the muscles builds to dangerous levels. Compartment syndrome is prevented by controlling edema by elevating and applying ice to the affected extremity. These measures encourage venous blood return and help reduce edema through vasoconstriction. A horizontal or dependent position will not assist in circulation, and the application of heat will vasodilate the blood vessels, thus adding to the edema.
Priority Nursing Tip: A casted extremity requires frequent assessment of circulation, sensation, and mobility.

Test-Taking Strategy: Focus on the **subject**, prevention of compartment syndrome. Knowing that edema is controlled or prevented with limb elevation helps eliminate options 3 and 4. From the remaining options, think about the effects of ice as compared with bath blankets. Ice further controls edema, whereas bath blankets produce heat and prevent the air circulation needed for the cast to dry. This will direct you to the correct option.

---

126. An 8-year-old child with a history of sexual abuse by an adult family member is noted to be withdrawn and appears frightened. What statement would the nurse make **initially** to convey concern and support?
1 "I want you to know that you are safe here."
2 "I would like to just sit here with you for a while."
3 "Tell me how you feel about what has happened to you."
4 "I'd like you to use the doll to show me what happened to you."

Answer: 2
Rationale: The initial role of the nurse working with an abused victim is to establish trust. This is accomplished by providing a nonthreatening, stable, and safe environment. Establishing trust takes time. Victims of sexual abuse may exhibit fear and anxiety because of the recent incident. In addition, they may fear further abuse. When initiating contact with a child victim of sexual abuse who demonstrates a fear of others, it is best to convey a willingness to spend time and to move slowly to initiate activities that may be perceived as threatening. After a rapport has been established, the nurse may explore the child's feelings or use various therapeutic modalities to encourage a recounting of the offensive experience.
Priority Nursing Tip: The prevalence of child sexual abuse is difficult to determine because it is often unreported. A nurse is required to report a suspicion of child abuse.

Level of Cognitive Ability: Applying
Client Needs: Safe and Effective Care Environment
Clinical Judgment/Cognitive Skills: Take Action
Integrated Process: Nursing Process/Implementation
Content Area: Mental Health
Health Problem: Mental Health: Violence

Test-Taking Strategy: Note the **strategic word,** *initially,* and focus on the **subject,** conveying concern and support. The correct option explains how to establish trust during an initial encounter by spending time with the child in a nonthreatening, nonjudgmental atmosphere. Options 3 and 4 may be implemented after trust and rapport are established. Option 1 may be appropriate but does not convey concern and support on the part of the nurse.

---

127. A physician is about to defibrillate a client and says, in a loud voice, "CLEAR!" What action does the nurse take **immediately**?

1 Removes the backboard
2 Steps away from the bed
3 Shuts off the intravenous (IV) infusion going into the client's arm
4 Places the conductive gel pads for defibrillation on the client's chest

Answer: 2

Rationale: For the safety of all personnel, everyone needs to stand back and be clear of all contact with the client and the client's bed when the defibrillator paddles are being discharged. It is the primary responsibility of the person using the defibrillator paddles to communicate the "clear" message loudly enough for all to hear and to ensure everyone's compliance. All personnel need to comply with this command. The gel pads would have been placed on the client's chest before the defibrillator paddles were applied. The backboard is left in place for resuming cardiopulmonary resuscitation, if necessary. Shutting off the IV infusion has no useful purpose.

Priority Nursing Tip: An automated external defibrillator, also known as AED, is a machine that makes the decision about whether to shock and how strong the shock needs to be.

Level of Cognitive Ability: Applying
Client Needs: Safe and Effective Care Environment
Clinical Judgment/Cognitive Skills: Take Action
Integrated Process: Nursing Process/Implementation
Content Area: Foundations of Care: Safety
Health Problem: Adult Health: Cardiovascular: Dysrhythmias

Test-Taking Strategy: Focus on the **subject** of the question, safety during defibrillation. Note the **strategic word,** *immediately.* Applying your understanding of the defibrillation process and the possible risks created will help you select the option that identifies the need to avoid conduction of the electrical current being used.

---

128. The nurse reviews laboratory results and notes that a client's urine culture identifies the presence of several different organisms. What is the **most likely** cause for this result?

1 The specimen was contaminated.
2 The client has a kidney infection.
3 The client has a bladder infection.
4 The specimen was mishandled in the laboratory.

Answer: 1

Rationale: The presence of several different organisms in a urine culture usually indicates that contamination has occurred. The urinary tract is normally sterile, and infection, if it occurs, is usually with one organism. There is no information in the question that indicates that the laboratory personnel mishandled the specimen. A urine culture will not discriminate between bladder or kidney infection. A repeat of the urine culture is indicated.

Priority Nursing Tip: Most urinary tract infections are caused by a single organism, such as *Escherichia coli.*

Level of Cognitive Ability: Analyzing
Client Needs: Safe and Effective Care Environment
Clinical Judgment/Cognitive Skills: Analyze Cues
Integrated Process: Nursing Process/Analysis
Content Area: Foundations of Care: Diagnostic Tests
Health Problem: N/A

Test-Taking Strategy: Focus on the **data in the question,** and note the **strategic words,** *most likely.* There is no information in the question that indicates that the laboratory personnel mishandled the specimen. A urine culture will not discriminate between bladder or kidney infection; the clinical picture would help differentiate this. Remember that specimen contamination is the most frequent reason that several different organisms are cultured.

---

129. The nurse is evaluating the client's safe use of a cane for left-sided weakness. What action by the client **requires further teaching** by the nurse?

1 Holding the cane on the right side
2 Moving the cane when the right leg is moved
3 Leaning on the cane when the right leg swings through
4 Keeping the cane 6 inches out to the side of the right foot

Level of Cognitive Ability: Evaluating
Client Needs: Safe and Effective Care Environment
Clinical Judgment/Cognitive Skills: Evaluate Outcomes
Integrated Process: Teaching and Learning
Content Area: Skills: Activity/Mobility
Health Problem: N/A

Answer: 2

Rationale: The cane is held on the stronger side to minimize stress on the affected extremity and to provide a wide base of support. The cane is held 6 inches lateral to the fifth toe and moved forward with the affected leg. The client leans on the cane for added support while the stronger side swings through.

Priority Nursing Tip: To teach a client how to come down stairs using a cane, instruct the client to place the cane on the step first, then the affected leg and then, finally, the strong leg, which carries the body weight.

Test-Taking Strategy: Focus on the **subject,** safe use of a cane, and note the **strategic words,** *requires further teaching.* These words indicate a **negative event query** and the need to select the incorrect client statement. Knowing that the cane is held on the stronger side helps you eliminate options 1 and 4 first. To select between the remaining options, recall that the client moves the cane with the weaker leg and leans on it for support when the stronger leg swings through.

---

130. The nurse reinforces instructions to the parent of an infant diagnosed with acute infectious diarrhea about measures to prevent the spread of pathogens. Which action by the parent indicates a **need for further teaching?**

1 Washes the infant's hands after changing the diaper
2 Restrains the infant's hands when changing the diaper
3 Places the soiled diaper in a sealed, double plastic bag
4 Applies a cloth diaper snugly after cleaning the perineum

Level of Cognitive Ability: Evaluating
Client Needs: Safe and Effective Care Environment
Clinical Judgment/Cognitive Skills: Evaluate Outcomes
Integrated Process: Teaching and Learning
Content Area: Foundations of Care: Infection Control
Health Problem: N/A

Answer: 4

Rationale: Cloth diapers do not have elastic in the legs; this could allow for seepage of the infectious stool and cause the spread of pathogens. Also, liquid stool makes the diaper wet, which also promotes the spread of disease. Disposable plastic diapers have elastic in the legs, high absorbency, and plastic on the outside; these features decrease the transmission of pathogens. Option 1 prevents the spread of pathogens through hand washing. Option 2 prevents the infant from coming into contact with the infectious material. Option 3 identifies the appropriate disposal of infectious waste.

Priority Nursing Tip: Gastroenteritis, also known as infectious diarrhea, is inflammation of the gastrointestinal tract involving the stomach and small intestine. Symptoms may include vomiting, diarrhea, and abdominal pain.

Test-Taking Strategy: Focus on the **subject,** preventing the spread of infection via stool, and note the **strategic words,** *need for further teaching.* These words indicate a **negative event query** and ask you to select an option that is an incorrect action by the parent. Use the principles of standard precautions, which include hand washing, the proper disposal of body fluids and waste, and avoiding contact with body fluid. The only option that does not accurately reflect these precautions is the correct option.

---

131. After giving medications to the wrong client, it was determined that the nurse failed to check the client's identification bracelet before administering the medications. What is the basis for determining whether the nurse is guilty of negligence?

1 The nurse failed to meet established standards of care.
2 The incident could have resulted in the injury of the client.
3 The nurse demonstrated poor understanding of client safety needs.
4 The nurse ignored hospital policies about medication administration.

Level of Cognitive Ability: Evaluating
Client Needs: Safe and Effective Care Environment
Clinical Judgment/Cognitive Skills: Evaluate Outcomes
Integrated Process: Nursing Process/Evaluation
Content Area: Leadership/Management: Ethical/Legal
Health Problem: N/A

Answer: 1
Rationale: The legal definition of negligence is the failure to meet accepted standards of care. None of the other options accurately define negligence.
Priority Nursing Tip: All nurses are responsible for knowing the provisions of the nurse practice act of the state or province in which they work.

Test-Taking Strategy: Focus on the **subject,** negligence. Options 3 and 4 are true in that the purpose of the nurse practice act and of the institutional policies and procedures is to protect the public from harm. From the remaining options, select option 1 because it is the **umbrella option.**

---

132. The nurse is assigned a client diagnosed with acquired methicillin-resistant *Staphylococcus aureus* (MRSA). In addition to standard precautions, the nurse places the client on which type of transmission-based precautions?

1 Droplet precautions
2 Contact precautions
3 Airborne precautions
4 Isolation precautions

Level of Cognitive Ability: Applying
Client Needs: Safe and Effective Care Environment
Clinical Judgment/Cognitive Skills: Take Action
Integrated Process: Nursing Process/Implementation
Content Area: Foundations of Care: Infection Control
Health Problem: N/A

Answer: 2
Rationale: Contact precautions are precautions that include standard precautions and the use of barrier precautions such as gloves and impermeable gowns. Contact precautions are used for clients with diarrhea, antibiotic-resistant infections, or draining wounds that are not contained by sterile dressings. Airborne precautions and droplet precautions are relevant to infections spread via the air. Isolation precautions are special precautionary measures, practices, and procedures used in the care of clients with contagious or communicable diseases.
Priority Nursing Tip: Most hospitals routinely screen clients for methicillin-resistant *Staphylococcus aureus* (MRSA).

Test-Taking Strategy: Focus on the **subject,** precautions to prevent the transmission of MRSA. Apply your knowledge of MRSA, especially the method of transmission of the infection to others. Eliminate options 1 and 3 first because they are **comparable or alike** in that both relate to transmission of infection in the air. Recalling that MRSA can be transmitted by contact with the infecting organism will assist with directing you to the correct option.

---

133. A prenatal client diagnosed with *Condyloma acuminatum* caused by **human papillomavirus (HPV)** asks the nurse to again explain the treatment for the infection. The nurse would provide information about which possible treatment with this client?

1. Laser therapy
2. Interferon therapy
3. Cytotoxic medications
4. No therapy is available

Level of Cognitive Ability: Applying
Client Needs: Safe and Effective Care Environment
Clinical Judgment/Cognitive Skills: Take Action
Integrated Process: Nursing Process/Implementation
Content Area: Maternity: Antepartum
Health Problem: Maternity: Infections/Inflammations

Answer: 1

Rationale: *Condyloma acuminatum* refers to genital warts, which are an infection spread through skin-to-skin contact during sexual activity. The warts are caused by the human papillomavirus (HPV). For the pregnant client, laser therapy is the most effective method of destroying human papillomavirus. This therapy is localized, whereas medications (which are considered toxic to the fetus) would have a systemic effect and so are contraindicated at this time.

Priority Nursing Tip: The human papillomavirus (HPV) can be transmitted through skin-to-skin contact or through sexual activity. A vaccine is available and can protect children and adults from HPV-related diseases.

Test-Taking Strategy: Focus on the **subject,** *Condyloma acuminatum* treatment. Note that the client is pregnant. Applying your understanding of this infection would lead you to eliminate option 4. Options that are **comparable or alike** are unlikely to be correct and would be eliminated. With this in mind, eliminate options 2 and 3 next because they are both medications, a potential problem for the fetus.

---

134. A newly licensed practical nurse (LPN) has been instructed on the appropriate way to transfer a client from the bed to a chair one day after a total knee replacement. The teaching has been **effective** if the LPN completes which task prior to the transfer?

1. Applies a compression bandage around the dressing while the client is seated
2. Applies a knee immobilizer before moving the client from the bed
3. Obtains a walker to minimize weight bearing by the client on the affected leg
4. Lifts the client to the bedside chair, leaving the continuous passive motion (CPM) machine in place

Level of Cognitive Ability: Evaluating
Client Needs: Safe and Effective Care Environment
Clinical Judgment/Cognitive Skills: Evaluate Outcomes
Integrated Process: Teaching and Learning
Content Area: Skills: Activity/Mobility
Health Problem: Adult Health: Musculoskeletal: Skeletal Injury

Answer: 2

Rationale: On the first postoperative day, the nurse assists the client with getting out of bed after stabilizing the affected joint with a knee immobilizer. The surgeon prescribes weight-bearing limits on the affected leg. The leg is elevated while the client is sitting in the chair to minimize edema. A compression dressing would already be in place on the wound. The CPM machine is used only while the client is in bed. Ambulation is not started until the second postoperative day.

Priority Nursing Tip: A knee CPM machine helps decrease swelling, decrease pain, and increase range of motion.

Test-Taking Strategy: Focus on the **data in the question** and the **subject,** the protection of the knee joint. Note the **strategic word,** *effective*. Applying your knowledge related to knee replacement surgery and the potential risks to the knee in the recovery phase will help you eliminate options that are medically unsafe or unnecessary. Reviewing each option for its benefit to the knee will help direct you to the correct option.

---

135. The nurse collecting information about a client's suicide potential would consider what assessment question as **most important initially?**

1 "Do you have a plan to commit suicide?"
2 "Can we talk about your need to hurt yourself?"
3 "Has anyone in your family committed suicide?"
4 "Can you describe how you are feeling right now?"

Level of Cognitive Ability: Applying
Client Needs: Safe and Effective Care Environment
Clinical Judgment/Cognitive Skills: Recognize Cues
Integrated Process: Nursing Process/Data Collection
Content Area: Mental Health
Health Problem: Mental Health: Suicide

Answer: 1
Rationale: When collecting information about suicide risk, the nurse needs to determine whether the client has a suicide plan. Clients who have a definitive plan pose a greater risk for suicide. Options 2, 3, and 4 do not directly provide this information but are appropriate for future assessments.
Priority Nursing Tip: Potentially dangerous behavior, such as reckless driving, engaging in unsafe sex, and increased use of medications and/or alcohol, might indicate that the person no longer values his or her life.

Test-Taking Strategy: Focus on the **subject**, assessing for suicidal potential, and note the **strategic words,** *most important initially.* The correct option is the only one that directly questions the client about the presence of a suicide plan.

---

136. The nurse overhears an assistive personnel (AP) providing information about the client's condition to a visitor that the AP assumes to be a family member. What legal concept does the AP **require further education** on by the nurse?

1 Incompetency
2 Invasion of privacy
3 Communication techniques
4 Teaching and learning principles

Level of Cognitive Ability: Evaluate
Client Needs: Safe and Effective Care Environment
Clinical Judgment/Cognitive Skills: Evaluate Outcomes
Integrated Process: Nursing Process/Evaluation
Content Area: Leadership/Management: Ethical/Legal
Health Problem: N/A

Answer: 2
Rationale: Discussing a client's condition without the client's permission violates the client's rights and places the AP in legal jeopardy. This action is an invasion of privacy and affects the client's confidentiality. Incompetence could lead to negligence, but this legal concept is unrelated to the subject identified in the question. Communication techniques relate to the nurse–client relationship. Teaching and learning principles are considered concepts of standards of practice.
Priority Nursing Tip: Typically, a patient's bill of rights guarantees clients information, fair treatment, and autonomy over medical decisions, among other rights.

Test-Taking Strategy: Focus on the **subject,** the sharing of client information. Note the **strategic words,** *require further education.* Apply your understanding of a nurse's responsibility to preserve a client's right to confidentiality and of the ways in which confidentiality can be breached. This will direct you to the correct option.

---

137. A client with a seizure disorder has a prescription for valproic acid 250 mg once daily. To maximize the client's safety, when would the nurse plan to schedule the medication?

1 With lunch
2 At bedtime
3 After breakfast
4 Before breakfast

Answer: 2
Rationale: Valproic acid is an anticonvulsant that causes central nervous system (CNS) depression. Its side effects include sedation, dizziness, ataxia, and confusion. When the client is taking this medication as a single daily dose, administering it at bedtime negates the risk of injury from sedation and enhances client safety. All other options suggest times when the client has the potential to be physically active.
Priority Nursing Tip: Conventional antiseizure medications may block sodium channels or enhance γ-aminobutyric acid (GABA) function.

Level of Cognitive Ability: Applying
Client Needs: Safe and Effective Care Environment
Clinical Judgment/Cognitive Skills: Generate Solutions
Integrated Process: Nursing Process/Planning
Content Area: Foundations of Care: Safety
Health Problem: Adult Health: Neurological: Seizure Disorder/Epilepsy

Test-Taking Strategy: Focus on the **subject,** valproic acid and client safety. Recalling that this medication is an anticonvulsant with CNS depressant properties would lead you to consider its sedation as a side effect. Select the correct option because it allows the sedative effects of the medication to occur at a time when the client is less likely to be physically active; therefore, the client is less likely to become injured.

---

138. A client who had a synthetic cast placed on the right arm 24 hours ago to treat a fractured ulna wants to take a shower. Based on the review of the data related to the injury and the type of cast, what intervention **best** ensures a safe environment for this request?

1 "I'll get a shower chair for you."
2 "Okay, but don't let the cast get wet."
3 "Showering may lead to a serious infection."
4 "Exposing the cast to hot water may soften it."

Level of Cognitive Ability: Applying
Client Needs: Safe and Effective Care Environment
Clinical Judgment/Cognitive Skills: Generate Solutions
Integrated Process: Nursing Process/Implementation
Content Area: Foundations of Care: Safety
Health Problem: Adult Health: Musculoskeletal: Skeletal Injury

Answer: 1
Rationale: It may be unsafe for the client to shower with a cast on the arm because the client could slip and fall, so providing a shower chair will allow for stability and safety. Water does not damage the synthetic cast. Water may soften a plaster cast, but it has no effect on a synthetic cast. A shower is unlikely to cause an infection.
Priority Nursing Tip: The ulna is a long bone found in the forearm that stretches from the elbow to the smallest finger.

Test-Taking Strategy: Focus on the **subject,** care of a client with a synthetic arm cast, and note the **strategic word,** *best.* Eliminate options that are **comparable or alike**; options 2 and 4 both involve the effects of water. Next, recalling the causes of infection will assist in eliminating option 3.

---

139. A client is prepared to receive elective cardioversion to treat atrial fibrillation. Which assessment **requires further follow-up** before cardioversion to ensure client safety?

1 The client's digoxin has been withheld for the last 48 hours.
2 The client has received an intravenous (IV) dose of midazolam.
3 The defibrillator has the synchronizer turned on and is set at 50 joules.
4 The client is wearing a nasal cannula that is delivering oxygen at 2 L/min.

Level of Cognitive Ability: Analyzing
Client Needs: Safe and Effective Care Environment
Clinical Judgment/Cognitive Skills: Recognize Cues
Integrated Process: Nursing Process/Data Collection
Content Area: Foundations of Care: Safety
Health Problem: Adult Health: Cardiovascular: Dysrhythmias

Answer: 4
Rationale: During the procedure, any oxygen is removed temporarily because oxygen supports combustion, and a fire could result from electrical arcing. Digoxin may be withheld for up to 48 hours before cardioversion because it increases ventricular irritability and may cause ventricular dysrhythmias after countershock. The client typically receives an IV dose of a sedative or antianxiety agent. The defibrillator is switched to synchronizer mode to time the delivery of the electrical impulse, and the energy level is typically set at 50 to 100 joules.
Priority Nursing Tip: Cardioversion is usually done by sending electric shocks to the heart through electrodes placed on the chest in order to normalize the heart's rhythm.

Test-Taking Strategy: Focus on the **subject,** safety related to a cardioversion, and note the **strategic words,** *requires further follow-up.* These words indicate a **negative event query** and the need to select the incorrect client intervention. Applying your knowledge related to this procedure and its possible risks will help direct you to the correct option.

---

140. It is determined that the nurse did not note the client's heart rate of 45 beats per minute before administering a prescribed dose of digoxin to a client with heart failure. Failure to adequately collect data in this event is addressed under which function of the nurse practice act?

1 Defining the educational requirements for licensure in the state
2 Describing the scope of practice of licensed and assistive personnel
3 Identifying the process for disciplinary action if standards of care are not met
4 Recommending specific terms of incarceration for nurses who violate the law

Answer: 3

Rationale: In this scenario, acceptable standards of care were not met (i.e., the nurse failed to adequately assess the client before administering a medication). Option 3 refers specifically to the event described in the question, whereas options 1, 2, and 4 do not.

Priority Nursing Tip: In adults and older children, the first signs of digoxin toxicity usually include abdominal pain, anorexia, nausea, vomiting, visual disturbances, bradycardia, and other arrhythmias.

Test-Taking Strategy: Focus on the **subject,** failure to collect proper data. This information will direct you to option 3, which refers specifically to the event described in the question.

Level of Cognitive Ability: Analyzing
Client Needs: Safe and Effective Care Environment
Clinical Judgment/Cognitive Skills: Recognize Cues
Integrated Process: Nursing Process/Data Collection
Content Area: Leadership/Management: Ethical/Legal
Health Problem: Adult Health: Cardiovascular: Heart Failure

---

141. The nurse identifies a **need for further teaching** if the assistive personnel (AP) is observed engaging in what action while communicating with a hearing-impaired client?

1 Speaking in a normal tone
2 Speaking clearly to the client
3 Facing the client when speaking
4 Speaking directly into the impaired ear

Answer: 4

Rationale: Moving closer to the client and toward the better ear may facilitate communication, but the AP would avoid talking directly into the impaired ear. When communicating with a hearing-impaired client, the AP needs to speak in a normal tone to the client and not shout. The AP would talk directly to the client while facing him or her and speak clearly. If the client does not seem to understand what is said, the AP needs to express the statement differently.

Priority Nursing Tip: Hearing loss, also known as hearing impairment, is a partial or total inability to hear. A deaf person has little to no hearing. Hearing loss may occur in one or both ears.

Test-Taking Strategy: Focus both on the **subject,** communicating with a hearing-impaired client, and the **strategic words,** *need for further teaching*. These words indicate a **negative event query** and the need to select the incorrect intervention. Understanding the needs of the hearing impaired and the techniques needed to meet those needs will direct you to the correct option. Review the potential outcome of each option to determine its effect on the efforts to communicate.

Level of Cognitive Ability: Evaluating
Client Needs: Safe and Effective Care Environment
Clinical Judgment/Cognitive Skills: Evaluate Outcomes
Integrated Process: Teaching and Learning
Content Area: Leadership/Management: Delegating/Supervising
Health Problem: Adult Health: Ear: Hearing Loss

142. A nursing student has been assigned a client with a history of unsuccessful suicide attempts and suicidal ideation. Which statement made by the nursing student indicates an understanding on the topic?

1 "Only psychotic individuals commit suicide."
2 "Suicide attempts are just attention-seeking behaviors."
3 "Suicide is hereditary, so there is little health care personnel can do about it."
4 "Individuals who are serious often talk about their suicidal intentions to others."

Level of Cognitive Ability: Evaluating
Client Needs: Safe and Effective Care Environment
Clinical Judgment/Cognitive Skills: Evaluate Outcomes
Integrated Process: Teaching and Learning
Content Area: Mental Health
Health Problem: Mental Health: Suicide

Answer: 4
Rationale: Most people who commit suicide have given definite clues or warnings about their intentions. The individual who is suicidal is not necessarily psychotic or even mentally ill. A suicide attempt is not an attention-seeking behavior, and each act needs to be taken very seriously. Suicide is not an inherited condition; it is an individual condition, although there is an increased risk when there is a family history.
Priority Nursing Tip: Passive suicidal ideation involves a desire to die but without a specific plan for carrying out the death.

Test-Taking Strategy: Focus on the **subject**, suicidal ideations. Eliminate option 1 because of the **closed-ended word** *only*. Next, apply your knowledge related to suicide and suicide prevention when evaluating the accuracy of each option. This understanding would help you eliminate options that suggest characteristics or motivations that are not generally associated with depressed or suicidal individuals.

---

143. The nurse working in a crisis center receives a telephone call from a client who states the desire to commit suicide and who has a loaded gun on the table. Which intervention would be the nurse's **initial** response?

1 Ask the client why suicide is the only option.
2 Try to contact the primary health care provider.
3 Insist that the client give you an address so that the police can respond immediately.
4 Keep the client talking, and ask for consent to send medical assistance.

Level of Cognitive Ability: Applying
Client Needs: Safe and Effective Care Environment
Clinical Judgment/Cognitive Skills: Take Action
Integrated Process: Nursing Process/Implementation
Content Area: Mental Health
Health Problem: Mental Health: Suicide

Answer: 4
Rationale: During a crisis, the nurse needs to take an authoritative, active role to promote the client's safety. When a client verbalizes that he has a loaded gun in his home and wants to kill himself, the client's safety is the primary concern. Keeping the client on the phone and asking the client for consent to send medical assistance is the initial intervention. Insisting may anger the client and cause him to hang up. Asking the client why he wants to kill himself is not the initial intervention, nor is contacting the primary health care provider, because neither is related to assuring client safety at this time.
Priority Nursing Tip: Recent evidence suggests that the mixed-depressive form of bipolar disorder can be a particularly dangerous condition that can often go undetected or masquerade as general depression and irritability.

Test-Taking Strategy: Focus on the **subject,** a suicidal client's safety, and note the **strategic word,** *initial*. Eliminate any option that is likely to anger the client or that has little relevance to initial client safety. The correct option focuses on attempting to control the situation by addressing client safety.

---

144. The nurse in a long-term care facility determines that a cognitively impaired client's aggressive behavior is a risk for injury to other clients and staff. What intervention would the nurse implement **initially** to maximize milieu safety?

1 Apply one wrist restraint.
2 Assign staff to monitor the client continuously.
3 Place the client in an unlocked seclusion room.
4 Medicate the client with an as-needed chemical restraint.

Level of Cognitive Ability: Applying
Client Needs: Safe and Effective Care Environment
Clinical Judgment/Cognitive Skills: Take Action
Integrated Process: Nursing Process/Implementation
Content Area: Foundations of Care: Safety
Health Problem: N/A

Answer: 2
Rationale: The use of restraints would be avoided unless all other options have been exhausted. The initial intervention would be to provide the client with continuous supervision in order to manage aggressive behavior. All other options are forms of restraints.
Priority Nursing Tip: Clients have the right to refuse treatment, and alternate methods would be incorporated to promote client safety.

Test-Taking Strategy: Focus on the **subject,** managing an aggressive client, and note the **strategic word,** *initially.* Eliminate options 1, 3, and 4 as **comparable or alike** options, because all include a form of restraint and would be avoided until all other options have been exhausted.

---

145. The nurse is reinforcing instructions with the client and family about oxygen safety measures in the home. Which statement indicates that the client **requires further instruction?**

1 "I will turn my oxygen tank off if a visitor wants to smoke."
2 "I will not sit in front of my wood-burning fireplace with my oxygen on."
3 "I realize that I need to check the oxygen level of the portable tank frequently."
4 "I know I can't have lighted candles anywhere near my oxygen delivery system."

Level of Cognitive Ability: Evaluating
Client Needs: Safe and Effective Care Environment
Clinical Judgment/Cognitive Skills: Evaluate Outcomes
Integrated Process: Teaching and Learning
Content Area: Skills: Client Teaching
Health Problem: N/A

Answer: 1
Rationale: Oxygen is a highly combustible gas. Although it will not spontaneously burn or cause an explosion, oxygen can easily cause a fire to ignite in a client's room if it comes in contact with a spark from a cigarette, a candle, or electrical equipment. All remaining options demonstrate an understanding of oxygen safety measures.
Priority Nursing Tip: People diagnosed with asthma, emphysema, chronic bronchitis, occupational lung disease, lung cancer, cystic fibrosis, or congestive heart failure may use oxygen therapy at home.

Test-Taking Strategy: Focus on the **subject,** oxygen safety, and note the **strategic words,** *requires further instruction.* These words indicate a **negative event query** and ask you to select an option that is an incorrect client statement. Remembering that oxygen is a highly combustible gas will direct you to the correct option.

---

146. The licensed practical nurse (LPN) is assisting with planning care for a client diagnosed with deep vein thrombosis (DVT) of the left leg. What statement verbalized by the LPN indicates the **need for further instruction?**

1 "I will regularly elevate the client's left leg."
2 "Applying moist heat to the client's left leg is beneficial."
3 "I will ambulate the client in the hall at least once per shift."
4 "The client will benefit from regular doses of acetaminophen."

Level of Cognitive Ability: Evaluating
Client Needs: Safe and Effective Care Environment
Clinical Judgment/Cognitive Skills: Evaluate Outcomes
Integrated Process: Teaching and Learning
Content Area: Leadership/Management: Delegating/Supervising
Health Problem: Adult Health: Hematological: Clotting Disorders

Answer: 3
Rationale: Standard management of the client with DVT includes bed rest for the length of time prescribed; limb elevation; relief of discomfort with warm, moist heat and analgesics, as needed; anticoagulant therapy; and monitoring for signs of pulmonary embolism. Ambulation is usually contraindicated because it increases the likelihood of dislodgment of the thrombus, which could possibly travel to the lungs and become a pulmonary embolism.
Priority Nursing Tip: Signs and symptoms of a DVT generally include pain, redness, and swelling in the area around the blood clot.

Test-Taking Strategy: Focus on the **subject,** care of a client with a DVT, and note the **strategic words,** *need for further instruction;* this indicates a **negative event query** and asks you to select an option that is an incorrect action. Applying your understanding of appropriate care will help you identify that the reduction of inflammation and edema suggested by options 1 and 2 are appropriate. Acetaminophen relieves discomfort and is also indicated. This will direct you to the inappropriate intervention.

---

147. Knowing that a client in labor has a high risk for sickling crisis, the nurse would give **priority** to implementing which safe nursing action to prevent a crisis from occurring?

1 Reassure and encourage the client.
2 Maintain strict hand-washing technique.
3 Ensure that the client uses oxygen during labor.
4 Remind the client to not bear down for more than 3 seconds.

Level of Cognitive Ability: Applying
Client Needs: Safe and Effective Care Environment
Clinical Judgment/Cognitive Skills: Take Action
Integrated Process: Nursing Process/Implementation
Content Area: Maternity: Intrapartum
Health Problem: Adult Health: Cardiovascular: Vascular Disorders

Answer: 3
Rationale: Sickle cell anemia is a severe hereditary form of anemia in which a mutated form of hemoglobin distorts the red blood cells into a crescent shape at low oxygen levels. Administering oxygen as needed is an effective intervention to prevent sickle cell crisis during labor. The client is at high risk for being unable to meet the oxygen demands of labor and thus unable to prevent sickling. Option 1 is a generally helpful nursing measure, but it is not related to the prevention of sickling crisis. Option 2 is a safe nursing action, but it does nothing to prevent sickling crisis. Option 4 is unrealistic and would not prevent sickling crisis.
Priority Nursing Tip: A severe attack, known as sickle cell crisis, can cause pain because blood vessels can become blocked or the defective red blood cells can damage organs in the body.

Test-Taking Strategy: Focus on the **subject** of the question, preventing sickling crisis. Note that the question contains the **strategic word,** *priority.* Apply your understanding of the condition and review the options based on their impact on preventing the potential crisis.

---

148. A client admitted to the labor and delivery unit in labor has active genital herpes lesions present in the genital tract. The nurse would reinforce the teaching about what **immediate** plan of care for the client to help ensure a safe delivery?

1 Placement on protective isolation
2 Preparation for a cesarean delivery
3 Preparation for spontaneous vaginal delivery
4 Imminent artificial rupture of the membranes

Level of Cognitive Ability: Applying
Client Needs: Safe and Effective Care Environment
Clinical Judgment/Cognitive Skills: Take Action
Integrated Process: Teaching and Learning
Content Area: Maternity: Intrapartum
Health Problem: Maternity: Infections/Inflammation

Answer: 2
Rationale: Genital herpes is a sexually transmitted infection (STI) caused by a herpes simplex virus (HSV). The infant comes into contact with herpes blisters in the birth canal, which can cause the infant to become infected. Cesarean delivery reduces the risk of neonatal infection from a parent in labor who has either herpetic genital tract lesions or ruptured membranes. Options 3 and 4 would expose the fetus to the virus. Standard precautions are necessary, but protective isolation is not.
Priority Nursing Tip: The "classic" symptoms that most people associate with genital herpes are sores, vesicles, or ulcers—all of which can also be called "lesions."

Test-Taking Strategy: Note the **strategic word,** *immediate,* while focusing on the **subject,** genital herpes. Use your knowledge of the labor process and disease transmission to reason that the infant would not be born vaginally; this would help you eliminate option 3. Eliminate option 4 next, knowing that this could also expose the fetus to the virus. Eliminate option 1 because standard precautions are needed but protective isolation is not.

---

149. A client with possible renal disease is scheduled for an intravenous pyelogram (IVP). To ensure client safety, the nurse would be certain to collect data from this client concerning what aspect of their medical history?

1 Allergy to shellfish or iodine
2 Family incidences of renal disease
3 Frequent and chronic antibiotic use
4 Long-term use of diuretic medications

Level of Cognitive Ability: Applying
Client Needs: Safe and Effective Care Environment
Clinical Judgment/Cognitive Skills: Recognize Cues
Integrated Process: Nursing Process/Data Collection
Content Area: Foundations of Care: Safety
Health Problem: Adult Health: Renal and Urinary: Acute Kidney Injury and Chronic Kidney Disease

Answer: 1
Rationale: An IVP is an x-ray examination of the kidneys, ureters, and urinary bladder that uses iodinated contrast material injected into veins. A client undergoing diagnostic testing that involves the use of a contrast medium would be questioned about allergy to shellfish, seafood, or iodine; this would identify a potential allergic reaction to the contrast dye that may be used in such a test. The other items are useful as part of the general health history, but they are not as critical as the allergy determination in addressing risks presented by the test.
Priority Nursing Tip: Moderate allergic reactions to contrast dye, including severe vomiting, hives, and swelling, occur in 1% of clients receiving contrast media and frequently require treatment.

Test-Taking Strategy: Focus on the **subject,** risks related to IVP test. Apply your knowledge related to this test and the possible risks it presents. Recognizing that it requires the introduction of contrast dye will help direct you to the correct option.

---

150. The nephrologist prescribes 24-hour urine collection for a client with a suspected renal disorder. Which actions, if performed by the nurse, would identify a **need for further teaching** regarding proper collection technique?

1 Refrigerating the collection container
2 Discarding the first voiding during the prescribed 24-hour period
3 Asking the client to avoid fruit juices during the testing period
4 Instructing the client to void as close to the end of the testing period as possible

Level of Cognitive Ability: Evaluating
Client Needs: Safe and Effective Care Environment
Clinical Judgment/Cognitive Skills: Evaluate Outcomes
Integrated Process: Teaching and Learning
Content Area: Skills: Specimen Collection
Health Problem: Adult Health: Renal and Urinary: Acute Kidney Injury & Chronic Kidney Disease

Answer: 4
Rationale: Although a client would avoid caffeinated beverages for 48 hours prior to collection, there are no restrictions on fruit juices. To collect a 24-hour urine specimen, the nurse would ask the client to void at the beginning of the collection period and then discard this urine sample. This is done because the urine in that voiding has been in the bladder for an unknown period of time. All subsequent voided urine is saved in a container, which is placed on ice or refrigerated. The nurse would ask the client to void at the finish time and then add this sample to the collection. The nurse labels the container, places it on fresh ice if prescribed, and sends it to the laboratory immediately.
Priority Nursing Tip: Urine is made up of water and dissolved chemicals, such as sodium and potassium.

Test-Taking Strategy: Note the **strategic words,** *need for further teaching;* these words indicate a **negative event query** and ask you to select an option that is an incorrect nursing action. Focus on the **subject** of the question, proper collection technique for a 24-hour urine specimen. Visualize the procedure, and use your knowledge of this basic procedure to answer the question correctly.

---

151. A licensed practical nurse (LPN) assisting with care for a client in active labor would implement which intervention to **best** prevent fetal heart rate decelerations? **Select all that apply.**

❒ 1 Supporting the client's wish to stand upright when possible
❒ 2 Encouraging a side-lying maternal position when the client is in bed
❒ 3 Measuring and recording maternal and fetal vital signs every 30 minutes
❒ 4 Suggesting that the client and support person ambulate before the membranes rupture
❒ 5 Agreeing with the client that squatting will help during the pushing phase of the labor

Level of Cognitive Ability: Applying
Client Needs: Safe and Effective Care Environment
Clinical Judgment/Cognitive Skills: Take Action
Integrated Process: Nursing Process/Implementation
Content Area: Maternity: Intrapartum
Health Problem: N/A

Answer: 1, 2, 4, 5
Rationale: Side-lying and upright positions (e.g., walking, standing, squatting) can improve venous return and encourage effective uterine activity, which in turn will reduce the likelihood of fetal heart rate decelerations. Measuring the vital signs every 30 minutes will do nothing to prevent decelerations.
Priority Nursing Tip: A normal fetal heart rate at term is between 120 to 160 beats per minute.

Test-Taking Strategy: Note the **strategic word,** *best.* Focus on the **subject,** preventing fetal heart rate decelerations. Apply your understanding of fetal heart rate and the physiology of decelerations to each option to evaluate its effect on preventing this event. Identifying actions that will not prevent decelerations will lead you to the correct option.

---

152. The nurse is assisting with the care of a client diagnosed with diabetes mellitus who is 36 weeks pregnant. The results of three previous weekly nonstress tests have been reactive, but this week the test was nonreactive after 40 minutes. The nurse would expect that the obstetrician will prescribe which intervention to safely monitor this client?

1 An immediate contraction stress test
2 Admission to the hospital for continuous fetal monitoring
3 Admission to the hospital for immediate induction of labor
4 A follow-up appointment in 3 days to repeat the nonstress test

Level of Cognitive Ability: Analyzing
Client Needs: Safe and Effective Care Environment
Clinical Judgment/Cognitive Skills: Analyze Cues
Integrated Process: Nursing Process/Planning
Content Area: Maternity: Antepartum
Health Problem: Maternity: Diabetes

Answer: 1
Rationale: A nonstress test (NST), also known as fetal heart rate monitoring, is a common prenatal test used to check on a baby's health. During a nonstress test, a baby's heart rate is monitored to see how it responds to the baby's movements. A nonreactive stress test requires further evaluation of the baby's heart rate, thus indicating the need for a contraction stress test. Sending the client home for 3 days could place the fetus in jeopardy. Hospitalizing the client for either induction of labor or continuous fetal monitoring is premature without further diagnostic test data.
Priority Nursing Tip: During a nonstress test, a baby's heart rate is monitored to see how it responds to the baby's movements. A nonstress test may be done after 26 to 28 weeks of pregnancy.

Test-Taking Strategy: Focus on the **subject,** nonreactive nonstress test. Apply your knowledge of this test to the various options, and eliminate options 2 and 3 because they are unnecessary at this time. Choose correctly between the remaining options by selecting the one that provides further evaluation.

---

153. The nurse who begins to administer medications to a client via a nasogastric (NG) feeding tube suspects that the tube has become clogged. Which action would the nurse take **first**?

1 Aspirate the tube.
2 Flush the tube with warm water.
3 Prepare to remove and replace the tube.
4 Flush the tube with a carbonated liquid such as cola.

Level of Cognitive Ability: Applying
Client Needs: Safe and Effective Care Environment
Clinical Judgment/Cognitive Skills: Take Action
Integrated Process: Nursing Process/Implementation
Content Area: Skills: Tube Care
Health Problem: N/A

Answer: 1
Rationale: The nurse would first attempt to unclog the feeding tube by aspirating it. If this does not work, the nurse needs to try to flush the tube with warm water. Carbonated liquids such as cola may also be used, but only if agency policy identifies this practice as acceptable. There is no research evidence to support this practice. The replacement of the tube is the last step if others are unsuccessful.
Priority Nursing Tip: Pulmonary aspiration is the entry of material (such as pharyngeal secretions, food or drink, or stomach contents) from the oropharynx or gastrointestinal tract into the larynx (voice box) and lower respiratory tract.

Test-Taking Strategy: Focus on the **subject,** managing a potentially clogged NG tube, and note the **strategic word,** *first.* Apply your knowledge of the principles of NG tube management, and select the intervention that is least invasive and generally supported by most institutes.

---

154. A client admitted with severe depression 2 days ago suddenly begins smiling and stating that the current episode of depression has lifted. The client continues to be talkative and engages in conversation with other clients on the unit. The licensed practical nurse (LPN) consults with the registered nurse (RN), knowing that which change would be made to the client's treatment plan?

1 Allowing increased in-room activities
2 Increasing the level of suicide precautions
3 Allowing the client to spend time off of the unit
4 Reducing the dosage of antidepressant medication

Level of Cognitive Ability: Analyzing
Client Needs: Safe and Effective Care Environment
Clinical Judgment/Cognitive Skills: Recognize Cues
Integrated Process: Nursing Process/Planning
Content Area: Mental Health
Health Problem: Mental Health: Suicide

Answer: 2
Rationale: A depressed client who has been hospitalized for only 1 day is unlikely to have a dramatic reversal of mood. A sudden elevation in mood probably indicates that the client has decided to harm himself or herself, so an increase in the level of suicide precautions is indicated to keep the client safe. With this information in mind, option 1 is nontherapeutic, and options 3 and 4 could place the client at increased risk.
Priority Nursing Tip: When suicide risk is higher, staff will initiate precautionary measures and interventions immediately. Treatment is aimed at assisting the client through the stressful situation.

Test-Taking Strategy: Focus on the **subject**, care for the client with depression. Applying your understanding of the actions of a clinically depressed individual to the information provided in the question will help you arrive at the conclusion that the client is potentially contemplating suicide. Each of the incorrect options supports the client's idea that the depression has resolved. Keeping in mind that safety is of the utmost importance, eliminate each of the incorrect options.

---

155. The initial testing for human immunodeficiency virus (HIV) suggests that a child has been exposed to HIV infection. Which home-care instruction would the nurse reinforce to the parents of the child to minimize risk to others in the family? **Select all that apply.**

❒ **1** Wash the child's clothes in an antibacterial soap preparation.
❒ **2** Discourage others from kissing the affected child.
❒ **3** Clean any surface that comes in contact with the child's blood with a bleach and water solution.
❒ **4** Wash the hands with soap and water if they have touched the child's blood.
❒ **5** Serve the child's food using disposable plates and utensils.

Level of Cognitive Ability: Applying
Client Needs: Safe and Effective Care Environment
Clinical Judgment/Cognitive Skills: Take Action
Integrated Process: Teaching and Learning
Content Area: Foundations of Care: Infection Control
Health Problem: Pediatric-Specific: Immunodeficiency Disease

Answer: 3, 4
Rationale: HIV can only be transmitted from an infected person to another through direct contact of bodily fluids such as blood (including menstrual blood), semen, vaginal secretions, and breast milk. Blood spills are wiped up with a paper towel; the area is then washed with soap and water, rinsed with bleach and water, and allowed to air dry. Parents are instructed that neither hugging nor kissing will spread the infection. The disease is not transferred via cutlery or food service containers. Unless blood-stained, the child's clothes would be washed as is typical for the family. The hands are washed with soap and water if they come in contact with blood.
Priority Nursing Tip: Immunodeficiency is the failure of the immune system to protect the body adequately from infection due to the absence or insufficiency of some component process or substance.

Test-Taking Strategy: Focus on the **subject**, HIV precautions. Apply your understanding of the mode of transmission for HIV to eliminate options that are not directly associated with blood, breast milk, or body fluids.

---

156. The primary health care provider tells the nurse that a client admitted with a neurological problem will be scheduled for magnetic resonance imaging (MRI). The nurse questions the primary health care provider about this procedure based on a client history of which condition?

1 Heart failure
2 Cardiac dysrhythmias
3 Chronic airflow limitations
4 Mechanical valve replacement

Level of Cognitive Ability: Applying
Client Needs: Safe and Effective Care Environment
Clinical Judgment/Cognitive Skills: Analyze Cues
Integrated Process: Nursing Process/Data Collection
Content Area: Foundations of Care: Safety
Health Problem: N/A

Answer: 4

Rationale: The client scheduled for MRI removes all metallic objects because of the magnetic field generated by the device. A careful history is done to determine whether any metal objects have been implanted in the client, such as orthopedic hardware, pacemakers, artificial mechanical heart valves, aneurysm clips, or intrauterine devices. The remaining options pose no risk to the client scheduled for MRI because none involves a metallic implant.

Priority Nursing Tip: When heart valve disease progresses to the point that treatment by medicine does not provide relief from symptoms, surgery to repair or replace the valve may be recommended.

Test-Taking Strategy: Focus on the **subject,** contraindications to MRI. Applying your knowledge of the test and the technology involved while also noting the word *magnetic* in the name of the test will help direct you to the correct option.

---

157. A clinic nurse is providing instructions to a parent whose child was diagnosed with rubeola (red measles). To prevent the infection from spreading to their other children, the parent asks the nurse how measles is transmitted. The nurse educates the parent that rubeola is transmitted by which method?

1 Airborne mode
2 The fecal–oral route
3 Contact with infected saliva
4 Contact with the child's sweat

Level of Cognitive Ability: Applying
Client Needs: Safe and Effective Care Environment
Clinical Judgment/Cognitive Skills: Take Action
Integrated Process: Teaching and Learning
Content Area: Skills: Client Teaching
Health Problem: Pediatric-Specific: Communicable Diseases

Answer: 1

Rationale: Rubeola is transmitted via airborne particles or by direct contact with infectious droplets. This information makes clear that all the other options are incorrect.

Priority Nursing Tip: Saliva is a watery liquid secreted into the mouth by glands, providing lubrication for chewing and swallowing and aiding digestion.

Test-Taking Strategy: Focus on the **subject,** rubeola transmission. Knowledge regarding the route of transmission of rubeola is required to answer this question. Remembering that rubeola is transmitted via airborne particles or by direct contact with infectious droplets will help you select the correct option.

---

158. The nurse is notified that a trash-basket fire has occurred in a client's room. Upon arriving, the nurse notes that a staff member is in the process of removing the client from the room. What is the **next priority** action?

1 Confining the fire
2 Evacuating the unit
3 Extinguishing the fire
4 Activating the fire alarm

Level of Cognitive Ability: Applying
Client Needs: Safe and Effective Care Environment
Clinical Judgment/Cognitive Skills: Take Action
Integrated Process: Nursing Process/Implementation
Content Area: Foundations of Care: Safety
Health Problem: N/A

Answer: 4
Rationale: Remember the acronym *RACE* to set priorities when a fire occurs: **R**emove the victim; **A**ctivate the alarm; **C**ontain the fire; and **E**xtinguish as needed. In this event, the client has already been rescued from the immediate vicinity of the fire. The next action is to activate the fire alarm.
Priority Nursing Tip: The primary concern in the case of a fire is client and staff safety.

Test-Taking Strategy: Note the **strategic words,** *next priority.* Focus on the **subject,** fire safety. Remembering the order of the *RACE* acronym and using it to set priorities will help you answer the question correctly.

---

159. A licensed practical nurse (LPN) demonstrates responsibility as a team leader when engaging in what activity regarding nursing tasks?

1 Suggesting how to complete a task correctly
2 Checking to be sure the task is complete on time
3 Completing the task for a team member needing help
4 Getting a report from the assistive personnel (AP) concerning the completion of tasks

Level of Cognitive Ability: Applying
Client Needs: Safe and Effective Care Environment
Clinical Judgment/Cognitive Skills: Take Action
Integrated Process: Nursing Process/Implementation
Content Area: Leadership/Management: Delegating/Supervising
Health Problem: N/A

Answer: 4
Rationale: Authority for task completion is not given to the team member by directing or participating but by allowing the team member to be responsible for completing the task on his or her own. Options 1, 2, and 3 do not delegate authority and responsibility to the person performing the task.
Priority Nursing Tip: Good communication is an essential component of teamwork.

Test-Taking Strategy: Focus on the **subject,** giving authority and responsibility to a team member. Note that options 1, 2, and 3 are **comparable or alike** in that they all have the LPN involved in task completion.

---

160. Which action demonstrated by the nurse identifies a **need for further instruction** regarding the insertion and care of an indwelling urinary catheter? **Select all that apply.**

❒ 1 Coiling the tubing of the collection bag
❒ 2 Lubricating the catheter tip with water-soluble jelly
❒ 3 Inflating the balloon after the catheter is in the bladder
❒ 4 Using clean technique for the insertion of the catheter
❒ 5 Stopping catheter advancement just as urine appears in the catheter tubing

Answer: 4, 5
Rationale: The catheter would be advanced 1 to 2 inches beyond the point where the flow of urine is first noted; this ensures that the balloon is fully in the bladder before it is inflated. Each of the other options represents correct procedure. The catheter tip is lubricated for easier insertion. The balloon is inflated after the catheter is in the bladder. The tubing would be coiled (not kinked), and the collection bag would be placed lower than the level of the bladder. This is a sterile procedure, which needs to be completed under aseptic technique.
Priority Nursing Tip: In urinary catheterization, a latex, polyurethane, or silicone tube known as a urinary catheter is inserted into a client's bladder via the urethra.

Level of Cognitive Ability: Evaluating
Client Needs: Safe and Effective Care Environment
Clinical Judgment/Cognitive Skills: Evaluate Outcomes
Integrated Process: Teaching and Learning
Content Area: Skills: Safety
Health Problem: N/A

Test-Taking Strategy: Note the **strategic words,** *need for further instruction;* these words indicate a **negative event query** and ask you to select the option that is an incorrect nursing action. Visualizing this procedure and applying your understanding of the potential for risk of infection will help direct you to the correct options.

---

161. A licensed practical nurse (LPN) is asked to assist with preparing a forensic client who was admitted for a gunshot wound. The LPN removes the client's clothing and places a hospital gown on the client. Which intervention indicates the appropriate nursing action regarding the client's clothing, which is stained with blood?

1 Discard the clothing as biohazard waste.
2 Place the clothing in a paper bag.
3 Place the clothing in a plastic bag.
4 Give the clothing to a family member or significant other.

Level of Cognitive Ability: Applying
Client Needs: Safe and Effective Care Environment
Clinical Judgment/Cognitive Skills: Take Action
Integrated Process: Nursing Process/Implementation
Content Area: Leadership/Management: Ethical/Legal
Health Problem: N/A

Answer: 2
Rationale: Any evidence of crime discovered during an examination is saved and recorded to be handed off to police. The clothing is not given to a family member or significant other. Clothing is stored in a paper bag instead of plastic to prevent decomposition.
Priority Nursing Tip: The term *forensic* actually means relating to law and science.

Test-Taking Strategy: Focus on the **subject** of the question, the legal consideration of evidence related to a crime. Apply your understanding of the legal chain of possession when reviewing these options. Options that do not preserve the condition of the clothing can be eliminated first. From the remaining options, recalling that articles can decompose in a plastic bag will direct you to the correct option.

---

162. At the beginning of the day shift, a client consistently reports severe pain, even though pain medication was administered several times during the night by the regular night nurse. The nurse suspects that the night nurse is not administering the pain medication to the client as prescribed. According to the nurse practice act, which action is the nurse who discovered this situation required to perform?

1 Call the police to report the events.
2 Notify the state board of nursing.
3 Report the information to the nursing supervisor.
4 Wait until the next morning and talk to the night nurse.

Answer: 3
Rationale: The impaired nurse has cognitive, interpersonal, or psychomotor skills affected by psychiatric illness and/or medication or alcohol abuse or addiction. The nurse practice acts require reporting the suspicion of impaired nurses to the nursing supervisor, who then notifies the board of nursing. Option 4 prolongs the time in which the client receives inadequate pain relief. Options 1 and 2 will not alert the health care agency to the problem, which could result in client injury.
Priority Nursing Tip: The board of nursing has jurisdiction over the practice of nursing and may develop plans for treatment and supervision.

Level of Cognitive Ability: Applying
Client Needs: Safe and Effective Care Environment
Clinical Judgment/Cognitive Skills: Take Action
Integrated Process: Nursing Process/Implementation
Content Area: Leadership/Management: Ethical/Legal
Health Problem: N/A

Test-Taking Strategy: Focus on the **subject,** *ethical and legal responsibilities.* Your understanding of the issues related to the impaired nurse will help you prioritize safety as the prime concern. Review the options to evaluate which one is most focused on safety and addresses the agency's chain of command.

---

163. A client is receiving antibiotics by intramuscular (IM) injection. Because this client is also on anticoagulant therapy, the nurse knows that safety for this client would include what intervention?

1 Decreasing the IM needle size
2 Doubling the dose of the IM medication
3 Prolonging the pressure applied to the IM site after each injection
4 Applying a sterile bandage to the injection site after each IM injection

Level of Cognitive Ability: Applying
Client Needs: Safe and Effective Care Environment
Clinical Judgment/Cognitive Skills: Take Action
Integrated Process: Nursing Process/Implementation
Content Area: Skills: Medication Administration
Health Problem: N/A

Answer: 3
Rationale: An IM injection is given through the skin and into a muscle. This procedure can result in some degree of bleeding. Anticoagulants place the client at risk for bleeding. Prolonged pressure over the site of an IM injection will assist with preventing bleeding into the tissues that surround the injection site. Doubling the dose of the antibiotic is incorrect as well as dangerous, and a sterile bandage is unnecessary because infection is not the concern. Decreasing the IM needle size is an inappropriate action and can result in the medication not actually entering a muscle.
Priority Nursing Tip: An anticoagulant is used to prevent the formation of blood clots.

Test-Taking Strategy: Focus on the **subject,** safety of the client on anticoagulation. First, eliminate option 2, which suggests inappropriate administration of medication. Recalling the side effects of anticoagulant therapy will help in identifying the correct option.

---

164. When a medication is being administered, what actions would the nurse take to ensure client safety? **Select all that apply.**

❒ 1 Confirm the client's personal information on the medication administration record (MAR).
❒ 2 Ask the client to state his or her full name.
❒ 3 Check the name on the client's identification band.
❒ 4 Ask another nurse to verify the client's identity.
❒ 5 Ask the client to confirm his or her date of birth.

Level of Cognitive Ability: Applying
Client Needs: Safe and Effective Care Environment
Clinical Judgment/Cognitive Skills: Take Action
Integrated Process: Nursing Process/Implementation
Content Area: Skills: Medication Administration
Health Problem: N/A

Answer: 1, 2, 3, 5
Rationale: One of the rights of medication administration is the right client. This can be accurately verified by checking two forms of client identity such as identity band, asking the client to state his/her full name and date of birth, and checking the date of birth on the identification band against the MAR. Option 4 can result in medication errors because it does not involve objective comparison of identification information.
Priority Nursing Tip: A medication error is "a failure in the treatment process that leads to, or has the potential to lead to, harm to the client."

Test-Taking Strategy: Focus on the **subject,** identity of the client. Use your knowledge of the rights of medication administration to select the correct options after reviewing each for their effectiveness in identifying the client correctly.

---

165. After reviewing the client's medical record, the nurse notes a history of stroke and residual left-sided hemiplegia. Before ambulation, the nurse discusses with the assistive personnel (AP) what portion of client care?
 1 Safety
 2 Hygiene
 3 Hydration
 4 Elimination

Level of Cognitive Ability: Applying
Client Needs: Safe and Effective Care Environment
Clinical Judgment/Cognitive Skills: Generate Solutions
Integrated Process: Nursing Process/Planning
Content Area: Foundations of Care: Safety
Health Problem: Adult Health: Neurological: Stroke

Answer: 1
Rationale: Hemiplegia (sometimes called hemiparesis) is a condition that affects motor control and strength on one side of the body. Safety is the primary concern when the client is ambulating. Although hydration, hygiene, and elimination are also concerns in the plan of care, safety is the priority.
Priority Nursing Tip: Residual hemiplegia means that the person has recovered some function but not all.

Test-Taking Strategy: Noting the **data in the question** and your understanding of the needs of a client experiencing hemiplegia will direct you to the primary nursing concern.

---

166. The nurse demonstrates awareness of the single **most important** infection control technique when demonstrating what behavior?
 1 Using gloves when giving a bed bath
 2 Using sterile gloves when providing perineal care
 3 Washing hands before and after every client contact
 4 Using sterile technique for an abdominal dressing change

Level of Cognitive Ability: Applying
Client Needs: Safe and Effective Care Environment
Clinical Judgment/Cognitive Skills: Take Action
Integrated Process: Nursing Process/Implementation
Content Area: Foundations of Care: Infection Control
Health Problem: N/A

Answer: 3
Rationale: The most important infection control measure is the prevention of the spread of infection, which is accomplished by frequent hand washing. Options 1 and 4 are correct techniques, but they are not the most important infection control technique. Using sterile gloves for perineal care is unnecessary and is costly; clean gloves are sufficient for this procedure.
Priority Nursing Tip: Infection control is the discipline concerned with preventing nosocomial, or health care–associated, infection, a practical subdiscipline of epidemiology.

Test-Taking Strategy: Focus on the **subject,** infection control, and note the **strategic words,** *most important.* Recalling the basics of infection control will direct you to the correct option.

---

167. To prevent the spread of infection, the nurse would implement what intervention when a client is placed on contact precautions?
 1 Place strict restrictions on visitors.
 2 Perform meticulous hand washing frequently.
 3 Wear a mask and a gown with all client contacts.
 4 Wear sterile gloves for all contacts with the client.

Answer: 2
Rationale: Contact precautions apply to specified clients known or suspected to be infected or colonized with epidemiologically important microorganisms that can be transmitted by direct or indirect contact. Meticulous and frequent hand washing is necessary and has been proven to be a deterrent to the transfer of organisms. When the client is on contact precautions, a mask is unnecessary. However, a mask is necessary for respiratory precautions. Sterile gloves are not required for all client contacts, although clean (medical) gloves may be worn. All visitors need not be restricted from visiting if they are instructed in the measures that prevent infection.

Level of Cognitive Ability: Applying
Client Needs: Safe and Effective Care Environment
Clinical Judgment/Cognitive Skills: Take Action
Integrated Process: Nursing Process/Implementation
Content Area: Foundations of Care: Infection Control
Health Problem: N/A

Priority Nursing Tip: Medical gloves are disposable gloves used during medical examinations and procedures to help prevent cross-contamination between caregivers and clients.

Test-Taking Strategy: Focus on the **subject**, contact precautions. Apply your knowledge of contact precautions when reviewing each option for relevance or appropriateness related to infection control. Eliminate options 3 and 4 because of the **closed-ended word** "all."

---

168. When assisting with the care of a client diagnosed with hyperparathyroidism, the nurse implements what intervention to help safely minimize the effects of the disease process?

1. Restricts fluids to 1000 mL per day
2. Explains the benefits of a diet that is high in milk products
3. Encourages the liberal use of a calcium carbonate antacid
4. Assists the client to ambulate in the hall 3 times a day for 15 minutes

Level of Cognitive Ability: Applying
Client Needs: Safe and Effective Care Environment
Clinical Judgment/Cognitive Skills: Take Action
Integrated Process: Nursing Process/Implementation
Content Area: Adult Health: Endocrine
Health Problem: Adult Health: Endocrine: Parathyroid Disorders

Answer: 4
Rationale: The client with hyperparathyroidism is predisposed to hypercalcemia and to renal calculi formation; therefore, ambulation is important. A diet high in milk products would add to the client's calcium load. Calcium carbonate contains calcium and is therefore not the best choice as an antacid. Fluids would not be restricted because fluids aid in the excretion of calcium via the kidneys and prevent the formation of calcium-containing renal stones.
Priority Nursing Tip: Clients with hyperparathyroidism are at higher risk for fracture.

Test-Taking Strategy: Focus on the **subject**, care for client with hyperparathyroidism. Recalling that the client is predisposed to hypercalcemia will help you eliminate options that suggest increasing calcium consumption. Recalling that fluid will help reduce the likelihood of the development of renal stones will direct you to the correct option.

---

169. The nurse evaluating a client's readiness for discharge is performing a home safety assessment to determine whether there are any environmental hazards present. Which statement made by the client **requires need for follow-up** by the nurse?

1. "I live in a one-story house."
2. "I use smoke detectors in my home."
3. "I've lived alone since my partner's death."
4. "I've just had the bedroom rewired."

Level of Cognitive Ability: Evaluating
Client Needs: Safe and Effective Care Environment
Clinical Judgment/Cognitive Skills: Evaluate Outcomes
Integrated Process: Nursing Process/Evaluation
Content Area: Foundations of Care: Safety
Health Problem: N/A

Answer: 3
Rationale: An environmental hazard is a substance, state, or event that has the potential to threaten the surrounding natural environment or adversely affect people's health. Living alone can present issues if an emergency arises. The nurse would investigate further to determine the way the client would contact help if the need arises. The risk for falls is minimized by the absence of steps, whereas rewiring implies the risk of electrical fires and poor lighting in the bedroom has been addressed. A smoke detector is a positive factor in minimizing the dangers associated with fires.
Priority Nursing Tip: Tobacco smoke is a major source of indoor carbon monoxide exposure.

Test-Taking Strategy: Focus on the **strategic words,** *requires need for follow-up.* Apply your understanding of environmental safety when reviewing the options. Look for the option that identifies an environmental hazard to the client; this will direct you to the correct option.

---

170. The nurse is caring for a client diagnosed with a hiatal hernia. To prevent tracheal aspiration, the nurse would implement what intervention?

1. Administering antacids as needed
2. Encouraging the client to not smoke
3. Educating the client on the benefits of losing weight
4. Elevating the head of the bed on 4- to 6-inch blocks

Level of Cognitive Ability: Applying
Client Needs: Safe and Effective Care Environment
Clinical Judgment/Cognitive Skills: Take Action
Integrated Process: Nursing Process/Implementation
Content Area: Adult Health: Gastrointestinal
Health Problem: Adult Health: Gastrointestinal: Upper GI Disorders

Answer: 4
Rationale: Regurgitation with tracheal aspiration is a major complication of a hiatal hernia. Sleeping in an elevated position will help minimize the risk of aspiration. Although antacids, the avoidance of smoking, and losing weight will assist with alleviating the discomfort that can occur, these measures will not prevent aspiration.
Priority Nursing Tip: A hiatal hernia occurs when part of the stomach bulges into the chest. It can cause severe heartburn but is treatable.

Test-Taking Strategy: Note the **subject** of the question, preventing tracheal aspiration. Apply your knowledge related to the process and prevention of aspiration as you review each option for its possible effects. Options 1, 2, and 3 are all interventions that may be used with the client with a hiatal hernia, but they do not prevent regurgitation and aspiration.

---

171. The nurse is discussing the home environment with a client preparing for discharge to determine whether there are any fire hazards in the home. Which statement by the client **requires follow-up** by the nurse?

1. "I don't burn candles in my house."
2. "I need to plan and practice escape routes in case of a fire."
3. "I use smoke detectors and check the batteries faithfully every 2 years."
4. "My space heaters are located at least 3 feet from any items or furniture."

Level of Cognitive Ability: Evaluating
Client Needs: Safe and Effective Care Environment
Clinical Judgment/Cognitive Skills: Evaluate Outcomes
Integrated Process: Teaching and Learning
Content Area: Foundations of Care: Safety
Health Problem: N/A

Answer: 3
Rationale: Smoke detectors should be used; however, clients need to be instructed to test the batteries monthly and to change the batteries every 6 months. The client would also be instructed to keep a multipurpose fire extinguisher on hand in case of fire. Options 1, 2, and 4 identify correct actions regarding fire safety in the home.
Priority Nursing Tip: A smoke detector is a device that senses smoke, typically as an indicator of fire.

Test-Taking Strategy: Focus on the **subject,** fire hazards, and note the **strategic words,** *requires follow-up;* these words indicate a **negative event query** and ask you to select an option that is an incorrect client statement. Recalling that smoke detector batteries need to be checked monthly and changed every 6 months will direct you to the correct option.

---

172. Spironolactone is prescribed for a client. To ensure safety and minimize the risk for injury, the licensed practical nurse (LPN) would consult with the registered nurse (RN) before giving which medication that has already been prescribed for the client?

1 Digoxin
2 Warfarin sodium
3 Docusate sodium
4 Potassium chloride

Level of Cognitive Ability: Applying
Client Needs: Safe and Effective Care Environment
Clinical Judgment/Cognitive Skills: Take Action
Integrated Process: Nursing Process/Implementation
Content Area: Pharmacology: Cardiovascular: Diuretics
Health Problem: N/A

Answer: 4
Rationale: Spironolactone is a potassium-sparing diuretic that places the client at risk for hyperkalemia. If a potassium supplement were prescribed, the nurse would question the prescription. Docusate sodium is a stool softener, and warfarin sodium is an anticoagulant. Digoxin is a cardiac glycoside. None of these medications would contribute to an electrolyte imbalance.
Priority Nursing Tip: The most common cause of ascites is cirrhosis of the liver. Monitor serum potassium levels frequently in clients who have impaired renal function or who are currently taking potassium supplements because hyperkalemia is a common complication of spironolactone therapy.

Test-Taking Strategy: Focus on the **subject,** prescribed spironolactone. Use your knowledge of the medication classification of spironolactone to recall its classification, function, and possible adverse reactions. Keep this information in mind as you review the options to identify possible contraindications in function and adverse reactions.

---

173. The nurse discovers a dosage error while charting on digoxin medication administration. The nurse completes an irregular occurrence report and notifies the cardiologist of the incident. Which additional nursing actions need to be performed to ensure client safety as generally required? **Select all that apply.**

❒ 1 Documenting the incident in the client's record
❒ 2 Placing the irregular occurrence report in the client's record
❒ 3 Taking and recording a set of baseline vital signs
❒ 4 Sending a copy of the irregular occurrence report to the cardiologist's office
❒ 5 Monitoring the client's heart rate hourly to monitor for adverse effects

Level of Cognitive Ability: Applying
Client Needs: Safe and Effective Care Environment
Clinical Judgment/Cognitive Skills: Take Action
Integrated Process: Nursing Process/Implementation
Content Area: Leadership/Management: Ethical/Legal
Health Problem: N/A

Answer: 1, 3, 5
Rationale: The onset of action of oral digoxin is 1 to 2 hours, so the nurse would establish the baseline vital signs, particularly heart rate, so that there is a basis for comparison later. The irregular occurrence report is confidential and privileged information. It would not be copied, placed in the client's record, or have any reference to the actual report in the client's record. A copy would not be made or sent to the primary cardiologist's office.
Priority Nursing Tip: Digoxin is one of the oldest cardiac medications, most commonly used to treat atrial fibrillation and heart failure.

Test-Taking Strategy: Focus on the **subject,** administration of wrong dosage of medication. Apply your understanding regarding error reporting and the effects of digoxin when reviewing the options provided. Recalling the nurse's responsibilities regarding the client's safety, incident reporting, and documentation will direct you to options 1, 3, and 5.

---

174. A pregnant client diagnosed with acquired immunodeficiency syndrome (AIDS) is exhibiting signs of fever, weight loss, and candidiasis. The nurse would place **highest priority** on which intervention to meet the client's needs?

1 Providing emotional support to the parent
2 Assessing the parent's history for AIDS risk factors
3 Using disposable gloves when in contact with nonintact skin
4 Providing clear information about the consequences of AIDS on the unborn child

Level of Cognitive Ability: Applying
Client Needs: Safe and Effective Care Environment
Clinical Judgment/Cognitive Skills: Take Action
Integrated Process: Nursing Process/ Implementation
Content Area: Foundations of Care: Infection Control
Health Problem: Maternity: Infections/ Inflammations

Answer: 3
Rationale: Standard precautions would be used when caring for a pregnant client with AIDS. Options 1 and 4 are part of the plan of care, but they have a lesser priority than does staff and client safety. Option 2 is not a timely intervention because the client has already acquired the virus.
Priority Nursing Tip: Candidiasis is a fungal infection that presents with white patches on the tongue or other areas of the mouth and throat.

Test-Taking Strategy: Focus on the **subject,** care of the AIDS client, and note the **strategic words,** *highest priority.* Use **Maslow's Hierarchy of Needs theory** to eliminate options 1 and 4. From the remaining options, noting that the client has AIDS will eliminate option 2.

---

175. The nurse would put on gloves to perform which nursing interventions when working with a neonate?

1 Feeding the infant
2 Providing cord care
3 Discharging the infant
4 Changing the infant's clothes

Level of Cognitive Ability: Applying
Client Needs: Safe and Effective Care Environment
Clinical Judgment/Cognitive Skills: Take Action
Integrated Process: Nursing Process/ Implementation
Content Area: Foundations of Care: Infection Control
Health Problem: N/A

Answer: 2
Rationale: Standard precautions indicate that unsterile, clean gloves would be worn when touching nonintact skin. The nurse wears gloves when changing the baby's diaper and providing cord care. Gloves are unnecessary for the activities in options 1, 3, and 4 because these activities present little chance of bacterial transfer.
Priority Nursing Tip: A newborn baby, specifically a baby in the first 4 weeks after birth, is prone to infections, and a fever would be considered an emergency.

Test-Taking Strategy: Focus on the **subject,** the use of gloves when caring for a client. Recalling the principles of standard precautions related to wearing gloves and the likely situations for the transfer of bacteria will direct you to the correct option.

176. Which intervention in the general plan of care for a hospitalized client is specifically focused on assuring the client's rights as stated in the patient's (client's) bill of rights?

1 Maintaining accurate and current client information
2 Acting in a manner that reinforces the client's dignity
3 Incorporating available and appropriate teaching reference materials
4 Consulting with other health care team members about discharge planning

Level of Cognitive Ability: Applying
Client Needs: Safe and Effective Care Environment
Clinical Judgment/Cognitive Skills: Take Action
Integrated Process: Nursing Process/Implementation
Content Area: Leadership/Management: Ethical/Legal
Health Problem: N/A

Answer: 2
Rationale: Assuring dignity reflects one of the items identified in the patient's (client's) bill of rights. The other answer options relate to nursing interventions that reflect competent care but are not directly focused on client's rights.
Priority Nursing Tip: Client's rights include the right to make decisions regarding medical care and the right to accept or refuse treatment.

Test-Taking Strategy: Focus on the **subject** of the question, the patient's (client's) bill of rights. Applying your understanding of the client's rights as you evaluate each option's effect on these rights will help direct you to the correct option.

---

177. The nurse caring for a client diagnosed with hypoparathyroidism needs to focus **primarily** on what intervention to maintain a safe environment for this client?

1 Implementing seizure precautions
2 Keeping the client comfortably cool
3 Positioning the bed in a modified Trendelenburg's position
4 Applying a nonscented lotion to the client's hands and feet twice daily

Level of Cognitive Ability: Applying
Client Needs: Safe and Effective Care Environment
Clinical Judgment/Cognitive Skills: Take Action
Integrated Process: Nursing Process/Implementation
Content Area: Foundations of Care: Safety
Health Problem: Adult Health: Endocrine: Parathyroid Disorders

Answer: 1
Rationale: Hypoparathyroidism causes a deficiency of parathyroid hormone that leads to low serum calcium levels. Untreated hypocalcemia can cause tetany and seizure activity. The nurse would anticipate such a complication and institute seizure precautions to maintain a safe environment. The client's temperature does not elevate, nor does the skin tend to dry with this disorder. In addition, this disorder does not cause hypotension and does not require the modified Trendelenburg's position.
Priority Nursing Tip: Chronic moderate hypocalcemia may be completely asymptomatic.

Test-Taking Strategy: Focus on the **subject,** hypoparathyroidism and safety issues. Note the **strategic word,** *primarily.* Applying your understanding of the pathophysiology associated with hypoparathyroidism and its possible adverse reactions will help direct you to the correct option.

---

178. The nurse is beginning an intermittent enteral tube feeding via nasogastric (NG) tube. Which nursing action has the **highest priority** when considering client safety?

1. Weighing the client beforehand
2. Determining proper tube placement
3. Measuring intake and output each shift
4. Preparing the amount of formula needed

Level of Cognitive Ability: Applying
Client Needs: Safe and Effective Care Environment
Clinical Judgment/Cognitive Skills: Take Action
Integrated Process: Nursing Process/Implementation
Content Area: Skills: Tube Care
Health Problem: N/A

Answer: 2

Rationale: The highest priority is to determine tube placement. Initiating a tube feeding without checking tube placement places the client at risk for aspiration, which can lead to pneumonia. Options 1, 3, and 4 are routine care items for a client receiving enteral feedings, but they are not the highest priority because they are not associated with an acute problem that could be life-threatening.

Priority Nursing Tip: An NG tube can be used to drain gastric contents, decompress the stomach, obtain a specimen of gastric contents, or introduce a passage into the gastrointestinal tract.

Test-Taking Strategy: Note the **strategic words,** *highest priority,* and focus on the **subject,** client safety. Apply your understanding of the purpose and positioning of an NG tube while evaluating the options for their acute effect on client safety. Airway and breathing issues are priority concerns and will direct you to the correct option.

---

179. A client is being discharged to return home after a spinal fusion. The nurse would suggest a consultation with the continuing-care nurse regarding the need for modification of the home environment if the client makes what statement?

1. "I prefer showering to taking a bath."
2. "There are three steps to get up to the front door."
3. "The family has arranged for a bedside commode."
4. "There is carpeting on the steps to the upstairs bedrooms."

Level of Cognitive Ability: Applying
Client Needs: Safe and Effective Care Environment
Clinical Judgment/Cognitive Skills: Evaluate Outcomes
Integrated Process: Nursing Process/Planning
Content Area: Leadership/Management: Interprofessional Collaboration
Health Problem: Adult Health: Musculoskeletal: Skeletal Injury

Answer: 4

Rationale: Stair-climbing may be restricted or limited for several weeks after spinal fusion. The fact that the house is at least two stories with the bedrooms on the upper floor requires a modification, such as setting up a bedroom on the first floor. Three steps up to the front door would likely be manageable after spinal fusion and would adhere to stair-climbing restrictions. The other options will assist the client during the recovery.

Priority Nursing Tip: Spinal fusion is a surgical procedure used to correct problems with the small bones of the spine (vertebrae). The basic idea is to fuse together the painful vertebrae so that they heal into a single solid bone.

Test-Taking Strategy: Focus on the **subject,** challenges provided by the home environment. Use your understanding of the challenges associated with recovery after a spinal fusion when evaluating the client statements. Eliminate options that are actually helpful to the client first. To select between the options that involve stairs, you would consider which would be most problematic in day-to-day recovery.

---

180. What precautions will the nurse institute when providing direct client care until the diagnosis of scabies is ruled out?

1 Putting on a pair of gloves
2 Donning a mask and gloves
3 Putting on a gown and gloves
4 Donning gloves, mask, and gown

Level of Cognitive Ability: Applying
Client Needs: Safe and Effective Care Environment
Clinical Judgment/Cognitive Skills: Take Action
Integrated Process: Nursing Process/Implementation
Content Area: Skills: Infection Control
Health Problem: Adult Health: Integumentary: Inflammations/Infections

Answer: 3
Rationale: Scabies is a contagious skin disease marked by itching and small raised red spots, caused by the itch mite. The nurse would wear a gown and gloves during close contact with a person infested with scabies, because transmission is by skin-to-skin contact or contact with contaminated items of clothing or bedding. Masks are unnecessary because transmission is not air-related.
Priority Nursing Tip: Scabies symptomatology occurs as the mites burrow and lay eggs inside the skin; the infestation leads to relentless itching and an angry rash.

Test-Taking Strategy: Focus on the **subject,** minimizing scabies transmission. Considering the mode of transmission of scabies as you review the protection afforded by each of the options will help direct you to the correct option.

---

181. When charting the morning dose of digoxin, the nurse discovers that a dose of 0.25 mg was administered rather than the prescribed dose of 0.125 mg. Which action would the nurse take to assist in preventing future medication errors?

1 Complete an irregular occurrence report.
2 Administer an additional 0.125 mg.
3 Inform the client that a medication error was made.
4 Correct the mistake with a dosage adjustment with the next scheduled dose.

Level of Cognitive Ability: Applying
Client Needs: Safe and Effective Care Environment
Clinical Judgment/Cognitive Skills: Take Action
Integrated Process: Nursing Process/Implementation
Content Area: Leadership/Management: Ethical/Legal
Health Problem: N/A

Answer: 1
Rationale: In accordance with the agency's policies, nurses are required to file irregular occurrence reports when an event arises that could or did cause client harm. If a dose of 0.125 mg was prescribed and a dose of 0.25 mg was administered, then the client received too much medication; additional medication is not required and in fact could be detrimental. The client needs to be informed when an error has occurred but in a professional manner so as not to cause fear and concern in the client; however, this option does not help to prevent future medication errors. In many situations, the primary health care provider will discuss these issues with the client. The dosage changes require a prescription.
Priority Nursing Tip: All errors related to client care need to be reported.

Test-Taking Strategy: Focus on the **subject,** medication error. Apply your understanding of medication administration and error reporting and focus on the option that will assist in preventing future medication errors. Incident reporting will allow for a root cause analysis to be conducted. Recalling that information as you evaluate the options for compliance will help you arrive at the correct option.

---

182. The registered nurse determines that the assistive personnel (AP) **needs further instructions** about the care of the client with an indwelling catheter when the AP is observed engaging in what action? **Select all that apply.**

❒ 1 Removing kinks out of the tubing
❒ 2 Using soap and water to cleanse the perineal area
❒ 3 Letting the drainage tubing rest under the client's leg
❒ 4 Keeping the drainage bag below the level of the bladder
❒ 5 Holding the drainage bag at the level of the bed when emptying the drainage bag

Answer: 3, 5
Rationale: Proper care of an indwelling catheter is especially important to prevent infection. All caregivers need to use strict aseptic technique when emptying the drainage bag or obtaining urine specimens. The perineal area is cleansed thoroughly with mild soap and water at least twice a day and after a bowel movement. The drainage bag is kept below the level of the bladder to prevent urine from being trapped in the bladder, and, for the same reason, the drainage tubing is not placed under the client's leg or elevated to the level of the bed when emptying to prevent backflow of urine into the bladder from the tubing. The tubing needs to be allowed to drain freely at all times.
Priority Nursing Tip: An indwelling bladder catheter is a flexible plastic tube (a catheter) inserted into the bladder that remains ("dwells") there to provide continuous urinary drainage.

Level of Cognitive Ability: Evaluating
Client Needs: Safe and Effective Care Environment
Clinical Judgment/Cognitive Skills: Evaluate Outcomes
Integrated Process: Teaching and Learning
Content Area: Leadership/Management: Delegating/Supervising
Health Problem: N/A

Test-Taking Strategy: Focus on the **subject,** care of an indwelling catheter, and note the **strategic words,** *needs further instructions;* this indicates a **negative event query** and asks you to select an option that is an incorrect action. Applying your knowledge of the process and visualizing the steps involved will help you identify the incorrect actions. Eliminate options that suggest appropriate actions consistent with basic standard of care and effective functioning. Options that impede drainage would be identified as correct options for this question.

---

183. What is the nursing **priority** with preoperative care of a client scheduled for a bronchoscopy?

1 Asking the client about allergies to shellfish
2 Restricting the diet to clear liquids on the day of the test
3 Assuring that an informed consent for the procedure is signed
4 Securing a prescription for preprocedure prophylactic antibiotics

Answer: 3
Rationale: Bronchoscopy requires that an informed consent be obtained from the client before the procedure. The client receives nothing by mouth for at least 6 hours before the procedure. It is unnecessary to inquire about allergies to shellfish before this procedure because no contrast dye is injected. There is also no need for prophylactic antibiotics.
Priority Nursing Tip: A medical procedure is defined as invasive when there is a break in the skin, or there is contact with the mucosa or internal body cavity beyond a natural or artificial body orifice.

Level of Cognitive Ability: Applying
Client Needs: Safe and Effective Care Environment
Clinical Judgment/Cognitive Skills: Prioritize Hypotheses
Integrated Process: Nursing Process/Implementation
Content Area: Leadership/Management: Ethical/Legal
Health Problem: N/A

Test-Taking Strategy: Focus on the **subject,** preprocedure care for a bronchoscopy, and the **strategic word,** *priority.* Applying your understanding of a bronchoscopy will identify it as an invasive procedure, as well as suggesting necessary preparations. Using this knowledge when evaluating each option will direct you to the correct option.

---

184. A client diagnosed with both acquired immunodeficiency syndrome (AIDS) and cytomegalovirus retinitis is prescribed ganciclovir sodium. The nurse would implement what intervention to minimize the client's risk for associated injury?

1 Monitor blood glucose levels for elevation.
2 Administer the medication on an empty stomach only.
3 Apply pressure to venipuncture sites for at least 2 minutes.
4 Provide the client with a soft toothbrush and an electric razor.

Answer: 4
Rationale: Ganciclovir is an antiviral used to treat infections caused by viruses. Ganciclovir sodium causes neutropenia and thrombocytopenia as the most frequent side effects. For this reason, the nurse monitors the client for signs and symptoms of bleeding and implements the same precautions that are used for a client receiving anticoagulant therapy. These include providing a soft toothbrush and an electric razor to minimize the risk of trauma that could result in bleeding. The medication may cause hypoglycemia but not hyperglycemia, and it does not have to be taken on an empty stomach. Venipuncture sites would be held for approximately 10 minutes.
Priority Nursing Tip: Ganciclovir is used to treat complications from AIDS-associated cytomegalovirus infections.

Level of Cognitive Ability: Applying
Client Needs: Safe and Effective Care Environment
Clinical Judgment/Cognitive Skills: Take Action
Integrated Process: Nursing Process/Planning
Content Area: Pharmacology: Immune: Antivirals
Health Problem: Adult Health: Immune: Infections

Test-Taking Strategy: Focus on the **subject**, risks associated with ganciclovir therapy. Using your knowledge of ganciclovir and its effect on blood clotting as you review each option will direct you to the correct option.

---

185. A client is scheduled to have an inferior vena cava (IVC) filter inserted. The nurse would place **highest priority** on determining whether the surgeon will likely prescribe what medication held during the preoperative period?

1 Furosemide
2 Famotidine
3 Warfarin sodium
4 Multivitamin with minerals

Level of Cognitive Ability: Analyzing
Client Needs: Safe and Effective Care Environment
Clinical Judgment/Cognitive Skills: Analyze Cues
Integrated Process: Nursing Process/Data Collection
Content Area: Pharmacology: Cardiovascular: Anticoagulants
Health Problem: Adult Health: Cardiovascular: Vascular Disorders

Answer: 3
Rationale: The nurse is careful to question the surgeon about whether warfarin sodium would be administered during the preoperative period before the insertion of an IVC filter. This medication is often withheld during the preoperative period to minimize the risk of hemorrhage during surgery. The other medications may also be withheld if specifically prescribed, but they are usually discontinued as part of a prescription for nothing by mouth after midnight and, as importantly, none are likely to affect bleeding postprocedure.
Priority Nursing Tip: Furosemide is a diuretic; famotidine belongs to a class of medications known as H2 blockers; multivitamins with minerals are used to supplement the diet.

Test-Taking Strategy: Focus on the **subject,** preoperative medication administration prescriptions, and note the **strategic words,** *highest priority.* To choose the correct option, you would apply your knowledge of the procedure, including indications and expected results, as you evaluate each option. It is also necessary to understand the function of each of the medications identified for their effect on the client.

---

186. A client is receiving enteral feedings via a nasogastric tube. The nurse aspirates 40 mL of undigested formula from a client's nasogastric tube to assess for residual feeding content. Before administering the tube feeding, what would the nurse do with the 40 mL of gastric aspirate?

1 Pour it into the nasogastric tube through a syringe with the plunger removed.
2 Discard it properly and record it as output on the client's intake and output record.
3 Dilute it with water and inject it into the nasogastric tube by putting pressure on the plunger.
4 Mix it with the formula and pour it into the nasogastric tube through a syringe without a plunger.

Level of Cognitive Ability: Applying
Client Needs: Safe and Effective Care Environment
Clinical Judgment/Cognitive Skills: Take Action
Integrated Process: Nursing Process/Implementation
Content Area: Skills: Tube Care
Health Problem: N/A

Answer: 1
Rationale: After checking residual feeding contents, gastric contents are reinstilled into the stomach by removing the syringe bulb or plunger and pouring the gastric contents via the syringe into the nasogastric tube. Gastric contents would be reinstilled to maintain the client's electrolyte balance. The gastric aspirate does not need to be mixed with water or formula, and it would not be discarded or injected by putting pressure on the plunger.
Priority Nursing Tip: Nasogastric intubation is a medical process involving the insertion of a plastic tube (nasogastric tube or NG tube) through the nose, past the throat, and down into the stomach.

Test-Taking Strategy: Focus on the **subject,** care for the client with nasogastric tube. Apply your knowledge of the effects nasogastric feedings have on a client's electrolyte balance to the suggested options. Remembering that the removal of the gastric contents could disturb the client's electrolyte balance will assist you with eliminating option 2. Eliminate option 3 because of the word *pressure.* Recalling that aspirated gastric contents would be immediately replaced will direct you to the correct option.

---

187. Which action by the nurse obtaining a urinary sample from a client with an indwelling catheter **requires follow-up** to prevent the contamination of the specimen?

1 Clamping the tubing of the drainage bag
2 Obtaining the specimen from the urinary drainage bag
3 Aspirating a sample from the port on the drainage system
4 Wiping the port on the drainage system with an alcohol swab before inserting the syringe

Level of Cognitive Ability: Evaluating
Client Needs: Safe and Effective Care Environment
Clinical Judgment/Cognitive Skills: Evaluate Outcomes
Integrated Process: Teaching and Learning
Content Area: Skills: Specimen Collection
Health Problem: N/A

Answer: 2
Rationale: A urine specimen is not taken from the urinary drainage bag. Because it undergoes chemical changes, the urine sitting in the bag does not necessarily reflect the client's current status. In addition, it may become contaminated with bacteria from the opening of the system. The other actions are appropriate and would not contribute to sample contamination.
Priority Nursing Tip: The principal type of indwelling bladder catheter is the "Foley," which has a balloon on the bladder end.

Test-Taking Strategy: Note the **strategic words,** *requires follow-up;* these words indicate a **negative event query** and ask you to select an option that is an incorrect action. Focus on the **subject,** preventing contamination. Apply your knowledge of this procedure as you review the options. The correct option is the one that describes incorrect accepted practice.

---

188. What step is the nurse expected to take **immediately** after administering the intramuscular (IM) injection?

1 Recap the needle.
2 Place the syringe on the overbed table.
3 Assist the client to ambulate to aid in absorption.
4 Apply gentle pressure to the site with an alcohol swab.

Level of Cognitive Ability: Applying
Client Needs: Safe and Effective Care Environment
Clinical Judgment/Cognitive Skills: Take Action
Integrated Process: Nursing Process/Implementation
Content Area: Skills: Medication Administration
Health Problem: N/A

Answer: 4
Rationale: After administering an IM injection, the nurse would next apply gentle pressure to the site with an alcohol swab to prevent bleeding and to assist with medication absorption. The needle is not recapped or placed on the overbed table; rather, the needle and syringe are placed in the appropriate puncture-resistant receptacle to prevent unintentional injury by the needle. The client who is in pain would not be ambulated to aid in medication absorption, nor is it necessary under usual circumstances.
Priority Nursing Tip: An IM injection is a technique used to deliver a medication deep into the muscles. This allows the medication to be absorbed quickly.

Test-Taking Strategy: Note the **strategic word,** *immediately.* Focus on the **subject,** IM injection. Visualize this procedure, and use your knowledge of the principles related to the safe administration of IM medication to direct you to the correct option.

---

189. The nurse in a well-baby clinic is reinforcing safety instructions to a parent of a 4-month-old infant. Which safety instruction is **most appropriate** at this age?

1 Lock up all poisons.
2 Cover all electrical outlets.
3 Do not shake the infant's head.
4 Remove hazardous objects from low places.

Answer: 3
Rationale: The most important age-appropriate instruction is to not shake or vigorously jiggle the infant's head. Options 1, 2, and 4 become important instructions to provide to the parent as the child reaches the age of 6 months and begins to have the physical control and mobility to explore the environment.
Priority Nursing Tip: Most cases of shaken baby syndrome occur among infants that are 6 to 8 weeks old, which is when babies tend to cry the most.

Level of Cognitive Ability: Applying
Client Needs: Safe and Effective Care Environment
Clinical Judgment/Cognitive Skills: Take Action
Integrated Process: Teaching and Learning
Content Area: Developmental Stages: Infant
Health Problem: N/A

Test-Taking Strategy: Focus on the **subject,** instructions for care of a 4-month-old infant. Applying your understanding of developmental tasks associated with a 4-month-old infant to the various options will help you eliminate options 1, 2, and 4.

---

190. Which statement, if made by the client, indicates the **need for further teaching** regarding safety measures for their 9-month-old baby?

1 "I keep all my pots and pans in my lower cabinets."
2 "I will not use the microwave to heat my baby's formula."
3 "I have locks on all of the cabinets that hold my cleaning supplies."
4 "I have a car seat that I will put in the front seat to keep my baby safe."

Level of Cognitive Ability: Evaluating
Client Needs: Safe and Effective Care Environment
Clinical Judgment/Cognitive Skills: Evaluate Outcomes
Integrated Process: Teaching and Learning
Content Area: Maternity: Newborn
Health Problem: N/A

Answer: 4
Rationale: A baby car seat would never be placed in the front seat because of the potential for injury on impact. Infants would travel in federally approved, rear-facing car seats secured in the back seat of the car. All infants and toddlers would ride in a rear-facing seat until they are at least 2 years of age. Any cabinets that contain dangerous items that the baby could swallow would be locked. Microwaves would never be used to heat bottle formula because the formula could burn or even scald the baby's mouth. Although the bottle may only feel warm, it could contain hot spots that could severely damage the baby's mouth. It is perfectly safe to leave pots and pans in the lower cabinets for the baby to investigate when he or she begins to explore the environment, as long as they are not made of glass; glass items, if broken, could harm the baby.
Priority Nursing Tip: There are specific rules regarding car seat safety, and the rules and laws vary by region.

Test-Taking Strategy: Focus on the **subject,** child safety education, and note the **strategic words,** *need for further teaching;* these words indicate a **negative event query** and ask you to select an option that is an incorrect client statement. Apply your understanding of child safety measures as you evaluate the options for their ability to provide a safe environment.

---

191. The nurse, caring for a 9-month-old child after cleft palate repair, has applied elbow stabilizers to the child. The parent visits the child and asks the nurse to remove the restraints. Which is the **most appropriate** nursing action in response to the parent's request?

1 Remove both restraints because it is the parent's right to refuse treatment for the child.
2 Remove a restraint from one arm if she agrees to stay with the child.
3 Tell the parent that the restraints cannot be removed for 24 hours postsurgery.
4 Loosen the restraints, but explain to the parent that they cannot be completely removed.

Answer: 2
Rationale: Elbow stabilizers prevent the elbows from bending while permitting other movements of the arms and are used after cleft palate repair to prevent the child from touching the repair site, which could cause accidental rupture and tearing of the sutures. The restraints can be removed one at a time only if a parent or nurse is in constant attendance. Although it is the parent's right to refuse treatment, a thorough explanation of the purpose of the treatment and possible alternatives needs to be provided. Neither of the remaining options provide accurate information about the appropriate use of this method of restraint.
Priority Nursing Tip: A cleft palate is when the roof of the mouth contains an opening into the nose. These disorders can result in feeding problems, speech problems, hearing problems, and frequent ear infections.

Level of Cognitive Ability: Applying
Client Needs: Safe and Effective Care Environment
Clinical Judgment/Cognitive Skills: Take Action
Integrated Process: Nursing Process/Implementation
Content Area: Skills: Perioperative Care
Health Problem: Pediatric-Specific: Developmental GI defects

Test-Taking Strategy: Focus on the **subject,** elbow stabilizers, and note the **strategic words,** *most appropriate.* Eliminate options 3 and 4 first because they are **comparable or alike** in that the restraints are not removed. From the remaining options, recall the purpose of the restraints after this surgical procedure; this will direct you to the correct option, which is the safest nursing action.

---

192. The nurse is caring for a hospitalized child diagnosed with rubella. Which type of precautions would the nurse institute while caring for this child?

1 Droplet
2 Contact
3 Reverse
4 Protective isolation

Level of Cognitive Ability: Applying
Client Needs: Safe and Effective Care Environment
Clinical Judgment/Cognitive Skills: Take Action
Integrated Process: Nursing Process/Implementation
Content Area: Pediatrics: Infectious and Communicable Diseases
Health Problem: Pediatric-Specific: Communicable Diseases

Answer: 1
Rationale: The care of a child with rubella involves droplet precautions and contact precautions. Droplet precautions require the use of masks. Contact precautions require the use of gowns and gloves for contact with any infectious material. Contaminated articles need to be bagged and labeled before reprocessing. Reverse (protective) isolation procedures are designed to protect a client from infectious organisms that might be carried by the staff, other clients, or visitors; on droplets in the air; or on equipment or materials. Contact precautions are used for clients who have active infection with *C. difficile,* rotavirus, or norovirus.
Priority Nursing Tip: Isolation represents one of several measures that can be taken to implement infection control: the prevention of contagious diseases from being spread from a client to other clients, health care workers, and visitors, or from outsiders to a particular client.

Test-Taking Strategy: Focus on the **subject,** transmission of rubella. Applying your knowledge regarding this disease and the various forms of isolation will help you to evaluate the various options for appropriate protection and to select the correct option.

---

193. The nurse is caring for a child who was diagnosed with *Erythema infectiosum* (fifth disease). The child's parent asks the nurse how this disease is transmitted. The nurse informs the parent that fifth disease is transmitted by which route?

1 Saliva
2 Droplet particles
3 Fecal–oral route
4 Contact with sweat

Level of Cognitive Ability: Applying
Client Needs: Safe and Effective Care Environment
Clinical Judgment/Cognitive Skills: Take Action
Integrated Process: Teaching and Learning
Content Area: Pediatrics: Infectious and Communicable Diseases
Health Problem: Pediatric-Specific: Communicable Diseases

Answer: 2
Rationale: *Erythema infectiosum* (fifth disease) is transmitted via droplet particles, respiratory droplets, blood, blood products, or transplacental means. This information confirms that none of the remaining options is correct.
Priority Nursing Tip: Fifth disease is caused by infection with the human parvovirus.

Test-Taking Strategy: Focus on the **subject,** precautions needed to prevent transmission of *Erythema infectiosum.* Applying your knowledge regarding the mode of transmission of fifth disease will help you answer this question.

---

194. The nurse is giving a bed bath to a cognitively impaired client and notes the need for another towel. Which nursing action would the nurse take to meet the client's needs while maximizing safety?

1. Dry the client with an available pillowcase.
2. Use a towel originally intended for the roommate.
3. Instruct the client to wait quietly while you get the towel.
4. Use the call bell to ask a staff member to bring a towel.

Level of Cognitive Ability: Applying
Client Needs: Safe and Effective Care Environment
Clinical Judgment/Cognitive Skills: Take Action
Integrated Process: Nursing Process/Implementation
Content Area: Skills: Hygiene
Health Problem: Mental Health: Neurocognitive Impairment

Answer: 4
Rationale: Client safety is a priority, so the nurse would enlist the assistance of another staff member to acquire the additional towel rather than leave a client in this situation. It is never appropriate to borrow other clients' supplies because this will spread germs. It is inappropriate to assume that a cognitively impaired client will be able to understand or follow such instructions.
Priority Nursing Tip: Some clients with dementia may have brain damage that results in confusion between hot and cold temperature or in different sensations on contact with water.

Test-Taking Strategy: Focus on the **subject,** maintaining client safety. Apply your knowledge regarding the basic principles related to managing such a situation with a client. As you review each option, evaluate that it adheres to the relevant principles and its appropriateness for a client who has any degree of cognitive impairment.

---

195. The nurse is determining a family member's ability to use sterile gloves to perform a dressing change. Which statement indicates to the nurse that the family member **requires need for follow-up?**

1. "I'm more comfortable putting on the left-hand glove first."
2. "I'll use the inner wrapper of the gloves as a sterile field."
3. "If I touch the glove on the counter, I should open another pair and start over."
4. "I don't have to worry about washing my hands because I have sterile gloves."

Level of Cognitive Ability: Evaluating
Client Needs: Safe and Effective Care Environment
Clinical Judgment/Cognitive Skills: Evaluate Outcomes
Integrated Process: Teaching and Learning
Content Area: Skills: Infection Control
Health Problem: Adult Health: Integumentary: Wounds

Answer: 4
Rationale: The hands need to be washed—even when sterile gloves are used—to keep germs from spreading. The inner wrapper makes an excellent area for use because it is sterile. If the gloves touch anything unsterile, they need to be considered contaminated, and a new package of sterile gloves needs to be used. Which glove is put on first is up to the individual if sterile technique is not compromised.
Priority Nursing Tip: Hand washing precedes every procedure that involves client contact.

Test-Taking Strategy: Focus on the **subject,** sterile gloving, and note the **strategic words,** *requires need for follow-up;* these words indicate a **negative event query** and ask you to select an option that is an incorrect statement. Applying your understanding of the principles of sterile technique will direct you to the correct option.

---

196. Which action could lead to the spread of infection when removing personal protective equipment (PPE)?

1 Taking the gloves off first, then removing the gown
2 Rolling the removed gown with the outside surface out
3 Using ungloved hands to unfasten the gown's neck ties
4 Washing the hands after the entire procedure has been completed

Level of Cognitive Ability: Applying
Client Needs: Safe and Effective Care Environment
Clinical Judgment/Cognitive Skills: Take Action
Integrated Process: Nursing Process/ Implementation
Content Area: Foundations of Care: Infection Control
Health Problem: N/A

Answer: 2
Rationale: The gown needs to be rolled from inside out to prevent the organisms on the outside of the gown from contaminating other areas. Gloves are considered the most contaminated protective items that the nurse wears and therefore would be removed first. The hands would be washed after removing the protective items to eliminate any germs that are still present. Ungloved hands would be used to remove the gown to prevent contaminating the back of the gown with germs from the gloves.
Priority Nursing Tip: Personal protective equipment includes protective laboratory clothing, disposable gloves, eye protection, and face masks.

Test-Taking Strategy: Focus on the **subject,** steps necessary to complete the removal of PPE. Apply your knowledge of PPE removal to evaluate each option. The option that suggests an action contrary to the approved method of removal will be the one most likely to allow for the spread of infection.

---

197. The nurse caring for a hospitalized child diagnosed with rubeola would implement what intervention to minimize the transmission of the infection?

1 Wearing gloves
2 Wearing a gown
3 Wearing a mask
4 Wearing goggles

Level of Cognitive Ability: Applying
Client Needs: Safe and Effective Care Environment
Clinical Judgment/Cognitive Skills: Take Action
Integrated Process: Nursing Process/ Implementation
Content Area: Pediatrics: Infectious and Communicable Diseases
Health Problem: Pediatric-Specific: Communicable Diseases

Answer: 3
Rationale: Rubeola is transmitted via airborne particles or direct contact with infectious droplets. The treatment of rubeola is symptomatic, whether the child is hospitalized or remains at home. If hospitalized, however, airborne isolation precautions are required. Respiratory isolation for a child with rubeola requires masks for those in close contact with the child. Gowns, gloves, or goggles are not specifically indicated because the mode of transmission is not by direct contact.
Priority Nursing Tip: Rubeola starts with fever, runny nose, cough, red eyes, and sore throat. It is followed by a rash that spreads over the body.

Test-Taking Strategy: Focus on the **subject,** transmission of rubeola. Applying your understanding of the mode of transmission for rubeola will direct you to the correct option.

---

198. The nurse is reinforcing safety needs related to sight deficits resulting from normal age-related changes. Which statement by the older adult client indicates the **need for further teaching** about safety?

1 "I need to avoid nighttime driving."
2 "I need to have bright orange strips of tape installed at the edge of stairs."
3 "I need to keep the lights turned on in the stairways and hallways at night."
4 "I need to have a high-gloss paint put on the walls to increase light reflection."

Level of Cognitive Ability: Evaluating
Client Needs: Safe and Effective Care Environment
Clinical Judgment/Cognitive Skills: Evaluate Outcomes
Integrated Process: Teaching and Learning
Content Area: Foundations of Care: Safety
Health Problem: Adult Health: Eye: Visual Problems/Refractive Errors

Answer: 4
Rationale: Age-related changes in the eye (e.g., diminished or absent pupillary response, decreased retinal blood supply) can cause night blindness, the inability to see because of glare, and deficits of depth and color perception. Using high-gloss paint on the walls will increase glare and make it more difficult for the client to see. All the other options are appropriate safety measures that will help with age-related sight deficits.
Priority Nursing Tip: Although cataracts can be considered an age-related disease, they are extremely common among seniors and can be readily corrected with cataract surgery.

Test-Taking Strategy: Note the **strategic words,** *need for further teaching.* These words indicate a **negative event query** and ask you to select an option that is an incorrect intervention. Focus on the **subject,** age-related sight changes. Applying your understanding of the physiological changes in sight associated with aging will help you arrive at the problem commonly referred to as "night blindness." Review the options related to their ability to minimize the effect of "night blindness." The option that fails to help is the correct option.

---

199. The nurse is caring for an 8-month-old infant with a diagnosis of febrile seizures. When assisting with the planning of this infant's care, the nurse would anticipate the need for what item to help ensure the child's safety?

1 Restraints
2 Padded sides on the crib
3 A code cart at the bedside
4 A padded tongue blade taped to the head of the bed

Level of Cognitive Ability: Applying
Client Needs: Safe and Effective Care Environment
Clinical Judgment/Cognitive Skills: Recognize Cues
Integrated Process: Nursing Process/Planning
Content Area: Foundations of Care: Safety
Health Problem: Pediatric-Specific: Seizures

Answer: 2
Rationale: Padded crib sides will protect the child from injury during seizure activity. A padded tongue blade should never be used. During a seizure, nothing should be placed in a child's mouth; the child needs to be placed in a side-lying position after the seizure but should not be restrained. A code cart should be available but need not be placed at the bedside.
Priority Nursing Tip: Febrile seizures most commonly occur in children between the ages of 6 months and 5 years.

Test-Taking Strategy: Focus on the **subject,** the safety of a client with seizures. Applying your understanding of the safety risks associated with seizures, especially those experienced by an infant, while evaluating each option will help in selecting the one appropriate in this situation.

---

200. A licensed practical nurse (LPN) has been asked to do a safety survey at a children's day care center. The children cared for at the center are between the ages of 1 and 3 years. What situation presents the **primary** hazard to a toddler at the center?

1 A hot water heater set above 120° F
2 Toys with small, loose parts in the playroom
3 A swimming pool in the neighbor's gated yard
4 Toxic plants located in the front yard of the center

Level of Cognitive Ability: Analyzing
Client Needs: Safe and Effective Care Environment
Clinical Judgment/Cognitive Skills: Recognize Cues
Integrated Process: Nursing Process/Data Collection
Content Area: Developmental Stages: Toddler
Health Problem: N/A

Answer: 2
Rationale: Toys in the playroom would be the first concern because the toddlers will play in this area. Options 3 and 4 identify safety hazards that are not in the toddlers' play area and would not be the priority. Water temperature would be a priority in a toddler's home, where scalding could occur during bathing; this would be a secondary consideration in a day care setting.
Priority Nursing Tip: Keep in mind that it is common for toddlers to put things in their mouths.

Test-Taking Strategy: Note the **strategic word,** *primary,* and focus on the **subject,** safety in a day care center. An understanding of the developmental stage of toddlers and the risks that are involved in the day care setting will help you determine the primary safety risk.

CHAPTER 7

Health Promotion and Maintenance Practice Questions

1. The nurse is assisting in performing a neurovascular check on a client. Which is the **best** method to use when checking a client's pupillary reaction to light?
   1 Turn the light on directly in front of the eye and watch for a response.
   2 Ask the client to follow the light through the six cardinal positions of gaze.
   3 Check the pupil size and then have the client alternate between watching the light and watching the examiner's finger.
   4 Instruct the client to look straight ahead and then shine the light on the client, moving it from the temporal area to the eye.

Level of Cognitive Ability: Applying
Client Needs: Health Promotion and Maintenance
Clinical Judgment/Cognitive Skills: Take Action
Integrated Process: Nursing Process/Data Collection
Content Area: Health Assessment: Physical Exam: Neurological
Health Problem: N/A

Answer: 4
Rationale: Instructing the client to look straight ahead and then shining the light on the client, moving the light from the temporal area to the eye, identifies the correct procedure for checking a client's pupillary reaction to light. Turning the light on directly in front of the eye and watching for a response relates to the pupillary response to light, but shining the light directly into the client's eye without asking the client to focus on a distant object is an inappropriate technique. Asking the client to follow the light through the six cardinal positions of gaze assesses for eye movement related to cranial nerves III, IV, and VI. Checking the pupil size and having the client alternate between watching the light and watching the examiner's finger assesses the accommodation of the eye rather than the eye's response to light.
Priority Nursing Tip: Light causes the pupil to become smaller, whereas darkness causes it to expand.

Test-Taking Strategy: Focus on the **subject**, pupillary assessment and reaction to light, and note the **strategic word**, *best*. Visualize this technique and each description given in the options to answer the question.

---

2. A client is asked to describe how they perform a breast self-examination (BSE). Which statement made by the client would indicate the client **requires further instruction** regarding BSE?
   1 "I do the exam while taking a shower."
   2 "I avoid doing the exam during my period."
   3 "I concentrate the exam on my nipples and around it."
   4 "I do the exam usually about 7 days after the start of my period."

Answer: 3
Rationale: When performing BSE, the entire breast needs to be examined for abnormalities, not just the nipples and areolas. The client would do the exam about 7 days after the start of their period (not during their period) because of the hormonal changes that occur in the reproductive system during the period. These hormonal changes can affect the breast tissue. Doing the exam during a shower is helpful because it is easier to feel for abnormalities when the breast is wet and soapy.
Priority Nursing Tip: It is important to teach the client to look in the mirror for any changes in the breast before manually checking for changes.

Level of Cognitive Ability: Evaluating
Client Needs: Health Promotion and Maintenance
Clinical Judgment/Cognitive Skills: Evaluate Outcomes
Integrated Process: Teaching and Learning
Content Area: Adult Health: Oncology
Health Problem: Adult Health: Cancer: Breast

Test-Taking Strategy: Focus on the **subject**, the correct procedure for a BSE. Note the **strategic words**, *requires further instruction*. These words indicate a **negative event query** and the need to select the incorrect client statement. An effective BSE includes assessment of the entire breast and axilla area. The other statements are correct related to this procedure.

---

3. The nurse is reviewing the record of a client with a suspected malignant melanoma. Which assessment finding would support this diagnosis?
1 Genital warts
2 Dimpling of the skin
3 A mole that has turned blue
4 A mole with round, smooth borders

Answer: 3
Rationale: Shades of blue in a mole are considered ominous for malignant melanoma. Genital warts are associated with cancer of the cervix. The dimpling of the skin of the breast is associated with breast cancer. A mole with round, smooth borders would be a normal finding.
Priority Nursing Tip: Melanoma is usually located on the skin and has an irregular surface and notched border.

Level of Cognitive Ability: Applying
Client Needs: Health Promotion and Maintenance
Clinical Judgment/Cognitive Skills: Analyze Cues
Integrated Process: Nursing Process/Data Collection
Content Area: Adult Health: Oncology
Health Problem: Adult Health: Cancer: Skin

Test-Taking Strategy: Focus on the **subject**, malignant melanoma. Think about the pathophysiology associated with this condition. Recalling the characteristics of malignant melanoma will direct you to the correct option.

---

4. The nurse is auscultating the breath sounds of a client. Which technique, if used by the nurse, would indicate a **need for further teaching** in the use of the stethoscope?
1 Using the bell of the stethoscope
2 Asking the client to sit straight up
3 Placing the stethoscope directly on the client's skin
4 Having the client breathe slowly and deeply through the mouth

Answer: 1
Rationale: The bell of the stethoscope is not used to auscultate breath sounds. The client would ideally sit up and breathe slowly and deeply through the mouth. The diaphragm of the stethoscope, which is warmed before use, is placed directly on the client's skin rather than over a gown or clothing.
Priority Nursing Tip: The bell of the stethoscope is used for assessing heart sounds, specifically when checking for heart murmurs.

Level of Cognitive Ability: Evaluating
Client Needs: Health Promotion and Maintenance
Clinical Judgment/Cognitive Skills: Evaluate Outcomes
Integrated Process: Teaching and Learning
Content Area: Health Assessment: Physical Exam: Thorax and Lungs
Health Problem: N/A

Test-Taking Strategy: Focus on the **subject**, auscultation of breath sounds. Note the **strategic words**, *need for further teaching*. These words indicate a **negative event query** and the need to select the incorrect technique. Read each option carefully and visualize this procedure to assist in answering correctly.

---

5. Which assessment data suggest that the client is at risk for coronary artery disease (CAD)?
   1 Age of 39 years
   2 A total cholesterol level of 180 mg/dL
   3 Fasting blood glucose level of 80 mg/dL
   4 Resting blood pressure of 139/89 mm Hg

Level of Cognitive Ability: Analyzing
Client Needs: Health Promotion and Maintenance
Clinical Judgment/Cognitive Skills: Recognize Cues
Integrated Process: Nursing Process/Data Collection
Content Area: Adult Health: Cardiovascular
Health Problem: Adult Health: Cardiovascular: Coronary Artery Disease

Answer: 4
Rationale: Hypertension is a modifiable risk factor of CAD. Age is a nonmodifiable risk factor. The client's total cholesterol and blood glucose levels fall within the normal range.
Priority Nursing Tip: Stage 1 hypertension is characterized as a systolic pressure between 130 and 139 mm Hg or a diastolic pressure between 80 and 89 mm Hg, and is often seen with CAD.

Test-Taking Strategy: Focus on the **subject**, identifying the risk factor for this client associated with CAD. Option 1 can be eliminated first because age is a nonmodifiable risk factor. From the remaining options, note that the blood pressure is the only abnormal finding.

---

6. The nurse reviewing the health records of prenatal clients determines that which client is at risk for gestational hypertensive disorder? **Select all that apply.**
   ❒ 1 A client pregnant with a singleton
   ❒ 2 A client diagnosed with a hydatidiform mole
   ❒ 3 A client with a past medical history of hypertension
   ❒ 4 A client who is 20 years old, gravida 2, weighing 115 pounds
   ❒ 5 A client who was diagnosed with diabetes mellitus 10 years previously

Level of Cognitive Ability: Analyzing
Client Needs: Health Promotion and Maintenance
Clinical Judgment/Cognitive Skills: Analyze Cues
Integrated Process: Nursing Process/Data Collection
Content Area: Maternity: Antepartum
Health Problem: Maternity: Gestational Hypertension/Preeclampsia and Eclampsia

Answer: 2, 3, 5
Rationale: Gestational hypertension is the development of mild hypertension during pregnancy in a previously normotensive client without proteinuria or pathological edema. The client with a hydatidiform mole, a client with a past medical history of hypertension, and a client diagnosed with diabetes mellitus 10 years previously are at high risk for the development of gestational hypertension because of the health history and current health issues. In option 4, if the client had been younger than 18 or older than 35 years old and underweight or overweight, then she would have been at risk; however, she falls within normal age and weight criteria. Having a singleton pregnancy is not a risk factor for gestational hypertension.
Priority Nursing Tip: Those who are pregnant with twins or multiples have an elevated risk for gestational hypertension.

Test-Taking Strategy: Focus on the **subject**, risks for gestational hypertension. Note that the incorrect options are the only options that identify a client who does not have a preexisting health problem or a risk factor related to the pregnancy.

---

7. A child is to receive a measles, mumps, and rubella (MMR) vaccine. During data collection, the nurse notes that the child is allergic to eggs. Which intervention would the nurse anticipate being prescribed for this child?

Answer: 1
Rationale: Live measles vaccine is produced from chick embryo cell culture, so the possibility of anaphylactic hypersensitivity in children with egg allergies would be considered. If there is a question of sensitivity, children would be tested before the administration of the MMR vaccine. If a child tests positive for sensitivity,

1 Administration of an attenuated measles vaccine
2 Elimination of this vaccine from the immunization schedule
3 Administration of epinephrine before the administration of the MMR vaccine
4 Administration of diphenhydramine and acetaminophen before the administration of the MMR vaccine

Level of Cognitive Ability: Applying
Client Needs: Health Promotion and Maintenance
Clinical Judgment/Cognitive Skills: Generate Solutions
Integrated Process: Nursing Process/Planning
Content Area: Pharmacology: Immune: Vaccines
Health Problem: Pediatric-Specific: Immunizations

the attenuated (less virulent) measles vaccine may be given as an alternative. The use of medications before the administration of a vaccine is not a normal procedure. A vaccine would not be eliminated from the immunization schedule.
Priority Nursing Tip: Children would get two doses of MMR vaccine, with the first dose at 12 to 15 months of age and the second dose at 4 through 6 years of age.

Test-Taking Strategy: Focus on the **subject,** allergy to the MMR vaccine. A vaccine would not be eliminated from the immunization schedule, so remove this option first. Eliminate administering epinephrine and administering diphenhydramine and acetaminophen next because they are **comparable or alike.** The use of medications before a vaccine is not recommended procedure. Recalling that live measles vaccine is produced from chick embryo cell culture will direct you to the correct option.

---

8. A parent asks the nurse about the safety of attenuated or inactivated vaccines. The nurse would provide which statement to **best** address the parent's concern?
1 "All bacterial toxins have been made inactive by being exposed to high heat."
2 "This form of vaccine contains pathogens that have been made inactive by either chemicals or heat."
3 "These vaccines have their virulence (potency) diminished so that they do not produce a full-blown clinical illness."
4 "Such vaccines have been obtained from the pooled blood of many people, and that provides antibodies to a variety of diseases."

Level of Cognitive Ability: Applying
Client Needs: Health Promotion and Maintenance
Clinical Judgment/Cognitive Skills: Take Action
Integrated Process: Teaching and Learning
Content Area: Pharmacology: Immune: Vaccines
Health Problem: Pediatric-Specific: Immunizations

Answer: 2
Rationale: Killed or inactivated vaccines contain pathogens that have been made inactive by either chemicals or heat. These vaccines, which are noninfectious, cause the body to produce antibodies. Their disadvantage is that they elicit a limited immune response from the body, so several doses are necessary. Examples of this type of vaccine include the Salk polio vaccine, the rabies vaccine, and the pertussis vaccine. Option 1 identifies toxoids. Option 3 identifies live (attenuated) vaccines. Option 4 identifies human immunoglobulin.
Priority Nursing Tip: Killed vaccine or inactivated vaccines contain virus particles, not bacteria.

Test-Taking Strategy: Note the **strategic word,** *best.* Focus on the **subject,** safety of inactivated or attenuated vaccines. Note the relationship between the words *inactivated vaccines* in the question and the correct option.

---

9. The nurse is asked to monitor a client with cardiac disease for the presence of cyanosis. Which body area is the **best** site for checking for this condition?

Answer: 1
Rationale: The presence of cyanosis can best be seen in the nail beds, the conjunctivae, and the oral mucosa. Pallor is best seen in the buccal mucosa or the conjunctivae, particularly in

1 Nail beds
2 In the sclerae
3 Over the palms of the hands
4 At the junction of the hard and soft portions of the palate

Level of Cognitive Ability: Applying
Client Needs: Health Promotion and Maintenance
Clinical Judgment/Cognitive Skills: Recognize Cues
Integrated Process: Nursing Process/Data Collection
Content Area: Adult Health: Cardiovascular
Health Problem: Adult Health: Cardiovascular: Vascular Disorders

dark-skinned clients. Jaundice can be best assessed in the sclera, near the limbus at the junction of the hard and soft portions of the palate, and over the palms.
Priority Nursing Tip: Cyanosis refers to bluish discoloration of skin, nail beds, and mucous membranes.

Test-Taking Strategy: Focus on the **subject,** the site for assessing for cyanosis, and note the **strategic word,** *best.* Use your knowledge of data collection techniques related to the presence of cyanosis and recall the description of cyanosis to answer this question and direct you to the correct option.

---

10. The nurse is assisting with monitoring a client who has undergone shoulder arthroplasty for brachial plexus compromise. Which data collection technique would the nurse implement to check the status of the musculocutaneous nerve?
1 Ask the client to spread all the fingers wide and to resist pressure.
2 Ask the client to raise the forearm, and then check for the flexion of the biceps.
3 Ask the client to move the thumb toward the palm and then back to the neutral position.
4 Ask the client to grasp the nurse's hand; then note the strength of the client's first and second fingers.

Level of Cognitive Ability: Applying
Client Needs: Health Promotion and Maintenance
Clinical Judgment/Cognitive Skills: Take Action
Integrated Process: Nursing Process/Data Collection
Content Area: Adult Health: Musculoskeletal
Health Problem: Adult Health: Musculoskeletal: Tissue or Ligament Injury

Answer: 2
Rationale: To check musculocutaneous nerve status, the nurse checks for the flexion of the biceps by having the client raise the forearm. Poor biceps flexion may indicate compromise of the musculocutaneous nerve. The incorrect options are improper techniques and do not check the musculocutaneous nerve.
Priority Nursing Tip: The brachial plexus runs from the spine to the arm.

Test-Taking Strategy: Focus on the **subject,** checking the status of the musculocutaneous nerve. Recalling the anatomical location of the nerve and visualizing each of the techniques described in the options will direct you to the correct option.

---

11. A client is diagnosed with pernicious anemia. The nurse understands that which data collection question will **best** identify a risk factor associated with the development of this type of anemia?

Answer: 1
Rationale: Pernicious anemia results from a vitamin B_{12} deficiency. One major risk factor for the development of pernicious anemia is the physiology resulting from a gastric resection. Inadequate iron in the diet is not specifically associated with this

1 "Have you ever had gastric resection surgery?"
2 "How much iron do you regularly get in the diet?"
3 "Have you ever been diagnosed with a musculoskeletal disorder?"
4 "What, if any, central nervous system disorders have you experienced?"

Level of Cognitive Ability: Applying
Client Needs: Health Promotion and Maintenance
Clinical Judgment/Cognitive Skills: Generate Solutions
Integrated Process: Nursing Process/ Data Collection
Content Area: Adult Health: Hematological
Health Problem: Adult Health: Hematological/ Anemias

type of anemia; however, it is associated with iron-deficiency anemia. Central nervous system and musculoskeletal manifestations may occur because of pernicious anemia.
Priority Nursing Tip: A gastric resection decreases the amount of intrinsic factor needed to absorb vitamin B_{12} from the stomach, which in turn results in pernicious anemia.

Test-Taking Strategy: Focus on the **subject,** a risk factor associated with pernicious anemia, and note the **strategic word,** *best.* Recalling that the parietal cells of the stomach secrete the intrinsic factor necessary for vitamin B_{12} absorption and that pernicious anemia is caused by a deficiency of the intrinsic factor will direct you to the correct option.

---

12. The nurse is planning to assist with testing the function of a client's vestibulocochlear nerve. The nurse would gather which items to assist with the performance of the test? **Select all that apply.**
❒ 1 Flashlight
❒ 2 Audiometer
❒ 3 Tuning fork
❒ 4 Cotton wisp
❒ 5 Ophthalmoscope

Level of Cognitive Ability: Applying
Client Needs: Health Promotion and Maintenance
Clinical Judgment/Cognitive Skills: Generate Solutions
Integrated Process: Nursing Process/ Implementation
Content Area: Health Assessment: Physical Exam: Ear, Nose, Throat
Health Problem: Adult Health: Ear: Hearing Loss

Answer: 2, 3
Rationale: The vestibulocochlear nerve is responsible for auditory acuity as well as bone and air conduction. The audiometer assesses the client's hearing, and the tuning fork tests bone and air conduction. The remaining supplies are used for testing cranial nerves II, III, and V.
Priority Nursing Tip: The vestibulocochlear nerve is referred to as *cranial nerve VIII.*

Test-Taking Strategy: Focus on the **subject,** items needed to test the function of the vestibulocochlear nerve. Recalling the function of this nerve and that it is responsible for auditory acuity as well as bone and air conduction will direct you to the correct options.

---

13. The nurse is assisting with evaluating the deep tendon reflexes of a pregnant client who is receiving magnesium sulfate intravenously. The nurse exposes the woman's lower leg, places one hand under the woman's knee to raise it slightly off the bed, and uses the percussion hammer to strike the patellar tendon just below the

Answer: 3
Rationale: The normal response is extension and forward thrusting of the foot. A 1+ response indicates a diminished response, 2+ indicates a normal response, 3+ indicates an increased or brisker-than-average response, and 4+ indicates a very brisk or hyperactive response.
Priority Nursing Tip: The higher the assessment number in reflexes, the more hyperactive the nerve.

patella. The nurse identifies the response as 4+. How would the nurse document this response?
1 Normal
2 Diminished
3 Very brisk or hyperactive
4 Increased or brisker than average

Level of Cognitive Ability: Applying
Client Needs: Health Promotion and Maintenance
Clinical Judgment/Cognitive Skills: Evaluate Outcomes
Integrated Process: Nursing Process/Implementation
Content Area: Maternity: Antepartum
Health Problem: Maternity: Gestational Hypertension/Preeclampsia and Eclampsia

Test-Taking Strategy: Focus on the **subject,** documenting reflex assessment. It is necessary to know how to interpret these findings to answer correctly.

---

14. In order to accurately determine the developmental skills of a 1-year-old born 2 months prematurely, the nurse would anticipate that the child would be able to perform what activity?
1 Sit independently
2 Walk independently
3 Build a tower of three blocks
4 Indicate wants by pointing or grunting

Level of Cognitive Ability: Applying
Client Needs: Health Promotion and Maintenance
Clinical Judgment/Cognitive Skills: Analyze Cues
Integrated Process: Nursing Process/Implementation
Content Area: Developmental Stages: Toddler
Health Problem: N/A

Answer: 1
Rationale: For premature infants, the nurse needs to calculate the developmental age by deducting the time of prematurity from the age of the child until the child reaches the age of 2 years. In this case, subtracting 2 months from 1 year results in an adjusted age of 10 months. A 10-month-old infant can sit independently. By the age of 15 months, a child would walk independently and indicate wants by pointing and grunting. By the age of 18 months, a child would be able to build a tower of three blocks.
Priority Nursing Tip: Because growth and development are sequential and predictable, the nurse is able to determine whether a child is at a normal developmental stage.

Test-Taking Strategy: Focus on the **subject,** toddler developmental milestones. Note the words *1-year-old child who was born 2 months early.* Apply your knowledge of the psychomotor skills that would be present in a 10-month-old child to answer the question.

---

15. The nurse would plan which intervention as the **first** step in preparing to reinforce teaching a client about a new diagnosis of hypertension?
1 Decide on the teaching approach
2 Plan for the evaluation of the session
3 Gather all available resource materials
4 Identify the client's knowledge and needs

Answer: 4
Rationale: Determining what to teach a client begins with a determination of the client's own knowledge and learning needs. After these have been determined, the nurse can effectively plan a teaching approach and determine the actual content and resource materials that may be needed. The evaluation is performed after teaching is completed.
Priority Nursing Tip: The client's level of learning would be evaluated after information has been presented. Teach-back is an effective method of evaluation.

Level of Cognitive Ability: Applying
Client Needs: Health Promotion and Maintenance
Clinical Judgment/Cognitive Skills: Generate Solutions
Integrated Process: Teaching and Learning
Content Area: Skills: Client Teaching
Health Problem: Adult Health: Cardiovascular: Hypertension

Test-Taking Strategy: Note the **strategic word,** *first.* Use the **steps of the nursing process,** and remember that data collection is the first step. This will direct you to the correct option.

---

16. Which discharge instruction would the nurse provide to a client after elbow arthroplasty?
1 Do not lift anything that weighs more than 20 pounds.
2 Playing sports with the operative arm needs to be avoided.
3 Triceps and biceps strengthening exercises can be started in 6 weeks.
4 Elbow flexion and extension exercises are avoided for at least 2 weeks.

Level of Cognitive Ability: Applying
Client Needs: Health Promotion and Maintenance
Clinical Judgment/Cognitive Skills: Generate Solutions
Integrated Process: Teaching and Learning
Content Area: Adult Health: Musculoskeletal
Health Problem: Adult Health: Musculoskeletal: Tissue or Ligament Injury

Answer: 2
Rationale: After elbow arthroplasty, elbow flexion and extension exercises are allowed as tolerated. Clients would not lift more than 5 pounds, and they would not begin triceps and biceps strengthening exercises for 3 months. The client will not be able to use the operative arm to play sports.
Priority Nursing Tip: After elbow arthroplasty, the client would not use the extremity for contact sports due to the high risk of injury to the postsurgical site.

Test-Taking Strategy: Focus on the **subject,** discharge instructions after arthroplasty. Considering the involvement of this surgical procedure and the anatomical location will direct you to the correct option.

---

17. During a difficult vaginal delivery, a large-for-gestational-age (LGA) infant experiences a fracture of the left clavicle and is being discharged to home with an immobilizing sling. Which parent statement would indicate that **further instruction is needed**?
1 "I am so upset that my baby's arm will always be paralyzed."
2 "The primary purpose of the immobilization is to provide comfort."
3 "Our doctor explained that this is a complication associated with the delivery of a large infant."
4 "We understand that the final diagnosis was made by x-ray study and physical examination."

Answer: 1
Rationale: The complications of a vaginal LGA birth are associated with the need to assist the process with forceps, vacuum extraction, or both. Even without mechanical assistance, the clavicles may fracture during delivery if the infant is LGA. The diagnosis is made by physical examination of the infant and by x-ray study. Immobilization will provide comfort. The infant's arm will not be paralyzed, but immobilization is needed to facilitate healing.
Priority Nursing Tip: Macrosomia is birth weight >4000 g (8 pounds and 13 ounces) in a term infant.

Test-Taking Strategy: Note the **strategic words,** *further instruction is needed.* These words indicate a **negative event query** and ask you to select an option that is an incorrect statement. Recalling that the injury is temporary and treatable will direct you to the correct option.

Level of Cognitive Ability: Evaluating
Client Needs: Health Promotion and Maintenance
Clinical Judgment/Cognitive Skills: Evaluate Outcomes
Integrated Process: Teaching and Learning
Content Area: Maternity: Newborn
Health Problem: Newborn: Gestational Age Problems

---

18. The nurse reinforces home-care instructions to parents about their postmature infant's nutritional needs. Which parent statement indicates an understanding of the necessary care of the infant?

1. "Our baby is at risk for high blood sugar."
2. "Cold stress is unlikely to occur in our baby."
3. "Letting our baby sleep through feedings is OK."
4. "We need to anticipate that our baby will need frequent feedings."

Level of Cognitive Ability: Evaluating
Client Needs: Health Promotion and Maintenance
Clinical Judgment/Cognitive Skills: Evaluate Outcomes
Integrated Process: Nursing Process/Evaluation
Content Area: Maternity: Newborn
Health Problem: Newborn: Gestational Age Problems

Answer: 4
Rationale: A postmature infant has been poorly nourished in utero, resulting in wasting and growth restriction as a result of placental dysfunction. These infants need early and more frequent feedings to help compensate for the period of poor nutrition in utero. They are at risk for hypoglycemia and cold stress. It is best to not allow the infant to sleep through the scheduled feeding times because of the risk for hypoglycemia.
Priority Nursing Tip: Placental insufficiency puts the fetus at high risk for insufficient oxygenation in utero.

Test-Taking Strategy: Focus on the **subject,** the needs of a postmature infant. Knowledge of the nutritional needs of a postmature infant is necessary to answer this question. Noting that the correct option directly relates to feeding and nutritional needs will assist you in answering correctly.

---

19. When gathering data about the maternal history, the nurse asks which question to assess for a major risk factor that may result in a small-for-gestational-age (SGA) infant?

1. "Do you smoke?"
2. "How old are you?"
3. "Is your diet low in fat?"
4. "What is your blood type?"

Level of Cognitive Ability: Analyzing
Client Needs: Health Promotion and Maintenance
Clinical Judgment/Cognitive Skills: Recognize Cues
Integrated Process: Nursing Process/Data Collection
Content Area: Maternity: Antepartum
Health Problem: Newborn: Gestational Age Problems

Answer: 1
Rationale: Maternal smoking interferes with placental flow and oxygenation; this in turn impairs fetal growth and may result in an SGA infant. The other options are not factors that contribute to an SGA infant.
Priority Nursing Tip: Although some babies are small because of genetics (their parents are small), most SGA babies are small because of fetal growth problems that occur during pregnancy.

Test-Taking Strategy: Focus on the **subject,** major risk factors for SGA babies. Recalling the effects of smoking on the fetus will direct you to the correct option.

---

20. The nurse reinforces to the client with coronary artery disease who was placed on a low-cholesterol diet that which item is an appropriate dessert?

1 Apple pie
2 Ice cream
3 Pound cake
4 Frozen yogurt

Level of Cognitive Ability: Applying
Client Needs: Health Promotion and Maintenance
Clinical Judgment/Cognitive Skills: Take Action
Integrated Process: Teaching and Learning
Content Area: Foundations of Care: Therapeutic Diets
Health Problem: Adult Health: Cardiovascular: Coronary Artery Disease

Answer: 4
Rationale: Desserts that are higher in cholesterol include high-fat frozen desserts (e.g., ice cream) and high-fat cakes (e.g., frosted and pound cakes). Most store-bought pies and cookies are also high in fat. The best low-fat dessert choices include angel food cake; frozen desserts such as sorbet, sherbet, Italian ice, and frozen yogurt; and other desserts that are specifically labeled "low fat."
Priority Nursing Tip: Sherbet is made from mostly fruit, which is low in cholesterol.

Test-Taking Strategy: Focus on the **subject**, a low-cholesterol diet. Knowledge related to this diet and thinking about the nutritional components of each item in the options will direct you to option 4.

---

21. What behaviors in children are associated with the preoperational phase of cognitive development? **Select all that apply.**

❒ **1** Riding a broom like a horse
❒ **2** Role-playing mommy or daddy during play
❒ **3** Taking turns on the swings at a playground
❒ **4** Listening intently and complying with the rules of a board game
❒ **5** Picking a glass that looks fuller when the liquid amount in each is the same

Level of Cognitive Ability: Analyzing
Client Needs: Health Promotion and Maintenance
Clinical Judgment/Cognitive Skills: Recognize Cues
Integrated Process: Nursing Process/Data Collection
Content Area: Developmental Stages: Preschool and School Age
Health Problem: N/A

Answer: 1, 2, 5
Rationale: Children in the preoperational stage are increasing their play and pretending. Options 1 and 2 are examples of this action. Option 5 is an example of the concept of conservation as perceived by a child in the preoperational stage. Options 3 and 4 are examples of a child who has developed egocentrism, which is not common in the preschooler and preoperational stage. Development of this concept requires a higher form of thinking, and a preschooler is not able to demonstrate this until later.
Priority Nursing Tip: The preschooler is able to pretend and take on other roles but continues to be very self-centered or egocentric.

Test-Taking Strategy: Focus on the **subject**, the preoperational phase of cognitive development. Knowledge of characteristics of this phase is necessary to help you in selecting the correct options.

---

22. The nurse in a well-baby clinic is collecting data about the language and communication developmental milestones of a 7-month-old infant. The nurse determines that an appropriate milestone has been reached when observing the child engage in what behavior?

1 Making cooing sounds when being held

Answer: 4
Rationale: An increased interest in sounds occurs between the ages of 6 and 8 months, demonstrated by the infant's interest in who is talking. Between the ages of 1 and 3 months, the infant will produce cooing sounds. Babbling sounds begin between the ages of 3 and 4 months. The use of gestures and the imitation of sounds occur between the ages of 9 and 12 months.
Priority Nursing Tip: The stages of vocal development are progressive, so a child must coo and babble before turning to various sounds.

2 Using a hand gesture to get Mom's attention
3 Making babbling sounds as if talking to the nurse
4 Focusing attention on whoever is currently talking

Level of Cognitive Ability: Evaluating
Client Needs: Health Promotion and Maintenance
Clinical Judgment/Cognitive Skills: Analyze Cues
Integrated Process: Nursing Process/ Data Collection
Content Area: Developmental Stages: Infant
Health Problem: N/A

Test-Taking Strategy: Focus on the **data in the question.** Noting the age of the infant will help you eliminate options 1 and 3 because the developmental milestones cited in these options occur at an earlier age. From the remaining options, focus on the age of the child to direct you to the correct option, remembering that the use of gestures occurs later in infants.

---

23. The nurse obtains an older adult client's height and weight on admission to a long-term care facility. The nurse describes normal age-related changes in height and in the musculoskeletal system to the client. The client demonstrates an understanding of these changes if which client statement is made?
1 "I must have osteoporosis."
2 "I'm shorter because my cartilage is overgrown."
3 "We will use these results to determine my ideal body weight."
4 "I'm shorter because I don't have as much bone density as I used to."

Level of Cognitive Ability: Evaluating
Client Needs: Health Promotion and Maintenance
Clinical Judgment/Cognitive Skills: Evaluate Outcomes
Integrated Process: Nursing Process/Evaluation
Content Area: Developmental Stages: Early Adulthood to Later Adulthood
Health Problem: N/A

Answer: 4
Rationale: Age-related changes in the musculoskeletal system include decreased bone density, increased bony prominence, a kyphotic posture, cartilage degeneration, decreased range of motion, muscle atrophy, decreased strength, and slowed movement. Option 4 identifies correct information. Osteoporosis is not a normal age-related change. Although height and weight are used to determine ideal body weight, this is unrelated to age-related changes.
Priority Nursing Tip: As aging occurs, minerals needed to maintain bone strength are used by the body, thus depleting bone density.

Test-Taking Strategy: Focus on the **subject,** normal age-related changes. Noting the words *demonstrates an understanding* and thinking about changes that occur with the body in aging will direct you to the correct option.

---

24. The nurse is assisting with the development of a teaching plan for an older adult client diagnosed with hypertension. The client will be discharged to home and must learn to manage diet and medications. To facilitate the client's learning process, what would the nurse implement **first?**
1 Set priorities for the client.
2 Use only one teaching method.

Answer: 3
Rationale: Until the client is ready to learn, teaching sessions will be ineffective. Teaching would be performed in short sessions early in the day, when the client is well rested. It is important to include the client in the development of the teaching plan and to set priorities with the client. Varied teaching methods (e.g., verbal instruction) are best. Visual aids and written material would be provided for later reference.
Priority Nursing Tip: One of the first steps to teaching and learning is to assess the client for their current knowledge base.

3 Determine the client's readiness to learn.
4 Plan 30-minute teaching sessions only in the evening after visiting hours are over.

Test-Taking Strategy: Note the **strategic word,** *first,* and focus on the **subject,** teaching principles. Remembering that data collection is the first **step in the nursing process** will direct you to the correct option.

Level of Cognitive Ability: Applying
Client Needs: Health Promotion and Maintenance
Clinical Judgment/Cognitive Skills: Prioritize Hypotheses
Integrated Process: Teaching and Learning
Content Area: Skills: Client Teaching
Health Problem: Adult Health: Cardiovascular: Hypertension

---

25. The nurse has been reinforcing teaching to an older adult client about the influenza vaccine. The nurse determines that the client **needs further instruction** when the client makes what statement?
1 "I'll get the flu vaccine this fall."
2 "I need to get the vaccine every year."
3 "I need to get a flu vaccine even though I'm healthy."
4 "I don't need the vaccine this year because I had one last year."

Answer: 4
Rationale: New influenza vaccines are developed every year based on predictions of which strains of the virus will be active. Clients would be advised to get the vaccine every year. Options 1, 2, and 3 are correct statements about the influenza vaccine.
Priority Nursing Tip: Flu vaccines are administered annually starting in the fall.

Test-Taking Strategy: Note the **strategic words,** *needs further instruction.* These words indicate a **negative event query** and ask you to select an option that is an incorrect statement. Use your knowledge of this vaccine to answer the question. Recalling that the vaccine is administered yearly will direct you to the correct option.

Level of Cognitive Ability: Evaluating
Client Needs: Health Promotion and Maintenance
Clinical Judgment/Cognitive Skills: Evaluate Outcomes
Integrated Process: Teaching and Learning
Content Area: Foundations of Care: Infection Control
Health Problem: Adult Health: Respiratory: Viral, Bacterial, Fungal Infections

---

26. A client tells the nurse, "I did not take my heart medication today because I did not want to get that terrible headache again." The nurse would make which response to this client?
1 "If you are getting a headache, it is best to stand up when taking your heart medication."
2 "You were correct to not take your heart medication. Headaches are a sign of an allergic reaction."

Answer: 4
Rationale: Some cardiac medications, particularly the nitrates, dilate the body's arteries; this can increase blood flow to the brain and cause headaches. These headaches are usually transient and treatable with over-the-counter pain relievers (e.g., acetaminophen). Standing when taking the medication will not help. The client would not stop taking medication without advice from a health care provider.
Priority Nursing Tip: The effects of nitrate medications can result in orthostatic hypotension.

3 "Headaches are just something you'll have to get used to if you don't want to have another heart attack."
4 "The side effect of headaches will probably decrease in a few days. Let's discuss what analgesics you can take."

Level of Cognitive Ability: Applying
Client Needs: Health Promotion and Maintenance
Clinical Judgment/Cognitive Skills: Take Action
Integrated Process: Teaching and Learning
Content Area: Pharmacology: Cardiovascular: Antianginal Medications (Nitrates)
Health Problem: Adult Health: Cardiovascular: Coronary Artery Disease

Test-Taking Strategy: Focus on the **subject**, side effects of nitrates. Use your knowledge of this medication to eliminate option 2, because the client would always take the medication as prescribed. Option 1 will not relieve the headache. Option 3 is a nontherapeutic response.

---

27. The nurse is collecting information about weight loss from an obese client. What data collection method would the nurse use to **most accurately** determine the **effectiveness** of a weight-loss program?
1 Monitor the weight.
2 Review calorie counts.
3 Review laboratory results.
4 Monitor intake and output daily.

Level of Cognitive Ability: Applying
Client Needs: Health Promotion and Maintenance
Clinical Judgment/Cognitive Skills: Recognize Cues
Integrated Process: Nursing Process/Data Collection
Content Area: Foundations of Care: Therapeutic Diets
Health Problem: Adult Health: Gastrointestinal: Nutrition Problems

Answer: 1
Rationale: The most accurate weight-loss measurement entails weighing the client at the same time of day, while he or she is wearing the same clothes, on the same scale. Some health care providers recommend weekly weighing rather than daily weighing. The other options assist in measuring nutrition and hydration status.
Priority Nursing Tip: Weighing is an objective form of assessment in determining weight loss.

Test-Taking Strategy: Focus on the **subject,** assessing weight loss. Note the **strategic words,** *most accurately* and *effectiveness.* Note the similarity between the words *weight loss* in the question and *weight* in the correct option.

---

28. Which laboratory value identified during data collection would the nurse stress as being **most important** for a client to modify to lessen the risk for coronary artery disease (CAD)?
1 Elevated triglyceride levels
2 Elevated serum lipase levels
3 Elevated low-density lipoprotein (LDL) levels
4 Elevated high-density lipoprotein (HDL) levels

Answer: 3
Rationale: LDLs are the "bad" lipoproteins. LDL levels, along with cholesterol levels, have a higher associative and predictive value for CAD than triglyceride levels. In addition, HDLs are inversely associated with the risk of CAD. Lipase is a digestive enzyme that breaks down ingested fats in the gastrointestinal tract.
Priority Nursing Tip: LDL is a low-density lipoprotein.

Test-Taking Strategy: Note the **strategic words,** *most important,* and focus on the **subject,** lessening the risk of CAD. Remember that LDLs are the "bad" lipoproteins and are more directly associated with CAD than other lipoproteins.

Level of Cognitive Ability: Analyzing
Client Needs: Health Promotion and Maintenance
Clinical Judgment/Cognitive Skills: Prioritize Hypotheses
Integrated Process: Nursing Process/Data Collection
Content Area: Adult Health: Cardiovascular
Health Problem: Adult Health: Cardiovascular: Coronary Artery Disease

---

29. The parent of an adolescent whose child refuses to eat meat is concerned that the child will get sick from poor nutrition. Which response to the parent is **most** helpful for dealing with an adolescent vegetarian?

1 "You need to take your child to the doctor because eating this way causes health problems."
2 "This is just a phase. Keep preparing meals as you always have, and your child will come around."
3 "People follow vegetarian diets for many reasons. A vegetarian diet can provide needed nutrients if it is planned carefully."
4 "Your child will not eat meat, but I assume she is a lacto-ovo vegetarian. They will get adequate protein from dairy products."

Answer: 3
Rationale: A vegetarian diet can provide needed nutrients if it is planned carefully; the nurse would provide nutritional information about this type of diet to the parent. Option 3 provides the most helpful information. Option 1 will cause unnecessary alarm in the parent. Option 2 may not be accurate and is an assumption on the nurse's part. Option 4 makes an assumption that may not be accurate.
Priority Nursing Tip: The vegan or total vegetarian diet includes only foods from plants: fruits, vegetables, legumes (dried beans and peas), grains, seeds, and nuts.

Test-Taking Strategy: Note the **strategic words,** *most.* Read each option carefully and use **therapeutic communication techniques** to direct you to the correct option.

Level of Cognitive Ability: Applying
Client Needs: Health Promotion and Maintenance
Clinical Judgment/Cognitive Skills: Take Action
Integrated Process: Teaching and Learning
Content Area: Foundations of Care: Therapeutic Diets
Health Problem: Pediatric-Specific: Nutrition Problems

---

30. The nurse reinforces teaching to parents that preschool-age children have the developmental skills to be responsible for what preventive behavior?

1 Staying away from strange dogs
2 Knowing what is and is not harmful
3 Wearing a helmet when riding a bike
4 Making decisions about joining a gang

Answer: 3
Rationale: Preschool-age children are at risk for accidents because their judgment is overruled by curiosity. A preschooler has the developmental skills to be responsible for wearing a helmet when riding a bike. In addition, wearing a helmet can become a habit very quickly with parental insistence and behavioral training. Although these children may know safety rules, a strange dog may attract their attention. A preschool-age child may not have the developmental skill of knowing what is and is not harmful, and he or she cannot be expected to make sound decisions.

Level of Cognitive Ability: Applying
Client Needs: Health Promotion and Maintenance
Clinical Judgment/Cognitive Skills: Take Action
Integrated Process: Teaching and Learning
Content Area: Developmental Stages: Preschool and School Age
Health Problem: N/A

Priority Nursing Tip: Initiative vs. guilt is the stage of preschool development whereby the child takes initiative to learn safety rules and the results when they are not followed.

Test-Taking Strategy: Focus on the **subject,** development tasks, and note the age-group of the child. Use your knowledge of safety issues and the psychosocial development of this age-group to answer the question.

---

31. The nurse is reinforcing dietary home-care instructions to a client with coronary artery disease (CAD). Which statement by the client indicates an understanding of the recommended dietary practices?

1 "I need to become a strict vegetarian."
2 "I eliminate all cholesterol and fat from my diet."
3 "I need to use polyunsaturated oils, eat low-fat cheese, and drink skim milk."
4 "I need to substitute eggs and whole milk for meat to get adequate dietary protein."

Level of Cognitive Ability: Evaluating
Client Needs: Health Promotion and Maintenance
Clinical Judgment/Cognitive Skills: Evaluate Outcomes
Integrated Process: Nursing Process/Evaluation
Content Area: Adult Health: Cardiovascular
Health Problem: Adult Health: Cardiovascular/Coronary Artery Disease

Answer: 3
Rationale: A client with CAD needs to avoid foods that are high in saturated fat and cholesterol (e.g., eggs, whole milk, red meat) because they contribute to increases in low-density lipoproteins. The use of polyunsaturated oils, skim milk, and complex carbohydrates is recommended to control hypercholesterolemia. The client does not have to become a strict vegetarian or eliminate all cholesterol and fat from the diet to control the disorder.
Priority Nursing Tip: Symptoms occur when the coronary artery is occluded to the point that inadequate blood supply to the muscle occurs, causing ischemia.

Test-Taking Strategy: Focus on the **subject,** diet for CAD. Eliminate options 1 and 2 because of the **closed-ended words** "strict" and "all." Eliminate option 4 next because these items are high in cholesterol.

---

32. The nurse is collecting data from a client who has been diagnosed with coronary artery disease (CAD). Which data would the nurse educate the client on as modifiable risk factors for the development of CAD? **Select all that apply.**

❒ 1 Obesity
❒ 2 Gender
❒ 3 Ethnicity
❒ 4 Hypertension
❒ 5 Cigarette smoking

Level of Cognitive Ability: Applying
Client Needs: Health Promotion and Maintenance
Clinical Judgment/Cognitive Skills: Take Action
Integrated Process: Teaching and Learning
Content Area: Adult Health: Cardiovascular
Health Problem: Adult Health: Cardiovascular/Coronary Artery Disease

Answer: 1, 4, 5
Rationale: Nonmodifiable risk factors for CAD cannot be controlled; they include age, gender, family history, and ethnicity. Modifiable risk factors can be controlled; they include the cholesterol level, hypertension, cigarette smoking, and obesity.
Priority Nursing Tip: Risk factors that can be modified usually result in a need for lifestyle changes.

Test-Taking Strategy: Focus on the **subject,** risk factors for CAD. Note the word *modifiable.* Note that only options 1, 4, and 5 contain factors that can be controlled or changed.

33. The nurse is reinforcing home-care instructions to prevent recurrence of a pulmonary embolism (PE) with a client being discharged after treatment for the PE. The nurse determines that the instructions have been **effective** if the client states an intention to engage in what activity?

1 Limiting fluid intake
2 Wearing supportive hose
3 Sitting down whenever possible
4 Crossing the legs at the ankle and not at the knee

Level of Cognitive Ability: Evaluating
Client Needs: Health Promotion and Maintenance
Clinical Judgment/Cognitive Skills: Evaluate Outcomes
Integrated Process: Nursing Process/Evaluation
Content Area: Adult Health: Respiratory
Health Problem: Adult Health: Respiratory: Pulmonary Embolism

Answer: 2

Rationale: Recurrence of pulmonary embolism can be minimized by the wearing of elastic or supportive hose to enhance venous return. The client can also enhance venous return by avoiding crossing the legs at the knee or ankle, interspersing periods of sitting with walking, and doing active foot and ankle exercises. The client also needs to take in sufficient fluids to prevent hemoconcentration and hypercoagulability.

Priority Nursing Tip: Compression devices may be prescribed to facilitate circulation to decrease coagulability.

Test-Taking Strategy: Focus on the **subject,** preventing the recurrence of pulmonary embolism, and note the **strategic word,** *effective.* Recalling that prolonged immobilization and hypercoagulability can lead to pulmonary embolism will direct you to the correct option.

---

34. The nurse is reinforcing home-care instructions regarding the need to begin long-term anticoagulant therapy for a client who has atrial fibrillation. Which explanation would the nurse provide to describe the reasoning for this therapy?

1 "This dysrhythmia decreases the amount of blood flow from the heart, which can lead to blood clots forming in the brain."
2 "The antidysrhythmic medications you are taking cause blood clots as a side effect, so you need this medication to prevent them."
3 "Because of this dysrhythmia, blood backs up in the legs and puts you at risk for blood clots; this is also called *deep vein thrombosis.*"
4 "Because the atria are 'quivering,' blood flows sluggishly through them. Clots can form along the heart wall, which could then loosen and travel to the lungs or brain."

Level of Cognitive Ability: Applying
Client Needs: Health Promotion and Maintenance
Clinical Judgment/Cognitive Skills: Take Action
Integrated Process: Teaching and Learning
Content Area: Adult Health: Cardiovascular
Health Problem: Adult Health: Cardiovascular: Dysrhythmias

Answer: 4

Rationale: A severe complication of atrial fibrillation is the development of thrombi. The blood stagnates in the "quivering" atria because of the loss of organized atrial muscle contraction and "atrial kick," which can account for up to 30% of the cardiac output. The blood that pools in the atria can then clot, which increases the risk for pulmonary and cerebral emboli. Options 1, 2, and 3 are incorrect descriptions.

Priority Nursing Tip: When blood is allowed to pool in the atria, clots may form.

Test-Taking Strategy: Focus on the **data in the question** and the client's diagnosis: atrial fibrillation. Note the relationship between the words *fibrillation* in the question and *quivering* in the correct option.

---

35. A client with prostatitis asks the nurse, "Why do I need to take a stool softener? The problem is with my urine, not my bowels!" The nurse would provide which explanation to the client?

1 "This is a standard prescription for anyone with an abdominal problem."
2 "This will keep the bowel free of feces, which will decrease the swelling inside."
3 "Being constipated puts you at more risk for developing complications of prostatitis."
4 "This will help you avoid constipation, because straining is painful with prostatitis."

Level of Cognitive Ability: Applying
Client Needs: Health Promotion and Maintenance
Clinical Judgment/Cognitive Skills: Take Action
Integrated Process: Nursing Process/Implementation
Content Area: Adult Health: Renal and Urinary
Health Problem: Adult Health: Renal and Urinary: Inflammation/Infections

Answer: 4
Rationale: Prostatitis is an inflammation of the prostate gland. Stool softeners are prescribed for the client with prostatitis to prevent constipation, which can be painful. Stool softeners are not a standard medication prescription for anyone with an abdominal problem. Stool softeners have no direct effect on decreasing swelling, and they do not prevent complications (e.g., chronic prostatitis).
Priority Nursing Tip: Constipation increases pelvic pain in a client with prostatitis.

Test-Taking Strategy: Focus on the **data in the question** and the **subject,** prostatitis and stool softeners. The response in option 1 may be eliminated first because it is nonspecific and nonhelpful. The bowel is never "free of feces," so option 2 can be eliminated next. From the remaining options, recalling the action and purpose of stool softeners directs you to the correct option.

---

36. A client diagnosed with Parkinson's disease has begun therapy with carbidopa–levodopa. The nurse reinforces home-care instructions about the medication and determines that the client understands the action of the medication if the client verbalizes that results may not be apparent for which time period?

1 1 week
2 24 hours
3 2 to 3 days
4 2 to 3 weeks

Level of Cognitive Ability: Evaluating
Client Needs: Health Promotion and Maintenance
Clinical Judgment/Cognitive Skills: Evaluate Outcomes
Integrated Process: Nursing Process/Evaluation
Content Area: Pharmacology: Neurological: Antiparkinsonian
Health Problem: Adult Health: Neurological: Parkinson's Disease

Answer: 4
Rationale: Parkinson's disease is a debilitating disease that affects motor ability. Signs and symptoms of Parkinson's disease usually begin to resolve within 2 to 3 weeks of starting carbidopa–levodopa therapy, although marked improvement may not be seen for up to 6 months in some clients.
Priority Nursing Tip: Parkinson's disease is characterized by tremor, rigidity, akinesia (slow movement), and postural instability.

Test-Taking Strategy: Focus on the **subject,** expected effectiveness of carbidopa–levodopa. Remember that the effects of carbidopa–levodopa begin within 2 to 3 weeks of starting therapy, although marked improvement may not be seen for up to 6 months in some clients.

---

37. The nurse is participating in a prostate screening clinic and determines that a client understands the educational information when the client shares what information with another participant?

1 "A daily supplement of vitamin E prevents prostate problems."
2 "Cigarette smoking triples the chance of developing prostate problems."
3 "Increasing intake of green leafy vegetables prevents prostate problems."
4 "Annual rectal examinations need to begin at age 45 to detect possible prostate problems."

Level of Cognitive Ability: Evaluating
Client Needs: Health Promotion and Maintenance
Clinical Judgment/Cognitive Skills: Evaluate Outcomes
Integrated Process: Teaching and Learning
Content Area: Adult Health: Renal and Urinary
Health Problem: Adult Health: Renal and Urinary: Obstructive Problems

Answer: 4
Rationale: Benign prostatic hypertrophy (BPH) is thought to result from an alteration in the client's androgen levels, although the exact cause is still unknown. Increasing age is a risk factor for developing BPH, and an annual digital rectal examination and a prostate-specific antigen test need to be performed beginning at age 45. Increased intake of green leafy vegetables does not prevent BPH. Vitamin E and cigarette smoking have no known relationship with BPH.
Priority Nursing Tip: Prostate screening needs to begin at age 45 for those considered high risk, including those who had a brother or father diagnosed with prostate cancer before the age of 65.

Test-Taking Strategy: Focus on the **subject,** information about BPH. Recalling that advancing age is a primary risk factor assists you with eliminating the incorrect options. Also, the setting of the question is a prostate screening clinic, and so the focus would be on detection; this will guide you to option 4.

---

38. A client is being discharged home after a prostatectomy. The nurse reinforces home-care instructions by instructing the client to do what?

1 Wait 1 week before mowing the lawn.
2 Avoid lifting more than 50 pounds for 4 to 6 weeks after surgery.
3 Drink at least 15 glasses of water a day to minimize clot formation.
4 Notify the surgeon if fever, increased pain, or inability to void occurs.

Level of Cognitive Ability: Applying
Client Needs: Health Promotion and Maintenance
Clinical Judgment/Cognitive Skills: Take Action
Integrated Process: Teaching and Learning
Content Area: Adult Health: Renal and Urinary
Health Problem: Adult Health: Renal and Urinary: Obstructive Problems

Answer: 4
Rationale: A prostatectomy is the surgical removal of part of the prostate gland. Postoperatively, the client needs to notify the surgeon if there are any signs of infection, pain, bleeding, or urinary obstruction. Lifting more than 20 pounds is prohibited for 4 to 6 weeks after surgery. Other strenuous activities that could increase intra-abdominal tension are also restricted (e.g., mowing the lawn). The client needs to take in 6 to 8 glasses of water or nonalcoholic beverages per day to minimize the risk of clot formation. Drinking 15 glasses of water per day is excessive.
Priority Nursing Tip: A client is at high risk for infection after any surgical procedure.

Test-Taking Strategy: Focus on the **subject,** prostatectomy discharge instructions. Eliminate options 1, 2, and 3 because they are **comparable or alike** and are exaggerations of expected amounts. The client needs to notify the surgeon if signs of infection or obstruction occur.

---

39. The nurse is teaching a client with acute kidney injury to include high-quality proteins in the diet. The nurse educates the client to avoid which food item because it is a low-quality protein source?

Answer: 4
Rationale: Low-quality proteins are derived from plant sources and include vegetables and foods made from grains. The renal diet is limited in the amount of protein consumed; therefore it is important that high-quality proteins be ingested.

1 Fish
2 Eggs
3 Chicken
4 Broccoli

Level of Cognitive Ability: Applying
Client Needs: Health Promotion and Maintenance
Clinical Judgment/Cognitive Skills: Take Action
Integrated Process: Teaching and Learning
Content Area: Foundations of Care: Therapeutic Diets
Health Problem: Adult Health: Renal and Urinary: Acute Kidney Injury

Priority Nursing Tip: High-quality proteins come from animal sources and include such foods as eggs, meat, and fish.

Test-Taking Strategy: Focus on the **subject,** the food that is a low-quality protein. Note that options 1, 2, and 3 are **comparable or alike** protein sources. Note that broccoli is a plant.

---

40. A client is ready to be discharged from the hospital and will be changing a wound dressing at home. How can the nurse **best** evaluate the client's ability to care for the wound?
1 Ask the client to verbalize wound site care.
2 Review the entire discharge plan with the client again.
3 Observe the client while changing the wound dressing.
4 Demonstrate the dressing change for the client one last time before discharge.

Level of Cognitive Ability: Evaluating
Client Needs: Health Promotion and Maintenance
Clinical Judgment/Cognitive Skills: Evaluate Outcomes
Integrated Process: Teaching and Learning
Content Area: Skills: Wound Care: Dressings
Health Problem: Adult Health: Integumentary: Wounds

Answer: 3
Rationale: The acquisition of psychomotor skills is best evaluated by observing how a client carries out a procedure. This is known as teach-back. The client may be able to verbalize how to do the procedure yet be unable to perform the psychomotor functions required. Reviewing the entire plan and demonstrating it again will not evaluate the client's ability.
Priority Nursing Tip: Client-focused education would be presented in language the client is most likely to understand.

Test-Taking Strategy: Note the **strategic word,** *best,* and focus on the **subject,** the client's ability to perform wound care. The correct option would involve some type of active client participation. Having the client actively demonstrate a procedure is always the best method of evaluating a psychomotor skill.

---

41. The nurse reinforcing home-care instructions to a client being discharged with a peripherally inserted central catheter (PICC) line plans to teach the client which **most important** concept for preventing peripheral IV infections?
1 Change the IV tubing and fluid containers daily.
2 Redress the IV site daily and cleanse it with alcohol.

Answer: 4
Rationale: It is important for the client to realize the necessity of hand washing before working with IV fluids. Although the assessment of the IV site is important, it does not actively prevent infection. The IV site does not need to be redressed daily unless the dressing becomes wet, soiled, or loose. The IV containers would be changed daily, and the tubing would be changed every 48 to 72 hours, depending on the home-care agency policies.
Priority Nursing Tip: Nosocomial infections are those acquired while in a health care–providing environment.

3 Check the IV site carefully every day for redness and edema.
4 Carefully wash your hands with antibacterial soap before working with the IV site or equipment.

Level of Cognitive Ability: Applying
Client Needs: Health Promotion and Maintenance
Clinical Judgment/Cognitive Skills: Take Action
Integrated Process: Teaching and Learning
Content Area: Skills: Infection Control
Health Problem: N/A

Test-Taking Strategy: Focus on the **subject,** PICC care at home. Note the **strategic words,** *most important*. Read the question carefully, and note that infection prevention is the concept that would be taught to the client. Remember that the number-one priority of infection prevention always includes proper handwashing technique.

---

42. A client scheduled for the implantation of an automatic internal cardioverter-defibrillator (AICD) asks the nurse why there is a need to keep a diary after insertion. What would the nurse teach the client is the **primary** purpose of the diary?
1 Determining which activities to avoid
2 Documenting events that precipitate a countershock
3 Providing a count of the number of shocks delivered
4 Recording a variety of data that contribute to medical management

Level of Cognitive Ability: Applying
Client Needs: Health Promotion and Maintenance
Clinical Judgment/Cognitive Skills: Take Action
Integrated Process: Teaching and Learning
Content Area: Adult Health: Cardiovascular
Health Problem: Adult Health: Cardiovascular: Dysrhythmias

Answer: 4
Rationale: The client with an AICD maintains a log or diary that includes the date and time of the shock, activity that occurred before the shock, any symptoms that were experienced, the number of shocks delivered, and how the client felt after the shock. The information is used by the cardiologist to adjust the medical regimen (especially medication therapy), which must be maintained after AICD insertion.
Priority Nursing Tip: AICD delivers an electrical impulse or shock to the heart when it senses a life-threatening change in the heart's rhythm.

Test-Taking Strategy: Note the **strategic word,** *primary*, and focus on the **subject,** the primary purpose of the log or diary; this implies a comprehensive response. Each of the incorrect options lists one of the items that would be logged in the diary, but the correct option is the only one that can be considered a primary purpose. Option 4 is the **umbrella option** because it is an inclusive answer.

---

43. The nurse is determining a hypertensive client's understanding to control the disease process. The nurse evaluates a client's understanding of dietary modifications necessary for blood pressure management as satisfactory when the client selects what meal?
1 Corned beef, fresh carrots, and boiled potatoes
2 Hotdog on a bun, sauerkraut, and baked beans
3 Turkey, baked potato, and salad with oil and vinegar
4 Scallops, french fries, and salad with blue cheese dressing

Answer: 3
Rationale: A client with hypertension needs to avoid food products that are high in sodium content. Foods from the meat/protein group that are higher in sodium include bacon, luncheon meat, chipped or corned beef, kosher meat, smoked or salted meat or shellfish, peanut butter, and a variety of shellfish. Turkey as the entrée would be the best meal selection.
Priority Nursing Tip: Fruit canned in its own natural juice is an example of an acceptable food item.

Test-Taking Strategy: Focus on the **subject,** an appropriate diet to treat hypertension. Eliminate options 1 and 2 first because these are highly processed meats that are high in sodium. (The sauerkraut in option 2 is also high in sodium.) The shellfish and commercial dressing help you eliminate option 4.

Level of Cognitive Ability: Evaluating
Client Needs: Health Promotion and Maintenance
Clinical Judgment/Cognitive Skills: Evaluate Outcomes
Integrated Process: Nursing Process/Evaluation
Content Area: Foundations of Care: Therapeutic Diets
Health Problem: Adult Health: Cardiovascular: Hypertension

---

44. The nurse reinforces home-care instructions for a client who will be taking warfarin sodium indefinitely. The nurse determines that the client **needs further instruction** if the client states the intent to do what?

1 Use a soft toothbrush
2 Use a straight razor for shaving
3 Avoid drinking any form of alcohol
4 Carry identification about the medication being taken

Level of Cognitive Ability: Evaluating
Client Needs: Health Promotion and Maintenance
Clinical Judgment/Cognitive Skills: Evaluate Outcomes
Integrated Process: Teaching and Learning
Content Area: Pharmacology: Cardiovascular: Anticoagulants
Health Problem: Adult Health: Hematological: Bleeding/Clotting Disorders

Answer: 2
Rationale: Warfarin sodium is an oral anticoagulant. The client needs to notify all caregivers about the medication and carry a MedicAlert identification card. The client needs to use a soft toothbrush to prevent bleeding from the gums during tooth brushing and an electric razor rather than a straight razor because a straight razor can cause nicks and resultant bleeding. Alcohol needs to be avoided.
Priority Nursing Tip: The client prescribed an anticoagulant would be educated about the importance of adhering to the schedule for follow-up bloodwork.

Test-Taking Strategy: Focus on the **subject,** client instructions for warfarin sodium. Note the **strategic words,** *needs further instruction.* These words indicate a **negative event query** and ask you to select an option that is an incorrect statement. Measures to teach clients on anticoagulant therapy generally deal with the prevention of bleeding and the interference of medication effects. Only option 2 represents a danger in one of these areas; therefore it is the option to select.

---

45. The nurse has reinforced home-care instructions to a client being discharged from the hospital with an arterial ischemic leg ulcer. Which statement by the client indicates an understanding of these measures? **Select all that apply.**

❒ 1 "I need to wear shoes and socks."
❒ 2 "I need to apply lotion to my feet."
❒ 3 "I need to cut my toenails straight across."
❒ 4 "Crossing my legs for short periods of time is okay."
❒ 5 "I need to raise my legs above the level of my heart periodically."

Answer: 1, 2, 3
Rationale: Foot-care instructions for the client with peripheral arterial ischemia are the same as those given to the client with diabetes mellitus. This would include wearing shoes and socks, applying lotion to the feet, and cutting the toenails straight across. All these measures help minimize foot injury. To enhance blood flow, the client with arterial disease needs to avoid raising the legs above the level of the heart unless instructed to do so, and crossing the legs needs to always be avoided.
Priority Nursing Tip: Ischemia is the result of damage to the tissues.

Test-Taking Strategy: Focus on the **subject,** client instructions for treating arterial ischemic leg ulcer. Note the word *arterial* and think about the process of blood flow. Recalling the principles related to an arterial problem directs you to the correct options.

Level of Cognitive Ability: Evaluating
Client Needs: Health Promotion and Maintenance
Clinical Judgment/Cognitive Skills: Evaluate Outcomes
Integrated Process: Nursing Process/Evaluation
Content Area: Adult Health: Cardiovascular
Health Problem: Adult Health: Cardiovascular: Vascular Disorders

---

46. The nurse determines that the client diagnosed with diabetes understands dietary and insulin needs during pregnancy when the client states that she may require which intervention during the second half of the pregnancy?

1 Increased insulin
2 Decreased insulin
3 Increased caloric intake
4 Decreased caloric intake

Level of Cognitive Ability: Evaluating
Client Needs: Health Promotion and Maintenance
Clinical Judgment/Cognitive Skills: Evaluate Outcomes
Integrated Process: Nursing Process/Evaluation
Content Area: Maternity: Antepartum
Health Problem: Maternity: Diabetes

Answer: 1
Rationale: Glucose crosses the placenta, but insulin does not. High fetal demands for glucose in combination with the insulin resistance caused by hormonal changes during the last half of pregnancy can result in an elevation of maternal blood glucose levels. This increases the parent's demand for insulin and is referred to as the *diabetogenic effect of pregnancy.* Caloric intake is not affected by diabetes.
Priority Nursing Tip: The fetus produces its own insulin and pulls glucose from the parent, which predisposes the parent to hypoglycemic reactions.

Test-Taking Strategy: Focus on the **subject,** diabetes and pregnancy. Use your knowledge of the pathophysiology associated with diabetes to help you answer the question. Eliminate options 3 and 4 first because they are **comparable or alike** and deal with food intake. Diabetes does not change caloric needs. Recalling that the need for insulin may decrease during the first half of pregnancy and increase during the second half will direct you to option 1.

---

47. The nurse is monitoring a client at risk for preeclampsia for the presence of pitting edema. Which method would the nurse implement to check the edema level?

1 The nurse presses the fingertips of the index and middle finger against the shin and holds pressure for 2 to 3 seconds.
2 The nurse uses the fingertips of the index and middle finger and presses into the ankles for a period of 3 to 5 seconds.
3 The nurse uses the fingertips of the index and middle finger, presses against the upper arm, and holds pressure for 3 to 5 seconds.
4 The nurse uses the fingertips of the index and middle finger, presses against the abdomen, and holds pressure for 2 to 3 seconds.

Answer: 1
Rationale: To evaluate for the presence of pitting edema, the nurse uncovers the client's lower leg, presses the fingertips of the index and middle fingers against the shin, and holds the pressure for 2 to 3 seconds. The other options are inaccurate techniques for assessing the presence of pitting edema.
Priority Nursing Tip: An indentation in the skin results if pitting edema is present.

Test-Taking Strategy: Focus on the **subject,** the procedure for edema assessment. Visualize each technique described in the options to assist with selecting the correct option.

Level of Cognitive Ability: Applying
Client Needs: Health Promotion and Maintenance
Clinical Judgment/Cognitive Skills: Take Action
Integrated Process: Nursing Process/Data Collection
Content Area: Maternity: Antepartum
Health Problem: Maternity: Gestational Hypertension/Preeclampsia and Eclampsia

---

48. The nurse reinforces instructions to a pregnant woman regarding measures for relieving low back pain. Which statement by the client indicates an understanding of these measures?

1. "I will do the pelvic tilt exercises."
2. "I will wear an abdominal support."
3. "I need to wear shoes with a higher heel."
4. "I need to work at relaxing my abdominal muscles when I stand."

Level of Cognitive Ability: Evaluating
Client Needs: Health Promotion and Maintenance
Clinical Judgment/Cognitive Skills: Evaluate Outcomes
Integrated Process: Nursing Process/Evaluation
Content Area: Maternity: Antepartum
Health Problem: Adult Health: Musculoskeletal: Tissue or Ligament Injury

Answer: 1
Rationale: Pelvic tilt exercises decrease strain on the muscles of the abdomen and lower back; this strain is caused by the added weight of the abdomen and the shift in the center of gravity. An abdominal support would be worn only if recommended by the obstetrician. Relaxing the abdominal muscles adds to the problem. Wearing higher-heeled shoes adds to the muscle strain and exaggerates the shift in the center of gravity.
Priority Nursing Tip: Moving into a position in which the knees are flexed may help decrease back pain.

Test-Taking Strategy: Focus on the **subject,** measures for relieving low back pain. Visualize each option. Eliminate option 2 because an abdominal support needs to be prescribed by an obstetrician. Eliminate option 3 because higher-heeled shoes can cause an unsafe condition. Eliminate option 4 because relaxing the abdominal muscles while standing can increase back discomfort.

---

49. The parent of a 5-year-old child who has been newly diagnosed with diabetes mellitus is very concerned about the changes that will occur in the family's life. What would the nurse discuss with the parent to promote growth within the family?

1. Diabetes care is now the most important aspect of the family.
2. The child's growth and development will be slower with a chronic illness.
3. The child needs to learn coping mechanisms to deal with the diagnosis and the changes in life it will bring.
4. All members of the family need to accept that the child will be given special treatment.

Level of Cognitive Ability: Applying
Client Needs: Health Promotion and Maintenance

Answer: 3
Rationale: The family and the child need to integrate the care but not let it overtake the family. The child needs to learn coping mechanisms to deal with the changes of a chronic illness. The other options do not demonstrate the integration of the diagnosis but rather allow it to overtake the family.
Priority Nursing Tip: The diagnosis and integration of a chronic illness needs to become a part of the child's life so that normal growth and development can occur.

Test-Taking Strategy: Focus on the **subject,** promoting growth within the family. Helping the child develop coping mechanisms is the only option that deals with a method to promote growth within the family.

Clinical Judgment/Cognitive Skills: Generate Solutions
Integrated Process: Nursing Process/Planning
Content Area: Pediatrics: Metabolic and Endocrine
Health Problem: Pediatric-Specific: Diabetes Mellitus

---

50. The nurse is obtaining a health history from a client and is collecting data regarding the risk factors associated with osteoporosis. Which piece of data reported by the client places the client at low risk for osteoporosis?
1 Medicates to relieve stress
2 Gets 7 hours of sleep nightly
3 Consumes a high-calcium diet
4 Attends religious services regularly

Level of Cognitive Ability: Analyzing
Client Needs: Health Promotion and Maintenance
Clinical Judgment/Cognitive Skills: Analyze Cues
Integrated Process: Nursing Process/Data Collection
Content Area: Adult Health: Musculoskeletal
Health Problem: Adult Health: Musculoskeletal: Osteoporosis

Answer: 3
Rationale: Risk factors associated with osteoporosis include a diet that is deficient in calcium. Options 1, 2, and 4, although healthy lifestyle choices, are not associated with osteoporosis prevention. Additional risk factors include postmenopausal age, long-term use of corticosteroids, family history of osteoporosis, sedentary lifestyle, and long-term use of anticonvulsants and furosemide.
Priority Nursing Tip: Engaging in weight-bearing exercise, such as walking, is essential in helping prevent osteoporosis.

Test-Taking Strategy: Focus on the **subject,** risk factors associated with osteoporosis. Note the words *low risk.* Recalling the causes and risk factors associated with osteoporosis directs you to option 3.

---

51. A postpartum nurse is caring for a client who delivered a baby 2 hours ago. The nurse palpates the fundus and notes the expected character of the lochia. How would the nurse document the discharge as being normal?
1 Pink-colored lochia
2 White-colored lochia
3 Serosanguineous lochia
4 Dark red–colored lochia

Level of Cognitive Ability: Applying
Client Needs: Health Promotion and Maintenance
Clinical Judgment/Cognitive Skills: Take Action
Integrated Process: Nursing Process/Data Collection
Content Area: Maternity: Postpartum
Health Problem: N/A

Answer: 4
Rationale: When checking the perineum, the lochia is monitored for amount, color, and presence of clots. The color of the lochia during the fourth stage of labor (the first 1 to 4 hours after birth) is a dark red color, indicating "old" blood, not new active bleeding. Options 1, 2, and 3 are not expected characteristics of the lochia at this stage postpartum.
Priority Nursing Tip: Immediately after delivery the lochia color is known as *rubra,* which is dark red in color.

Test-Taking Strategy: Focus on the **subject**, the expected character of lochia after delivery. Note that the question refers to a client who delivered 2 hours previously; this would direct you to the correct option.

---

52. The nurse reinforces home-care instructions to a client diagnosed with systemic lupus erythematosus (SLE). Which statement by the client indicates the **need for further instruction** regarding the measures to use to manage fatigue?

1. "I need to sit whenever possible."
2. "I need to avoid long periods of rest."
3. "I need to take a hot bath in the evening."
4. "I need to engage in moderate- to low-impact exercise when not fatigued."

Level of Cognitive Ability: Evaluating
Client Needs: Health Promotion and Maintenance
Clinical Judgment/Cognitive Skills: Evaluate Outcomes
Integrated Process: Teaching and Learning
Content Area: Adult Health: Immune
Health Problem: Adult Health: Immune: Autoimmune Disease

Answer: 3

Rationale: To help reduce fatigue in the client with SLE, the nurse would instruct the client to sit whenever possible, avoid hot baths, schedule moderate- to low-impact exercises when not fatigued, and maintain a balanced diet. The client is not instructed to rest for long periods, because this promotes joint stiffness.

Priority Nursing Tip: Activities that result in vasoconstriction can contribute to fatigue.

Test-Taking Strategy: Focus on the **subject,** management of fatigue in SLE. Note the **strategic words,** *need for further instruction.* These words indicate a **negative event query** and ask you to select an option that is an incorrect client statement. Think about the effect of each item in the options; this would direct you to the correct option.

---

53. The nurse, as part of the teaching plan, reviews the process of involution with a postpartum client. Which statement made by the client demonstrates accurate knowledge of this process?

1. "Involution refers to the inverted uterus that is beginning to return to normal."
2. "Involution refers to the gradual reversal of the uterine muscle into the abdominal cavity."
3. "Involution refers to the descent of the uterus into the pelvic cavity occurring at a rate of 2 cm daily."
4. "Involution is the progressive descent of the uterus into the pelvic cavity, occurring at a rate of approximately 1 cm per day."

Level of Cognitive Ability: Evaluating
Client Needs: Health Promotion and Maintenance
Clinical Judgment/Cognitive Skills: Evaluate Outcomes
Integrated Process: Nursing Process/Evaluation
Content Area: Maternity: Postpartum
Health Problem: Maternity: Postpartum Uterine Problems

Answer: 4

Rationale: Involution is the progressive descent of the uterus into the pelvic cavity. After birth, descent occurs at a rate of approximately 1 fingerbreadth or 1 cm per day. The other options are incorrect descriptions of this process.

Priority Nursing Tip: After delivery it is important for the uterus to involute, or return to its prepregnant size to minimize the risk for bleeding.

Test-Taking Strategy: Focus on the **subject,** the description of uterine involution. Knowledge of the definition and process of involution is necessary to answer this question. Use medical terminology to assist you with defining the term and selecting the correct option.

---

54. A client admitted to labor and delivery with a low-lying placenta asks the nurse about the purpose of the placenta. What would be the nurse's response?

1 "It cushions and protects the fetus."
2 "It maintains the body temperature of the fetus."
3 "It prevents antibodies and viruses from passing to the fetus."
4 "It provides an exchange of nutrients and waste products between parent and fetus."

Level of Cognitive Ability: Applying
Client Needs: Health Promotion and Maintenance
Clinical Judgment/Cognitive Skills: Take Action
Integrated Process: Teaching and Learning
Content Area: Maternity: Intrapartum
Health Problem: Maternity: Placenta Previa

Answer: 4
Rationale: The placenta provides an exchange of nutrients and waste products between the parent and the fetus. The amniotic fluid surrounds, cushions, protects, and maintains the body temperature of the fetus. Nutrients, medications, antibodies, and viruses can pass through the placenta.
Priority Nursing Tip: The placenta is an organ that attaches to the maternal uterine wall.

Test-Taking Strategy: Focus on the **subject**, the placenta, and use your knowledge of the purpose of the placenta and the amniotic fluid to answer this question. Remember that the placenta provides nutrients.

---

55. The nurse is preparing to check the fetal heartbeat of a woman who is at 12 weeks' gestation. Which piece of equipment is **most appropriate** for the nurse to use?

1 Doppler ultrasound
2 A fetal heart monitor
3 An adult stethoscope
4 The bell of a stethoscope

Level of Cognitive Ability: Applying
Client Needs: Health Promotion and Maintenance
Clinical Judgment/Cognitive Skills: Generate Solutions
Integrated Process: Nursing Process/Data Collection
Content Area: Maternity: Antepartum
Health Problem: N/A

Answer: 1
Rationale: A Doppler ultrasound device can be used to check the fetal heartbeat, and if used, the fetal heart rate (FHR) can be detected as early as 10 weeks' gestation. Options 3 and 4 do not adequately assess the fetal heartbeat. A fetal heart monitor is used during labor or in other situations when the FHR requires continuous monitoring.
Priority Nursing Tip: A Doppler ultrasound is a medical device that is used to obtain information about the status of the fetus.

Test-Taking Strategy: Focus on the **subject,** monitoring fetal heartbeats. Eliminate options 3 and 4 first because they are **comparable or alike** and because neither is used for such an assessment. Knowing that a fetal heart monitor is used for continuous monitoring directs you to option 1.

---

56. A client arrives at the prenatal clinic for a first assessment. The client tells the nurse that the first day of the last menstrual period (LMP) was August 19, 2023. Using Naegele's rule, the nurse determines that which is the estimated date of delivery?

1 May 26, 2024
2 June 12, 2024
3 June 26, 2024
4 May 12, 2024

Level of Cognitive Ability: Applying
Client Needs: Health Promotion and Maintenance

Answer: 1
Rationale: The accurate use of Naegele's rule requires that the client it is being applied to have a regular 28-day menstrual cycle. Add 7 days to the first day of the LMP, subtract 3 months, and then add 1 year to that date to obtain the estimated date of delivery. In this case, the first day of the LMP was August 19, 2023; add 7 days to get August 26, 2023; subtract 3 months to get May 26, 2023; and then add 1 year to get May 26, 2024.
Priority Nursing Tip: The estimated date of delivery (EDD) is a term describing the estimated delivery date for a pregnant client.

Clinical Judgment/Cognitive Skills: Analyze Cues
Integrated Process: Nursing Process/Data Collection
Content Area: Maternity: Antepartum
Health Problem: N/A

Test-Taking Strategy: Focus on the **subject,** Naegele's rule, and follow the steps of Naegele's rule to determine the estimated date of delivery. Read all of the options carefully, and note the dates and years before selecting an option.

---

57. The nurse reinforces home-care instructions to a client with a muscle injury taking diazepam 5 mg orally three times daily. Which statement by the client indicates the **need for additional instruction**?

1 "A glass of wine every day with dinner helps me relax."
2 "I know I need to continue taking the medication until I see my doctor."
3 "I was very drowsy when I began to take this medication, but now I feel all right."
4 "I will call my doctor if I have a cold and want to purchase medicine at the pharmacy."

Level of Cognitive Ability: Evaluating
Client Needs: Health Promotion and Maintenance
Clinical Judgment/Cognitive Skills: Evaluate Outcomes
Integrated Process: Teaching and Learning
Content Area: Pharmacology: Musculoskeletal: Muscle Relaxants
Health Problem: Adult Health: Musculoskeletal: Tissue or Ligament Injury

Answer: 1
Rationale: Diazepam is a benzodiazepine. If a central nervous system depressant (e.g., alcohol) is taken with a benzodiazepine, additive effects can occur that may cause respiratory depression or even be lethal. Diazepam may cause initial drowsiness. It would not be discontinued abruptly because the client may develop withdrawal symptoms. Many over-the-counter medications that are used to treat the flu contain ingredients that interact with diazepam.
Priority Nursing Tip: A person drinking alcohol while taking a benzodiazepine may be more sensitive to the usual effects of alcohol.

Test-Taking Strategy: Note the **strategic words,** *need for additional instruction.* These words indicate a **negative event query** and ask you to select an option that is an incorrect statement. Recalling that alcohol needs to be avoided with the administration of medication directs you to option 1.

---

58. A client diagnosed with peripheral vascular disease (PVD) asks the nurse what home-care measures can be implemented to help manage the symptoms. The nurse shares what information with the client?

1 "There is no current treatment."
2 "The veins, not the arteries, are affected."
3 "Warmth, exercise, and smoking cessation are most helpful."
4 "Analgesics are primarily used to control the symptom of pain."

Level of Cognitive Ability: Applying
Client Needs: Health Promotion and Maintenance
Clinical Judgment/Cognitive Skills: Take Action
Integrated Process: Teaching and Learning
Content Area: Adult Health: Cardiovascular
Health Problem: Adult Health: Cardiovascular: Vascular Disorders

Answer: 3
Rationale: The main goal of treatment for PVD is to increase circulation. This is accomplished by enhancing vasodilation through warmth, exercise, and smoking cessation. The other options are incorrect statements.
Priority Nursing Tip: With PVD, there may be an elevation in blood pressure because of the vasoconstricting effects of this health problem.

Test-Taking Strategy: Focus on the **subject,** increasing circulation. Option 1 is not true. PVD disorder has both arterial and venous involvement, which eliminates option 2. Option 4 is of limited use because the pain is caused by ischemia.

---

59. A client is being discharged with a peripherally inserted central catheter (PICC) site for continued home intravenous (IV) therapy. When planning for the discharge, the nurse reinforces which home-care measure to help prevent phlebitis and infiltration?

1. Cleanse the site daily with alcohol.
2. Gently massage the area around the site daily.
3. Immobilize the extremity until the IV is discontinued.
4. Keep the cannula stabilized or anchored properly with a transparent dressing.

Level of Cognitive Ability: Applying
Client Needs: Health Promotion and Maintenance
Clinical Judgment/Cognitive Skills: Generate Solutions
Integrated Process: Teaching and Learning
Content Area: Skills: Wound Care: Dressings
Health Problem: N/A

Answer: 4

Rationale: The principles of maintaining IV therapy at home are the same as in the hospital. It is important to ensure that the IV site is anchored properly to reduce the risk of phlebitis and infiltration. Massaging the site may actually contribute to catheter movement and tissue damage. Dressings that surround PICC sites are changed and cleansed at various times (usually every 7 days), depending on facility protocols. Most dressings are to remain intact unless they become wet, soiled, or loose. Immobilizing the extremity is not routinely necessary for PICC sites. Arm boards for immobilization are used only if a site is near a joint and the IV is positional.

Priority Nursing Tip: Keeping the PICC line anchored with a transparent dressing will allow for frequent assessments of the site and surrounding tissue.

Test-Taking Strategy: Focus on the **subject**, preventing phlebitis and infiltration. Recalling what these complications are and reading each option carefully will direct you to the correct option. Option 4 is the only action that will prevent these complications.

---

60. Diltiazem hydrochloride is prescribed for the client with Prinzmetal's angina. The nurse reinforces home-care instructions to the client regarding this medication. Which statement made by the client indicates the **need for further instruction**?

1. "I will take the medication after meals."
2. "I will call my doctor if shortness of breath occurs."
3. "I will rise slowly when getting out of bed in the morning."
4. "I will avoid activities that require alertness until my body gets used to the medication."

Level of Cognitive Ability: Evaluating
Client Needs: Health Promotion and Maintenance
Clinical Judgment/Cognitive Skills: Evaluate Outcomes
Integrated Process: Teaching and Learning
Content Area: Pharmacology: Cardiovascular: Calcium Channel Blockers
Health Problem: Adult Health: Cardiovascular/Coronary Artery Disease

Answer: 1

Rationale: Diltiazem hydrochloride is a calcium channel blocker. It is administered before meals on an empty stomach as prescribed. Hypotension can occur, and the client is instructed to rise slowly. The client needs to avoid tasks that require alertness until a response to the medication is established. The client needs to call the primary health care provider if an irregular heartbeat, shortness of breath, pronounced dizziness, nausea, or constipation occurs.

Priority Nursing Tip: Diltiazem hydrochloride may be prescribed to treat hypertension, angina, and dysrhythmias.

Test-Taking Strategy: Note the **strategic words,** *need for further instruction.* These words indicate a **negative event query** and ask you to select an option that is an incorrect statement. Recalling that this medication is used for angina and using general medication guidelines may assist you with eliminating the incorrect options.

---

61. The nurse explains the risk factors associated with breast cancer to a client. The nurse determines that the client **requires further explanation** when the client identifies what as a risk factor?

1 Late age of menopause
2 Late age of menarche
3 A history of breast cancer
4 A family history of breast cancer

Level of Cognitive Ability: Evaluating
Client Needs: Health Promotion and Maintenance
Clinical Judgment/Cognitive Skills: Evaluate Outcomes
Integrated Process: Teaching and Learning
Content Area: Adult Health: Oncology
Health Problem: Adult Health: Cancer: Breast

Answer: 2
Rationale: Factors that increase the risk for breast cancer include an early age of menarche and a late age of menopause, or more than 40 years of menses. Options 1, 3, and 4 are risk factors.
Priority Nursing Tip: Menstrual cycles result in exposure of the breast tissue to hormones increasing the risk for breast cancer, making early menarche a risk factor.

Test-Taking Strategy: Focus on the **subject,** risk factors for breast cancer, and note the **strategic words,** *requires further explanation.* These words indicate a **negative event query** and ask you to select an option that is an incorrect statement. You can easily eliminate options 3 and 4 because they are known risk factors for breast cancer. From the remaining options, remembering that a greater number of years of menses increases the risk directs you to the correct option.

---

62. When caring for a client diagnosed with peripheral vascular disease (PVD), the nurse incorporates measures to help the client cope with the lifestyle changes that are required to control the disease process. The nurse initiates a referral to which resource to help the client achieve this goal?

1 Occupational therapist
2 Medical social worker
3 Pain management clinic
4 Smoking-cessation program

Level of Cognitive Ability: Applying
Client Needs: Health Promotion and Maintenance
Clinical Judgment/Cognitive Skills: Take Action
Integrated Process: Nursing Process/Implementation
Content Area: Adult Health: Cardiovascular
Health Problem: Adult Health: Cardiovascular: Vascular Disorders

Answer: 4
Rationale: Smoking is highly detrimental to clients with PVD, and they are advised to stop smoking completely. Given that smoking is a form of chemical dependency, referral to a smoking-cessation program may be helpful for many clients. For many clients, symptoms are relieved or alleviated after they stop smoking. The other resources listed are unnecessary for this client based on the information presented in the question.
Priority Nursing Tip: Smoking affects the cardiovascular system, resulting in a higher risk of vasoconstriction and thrombus formation.

Test-Taking Strategy: Focus on the **subject,** lifestyle changes to control PVD. Recalling that this disorder is characterized by the inflammation and thrombosis of the large arteries will direct you to the correct option.

---

63. The nurse has reinforced home-care instructions to a client being discharged to home after an abdominal aortic aneurysm (AAA) resection. The nurse determines that the client understands the instructions if the client identifies what as an appropriate activity?

1 Driving an automobile
2 Playing 18 holes of golf
3 Lifting objects up to 30 pounds in weight

Answer: 4
Rationale: The client can walk as tolerated after the repair or resection of an AAA, including walking outdoors. Walking is a healthy and beneficial activity during the postoperative period. The client needs to avoid lifting objects that weigh more than 15 to 20 pounds for 6 to 12 weeks or engage in any activities that involve pushing, pulling, or straining. Driving is also prohibited for several weeks.
Priority Nursing Tip: After abdominal aortic aneurysm resection surgery, exercise would gradually be increased in strenuousness and duration.

4 Taking daily walks outdoors when the weather permits

Level of Cognitive Ability: Evaluating
Client Needs: Health Promotion and Maintenance
Clinical Judgment/Cognitive Skills: Evaluate Outcomes
Integrated Process: Nursing Process/Evaluation
Content Area: Adult Health: Cardiovascular
Health Problem: Adult Health: Cardiovascular/ Vascular Disorders

Test-Taking Strategy: Focus on the **subject,** AAA resection. To answer this question, evaluate each option in terms of the strain it could put on the sutured graft; this directs you to the correct option.

---

64. The nurse is reinforcing home-care dietary instructions with a client with hypertension prescribed triamterene. The nurse plans to include which item in a list of acceptable foods?

1 Oranges
2 Bananas
3 Baked potatoes
4 Pears canned in water

Level of Cognitive Ability: Applying
Client Needs: Health Promotion and Maintenance
Clinical Judgment/Cognitive Skills: Generate Solutions
Integrated Process: Teaching and Learning
Content Area: Pharmacology: Cardiovascular: Diuretics
Health Problem: Adult Health: Cardiovascular: Hypertension

Answer: 4
Rationale: Triamterene is a potassium-sparing diuretic, and clients taking this medication need to be cautioned against eating foods that are high in potassium unless they are taking a potassium-losing diuretic with it. Many foods are high in potassium, especially unprocessed foods and many vegetables, fruits, potatoes, and fresh meats. Because potassium is very water soluble, foods that are prepared in water are often lower in potassium. Of the options provided, pears canned in water provide the lowest source of potassium.
Priority Nursing Tip: Potassium-sparing diuretics are medications used as adjunctive therapy in the treatment of hypertension and management of heart failure.

Test-Taking Strategy: Focus on the **subject,** triamterene, and recall that triamterene is a potassium-sparing diuretic. Next, determine which food item is lowest in potassium and thus acceptable for the client to consume; this will direct you to the correct option.

---

65. The nurse has reinforced home-care instructions to the parents of a child after heart surgery. Which parent statement indicates the **need for further instruction**?

1 "My child can return to school for full days 1 week after discharge."
2 "My child needs to avoid crowds and people for 1 week after discharge."
3 "My child needs to be allowed to play inside but not outside at this time."
4 "I need to call the doctor if my child develops faster or harder breathing than normal."

Level of Cognitive Ability: Evaluating
Client Needs: Health Promotion and Maintenance
Clinical Judgment/Cognitive Skills: Evaluate Outcomes

Answer: 1
Rationale: The child who has undergone heart surgery can usually return to school the third week after hospital discharge but would go for only half-days for the first week (depending on surgeon preference). Returning to school for full days 1 week after discharge will be too strenuous for the child and will place the child at risk for infection. Outdoor play needs to be omitted for several weeks, and indoor play would be allowed as tolerated. The child needs to avoid crowds for 1 week after discharge, including crowds at day care centers and churches. The parents need to notify the surgeon if any difficulty with breathing occurs.
Priority Nursing Tip: After a cardiac surgery the child will be at high risk for infection.

Test-Taking Strategy: Note the **strategic words,** *need for further instruction.* These words indicate a **negative event query** and ask you to select an option that is an incorrect statement. Recalling the principles related to the prevention of infection and the complications of surgery directs you to the correct option.

Integrated Process: Teaching and Learning
Content Area: Pediatrics: Cardiovascular
Health Problem: Pediatric-Specific: Congenital Cardiac Defects

---

66. The nurse teaching female clients how to prevent pelvic inflammatory disease (PID) would include what instructions?

1 Douche monthly.
2 Avoid unprotected intercourse.
3 Single sexual partners need to be avoided.
4 Consult with a gynecologist regarding the placement of an intrauterine device (IUD).

Level of Cognitive Ability: Applying
Client Needs: Health Promotion and Maintenance
Clinical Judgment/Cognitive Skills: Take Action
Integrated Process: Teaching and Learning
Content Area: Adult Health: Reproductive
Health Problem: Adult Health: Reproductive: Inflammatory: Infections Problems

Answer: 2
Rationale: PID is any inflammatory condition of the female pelvic organs, especially one caused by a bacterial infection. The primary prevention of PID includes avoiding the following: unprotected intercourse, multiple sexual partners, the use of an IUD, and douching.
Priority Nursing Tip: Having unprotected sex can result in contracting sexually transmitted infections.

Test-Taking Strategy: Focus on the **subject,** measures for preventing PID. Read each option carefully. Recalling that the pelvic area is the focus of infection will help eliminate the incorrect options.

---

67. The nurse in a well-baby clinic is collecting data about the motor development of an 18-month-old child. Which activity demonstrates the highest level of development that the nurse would expect to note in this child?

1 The child is able to ride a tricycle.
2 The child snaps together large snaps.
3 The child builds a tower of 4 to 5 blocks.
4 The child puts on simple clothes independently.

Level of Cognitive Ability: Applying
Client Needs: Health Promotion and Maintenance
Clinical Judgment/Cognitive Skills: Analyze Cues
Integrated Process: Nursing Process/Data Collection
Content Area: Developmental Stages: Toddler
Health Problem: N/A

Answer: 3
Rationale: A child is expected to be able to build a tower of 4 to 5 blocks at the age of 18 months. A child would be able to ride a tricycle by 3 years of age. A child is expected to be able to snap large snaps and put on simple clothes independently at the age of 30 months.
Priority Nursing Tip: Normal growth and development proceed in an orderly, systemic, and predictable pattern, which provides a basis for identifying and assessing a child's abilities.

Test-Taking Strategy: Focus on the **subject,** developmental tasks for an 18-month-old. Visualize each of the fine motor skills presented in the options to help you select the correct option. Noting the age of the child directs you to the correct option.

---

68. The nurse reinforces instructions to a new breast-feeding parent. Which statement by the parent indicates the **need for further instruction**?

1 "I need to turn my newborn infant on their side facing me."
2 "When my newborn opens their mouth, I need to draw them the rest of the way onto my breast."
3 "I need to tilt my nipple upward or squeeze the areola and push it into my newborn infant's mouth."
4 "I need to place a clean finger in the side of my newborn infant's mouth to break the suction before removing my baby from my breast."

Level of Cognitive Ability: Evaluating
Client Needs: Health Promotion and Maintenance
Clinical Judgment/Cognitive Skills: Evaluate Outcomes
Integrated Process: Teaching and Learning
Content Area: Maternity: Newborn
Health Problem: Newborn: Newborn Feeding

Answer: 3

Rationale: The parent is instructed to avoid tilting the nipple upward or squeezing the areola and pushing it into the baby's mouth. Options 1, 2, and 4 are correct procedures for breast-feeding.

Priority Nursing Tip: It is important to bring the newborn to the breast when feeding.

Test-Taking Strategy: Note the **strategic words,** *need for further instruction.* These words indicate a **negative event query** and ask you to select an option that is an incorrect statement. Visualize the descriptions given in each of the options; this will help you eliminate the incorrect options. Reading option 3 carefully and noting that the word *push* suggests force or resistance would direct you to this option.

---

69. The parents of a male newborn who is not circumcised request information about how to clean the newborn's penis. The nurse would provide the parents with which **best** information?

1 "Retract the foreskin and cleanse the glans once a week."
2 "Retract the foreskin during cleaning to prevent adhesions."
3 "Retract the foreskin and cleanse the glans when bathing your newborn."
4 "Retract the foreskin slightly, no farther than it will easily go, and replace it over the glans after cleaning."

Level of Cognitive Ability: Applying
Client Needs: Health Promotion and Maintenance
Clinical Judgment/Cognitive Skills: Take Action
Integrated Process: Teaching and Learning
Content Area: Maternity: Newborn
Health Problem: Newborn: Circumcision

Answer: 4

Rationale: In newborn boys, the prepuce is continuous with the epidermis of the glans and is nonretractable. Forced retraction may cause adhesions to develop. It is best to allow separation to occur naturally, which takes place between 3 years of age and puberty. Most foreskins are retractable by 3 years of age and need to be pushed back gently for cleaning once a week.

Priority Nursing Tip: Male circumcision is a surgical procedure that involves the removal of the foreskin of the penis.

Test-Taking Strategy: Focus on the **subject,** care of an uncircumcised newborn. Note the **strategic word,** *best.* Note that options 1, 2, and 3 are **comparable or alike** in that they indicate the need to retract the foreskin. Although option 4 also mentions retracting the foreskin, note the word *slightly* to direct you to this option.

---

70. The nurse is teaching a client with peripheral vascular disease (PVD) about interventions to use to control the disease process. Which comment by the client would indicate a **need for further instruction**?

1. "I need to keep my legs cool."
2. "I need to take nifedipine as directed."
3. "I need to inspect my legs for signs of infection."
4. "I need to inspect my legs for signs of ulceration."

Level of Cognitive Ability: Evaluating
Client Needs: Health Promotion and Maintenance
Clinical Judgment/Cognitive Skills: Evaluate Outcomes
Integrated Process: Teaching and Learning
Content Area: Adult Health: Cardiovascular
Health Problem: Adult Health: Cardiovascular/ Vascular Disorders

Answer: 1

Rationale: PVD is an occlusive disease that affects the large arteries. Interventions are directed at preventing progression of PVD. The client needs to maintain warmth in the extremities, especially by avoiding exposure to cold. Other interventions include conveying the need for immediate smoking cessation and providing the medications prescribed for vasodilation (e.g., the calcium channel blocker nifedipine). The client needs to inspect the extremities and report signs of infection or ulceration.

Priority Nursing Tip: The client with peripheral vascular disease needs to practice self-care measures that will promote vasodilation.

Test-Taking Strategy: Note the **strategic words,** *need for further instruction.* These words indicate a **negative event query** and ask you to select an option that is an incorrect measure. Recalling that the client with PVD disease needs to maintain warmth in the extremities directs you to option 1.

---

71. The nurse is reinforcing teaching to a client about the self-administration of betamethasone dipropionate and albuterol for the treatment of asthma. The nurse determines that teaching has been **effective** when the client makes what statement?

1. "I'll keep the inhalers in the refrigerator."
2. "I can use an inhaler for a week past the expiration date."
3. "I will take the bronchodilator first, then the corticosteroid."
4. "I will take the corticosteroid first, wait a few minutes, and then take the bronchodilator."

Level of Cognitive Ability: Evaluating
Client Needs: Health Promotion and Maintenance
Clinical Judgment/Cognitive Skills: Evaluate Outcomes
Integrated Process: Teaching and Learning
Content Area: Pharmacology: Respiratory: Restrictive Airway Disease Agents
Health Problem: Adult Health: Respiratory: Asthma

Answer: 3

Rationale: When betamethasone dipropionate and albuterol are taken together, the bronchodilator needs to be taken first to open the airways. This allows for better penetration of the corticosteroid into the bronchial tree. In addition, the client needs to wait 5 minutes after administering the bronchodilator before administering the corticosteroid. Inhalers do not need to be refrigerated, and medication would not be taken after the expiration date.

Priority Nursing Tip: The initial treatment goal with asthma is to open the airway and then decrease swelling.

Test-Taking Strategy: Note the **strategic word,** *effective.* Option 2 is eliminated first because medication would not be taken past the expiration date. From the remaining options, recalling that the airways need to be dilated first will direct you to the correct option.

---

72. The nurse reinforces instructions to a parent about measures to reduce the incidence of gastroesophageal reflux disease (GERD) in their child. Which statement by the client indicates an understanding of these measures?

1 "I need to buy bottle nipples that have smaller holes."
2 "I need to add a small amount of cereal to my child's formula."
3 "I need to keep the formula as thin as I can to prevent spitting up."
4 "I will give my child larger feedings less often throughout the day."

Level of Cognitive Ability: Evaluating
Client Needs: Health Promotion and Maintenance
Clinical Judgment/Cognitive Skills: Evaluate Outcomes
Integrated Process: Nursing Process/Evaluation
Content Area: Pediatrics: Gastrointestinal
Health Problem: Pediatric-Specific: Gastroesophageal Reflux Disease

Answer: 2
Rationale: In GERD, the transfer of gastric contents into the esophagus occurs. When feeding the child with this disorder, the bottle nipple holes need to be larger to allow for the easy flow of thicker formula. This child's formula will most likely be thickened with 1 teaspoon to 1 tablespoon of cereal per ounce of formula to increase the consistency and decrease the incidence of regurgitation. The child needs to receive smaller feedings throughout the day.
Priority Nursing Tip: Rice cereal is often used to increase the thickness of formula.

Test-Taking Strategy: Focus on the **subject,** GERD, and note the words *understanding of these measures.* You are being asked to select an option that is a correct statement. To prevent regurgitation, formula can be thickened. Options 1, 3, and 4 could all result in regurgitation.

---

73. A licensed practical nurse is assisting a registered nurse at a health screening clinic. Which client behavior is significant and indicates the **need for further teaching** of stroke (brain attack) prevention education?

1 Eats a bowl of high-fiber grain cereal with skim milk for breakfast
2 Has a blood pressure of 120/70 mm Hg and has lost 10 pounds recently
3 Uses oral contraceptives and condoms for pregnancy and disease prevention
4 Works as the manager of a busy medical-surgical unit and jogs 2 miles each day

Level of Cognitive Ability: Evaluating
Client Needs: Health Promotion and Maintenance
Clinical Judgment/Cognitive Skills: Evaluate Outcomes
Integrated Process: Teaching and Learning
Content Area: Adult Health: Neurological
Health Problem: Adult Health: Neurological: Stroke

Answer: 3
Rationale: Obesity, hypertension, hyperlipidemia, smoking, and the use of oral contraceptives are all modifiable risk factors associated with stroke. Oral contraceptive use may be discouraged because of the side effect of clot formation. In option 1, the client eats a fairly low-fat meal. In option 2, the client has a normal blood pressure and has made a change in lifestyle. In option 4, the client has a stressful job but uses a stress-reduction method.
Priority Nursing Tip: A side effect of oral contraceptives is thrombosis formation.

Test-Taking Strategy: Note the **strategic words,** *need for further teaching.* These words indicate a **negative event query** and ask you to select an option that is a high-risk behavior. Recalling that the use of oral contraceptives carries a risk of clot formation will direct you to this option.

74. The nurse caring for an adult client who had a stroke (brain attack) plans to check the plantar reflex. What is the **best** way to elicit this reflex?

1 Tap the Achilles tendon with a reflex hammer.
2 Gently prick the client's skin on the dorsum of the foot in two places.
3 Firmly stroke the lateral sole of the foot and under the toes with a blunt instrument.
4 Hold the sides of the client's great toe, and, while moving it, ask the client what position it is in.

Level of Cognitive Ability: Applying
Client Needs: Health Promotion and Maintenance
Clinical Judgment/Cognitive Skills: Generate Solutions
Integrated Process: Nursing Process/Data Collection
Content Area: Adult Health: Neurological
Health Problem: Adult Health: Neurological: Stroke

Answer: 3
Rationale: The plantar reflex is elicited by firmly stroking the lateral sole of the foot and under the toes with a blunt instrument. The toes plantarflex normally, but they dorsiflex and fan out when an abnormal response is present. Option 1 assesses gastrocnemius muscle contraction, option 2 assesses two-point discrimination, and option 4 assesses proprioception.
Priority Nursing Tip: The Babinski's reflex occurs after the sole of the foot has been firmly stroked. The big toe then moves upward or toward the top surface of the foot. The other toes fan out. This reflex is normal in children up to 2 years old. When it is present in a child older than 2 years or present in an adult, it could be an indication of a central nervous system disorder.

Test-Taking Strategy: Focus on the **subject,** assessing the plantar reflex. Note the **strategic word,** *best.* Read each option carefully. Note the relationship between the subject and the correct option.

---

75. The nurse is assigned to reinforce dietary measures to a client with coronary artery disease. The nurse would plan to take what action **first** if the client expresses frustration with the dietary regimen?

1 Notify the registered nurse (RN).
2 Leave the client alone for a while.
3 Continue with the dietary teaching.
4 Identify the cause of the frustration.

Level of Cognitive Ability: Applying
Client Needs: Health Promotion and Maintenance
Clinical Judgment/Cognitive Skills: Prioritize Hypotheses
Integrated Process: Nursing Process/Data Collection
Content Area: Adult Health: Cardiovascular
Health Problem: Adult Health: Cardiovascular: Coronary Artery Disease

Answer: 4
Rationale: The first action by the nurse would be to determine the cause of the frustration. Continuing to teach and leaving the client alone may block the communication and learning processes. The RN may need to be notified of the client's frustration, but the first action is to determine the cause.
Priority Nursing Tip: When reinforcing information, it is important to determine what the client already knows and whether the client is adherent, and if not, to identify a reason for nonadherence.

Test-Taking Strategy: Note the **strategic word,** *first,* and use the **steps of the nursing process;** remember that data collection is the first step. Options 1, 2, and 3 represent the implementation phases of the nursing process. The only data collection choice is option 4.

---

76. The nurse is trying to determine the client's adjustment to a new diagnosis of coronary heart disease. Which question would the nurse ask to elicit the **most** useful response from the client?

Answer: 4
Rationale: Option 4 is the only question that is open-ended and explores the client's feelings about the disease. It requires more than a "yes" or "no" answer.

1 "Do you understand the use of your new medications?"
2 "Are you going to schedule your follow-up doctor visit?"
3 "Do you have anyone at home to help with housework and shopping?"
4 "How do you feel about the lifestyle changes you are planning to make?"

Level of Cognitive Ability: Applying
Client Needs: Health Promotion and Maintenance
Clinical Judgment/Cognitive Skills: Take Action
Integrated Process: Communication and Documentation
Content Area: Adult Health: Cardiovascular
Health Problem: Adult Health: Cardiovascular: Coronary Artery Disease

Priority Nursing Tip: Open-ended questions will elicit an answer that is more than a "yes" or "no."

Test-Taking Strategy: Note the **strategic word,** *most.* Use **therapeutic communication techniques** to direct you to the correct option. Closed-ended questions such as options 1, 2, and 3 generally elicit a "yes" or "no" response exclusively and would be avoided.

---

77. A licensed practical nurse (LPN) is assisting a school nurse with the routine health assessment of 11-year-old children. The LPN expects to assist with screening for what common health issue observed in this population?
1 Scoliosis
2 Meningitis
3 Congenital hip disorder
4 Phenylketonuria (PKU)

Level of Cognitive Ability: Applying
Client Needs: Health Promotion and Maintenance
Clinical Judgment/Cognitive Skills: Recognize Cues
Integrated Process: Nursing Process/ Data Collection
Content Area: Health Assessment: Physical Exam: Musculoskeletal
Health Problem: Pediatric-Specific: Scoliosis

Answer: 1
Rationale: Scoliosis is a common deformity that affects children who have some degree of spinal curvature. Screening for the disorder generally begins in the fifth grade. There is no routine screening test for meningitis. Congenital hip disorder and PKU are screened for in newborns.
Priority Nursing Tip: Neuromuscular screening for scoliosis is usually done when the child is in the fifth grade.

Test-Taking Strategy: Focus on the **subject,** a common health issue in an 11-year-old. Knowledge of disorders common to school-age children and of routine screenings is needed to select the correct option. Eliminate option 2 because there is no routine screening for meningitis. PKU is screened for in newborns, and the word *congenital* in option 3 suggests that it is screened for in infancy.

---

78. The nurse is teaching a class on health screening for testicular cancer. What would the nurse include as a major risk factor associated with the diagnosis?
1 Age of the male
2 Number of sexual partners
3 Geographic location of residence
4 Marital status and number of children

Level of Cognitive Ability: Applying
Client Needs: Health Promotion and Maintenance

Answer: 1
Rationale: Age is a basic but important risk factor for testicular cancer. The disease is the most common malignancy in males between the ages of approximately 15 and 40 years. Other risk factors include a history of undescended testis and a family history of testicular cancer. Options 2 and 4 are unrelated risk factors. Although geographic location of residence can be a consideration, it is not a major risk factor.
Priority Nursing Tip: The cause of testicular cancer is unknown, but a history of undescended testicle and genetic predisposition have been associated with the development of testicular tumors.

Clinical Judgment/Cognitive Skills: Generate Solutions
Integrated Process: Nursing Process/Implementation
Content Area: Adult Health: Oncology
Health Problem: Adult Health: Cancer: Testicular

Test-Taking Strategy: Focus on the **subject,** risk factors for testicular cancer. Knowledge of these risk factors for testicular cancer is needed to answer correctly. Remember that age is a basic but important risk factor for testicular cancer.

---

79. The nurse is assisting at a health screening clinic and collecting data from clients about environmental risk factors for neurological disorders. Which factors place a client at risk for a neurological disorder? **Select all that apply.**

❒ 1 Exposure to pesticides
❒ 2 Adequate lighting in the work area
❒ 3 Adequate ventilation in the work area
❒ 4 Exposure to secondhand smoke while pregnant
❒ 5 Exposure to fumes from things such as paints or glues

Level of Cognitive Ability: Analyzing
Client Needs: Health Promotion and Maintenance
Clinical Judgment/Cognitive Skills: Recognize Cues
Integrated Process: Nursing Process/Data Collection
Content Area: Adult Health: Neurological
Health Problem: N/A

Answer: 1, 4, 5
Rationale: The nurse assesses the risk of exposure to neurotoxic fumes and chemicals, including paint, bonding agents, and pesticides. The nurse also inquires about the adequacy of ventilation in the home and work area. The adequacy of lighting in the work area is unrelated to an environmental risk factor for a neurological disorder. Exposure to secondhand smoke while pregnant has been linked to behavioral disorders in the offspring.
Priority Nursing Tip: Long-term exposure to environmental toxins can lead to neurological disorders.

Test-Taking Strategy: Focus on the **subject,** environmental risk factors for neurological disorders. Noting the word *adequate* in options 2 and 3 will assist in eliminating these options.

---

80. The nurse is assisting with checking the reflexes of a client who had a stroke. How does the nurse expect that the pharyngeal reflex will be tested?

1 Stroking the skin on an abdominal quadrant
2 Stimulating the back of the throat with a tongue depressor
3 Stroking the outer plantar surface of the foot from heel to toe
4 Stimulating the perianal skin or gently inserting a gloved finger into the rectum

Level of Cognitive Ability: Applying
Client Needs: Health Promotion and Maintenance
Clinical Judgment/Cognitive Skills: Generate Solutions
Integrated Process: Nursing Process/Data Collection
Content Area: Adult Health: Neurological
Health Problem: Adult Health: Neurological: Stroke

Answer: 2
Rationale: The pharyngeal reflex is tested by touching the back of the throat with an object such as a tongue depressor. The abdominal reflex, the plantar reflex, and the anal reflex are described in options 1, 3, and 4, respectively. A positive response to each of these reflexes is considered normal.
Priority Nursing Tip: Pharyngeal reflex is also referred to as the *gag reflex.*

Test-Taking Strategy: Focus on the **subject,** the pharyngeal reflex. Recalling that the word *pharyngeal* refers to the pharynx or the back of the throat directs you to the correct option.

---

81. How does the nurse caring for a client diagnosed with atrial fibrillation check for a pulse deficit?

1. Palpating the radial pulse for quality while auscultating the apical pulse volume
2. Auscultating the apical pulse for a lower rate than the apical rate
3. Auscultating the apical pulse for a regular rate while palpating the radial pulse for quality
4. Palpating the radial pulse for quality while auscultating the apical pulse for an irregular rate

Level of Cognitive Ability: Applying
Client Needs: Health Promotion and Maintenance
Clinical Judgment/Cognitive Skills: Recognize Cues
Integrated Process: Nursing Process/Data Collection
Content Area: Adult Health: Cardiovascular
Health Problem: Adult Health: Cardiovascular: Dysrhythmias

Answer: 2

Rationale: In clients with atrial fibrillation, the pulse is irregular. Pulse deficit is a condition in which the peripheral pulse rate is less than the ventricular contraction rate and is a characteristic of atrial fibrillation. When a pulse rate is irregular, the apical pulse would be auscultated for the irregularity and the radial pulse would be palpated for the pulse deficit. The descriptions in options 1, 3, and 4 are inaccurate.

Priority Nursing Tip: Clients with atrial fibrillation are at a high risk for clot formation.

Test-Taking Strategy: Focus on the **subject,** pulse deficit, and consider the nature of atrial fibrillation. Option 2 is the only option that addresses the assessment of both the apical and radial pulses.

---

82. A client is seen in the health care clinic 2 weeks after a segmental resection of the upper lobe of the left lung. The nurse is assisting with collecting information from the client and notes that the client is sitting stiffly in the examining room chair with the right arm held close to the chest. The nurse determines that it is **most important** to ask the client about what subject?

1. The client's ability to ambulate
2. Dietary habits and the effectiveness of support services
3. Adherence to the prescribed arm and shoulder exercises
4. The physical characteristics of the client's house and the number of steps

Level of Cognitive Ability: Applying
Client Needs: Health Promotion and Maintenance
Clinical Judgment/Cognitive Skills: Recognize Cues
Integrated Process: Nursing Process/Data Collection
Content Area: Adult Health: Respiratory
Health Problem: Adult Health: Musculoskeletal: Tissue or Ligament Injury

Answer: 3

Rationale: Failure of the client to perform active range-of-motion exercises as prescribed after lung surgery allows for the formation of adhesions of the incised muscle layer and leads to dysfunction syndrome. Only option 3 relates to the information in the question.

Priority Nursing Tip: After a variety of surgeries it is important for the client to perform appropriate exercises to prevent the formation of muscle adhesions, which can result in difficulty with movement.

Test-Taking Strategy: Focus on the **strategic words,** *most important.* Note the words *sitting stiffly.* Focus on the client **data in the question** to direct you to the correct option. Only option 3 relates to the nurse's observations.

83. The nurse is evaluating a client's understanding of health measures to prevent coronary artery disease (CAD). Which client statement indicates a **need for further teaching**?

1 "I need to restrict my intake of fried foods."
2 "I could bring on a heart attack if I exercise."
3 "I need to take my medicines at the same times each day."
4 "If I quit smoking, I will eventually lose my risk for heart disease caused by smoking."

Level of Cognitive Ability: Evaluating
Client Needs: Health Promotion and Maintenance
Clinical Judgment/Cognitive Skills: Evaluate Outcomes
Integrated Process: Teaching and Learning
Content Area: Adult Health: Cardiovascular
Health Problem: Adult Health: Cardiovascular: Coronary Artery Disease

Answer: 2
Rationale: CAD affects the arteries that provide blood, oxygen, and nutrients to the myocardium. A sedentary lifestyle is a major risk factor for the development of CAD. Exercise may reduce the risk of CAD by decreasing weight, reducing blood pressure, and elevating the high-density lipoprotein level. All the other options are health measures to prevent CAD.
Priority Nursing Tip: Being overweight or obese can raise your risk of CAD and a heart attack. This is mainly because overweight and obesity are linked to other CAD risk factors, such as high blood cholesterol and triglyceride levels, high blood pressure, and diabetes.

Test-Taking Strategy: Focus on the **subject,** CAD, and note the **strategic words,** *need for further teaching.* These words indicate a **negative event query** and ask you to select an option that is an incorrect statement. Remember that exercise is a key component of preventing this disease.

---

84. The nurse is providing dietary instructions to a client diagnosed with a uric acid renal stone. Which dietary instruction would the nurse provide to the client?

1 Seafood is allowed in the diet.
2 Increase your intake of legumes.
3 Increase your intake of cranberries and citrus fruits.
4 Organ meat–type foods can be included in the diet.

Level of Cognitive Ability: Applying
Client Needs: Health Promotion and Maintenance
Clinical Judgment/Cognitive Skills: Take Action
Integrated Process: Teaching and Learning
Content Area: Adult Health: Renal and Urinary
Health Problem: Adult Health: Renal and Urinary: Obstructive Problems

Answer: 2
Rationale: Dietary interventions may be important for the management of renal stones. Dietary instructions to the client with a uric acid stone include increasing the intake of legumes, green vegetables, and fruits (except prunes, grapes, cranberries, and citrus fruits) to increase the alkalinity of the urine. The client would also be instructed to decrease purine sources, which include organ meats, gravies, red wines, goose, venison, and seafood.
Priority Nursing Tip: Organ meats include brain, liver, and tongue.

Test-Taking Strategy: Focus on the **subject,** acid renal stones. Recalling that the goal of treatment is to increase the alkalinity of the urine will direct you to the correct option.

---

85. The nurse reinforces home-care instructions to a client with Bell's palsy about treatment measures for the disorder. Which statement by the client indicates a **need for further instruction?**

1 "I need to eat small meals and soft foods frequently."

Answer: 3
Rationale: Bell's palsy is an acute and temporary paralysis of cranial nerve VII (facial nerve). Therapeutic management for the client with this condition includes providing moist heat packs to the affected area. The client is instructed to eat small amounts of soft foods frequently and to protect the affected eye by using an eye patch. The client is also instructed to use artificial tears

2 "I need to protect my affected eye by using an eye patch."
3 "I need to apply ice packs to the affected side of my face."
4 "I need to place artificial tears into my affected eye 4 times daily."

Level of Cognitive Ability: Evaluating
Client Needs: Health Promotion and Maintenance
Clinical Judgment/Cognitive Skills: Evaluate Outcomes
Integrated Process: Teaching and Learning
Content Area: Adult Health: Neurological
Health Problem: Adult Health: Neurological: Bell's Palsy

4 times daily and to manually close the affected eye from time to time.
Priority Nursing Tip: Prolonged vasoconstriction can result in Bell's palsy becoming a chronic condition.

Test-Taking Strategy: Note the **strategic words,** *need for further instruction.* These words indicate a **negative event query** and ask you to select an option that is an incorrect statement. Read each option carefully and consider the anatomical area that is affected to assist you with answering the question; this would direct you to the correct option.

---

86. While reviewing the nursing care plan of a hospitalized 6-year-old child who is immobilized because of skeletal traction, a licensed practical nurse notes that the child has a delayed growth and development problem because of immobilization and hospitalization. Which evaluative statement indicates a positive outcome for this child?
1 The fracture heals without complications.
2 The caregivers verbalize safe and effective home care.
3 The child maintains normal joint and muscle integrity.
4 The child displays age-appropriate developmental behaviors.

Level of Cognitive Ability: Evaluating
Client Needs: Health Promotion and Maintenance
Clinical Judgment/Cognitive Skills: Evaluate Outcomes
Integrated Process: Nursing Process/Evaluation
Content Area: Developmental Stages: Preschool and School Age
Health Problem: Pediatric-Specific: Fractures

Answer: 4
Rationale: Delayed growth and development is the state in which an individual is not performing age-appropriate tasks. Regression and inappropriate developmental behaviors may be displayed in response to immobilization and hospitalization. Options 1, 2, and 3 are appropriate evaluative statements for an immobilized child, but they do not directly address the problem of delayed growth and development.
Priority Nursing Tip: Children usually progress in a natural, predictable sequence from one developmental milestone to the next. But each child grows and gains skills at his or her own pace.

Test-Taking Strategy: Focus on the **subject,** a positive outcome for a child with delayed growth and development. All options are evaluative statements, but only option 4 addresses this problem.

---

87. The nurse is caring for a client with deep vein thrombosis (DVT) being discharged to home and has reinforced teaching about the signs of pulmonary embolism (PE). Which client statement indicates that the client identifies the clinical manifestations of PE?

Answer: 4
Rationale: The occurrence of DVT presents a risk of PE, which is when a dislodged blood clot travels to the pulmonary artery. Of the clinical manifestations of a PE, chest pain is the most common; coughing, diaphoresis, dyspnea, and apprehension are the other clinical manifestations. Pleuritic chest pain (sudden onset and aggravated by breathing) is caused by an inflammatory

1 "I will call you if I begin to get dizzy."
2 "I will notify you if anything unusual occurs."
3 "I will notify the doctor immediately if I become nauseous, start vomiting, and have diarrhea."
4 "I will notify the doctor immediately if I develop coughing, difficulty breathing, or chest pain."

Level of Cognitive Ability: Evaluating
Client Needs: Health Promotion and Maintenance
Clinical Judgment/Cognitive Skills: Evaluate Outcomes
Integrated Process: Nursing Process/Evaluation
Content Area: Adult Health: Respiratory
Health Problem: Adult Health: Respiratory: Pulmonary Embolism

reaction of the lung parenchyma or when there is a pulmonary infarction or ischemia caused by an obstruction of the small pulmonary arterial branches. Options 1, 2, and 3 provide inaccurate clinical descriptions of PE.
Priority Nursing Tip: Efforts to prevent pulmonary embolism include beginning to move as soon as possible after surgery, lower leg exercises during periods of sitting, and the use of blood thinners after some types of surgery.

Test-Taking Strategy: Focus on the **subject** and use your knowledge of the clinical manifestations of PE to answer the question. Think about the pathophysiology of this disorder. Recall that of the clinical manifestations of a PE, chest pain is the most common; this will direct you to the correct option.

---

88. A client has a prescription to begin using nitroglycerin transdermal patches for the management of coronary artery disease. The nurse providing home-care instructions for using nitroglycerin transdermal patches would include what information about this medication administration system?
1 Apply a new system every 7 days under the arm.
2 Place the medication system in a skin fold to promote better adherence.
3 Wait 1 day to apply a new system if the current one becomes dislodged.
4 Apply the system in the morning and leave it in place for 12 to 14 hours.

Level of Cognitive Ability: Applying
Client Needs: Health Promotion and Maintenance
Clinical Judgment/Cognitive Skills: Take Action
Integrated Process: Teaching and Learning
Content Area: Pharmacology: Cardiovascular: Antianginal Medications (Nitrates)
Health Problem: Adult Health: Cardiovascular: Coronary Artery Disease

Answer: 4
Rationale: Nitroglycerin is a coronary vasodilator used for the management of coronary artery disease and angina pectoris. The client is generally advised to apply a new system each morning and to leave it in place for 12 to 14 hours, per primary health care provider or cardiology instructions; this prevents the client from developing tolerance, which happens with 24-hour use. The client needs to avoid placing the system in skin folds. The client can apply a new system if the current one becomes dislodged because the dose is released continuously in small amounts through the skin.
Priority Nursing Tip: As prescribed, a new nitroglycerin transdermal patch would be applied daily in an area that is free of excoriation and left in place for 12 to 14 hours.

Test-Taking Strategy: Focus on the **subject,** client instructions for nitroglycerin transdermal patches. Specific information about this type of medication administration system is needed to answer this question correctly. Remember that with a nitroglycerin transdermal patch, a new system is applied each morning and left in place for 12 to 14 hours, per primary health care provider or cardiology instructions.

---

89. The nurse reinforces teaching to the client with bronchitis to do what to help clear the bronchial secretions?

1 Get more exercise each day.
2 Use a dehumidifier in the home.
3 Take in increased amounts of fluids every day.
4 Administer an extra dose of medication before bedtime.

Answer: 3

Rationale: The client needs to take in increased fluids to make secretions less viscous and for help with expectorating them. This is standard advice given to clients receiving a bronchodilator unless the client has another health problem that could be worsened by increased fluid intake. A dehumidifier will dry secretions. The client is not advised to take additional medication. Additional exercise will not effectively clear bronchial secretions.

Priority Nursing Tip: Increasing fluids to 2000 to 3000 mL/day is helpful in making respiratory secretions less viscous.

Test-Taking Strategy: Focus on the **subject,** bronchial secretions, and use your knowledge of the measures that aid in effectively dealing with their removal. Recalling basic respiratory principles directs you to the correct option.

Level of Cognitive Ability: Applying
Client Needs: Health Promotion and Maintenance
Clinical Judgment/Cognitive Skills: Take Action
Integrated Process: Teaching and Learning
Content Area: Adult Health: Respiratory
Health Problem: Adult Health/Respiratory: Upper Airway

---

90. A client is taking an oral daily dose of amiloride hydrochloride to treat hypertension. The nurse gives the client which home-care instruction about its use?

1 Take the dose in the morning.
2 Take the dose on an empty stomach.
3 Withhold the dose if the blood pressure is high.
4 Eat foods with extra sodium while taking this medication.

Answer: 1

Rationale: Amiloride is a potassium-sparing diuretic used to treat edema or hypertension. A daily dose needs to be taken in the morning to avoid nocturia, and the dose would be taken with food to increase bioavailability. Sodium needs to be restricted if the medication is used as an antihypertensive. Increased blood pressure is not a reason to hold the medication, although it may be an indication for its use.

Priority Nursing Tip: Potassium-sparing diuretics have the potential to cause hyperkalemia.

Test-Taking Strategy: Focus on the **subject,** client instructions about amiloride hydrochloride. Recalling that this medication is a potassium-sparing diuretic will direct you to the correct option.

Level of Cognitive Ability: Applying
Client Needs: Health Promotion and Maintenance
Clinical Judgment/Cognitive Skills: Take Action
Integrated Process: Nursing Process/Implementation
Content Area: Pharmacology: Cardiovascular: Diuretics
Health Problem: Adult Health: Cardiovascular: Hypertension

---

91. The nurse reinforces home-care medication instructions to a client who is taking lithium carbonate to treat a mood disorder. The nurse determines that the client **requires further instruction** when the client states what intention?

1 To take the lithium with meals
2 To decrease fluid intake while taking the lithium
3 That lithium blood levels must be monitored very closely

Answer: 2

Rationale: Lithium carbonate is an antimanic and antidepressant medication. Because therapeutic and toxic dosage ranges are so close, lithium blood levels must be monitored very closely; they are reviewed more frequently at first and then once every several months. The client would be instructed to stop taking the medication if excessive diarrhea, vomiting, or diaphoresis occurs and to inform the psychiatrist. Lithium is irritating to the gastric mucosa, so it would be taken with meals. A normal diet and normal intake of salt and fluid need to be maintained because lithium decreases sodium reabsorption by the renal tubules, which could cause

4 To stop taking the medication if excessive diarrhea, vomiting, or diaphoresis occurs

Level of Cognitive Ability: Evaluating
Client Needs: Health Promotion and Maintenance
Clinical Judgment/Cognitive Skills: Evaluate Outcomes
Integrated Process: Teaching and Learning
Content Area: Pharmacology: Psychotherapeutic: Mood Stabilizers
Health Problem: Mental Health: Mood Disorders

sodium depletion. A low sodium intake causes a relative increase in lithium retention and could lead to toxicity.
Priority Nursing Tip: A fluid intake of 1500 to 3000 mL/day or six 12-oz glasses is considered normal.

Test-Taking Strategy: Focus on the **subject,** lithium carbonate, and note the **strategic words,** *requires further instruction.* These words indicate a **negative event query** and ask you to select an option that is an incorrect statement. Remembering that it is generally important that clients be taught to maintain an adequate fluid intake directs you to the correct option.

---

92. The nurse is reinforcing home-care instructions to a client with hypertension about quinapril hydrochloride. Which instruction would the nurse give to the client?

1 Take the medication with food only.
2 Discontinue the medication if nausea occurs.
3 Rise slowly from a lying to a sitting position.
4 A therapeutic effect will be seen immediately.

Level of Cognitive Ability: Applying
Client Needs: Health Promotion and Maintenance
Clinical Judgment/Cognitive Skills: Take Action
Integrated Process: Teaching and Learning
Content Area: Pharmacology: Cardiovascular: Angiotensin-Converting Enzyme (ACE) Inhibitor
Health Problem: Adult Health: Cardiovascular: Hypertension

Answer: 3
Rationale: Quinapril hydrochloride is an angiotensin-converting enzyme inhibitor used for the treatment of hypertension. The client would be instructed to rise slowly from a lying to a sitting position and to permit the legs to dangle from the bed momentarily before standing to reduce the hypotensive effect. The medication may be given without regard to food. The client would be instructed to take a noncola carbonated beverage and salted crackers or dry toast if nausea occurs. The full therapeutic effect may take place after 1 to 2 weeks.
Priority Nursing Tip: Orthostatic hypotension presents an increased risk for falls.

Test-Taking Strategy: Focus on the **subject,** client instructions for quinapril hydrochloride. Eliminate option 1 because of the **closed-ended word** *only* and option 4 because of the word *immediately.* From the remaining options, recalling that the medication is used for the treatment of hypertension directs you to the correct option.

---

93. The nurse is reinforcing instructions to the client about the antiparkinsonian medication benztropine mesylate. The nurse determines that the client **requires further instruction** if the client makes which statement?

1 "I will avoid driving if I become drowsy or dizzy."
2 "I will watch my urinary output and watch for signs of constipation."
3 "I will spend 1 hour each day sitting in the sun during quiet periods."
4 "I will call my doctor if I have difficulty swallowing or vomiting occurs."

Answer: 3
Rationale: The client taking benztropine mesylate needs to be instructed to avoid driving or operating hazardous equipment if drowsy or dizzy. Tolerance to heat may be reduced because of a diminished ability to sweat, and the client needs to be instructed to plan rest periods in cool places during the day. The client needs to be instructed to stop taking the medication if vomiting or difficulty swallowing or speaking occurs. The client needs to also inform the prescriber if central nervous system effects occur. The client needs to be instructed to monitor urinary output and to watch for signs of constipation.
Priority Nursing Tip: Parkinson's disease (PD) is a type of movement disorder. It happens when nerve cells in the brain do not produce enough of a brain chemical called *dopamine.*

Level of Cognitive Ability: Evaluating
Client Needs: Health Promotion and Maintenance
Clinical Judgment/Cognitive Skills: Evaluate Outcomes
Integrated Process: Teaching and Learning
Content Area: Pharmacology: Neurological: Antiparkinsonian
Health Problem: Adult Health: Neurological: Parkinson's Disease

Test-Taking Strategy: Focus on the **subject**, client instructions for benztropine mesylate, and note the **strategic words**, *requires further instruction*. These words indicate a **negative event query** and ask you to select an option that is an incorrect statement. Recalling that this medication causes a reduced tolerance to heat directs you to the correct option.

---

94. The nurse is reinforcing home-care instructions to a client after a corneal transplant. Which statement by the client indicates the **need for further instruction**?

1 "I need to avoid bending over and lifting heavy objects."
2 "I need to avoid crowded environments and smoke-filled areas."
3 "Within a week after surgery, I should be able to return to work."
4 "Depending on my rate of healing, the sutures should be removed in 3 days."

Level of Cognitive Ability: Evaluating
Client Needs: Health Promotion and Maintenance
Clinical Judgment/Cognitive Skills: Evaluate Outcomes
Integrated Process: Teaching and Learning
Content Area: Adult Health: Eye
Health Problem: Adult Health: Eye: Corneal Problems

Answer: 4
Rationale: A corneal transplant is the surgical removal of diseased corneal tissue followed by replacement with tissue from a human donor cornea. The client is told that the sutures are usually left in place for as long as 6 months or as prescribed by the surgeon. After the sutures are removed and complete healing has occurred, glasses or contact lenses will be prescribed. Options 1, 2, and 3 are correct discharge instructions for the client after corneal transplant.
Priority Nursing Tip: Corneal graft rejection is the most common cause of graft failure.

Test-Taking Strategy: Note the **strategic words**, *need for further instruction*. These words indicate a **negative event query** and ask you to select an option that is an incorrect statement. Focus on the **subject**, corneal transplant, and recall that any activities that tend to increase intraocular pressure are avoided; this will help you eliminate options 1 and 3. Knowing that crowded environments and smoke-filled areas increase the chance of inflammation and infection will assist you with eliminating option 2.

---

95. The registered nurse in charge of the clinic instructs the licensed practical nurse (LPN) to perform a voice test to assess the client's hearing. What action demonstrates that the LPN is appropriately performing the screening?

1 Whispering a question while the client blocks one ear canal
2 Facing the client and whispering a question while the client blocks both ears
3 Facing the back to the client, whispering a statement, and having the client repeat it
4 Standing 4 feet away from the client and then talking to determine whether the client can hear

Answer: 1
Rationale: The nurse would stand 1 to 2 feet away from the client and ask the client to block one external ear canal. The nurse then quietly whispers a statement and asks the client to repeat it. Each ear is tested separately. Options 2, 3, and 4 are incorrect.
Priority Nursing Tip: When performing a voice test screening, the examiner would quietly exhale before whispering to ensure as quiet a voice as possible.

Test-Taking Strategy: Focus on the **subject**, performing the whispered voice test. Eliminate options 2 and 3 because they are not measures that would effectively assess hearing. Eliminate option 4 because distance hearing is not the subject of the question. This leaves option 1 as the correct option.

Level of Cognitive Ability: Applying
Client Needs: Health Promotion and Maintenance
Clinical Judgment/Cognitive Skills: Evaluate Outcomes
Integrated Process: Nursing Process/Data Collection
Content Area: Health Assessment: Physical Exam: Head, Eyes, Ears, Nose, Throat
Health Problem: Adult Health: Ear: Hearing Loss

---

96. The nurse is reinforcing home-care instructions to a client after a hydrocelectomy. Which statement by the client indicates the **need for further instruction**?

1 "I need to avoid sexual intercourse now."
2 "I need to apply ice packs to the scrotum."
3 "The sutures will be removed by the doctor in 2 weeks."
4 "I need to keep the scrotum elevated until the swelling has gone away."

Level of Cognitive Ability: Evaluating
Client Needs: Health Promotion and Maintenance
Clinical Judgment/Cognitive Skills: Evaluate Outcomes
Integrated Process: Teaching and Learning
Content Area: Adult Health: Reproductive
Health Problem: Adult Health: Reproductive: Inflammatory/Infections/Problems

Answer: 3
Rationale: A hydrocele is an abnormal collection of fluid within the layers of the tunica vaginalis that surrounds the testis. It may be unilateral or bilateral, and it can occur in an infant or an adult. Hydrocelectomy is the excision of the fluid-filled sac in the tunica vaginalis. The client would be instructed that the sutures used during the hydrocelectomy are absorbable. The other options are correct.
Nursing Priority Tip: Hydrocele may be caused by an infection or by injury to the testicle, but many times the cause is unknown.

Test-Taking Strategy: Focus on the **subject,** hydrocelectomy, and note the **strategic words,** *need for further instruction.* These words indicate a **negative event query** and ask you to select an option that is an incorrect statement. Focus on the anatomical location of the surgical procedure to direct you to the correct option.

---

97. The nurse reinforces instructions to a client with coronary artery disease about administering nitroglycerin ointment. The nurse determines that the client is using the correct technique when demonstrating what action?

1 Reapplying the ointment after bathing
2 Gently rubbing the ointment into the skin
3 Applying additional ointment when chest pain occurs
4 Placing the ointment on a nonhairy area of the upper body

Level of Cognitive Ability: Evaluating
Client Needs: Health Promotion and Maintenance

Answer: 4
Rationale: Nitroglycerin ointment is used on a scheduled basis and is not prescribed specifically for chest pain. The ointment is applied to a nonhairy area of the upper body and is not rubbed into the skin. It is reapplied only as directed.
Priority Nursing Tip: Instruct the client to rotate sites and to avoid touching the ointment when applying.

Test-Taking Strategy: Focus on the **subject,** using the correct technique for administering nitroglycerin ointment. Recalling the medication principles related to the application of ointments will direct you to the correct option.

Clinical Judgment/Cognitive Skills: Evaluate Outcomes
Integrated Process: Nursing Process/Evaluation
Content Area: Pharmacology: Cardiovascular: Antianginal Medications (Nitrates)
Health Problem: Adult Health: Cardiovascular: Coronary Artery Disease

---

98. A client is being discharged to home after the application of a plaster leg cast. The nurse gives the client which instruction about cast care?

1 Avoid getting the cast wet.
2 Cover the casted leg with warm blankets.
3 Use the fingertips to lift and move the leg.
4 Use a soft knitting needle to scratch under the cast.

Level of Cognitive Ability: Applying
Client Needs: Health Promotion and Maintenance
Clinical Judgment/Cognitive Skills: Take Action
Integrated Process: Teaching and Learning
Content Area: Adult Health: Musculoskeletal
Health Problem: Adult Health: Musculoskeletal: Skeletal Injury

Answer: 1
Rationale: A plaster cast must remain dry to keep its strength. The cast needs to be handled with the palms of the hands (not the fingertips) until it is fully dry. Air needs to circulate freely around the cast to help it dry; the cast also gives off heat as it dries. The client would never scratch under the cast, although a hair dryer set at a cool setting may be used if the skin becomes itchy.
Priority Nursing Tip: A safety goal for plaster cast application is to promote drying of the plaster to avoid indenting, which can result in the development of skin breakdown and an infection.

Test-Taking Strategy: Focus on the **subject,** a plaster leg cast. Option 4 is dangerous to skin integrity and is immediately eliminated. Recalling that a wet cast can be dented with the fingertips, causing pressure underneath, will assist you with eliminating option 3. Knowing that the cast needs air circulation to dry helps you eliminate option 2. Option 1 is correct because getting the plaster cast wet would promote the formation of indentions.

---

99. A client with an acute gastric ulcer is being discharged to home with a prescription for sucralfate, 1 g by mouth 4 times daily. The nurse reinforces that the client needs to take the medication at what time?

1 With meals and at bedtime
2 Every 6 hours around the clock
3 1 hour after meals and at bedtime
4 1 hour before meals and at bedtime

Level of Cognitive Ability: Applying
Client Needs: Health Promotion and Maintenance
Clinical Judgment/Cognitive Skills: Take Action
Integrated Process: Teaching and Learning
Content Area: Pharmacology: Gastrointestinal: Gastric Protectants
Health Problem: Adult Health: Gastrointestinal: Upper GI Disorders

Answer: 4
Rationale: Sucralfate would be scheduled for administration 1 hour before meals and at bedtime. Administration at these times allows the medication to form a protective coating over the ulcer before food intake stimulates gastric acid production and mechanical irritation. The bedtime dose protects the stomach lining during sleep. All the other options are incorrect for these reasons.
Priority Nursing Tip: Taking sucralfate before meals will assist in protecting the ulcer because meals increase the production of gastric secretions.

Test-Taking Strategy: Focus on the **subject,** administration of sucralfate and the client's diagnosis. Recalling that sucralfate protects damaged mucosa from further destruction will direct you to the correct option.

100. When carbamazepine is prescribed to a client for the management of generalized tonic-clonic seizures, the nurse reinforces instructions to the client about the possible adverse effects associated with the medication. The nurse also conveys to the client the importance of informing the neurologist if what occurs?

1 Nausea
2 Dizziness
3 Drowsiness
4 Dark-colored urine

Level of Cognitive Ability: Applying
Client Needs: Health Promotion and Maintenance
Clinical Judgment/Cognitive Skills: Take Action
Integrated Process: Teaching and Learning
Content Area: Pharmacology: Neurological: Anticonvulsants
Health Problem: Adult Health: Neurological: Seizure Disorder/Epilepsy

Answer: 4
Rationale: Carbamazepine is an anticonvulsant, antineuralgic, antimanic, and antipsychotic medication. Drowsiness, dizziness, nausea, and vomiting are frequent side effects associated with the medication. Adverse reactions include blood dyscrasias, petechiae, and dark-colored urine; these need to be reported immediately because they could indicate bleeding.
Priority Nursing Tip: The development of a fever, sore throat, mouth ulcerations, or joint pain when the client is taking carbamazepine may indicate a blood dyscrasia has developed.

Test-Taking Strategy: Focus on the **subject,** adverse effects of carbamazepine. Review each item in the options and think about the difference between side effects and adverse effects. Recalling that blood dyscrasias can occur with the use of carbamazepine directs you to the correct option.

---

101. The nurse is collecting data from a client who was admitted to the hospital with reports of anorexia, weight loss, fever, night sweats, and a persistent cough; tuberculosis (TB) is suspected. Based on these symptoms, what is the nurse's **initial priority** nursing action?

1 Admitting the client in a private room
2 Checking the client's vital signs, including blood pressure
3 Contacting respiratory therapy to initiate any prescribed treatments
4 Inserting an intravenous (IV) catheter and beginning an infusion of fluids

Level of Cognitive Ability: Applying
Client Needs: Health Promotion and Maintenance
Clinical Judgment/Cognitive Skills: Prioritize Hypotheses
Integrated Process: Nursing Process/Implementation
Content Area: Foundations of Care: Infection Control
Health Problem: Adult Health: Respiratory: Tuberculosis

Answer: 1
Rationale: A diagnosis of TB would be considered for any client with a persistent cough or other symptoms that suggest TB, such as weight loss, anorexia, fatigue, night sweats, and fever. Based on the symptoms presented, it is important to isolate the client until a definitive diagnosis is achieved.
Priority Nursing Tip: Infection control is a high priority for a client with tuberculosis.

Test-Taking Strategy: Focus on the **data in the question.** Note the **strategic words,** *initial priority*. Recalling the pathophysiology associated with tuberculosis and its infectious nature will direct you to option 1. The question is also referring to the initial priority, which would include isolating the client as soon as admitted to the unit.

---

102. The nurse reinforces teaching to a pregnant client diagnosed with human immunodeficiency virus (HIV) about measures to prevent an opportunistic infection. Which client statement indicates an understanding of these measures?

1. "I plan to have a natural childbirth experience."
2. "Tomorrow I will go to my niece's sixth birthday party."
3. "I will always wash my hands before consuming any food."
4. "I know I must have a cesarean section to avoid infecting my baby."

Level of Cognitive Ability: Evaluating
Client Needs: Health Promotion and Maintenance
Clinical Judgment/Cognitive Skills: Evaluate Outcomes
Integrated Process: Nursing Process/Evaluation
Content Area: Maternity: Antepartum
Health Problem: Maternity: Infections/Inflammations

Answer: 3

Rationale: Attending a party with many preschool children may increase the client's exposure to colds and opportunistic infections. Clients need to always wash their hands before consuming any foods to prevent ingestion of any pathogens. A pregnant client with HIV may have a normal, spontaneous vaginal delivery; however, this is not related to methods of preventing infection.

Priority Nursing Tip: Individuals with a compromised immune system are at risk for opportunistic infections.

Test-Taking Strategy: Focus on the **subject,** measures to prevent an opportunistic infection. Option 1 is unrelated to infection. Option 2 exposes the client to the risk of infection. Option 4 is not a measure to prevent an opportunistic infection.

---

103. The nurse has reinforced home-care instructions to a client who is about to be discharged after a prostatectomy for cancer of the prostate. Which statement by the client indicates an understanding of the instructions?

1. "I can begin to drive my car in 1 week."
2. "I cannot lift anything that weighs more than 20 pounds."
3. "If I see any clots in my urine, I need to call my surgeon immediately."
4. "To prevent the dribbling of urine, I need limit my fluid intake to 4 glasses per day."

Level of Cognitive Ability: Evaluating
Client Needs: Health Promotion and Maintenance
Clinical Judgment/Cognitive Skills: Evaluate Outcomes
Integrated Process: Nursing Process/Evaluation
Content Area: Adult Health: Renal and Urinary
Health Problem: Adult Health: Cancer: Prostate

Answer: 2

Rationale: The client would be instructed to avoid lifting objects that weigh more than 20 pounds for at least 6 weeks. Small pieces of tissue or blood clots can be passed during urination for up to 2 weeks after surgery; if they are noticed, the surgeon does not need to be notified immediately. Driving a car and sitting for long periods are restricted for at least 3 weeks. A high daily fluid intake of 2 to 2.5 L/day needs to be maintained to limit clot formation and prevent infection.

Priority Nursing Tip: It is important to instruct the client to limit lifting after a major surgical procedure to prevent trauma to the surgical site.

Test-Taking Strategy: Focus on the **subject,** client instructions after prostatectomy. Option 4 can be eliminated first because of the word *limit.* Eliminate option 1 next because 1 week is a rather short period. Recalling that blood clots in the urine are expected after this type of surgery will help direct you to the correct option.

---

104. The nurse is reinforcing instructions to a client who will be discharged with an axillary drain in place after mastectomy. Which statement by the client indicates the **need for further instruction?**

1 "I need to keep my arm elevated when I sit or lie down."
2 "I can massage the area with lotion after the incision heals."
3 "I may feel pain in the breast even though it has been removed."
4 "I need to begin full range-of-motion (ROM) exercises to my upper arm immediately."

Level of Cognitive Ability: Evaluating
Client Needs: Health Promotion and Maintenance
Clinical Judgment/Cognitive Skills: Evaluate Outcomes
Integrated Process: Teaching and Learning
Content Area: Adult Health: Oncology
Health Problem: Adult Health: Cancer: Breast

Answer: 4
Rationale: The client would be instructed to limit upper-arm ROM to the level of the shoulder only. After the axillary drain is removed, the client can begin full ROM exercises of the upper arm if prescribed by the surgeon. Options 1, 2, and 3 are correct measures after a mastectomy.
Priority Nursing Tip: After mastectomy, care must be taken to prevent the ROM exercises from dislodging the axillary drain.

Test-Taking Strategy: Focus on the **subject**, care after mastectomy. Note the **strategic words,** *need for further instruction.* These words indicate a **negative event query** and ask you to select an option that is an incorrect statement. Also note the word *full* in the correct option.

---

105. Prescriptive glasses are prescribed for a client with bilateral aphakia, and the nurse reinforces instructions to the client about the use of the glasses. Which statement by the client indicates the **need for further instruction**?

1 "Objects that I look at may be distorted."
2 "It may be difficult to judge distances when I drive a car."
3 "The prescriptive glasses will correct my visual field of sight."
4 "The prescriptive glasses will magnify my central vision by 30%."

Level of Cognitive Ability: Evaluating
Client Needs: Health Promotion and Maintenance
Clinical Judgment/Cognitive Skills: Evaluate Outcomes
Integrated Process: Teaching and Learning
Content Area: Adult Health: Eye
Health Problem: Adult Health: Eye: Visual Problems/Refractive Errors

Answer: 3
Rationale: Aphakia can be corrected with prescriptive glasses, contact lenses, or intraocular lenses. Only central vision is corrected with prescriptive glasses; peripheral vision is distorted. There is a magnification of the central vision of approximately 30% with prescriptive glasses; this requires the adjustment of daily activities and safety precautions. Because of the magnification, objects viewed centrally appear distorted, and it is difficult to judge distances when driving a car.
Priority Nursing Tip: Aphakia is the absence of the lens of the eye.

Test-Taking Strategy: Note the **strategic words,** *need for further instruction.* These words indicate a **negative event query** and ask you to select an option that is an incorrect statement. Think about the use of glasses and the visual field as you answer the question; this will direct you to the correct option.

---

106. A client is brought to the ambulatory care department 1 day after a cataract extraction procedure. The client is diagnosed with hyphema resulting from the surgical procedure. The nurse reinforces home-care instructions that encourage what action?

1 Maintaining rest periods
2 Taking aspirin every 12 hours
3 Patching of both eyes for a period of at least 1 week
4 Resuming normal activities because the condition will self-resolve

Level of Cognitive Ability: Applying
Client Needs: Health Promotion and Maintenance
Clinical Judgment/Cognitive Skills: Take Action
Integrated Process: Teaching and Learning
Content Area: Adult Health: Eye
Health Problem: Adult Health: Eye: Cataracts

Answer: 1
Rationale: Hyphema is bleeding into the anterior chamber of the eye; it can occur postoperatively as a complication of cataract surgery. Treatment includes rest and the client should not resume normal activities until the condition resolves. Cycloplegics and corticosteroid drops may be prescribed. Aspirin is avoided because it can increase the risk of bleeding. Patching both eyes is not helpful. Therefore options 2, 3, and 4 are incorrect.
Priority Nursing Tip: Following cataract extraction, the client would be instructed to monitor for signs of increased intraocular pressure, which commonly causes sudden ocular pain.

Test-Taking Strategy: Focus on the **subject,** hyphema after cataract surgery. Recalling that hyphema is bleeding in the eye will assist in answering correctly.

---

107. The nurse reinforces home-care instructions to a client with Raynaud's phenomenon and encourages the client to engage in measures that will minimize the effects of the disorder. Which statement by the client indicates an understanding of these measures?

1 "I will take daily cool baths."
2 "I will cut down on smoking."
3 "I will eat a high-protein diet."
4 "I will keep my hands and feet warm and dry."

Level of Cognitive Ability: Evaluating
Client Needs: Health Promotion and Maintenance
Clinical Judgment/Cognitive Skills: Evaluate Outcomes
Integrated Process: Nursing Process/Evaluation
Content Area: Adult Health: Cardiovascular
Health Problem: Adult Health: Cardiovascular: Vascular Disorders

Answer: 4
Rationale: Raynaud's phenomenon is caused by the vasospasm of the arterioles and arteries of the upper and lower extremities. This disorder is managed by avoiding activities that promote vasoconstriction. The hands and feet are kept dry; gloves and warm fabrics need to be worn in cold weather; and the client needs to avoid exposure to nicotine and caffeine. The avoidance of situations that trigger stress is also helpful. A high-protein diet is of no use for managing the effects of this disorder.
Priority Nursing Tip: Severe cases of Raynaud's can lead to sores or gangrene (tissue death) in the fingers and toes.

Test-Taking Strategy: Focus on the **subject**, Raynaud's phenomenon. Recalling that the goal for managing the disorder is to avoid activities that promote vasoconstriction will direct you to the correct option.

---

108. Probenecid is prescribed to a client for the treatment of gout. The nurse reinforces home-care instructions about the medication to the client. Which statement by the client indicates the **need for further instruction**?

1 "I need to take the medication on an empty stomach."
2 "I need to avoid any medication that contains aspirin."
3 "I need to avoid alcohol because it will increase the uric acid levels."
4 "I need to increase my fluid intake to maintain an adequate urine output."

Level of Cognitive Ability: Evaluating
Client Needs: Health Promotion and Maintenance
Clinical Judgment/Cognitive Skills: Evaluate Outcomes
Integrated Process: Teaching and Learning
Content Area: Adult Health: Musculoskeletal
Health Problem: Adult Health: Musculoskeletal: Gout

Answer: 1
Rationale: Probenecid is a uricosuric medication. The client is instructed to administer the medication with milk or meals to prevent gastric distress. The client would be instructed to avoid alcohol because it increases the urate levels and to avoid medications that contain aspirin. Increased fluid intake is encouraged to maintain an adequate urine output and to prevent hematuria, renal colic, and stone development.
Priority Nursing Tip: The client diagnosed with gout would be encouraged to limit high-purine foods.

Test-Taking Strategy: Note the **strategic words,** *need for further instruction.* These words indicate a **negative event query** and ask you to select an option that is an incorrect statement. Using general principles related to medication therapy will direct you to the correct option. Thinking about the pathophysiology associated with gout will also direct you to the correct option.

---

109. Calcium carbonate has been prescribed for a client with a diagnosis of osteomalacia. The nurse is reinforcing home-care instructions to the client about the supplement. Which statement by the client indicates the **need for further instruction**?

1 "I need to drink an increased amount of water."
2 "I need to increase my intake of leafy green vegetables."
3 "Constipation can occur from the use of these supplements."
4 "I might experience a chalky taste in my mouth from the medication."

Level of Cognitive Ability: Applying
Client Needs: Health Promotion and Maintenance
Clinical Judgment/Cognitive Skills: Evaluate Outcomes
Integrated Process: Teaching and Learning
Content Area: Adult Health: Musculoskeletal
Health Problem: Adult Health: Musculoskeletal: Skeletal Injury

Answer: 2
Rationale: Osteomalacia is the softening of the bones, typically through a deficiency of vitamin D or calcium. The client is advised to limit their intake of soy and leafy green vegetables when taking a calcium supplement (such as calcium carbonate) because these foods decrease the absorption of the calcium. The client would be instructed to drink water while taking the supplements to prevent renal stones. Side effects include constipation, gastric irritation, a chalky taste in the mouth, nausea, and gastric bleeding.
Priority Nursing Tip: Most calcium supplements would be taken on an empty stomach to promote absorption, but food may be necessary if gastric irritation develops.

Test-Taking Strategy: Note the **strategic words,** *need for further instruction.* These words indicate a **negative event query** and ask you to select an option that is an incorrect statement. Use your nursing knowledge and general principles related to medication therapy to direct you to the correct option.

---

110. Fluoxetine hydrochloride daily is prescribed for a client with depression, and the nurse reinforces home-care instructions about its administration. Which client statement indicates an understanding of the administration of the medication?

1 "I need to take the medication right before bedtime."
2 "I need to take the medication with my evening meal."
3 "I need to take the medication at noontime with an antacid."
4 "I need to take the medication in the morning when I first arise."

Level of Cognitive Ability: Evaluating
Client Needs: Health Promotion and Maintenance
Clinical Judgment/Cognitive Skills: Evaluate Outcomes
Integrated Process: Nursing Process/Evaluation
Content Area: Pharmacology: Psychotherapeutic: Selective Serotonin Reuptake Inhibitors (SSRIs)
Health Problem: Mental Health: Mood Disorders

Answer: 4
Rationale: Fluoxetine hydrochloride is an antidepressant, antiobsessional, and antibulimic agent. A daily dose needs to be taken in the early morning at the same time each day, without consideration of meals. Options 1, 2, and 3 are incorrect.
Priority Nursing Tip: Fluoxetine hydrochloride would be given in the morning to prevent insomnia.

Test-Taking Strategy: Focus on the **subject,** fluoxetine hydrochloride. Knowledge of client instructions related to the use of fluoxetine hydrochloride is necessary to answer this question. Recalling that medications would generally not be administered with antacids will help you eliminate option 3. To select from the remaining options, remember that fluoxetine hydrochloride is administered in the early morning, without consideration of meals.

---

111. The nurse is preparing to reinforce teaching provided to a client on mixing regular and NPH insulin in the same syringe. What technique does the nurse reinforce?

1 Draw up the NPH insulin first into the syringe.
2 Remove all the air out of the bottles before mixing.
3 Keep both insulins refrigerated until just before mixing.
4 Rotate the NPH insulin bottle in the hands before mixing.

Level of Cognitive Ability: Applying
Client Needs: Health Promotion and Maintenance
Clinical Judgment/Cognitive Skills: Take Action
Integrated Process: Teaching and Learning
Content Area: Pharmacology: Endocrine: Insulin
Health Problem: Adult Health: Endocrine: Diabetes Mellitus

Answer: 4
Rationale: Before mixing different types of insulin, the bottle needs to be rotated for at least 1 minute between the hands; this resuspends the insulin and helps warm the medication. Insulin may be maintained at room temperature, but additional bottles need to be stored in the refrigerator for future use. Regular insulin is drawn up before NPH insulin. Air does not need to be removed from the insulin bottle.
Priority Nursing Tip: Shaking insulin bottles causes foaming and bubbles to form, which may trap particles of insulin and alter the dosage.

Test-Taking Strategy: Focus on the **subject,** mixing insulins. Knowledge of the procedure for mixing NPH and regular insulin in the same syringe is necessary to answer this question. Visualizing the procedure as you carefully read each option will direct you to the correct option.

112. Methylphenidate hydrochloride is prescribed for a child with attention-deficit/hyperactivity disorder (ADHD). The nurse reinforces that the parent needs to administer the medication at what time?

1 At bedtime
2 1 hour before bedtime
3 With the evening meal
4 With the noontime meal

Level of Cognitive Ability: Applying
Client Needs: Health Promotion and Maintenance
Clinical Judgment/Cognitive Skills: Take Action
Integrated Process: Teaching and Learning
Content Area: Pharmacology: Psychotherapeutics: Medications for Attention-Deficit/Hyperactivity Disorder (ADHD)
Health Problem: Pediatric-Specific: Attention Deficit/Hyperactivity Disorder

Answer: 4

Rationale: Methylphenidate hydrochloride is a central nervous system stimulant. Medications are best taken shortly before meals and not after noon or 1:00 PM for children or 6:00 PM for adults because the stimulating effect may keep the client awake. Options 1, 2, and 3 are incorrect.

Priority Nursing Tip: The primary features of attention-deficit/hyperactivity disorder include inattention and hyperactive-impulsive behavior. ADHD symptoms start before age 12, and in some children they are noticeable as early as 3 years of age. Early diagnosis is important to prevent impaired emotional and psychological development.

Test-Taking Strategy: Focus on the **subject,** the administration of methylphenidate hydrochloride. Recalling that methylphenidate hydrochloride is a central nervous system stimulant will direct you to the correct option.

---

113. Calcium carbonate chewable tablets are prescribed for a client with a history of duodenal ulcer. The nurse reinforces home-care instructions to the client and suggests that the medication will provide relief from which disorder?

1 Flatus
2 Heartburn
3 Rectal pain
4 Muscle twitching

Level of Cognitive Ability: Applying
Client Needs: Health Promotion and Maintenance
Clinical Judgment/Cognitive Skills: Take Action
Integrated Process: Teaching and Learning
Content Area: Pharmacology: Gastrointestinal: Antacids
Health Problem: Adult Health: Gastrointestinal: Upper GI Disorders

Answer: 2

Rationale: Calcium carbonate can be used as an antacid for the relief of heartburn and indigestion. It can also be used as a calcium supplement or to bind phosphorus in the gastrointestinal tract of clients with renal failure. The disorders identified in the other options are unrelated to the use of this medication.

Priority Nursing Tip: Calcium carbonate is classified as an antacid; it is effective for the treatment of gastroesophageal reflux disease (GERD). Instruct the client regarding this medication.

Test-Taking Strategy: Note the words *duodenal ulcer* and *relief from.* Next, focus on the **subject,** the action of calcium carbonate chewable tablets. Noting the relationship between the client's diagnosis and option 2 will direct you to this option.

---

114. Aluminum hydroxide tablets have been prescribed for a client with peptic ulcer disease. The nurse plans to teach about common side effects of the medication. What common side effect would the nurse include in the teaching plan?

1 Diarrhea
2 Stomach cramps
3 Muscle joint pain
4 Dizziness upon rising

Level of Cognitive Ability: Applying
Client Needs: Health Promotion and Maintenance
Clinical Judgment/Cognitive Skills: Generate Solutions
Integrated Process: Teaching and Learning
Content Area: Pharmacology: Gastrointestinal: Antacid
Health Problem: Adult Health: Gastrointestinal: Upper GI Disorders

Answer: 2
Rationale: Aluminum hydroxide is an antacid. It causes the side effect of stomach cramps because of its aluminum base. Hypophosphatemia, which is noted by monitoring serum laboratory studies, is the other possible side effect. Options 1, 3, and 4 are incorrect.
Priority Nursing Tip: Initially, stomach cramps are common with aluminum hydroxide tablets, but the cramps would subside with time.

Test-Taking Strategy: Focus on the **subject,** common side effects of aluminum hydroxide. Specific knowledge of this type of antacid and its side effects is needed to answer this question. Remember that aluminum hydroxide causes the side effect of stomach cramps because of its aluminum base.

---

115. The nurse is reinforcing home-care instructions to a client diagnosed with chronic venous insufficiency secondary to deep vein thrombosis. The nurse would tell the client to avoid which activity?

1 Sleeping with the foot of the bed elevated
2 Wearing elastic hose for at least 6 to 8 weeks
3 Elevating the head of the bed 6 inches during sleep
4 Sitting in chairs that allow the feet to touch the floor

Level of Cognitive Ability: Applying
Client Needs: Health Promotion and Maintenance
Clinical Judgment/Cognitive Skills: Take Action
Integrated Process: Teaching and Learning
Content Area: Adult Health: Cardiovascular
Health Problem: Adult Health: Cardiovascular: Vascular Disorders

Answer: 3
Rationale: Clients with chronic venous insufficiency are advised to avoid the following: crossing their legs, sitting in chairs in which their feet do not touch the floor, standing or sitting for prolonged periods, and wearing garters or sources of pressure above the legs (e.g., girdles). These clients need to wear elastic hose as prescribed, and they need to sleep with the foot of the bed (not the head of the bed) elevated to promote venous return during sleep.
Priority Nursing Tip: Venous return is improved with interventions aimed at elevating the lower body.

Test-Taking Strategy: Focus on the **subject,** deep vein thrombosis, and note the word *avoid.* This word asks you to select an option that is an incorrect home-care measure. Use the concept of gravity when answering questions that relate to peripheral vascular problems. Venous problems are characterized by the insufficient drainage of blood from the legs returning to the heart; thus, interventions would be directed toward promoting the flow of blood from the legs and to the heart. Only option 3 does not promote venous drainage, thereby making it the correct answer.

---

116. The nurse has reinforced home-care instructions to a hypertensive client about nonfood items that contain sodium. The nurse determines that the client understands the information presented if the client states that which may be used?

1 Toothpaste
2 Mouthwash
3 Cold remedies
4 Demineralized water

Level of Cognitive Ability: Evaluating
Client Needs: Health Promotion and Maintenance
Clinical Judgment/Cognitive Skills: Evaluate Outcomes
Integrated Process: Nursing Process/Evaluation
Content Area: Adult Health: Cardiovascular
Health Problem: Adult Health: Cardiovascular: Hypertension

Answer: 4

Rationale: Sodium intake can be increased with the use of several products, including toothpaste and mouthwashes; over-the-counter (OTC) medications such as analgesics, antacids, cough remedies, laxatives, and sedatives; and softened water, as well as some mineral waters. Clients are advised to read labels for sodium content. Water that is bottled, distilled, deionized, or demineralized may be used for drinking and cooking.

Priority Nursing Tip: Manufactured products will contain sodium unless identified on the label as low sodium or demineralized.

Test-Taking Strategy: Focus on the **subject,** sodium content. The wording of the question directs you to seek the item that is low in sodium. Remember that several OTC products contain significant levels of sodium; this will assist you with eliminating options 1, 2, and 3. Finally, look at the word *demineralized,* which means having the minerals removed. This option would be a good choice when selecting an item that is low in sodium.

---

117. The nurse is reinforcing instructions with a client with a cast about how to perform the 3-point gait with crutches. Which instruction would the nurse provide to the client?

1 Move both crutches forward and then swing both feet forward to the crutches.
2 Move the right crutch, the left foot, the left crutch, and then the right foot forward.
3 Advance the right crutch and the left foot forward, and then bring the right foot and left crutch forward.
4 Simultaneously move both crutches and the affected leg forward, and then move the unaffected leg forward.

Level of Cognitive Ability: Applying
Client Needs: Health Promotion and Maintenance
Clinical Judgment/Cognitive Skills: Take Action
Integrated Process: Teaching and Learning
Content Area: Adult Health: Musculoskeletal
Health Problem: Adult Health: Musculoskeletal: Skeletal Injury

Answer: 4

Rationale: A 3-point gait or orthopedic gait is used for amputees and orthopedic clients. It requires that the client have normal use of one leg and both arms. The client is instructed to simultaneously move both crutches and the affected leg forward, and then the unaffected leg would be moved forward. Option 1 identifies a swing-through gait. Options 2 and 3 identify a 4-point gait.

Priority Nursing Tip: A 3-point gait requires three maneuvers.

Test-Taking Strategy: Focus on the **subject,** a 3-point gait, and read the description in each option. This will assist you with eliminating options 1, 2, and 3 because these are not 3-point gaits.

118. The nurse is reinforcing instructions with a client with a skeletal injury about the use of crutches and teaching the client the method for ascending and descending stairs. When instructing the client about ascending and descending the stairs, the nurse gives the client what instruction?

1. Move the crutches and the unaffected leg down, followed by the affected leg.
2. Move the unaffected leg up first, followed by the affected leg and the crutches.
3. Move both crutches up the stair, followed by the unaffected leg and then the affected leg.
4. Move both crutches up the stair, followed by the affected leg and then the unaffected leg.

Level of Cognitive Ability: Applying
Client Needs: Health Promotion and Maintenance
Clinical Judgment/Cognitive Skills: Take Action
Integrated Process: Teaching and Learning
Content Area: Skills: Activity/Mobility
Health Problem: Adult Health: Musculoskeletal: Skeletal Injury

Answer: 2
Rationale: To go up the stairs, the client needs to move the unaffected leg up first, followed by the affected leg and the crutches. When going down the stairs, the client needs to move the crutches and the affected leg first, followed by the unaffected leg.
Priority Nursing Tip: To be most effective, crutches need to be specifically fitted for a client.

Test-Taking Strategy: Focus on the **subject,** crutch use up and down the stairs. When answering this question, visualize the process of going up and down the stairs while using crutches. Remember "good up and bad down," then you will be able to answer this question. When going up the stairs, the good or unaffected leg moves first. When going down the stairs, the bad or affected leg moves first.

---

119. A client being discharged to home after hip surgery is prescribed enoxaparin subcutaneously and will self-administer the medication. The nurse reinforcing the teaching would make what statement?

1. "Massage the skin after giving the injection."
2. "Aspirate the syringe before pushing down on the plunger."
3. "Push the skin flat and taut before injecting the medication."
4. "A 25- to 27-gauge, ⅝-inch needle is attached to the syringe."

Level of Cognitive Ability: Applying
Client Needs: Health Promotion and Maintenance
Clinical Judgment/Cognitive Skills: Take Action
Integrated Process: Teaching and Learning
Content Area: Skills: Medication Administration
Health Problem: Adult Health: Musculoskeletal: Skeletal Injury

Answer: 4
Rationale: Enoxaparin is an anticoagulant administered via the subcutaneous route. With the subcutaneous injection of enoxaparin, the administration technique is the same as for subcutaneous heparin. The nurse teaches the client that a 25- to 27-gauge needle is attached to the syringe to prevent hematoma formation at the injection site. The client would use a "bunching" technique to inject the medication deep into fatty abdominal tissue. The nurse teaches the client to not aspirate the syringe before injection and to not massage the injection site.
Priority Nursing Tip: Subcutaneous injections require a short needle so as to not inject into the intramuscular tissue.

Test-Taking Strategy: Focus on the **subject,** administrating enoxaparin. Note the word *subcutaneously.* Think about the procedure for subcutaneous injections. Knowing that subcutaneous injections require a short needle to not inject into the intramuscular tissue will help you select the correct option.

---

120. The nurse caring for a client who experiences frequent episodes of bronchial asthma is reinforcing home-care instructions about measures to reduce the exacerbation of the condition. Which statement by the client would indicate **further teaching is required**?

1 "I will buy a humidifier for use at home."
2 "I have already had my chimney cleaned this year."
3 "I will be damp dusting the furniture once a week."
4 "I will be having my furnace serviced as soon as I am discharged."

Level of Cognitive Ability: Evaluating
Client Needs: Health Promotion and Maintenance
Clinical Judgment/Cognitive Skills: Evaluate Outcomes
Integrated Process: Teaching and Learning
Content Area: Adult Health: Respiratory
Health Problem: Adult Health: Respiratory: Asthma

Answer: 1

Rationale: Environmental allergens and organisms that can cause infection are likely to exacerbate asthma. These irritants can be reduced by having the chimney cleaned and by dusting with a damp cloth. Having the furnace serviced will eliminate dirt and soot from the system and detect any carbon monoxide that is leaking or present. A humidifier will increase the moisture in the air, but it may also increase the growth of mold and mildew, which would not be helpful for this client.

Priority Nursing Tip: Bronchial asthma is an intermittent and reversible airflow obstruction that affects only the airways and not the alveoli.

Test-Taking Strategy: Focus on the **subject**, asthma, and note the **strategic words**, *further teaching is required.* These words indicate a **negative event query** and ask you to select an option that will not help the client's condition. Recalling the factors that contribute to asthma will direct you to the correct option.

---

121. A client diagnosed with obstructive respiratory disease is experiencing activity intolerance at home related to fatigue and dyspnea after physical exertion. The nurse suggests which health care measure to improve the client's functioning?

1 Reduce caloric intake by half to allow more energy for breathing.
2 Gradually increase ambulation and the completion of small tasks daily.
3 Stay in one room of the house to decrease episodes of fatigue and dyspnea.
4 Begin taking a light sedative medication each night to ensure a good night's sleep.

Level of Cognitive Ability: Applying
Client Needs: Health Promotion and Maintenance
Clinical Judgment/Cognitive Skills: Take Action
Integrated Process: Teaching and Learning
Content Area: Adult Health: Respiratory
Health Problem: Adult Health: Respiratory: Obstructive Pulmonary Disease

Answer: 2

Rationale: The client with activity intolerance related to fatigue and dyspnea after physical exertion needs to try to gradually increase activity and mobility each day. The client would not reduce caloric intake by half because the client will not have sufficient energy for respiration. Rather, the client needs to take in adequate calories but eat small, frequent meals each day. The client needs adequate rest, but relying on a sedative each night could foster dependence. Finally, the client would not stay in one room of the house because doing so will not increase endurance and will also foster feelings of seclusion and social isolation.

Priority Nursing Tip: Some conditions and factors that cause respiratory distress are sepsis, pneumonia, severe bleeding caused by an injury, an injury to the chest or head, breathing in harmful fumes or smoke, and inhaling vomited stomach contents.

Test-Taking Strategy: Focus on the **data in the question** and the **subject**, activity intolerance. The correct option is the only option that relates to activity.

---

122. Captopril has been prescribed for a hospitalized client with hypertension. The nurse reinforces home-care instructions to the client about the medication. The nurse determines that the client understands these instructions when the client makes which statement?

1 "I will stand and sit upright slowly."
2 "I will eat more foods high in fiber."
3 "I will drink larger amounts of water."
4 "I will eat foods that are high in potassium."

Level of Cognitive Ability: Evaluating
Client Needs: Health Promotion and Maintenance
Clinical Judgment/Cognitive Skills: Evaluate Outcomes
Integrated Process: Nursing Process/Evaluation
Content Area: Pharmacology: Cardiovascular: Angiotensin-Converting Enzyme (ACE) Inhibitors
Health Problem: Adult Health: Cardiovascular: Hypertension

Answer: 1
Rationale: Captopril is an antihypertensive medication (angiotensin-converting enzyme inhibitor). Orthostatic hypotension is a concern for clients taking antihypertensive medications. Clients are advised to change positions slowly and to avoid extreme warmth (e.g., shower, bath, weather). The other options are unnecessary, and option 3 could aggravate the hypertension.
Priority Nursing Tip: Clients would be taught to recognize the symptoms of orthostatic hypotension, including dizziness, lightheadedness, weakness, and syncope.

Test-Taking Strategy: Focus on the **subject,** client instructions for captopril. Recalling that captopril is an antihypertensive will direct you to the correct option because the risk of orthostatic hypotension is present with all types of antihypertensives.

---

123. A client is 39 years old, has three children, and is a server in a restaurant. During a routine visit to the primary health care provider the nurse recognizes that the client is **most** at risk for developing which peripheral vascular disorder?

1 Varicose veins
2 Thrombophlebitis
3 Arterial insufficiency
4 Acute arterial emboli

Level of Cognitive Ability: Analyzing
Client Needs: Health Promotion and Maintenance
Clinical Judgment/Cognitive Skills: Recognize Cues
Integrated Process: Nursing Process/Data Collection
Content Area: Adult Health: Cardiovascular
Health Problem: Adult Health: Cardiovascular: Vascular Disorders

Answer: 1
Rationale: Varicose veins are distended, protruding veins that appear darkened and tortuous. They are more common after the age of 30 years in clients who have occupations that require prolonged standing. There is no information in the question to indicate prolonged immobility (option 2), risk of arterial insufficiency (option 3), or added risk of cardiac thrombus (option 4).
Priority Nursing Tip: Varicose veins occur more frequently in pregnant women, obese individuals, and those with a positive family history of varicose veins or systemic problems (e.g., heart disease).

Test-Taking Strategy: Note the **strategic word,** *most.* Focus on the **subject,** risk for peripheral vascular disorders, and note the **data in the question,** specifically the age and occupation. Use your knowledge of the risk factors for development of varicose veins to answer correctly.

---

124. The nurse is giving a client with hypertension general information about acceptable foods to include on a sodium-restricted diet. The nurse tells the client that which item is lowest in sodium content?

1 Potatoes
2 Instant rice
3 Frozen bread dough
4 Commercial stuffing

Level of Cognitive Ability: Applying
Client Needs: Health Promotion and Maintenance
Clinical Judgment/Cognitive Skills: Take Action
Integrated Process: Teaching and Learning
Content Area: Foundations of Care: Therapeutic Diets
Health Problem: Adult Health: Cardiovascular: Hypertension

Answer: 1
Rationale: Clients on a sodium-restricted diet need to avoid the use of commercially prepared products, which often contain sodium as a preservative. Potatoes are a sodium free food.
Priority Nursing Tip: Foods that are commercially processed contain more salt than those prepared at home.

Test-Taking Strategy: Focus on the **subject,** the food item lowest in sodium. Recalling that many commercially prepared products contain sodium will direct you to the correct option.

---

125. A client diagnosed with hyperlipidemia at risk for coronary artery disease is advised to limit the intake of dietary cholesterol. The nurse reinforces dietary instructions by suggesting the client choose which food item?

1 Liver
2 Bacon
3 Spare ribs
4 Baked scrod

Level of Cognitive Ability: Applying
Client Needs: Health Promotion and Maintenance
Clinical Judgment/Cognitive Skills: Take Action
Integrated Process: Teaching and Learning
Content Area: Foundations of Care: Therapeutic Diets
Health Problem: Adult Health: Cardiovascular: Coronary Artery Disease

Answer: 4
Rationale: The best choices to lower the intake of cholesterol include lean cuts of beef with the fat trimmed, lamb, pork (except spare ribs), veal (except when ground), skinless poultry, and some types of fish. Meats that have larger amounts of cholesterol include prime grades of beef, pork spare ribs, goose, duck, organ meats (e.g., liver, brain, kidney), sausage, bacon, luncheon meats, frankfurters, and caviar.
Priority Nursing Tip: A low-fat diet is one that restricts fat and often saturated fat and cholesterol as well. Low-fat diets are intended to reduce diseases such as heart disease and obesity.

Test-Taking Strategy: Focus on the **subject,** a low-fat diet. Think about each food item in the options. Remember that liver, bacon, and spare ribs are high in fat.

---

126. The nurse has reinforced home-care instructions about body mechanics and low back care to the client with a herniated lumbar disk. Which statement by the client indicates the **need for further instruction**?

1 "I need to bend at the knees to pick up objects."
2 "I need to swim or walk to strengthen my back muscles."
3 "I need to increase the amount of fluid and fiber in my diet."
4 "I need to get out of bed by sitting up straight and swinging my legs over the side."

Level of Cognitive Ability: Evaluating
Client Needs: Health Promotion and Maintenance
Clinical Judgment/Cognitive Skills: Evaluate Outcomes
Integrated Process: Teaching and Learning
Content Area: Adult Health: Musculoskeletal
Health Problem: Adult Health: Musculoskeletal: Intervertebral Disk Herniation

Answer: 4
Rationale: Clients would get out of bed by sliding toward the mattress edge. The client needs to then roll onto one side and push up from the bed using one or both arms. The client needs to keep the back straight as the legs are swung over the side. Proper body mechanics includes bending at the knees rather than at the waist to lift objects. The client needs to increase dietary fiber and fluids to prevent straining during stooling, which could increase intraspinal pressure. Walking and swimming are excellent exercises for strengthening the lower back muscles.
Priority Nursing Tip: With low back pain it is important to use body mechanics that put very little strain directly on the back.

Test-Taking Strategy: Focus on the **subject**, herniated lumbar disk, and note the **strategic words**, *need for further instruction*. These words indicate a **negative event query** and ask you to select an option that is an incorrect client statement. Visualize each action in the options. Eliminate options 1 and 2 first because they are correct actions. Choose option 4 instead of option 3, knowing that sitting up straight causes strain on the lower back muscles or that straining during stooling increases intraspinal pressure.

---

127. The nurse has reinforced home-care instructions about energy conservation techniques with a client with chronic airflow limitation (CAL). Which statement by the client indicates the **need for further instruction**?

1 "I need to limit activities that involve much arm movement."
2 "I need to not hold my breath during activities that require exertion."
3 "I need to perform all activities early in the day when I am most rested."
4 "I need to sit when performing activities that do not require much movement."

Level of Cognitive Ability: Evaluating
Client Needs: Health Promotion and Maintenance
Clinical Judgment/Cognitive Skills: Evaluate Outcomes
Integrated Process: Teaching and Learning
Content Area: Adult Health: Respiratory
Health Problem: Adult Health: Respiratory: Obstructive Pulmonary Disease

Answer: 3
Rationale: The client diagnosed with CAL needs to alternate periods of activity with rest periods to conserve energy. The client needs to also sit when performing activities that do not require exertion (e.g., sewing, ironing). The client needs to limit activities that involve arm movements because these will increase dyspnea; the client would not hold the breath for the same reason.
Priority Nursing Tip: Energy conservation needs to have the highest priority with clients diagnosed with obstructive pulmonary disease.

Test-Taking Strategy: Focus on the **subject**, energy conservation techniques, and note the **strategic words**, *need for further instruction*. These words indicate a **negative event query** and ask you to select an option that is an incorrect client statement. Remember that clients with obstructive lung disease need to alternate periods of activity with rest periods to conserve energy.

---

128. The nurse has taught the client diagnosed with chronic airflow limitation (CAL) about positions that help breathing during dyspneic episodes. Which statement by the client indicates a **need for further instruction**?

1 "When I am standing, I lean against a wall."
2 "When I am sitting, I always lean on a table."
3 "When I sit in a chair, I rest my elbows on my knees."
4 "When I lie flat on my back, I prop myself up on a pillow."

Level of Cognitive Ability: Evaluating
Client Needs: Health Promotion and Maintenance
Clinical Judgment/Cognitive Skills: Evaluate Outcomes
Integrated Process: Teaching and Learning
Content Area: Adult Health: Respiratory
Health Problem: Adult Health: Respiratory: Obstructive Pulmonary Disease

Answer: 4
Rationale: The client with CAL needs to use the positions identified in options 1, 2, and 3. These allow for maximal chest expansion and the decreased use of the accessory muscles of respiration. The client would not lie flat on the back because this reduces movement of a large area of the client's chest wall. Sitting is better than standing for these clients whenever possible. If no chair is available, then leaning against a wall while standing allows accessory muscles to be used for breathing rather than posture control.
Priority Nursing Tip: The airflow limitation that defines chronic obstructive pulmonary disease (COPD) is the result of a prolonged time constant for lung emptying, caused by increased resistance of the small conducting airways as a result of emphysematous destruction.

Test-Taking Strategy: Note the **strategic words,** *need for further instruction.* These words indicate a **negative event query** and ask you to select an option that is an incorrect client statement. Visualize each position described, and note that options 1, 2, and 3 are **comparable or alike** in that they involve a position in which the client leans forward.

---

129. The nurse reinforces home-care instructions with a client who has depression regarding monoamine oxidase (MAO) inhibitor toxicity. Which statement by the client would indicate that the client understands the signs of toxicity?

1 "I will call if I have lethargy."
2 "I will call if I have excessive fatigue."
3 "I will call if I develop a low-grade fever."
4 "I will call if I have trouble sleeping at night."

Level of Cognitive Ability: Evaluating
Client Needs: Health Promotion and Maintenance
Clinical Judgment/Cognitive Skills: Evaluate Outcomes
Integrated Process: Nursing Process: Evaluation
Content Area: Pharmacology: Psychotherapeutic: Monoamine Oxidase Inhibitors (MAOIs)
Health Problem: Mental Health: Mood Disorders

Answer: 4
Rationale: Acute toxicity of MAO inhibitors is manifested by restlessness, anxiety, and insomnia. Dizziness and hypertension may also occur. Options 1, 2, and 3 are not signs of toxicity.
Priority Nursing Tip: Toxicity of monoamine oxidase inhibitors is characterized by symptoms related to the neurological system.

Test-Taking Strategy: Focus on the **subject,** MAO inhibitor toxicity. Options 1 and 2 can be eliminated first because they are **comparable or alike** and relate to energy levels. From the remaining options, it is necessary to know the signs of toxicity associated with these medications. Remember that acute toxicity of MAO inhibitors is manifested by restlessness, anxiety, and insomnia.

---

130. The nurse is reinforcing home-care instructions to the client diagnosed with chronic kidney disease regarding ways to reduce pruritus caused by uremia. The nurse tells the client to avoid which type of skin care product?

1 Bath oil
2 Mild soap
3 Lanolin-based lotion
4 Astringent facial cleansing pads

Level of Cognitive Ability: Applying
Client Needs: Health Promotion and Maintenance
Clinical Judgment/Cognitive Skills: Take Action
Integrated Process: Teaching and Learning
Content Area: Adult Health: Renal and Urinary
Health Problem: Adult Health: Renal and Urinary: Chronic Kidney Disease

Answer: 4

Rationale: The client with chronic kidney disease often has dry skin that is accompanied by pruritus caused by uremia. The client needs to use mild soaps, lotions, and bath oils to reduce dryness without increasing skin irritation. Products that contain perfumes or alcohol increase dryness and pruritus and need to be avoided.

Priority Nursing Tip: Uremia is a clinical syndrome associated with fluid, electrolyte, and hormone imbalances and metabolic abnormalities.

Test-Taking Strategy: Focus on the **subject,** pruritus, and note the word *avoid.* Options 1 and 3 are **comparable or alike** in that they enhance skin moisture and would therefore be eliminated. From the remaining options, select option 4 instead of option 2, knowing that the client would avoid putting irritating products on the skin.

---

131. The nurse has reinforced instructions to a client diagnosed with chronic kidney disease about medication therapy for increasing red blood cell (RBC) production. Which medication, if stated by the client, would indicate a **need for further instruction** about treatment for anemia?

1 Epoetin
2 Folic acid
3 Ferrous sulfate
4 Calcium carbonate

Level of Cognitive Ability: Evaluating
Client Needs: Health Promotion and Maintenance
Clinical Judgment/Cognitive Skills: Evaluate Outcomes
Integrated Process: Teaching and Learning
Content Area: Adult Health: Renal and Urinary
Health Problem: Adult Health: Renal and Urinary: Chronic Kidney Disease

Answer: 4

Rationale: Calcium carbonate is a calcium salt that is used as a phosphate binder in the client with chronic kidney disease; it has nothing to do with treatment of anemia. Folic acid is a vitamin that is needed for RBC production, and it is usually deficient in the client with chronic kidney disease. Iron supplements (ferrous sulfate) are needed to produce adequate hemoglobin. Epoetin stimulates the production of RBCs because it is an external source of erythropoietin.

Priority Nursing Tip: Anemia is a condition marked by a deficiency of red blood cells or of hemoglobin in the blood, resulting in pallor and weariness.

Test-Taking Strategy: Note the **strategic words,** *need for further instruction.* These words indicate a **negative event query** and the need to select the incorrect client statement. Focus on the **subject,** enhancing RBC production. Recalling the pathophysiology and medication therapy used for the treatment of anemia in the client with chronic kidney disease and the actions and uses of the medications presented in the options will direct you to the correct option.

---

132. The nurse is teaching about the action of the medication levothyroxine sodium to a client with hypothyroidism. Which outcome would the nurse describe as an expected effect of the medication?

1 Weight gain
2 Increased energy level
3 Decreased acid production
4 Lowered body temperature

Answer: 2

Rationale: Levothyroxine sodium is a synthetically prepared thyroid hormone that increases body metabolism; the client feels this effect as an increased energy level. Other effects are weight loss and increased body temperature. This medication does not affect acid production in the gastrointestinal tract.

Priority Nursing Tip: Clients diagnosed with hypothyroidism present with decreased energy levels.

Level of Cognitive Ability: Applying
Client Needs: Health Promotion and Maintenance
Clinical Judgment/Cognitive Skills: Take Action
Integrated Process: Teaching and Learning
Content Area: Pharmacology: Endocrine: Thyroid Hormones
Health Problem: Adult Health: Endocrine: Thyroid Disorders

Test-Taking Strategy: Focus on the **subject,** the expected effect of levothyroxine sodium, and recall that this medication replaces thyroid hormone. Knowledge of the pathophysiology of hypothyroidism and the effects of thyroid hormone will direct you to the correct option.

---

133. The nurse has taught a client about the dietary changes required to manage hyperaldosteronism. The nurse determines that the client understands the information presented if the client states a need to decrease which type of food?
1 Oranges
2 Red meats
3 Salty snacks
4 Whole-grain breads

Level of Cognitive Ability: Evaluating
Client Needs: Health Promotion and Maintenance
Clinical Judgment/Cognitive Skills: Evaluate Outcomes
Integrated Process: Nursing Process/Evaluation
Content Area: Adult Health: Endocrine
Health Problem: Adult Health: Endocrine: Adrenal Disorders

Answer: 3
Rationale: Hyperaldosteronism is a condition in which too much aldosterone is produced by the adrenal glands. Clients with hyperaldosteronism need to follow a low-sodium diet as an adjunct to medical management to decrease serum sodium levels. For this reason, salty foods are to be avoided. Potassium intake (e.g., oranges) needs to be maintained because the client is at risk for hypokalemia. The diet needs to have adequate protein, carbohydrates, and fat to maintain a normal body weight (options 2 and 4).
Priority Nursing Tip: The causes of primary hyperaldosteronism are adrenal hyperplasia and adrenal adenoma (Conn's syndrome). These cause hyperplasia of aldosterone-producing cells of the adrenal cortex, resulting in primary hyperaldosteronism.

Test-Taking Strategy: Focus on the **subject,** hyperaldosteronism. Recalling that aldosterone is a mineralocorticoid that helps regulate sodium and potassium levels will assist you with eliminating the incorrect options.

---

134. A client has undergone laser surgery to remove two nevi from the skin. The nurse includes which statement when reinforcing home-care instructions to the client?
1 "Scrub the affected areas daily to prevent infection."
2 "Protect the areas from direct sunlight for at least 3 months."
3 "Expect frequent episodes of discomfort after the procedure."
4 "Report any swelling or redness to the dermatologist immediately."

Level of Cognitive Ability: Applying
Client Needs: Health Promotion and Maintenance
Clinical Judgment/Cognitive Skills: Take Action
Integrated Process: Teaching and Learning
Content Area: Adult Health: Integumentary
Health Problem: Adult Health: Integumentary: Wounds

Answer: 2
Rationale: After the laser removal of any type of skin lesion, the skin needs to be protected from direct sunlight for at least 3 months. The area needs to be cleansed gently twice a day as prescribed after the initial dressing is removed 24 hours after the procedure. There would be minimal or no discomfort after the procedure, and if it is present, it would easily be relieved with acetaminophen. Redness and swelling are expected after this procedure.
Priority Nursing Tip: Nevi, also called *moles,* are growths on the skin that usually are flesh-colored, brown, or black.

Test-Taking Strategy: Focus on the **subject,** laser surgery to remove nevi. To answer this question correctly, you must be familiar with laser surgery and the elements of subsequent self-care. Read each option carefully. The words *scrub* in option 1, *frequent* in option 3, and *immediately* in option 4 would assist you with eliminating these options.

---

135. The nurse is reinforcing home-care measures with a client diagnosed with Addison's disease regarding ways to prevent addisonian crisis. The client is encouraged to implement which action?

1 "Eat a diet high in protein."
2 "Eat a diet high in glucose."
3 "Avoid stressful situations whenever possible."
4 "Stop medication therapy if infection or illness occurs."

Level of Cognitive Ability: Applying
Client Needs: Health Promotion and Maintenance
Clinical Judgment/Cognitive Skills: Take Action
Integrated Process: Teaching and Learning
Content Area: Adult Health: Endocrine
Health Problem: Adult Health: Endocrine: Adrenal Disorders

Answer: 3
Rationale: Addisonian crisis occurs when the need for cortisol and aldosterone is greater than the available supply. It is triggered by stressful events such as emotional crises, illness, injury, or surgery. The client needs to minimize the risk of infection and illness whenever possible. If the client becomes ill, doses of adrenocortical replacement medication are increased. No specific dietary alterations are used to manage this disorder.
Priority Nursing Tip: Addisonian crisis (acute adrenal insufficiency) is a life-threatening event.

Test-Taking Strategy: Focus on the **subject,** preventing addisonian crisis. Recalling that medication therapy would not be interrupted will assist you with eliminating option 4. Eliminate options 1 and 2 because they are **comparable or alike** in that they involve food intake. From the remaining options, recall that stressful events will cause a crisis.

---

136. A client who has been newly diagnosed with type 1 diabetes mellitus exercises daily. In reinforcing home-care instructions about medication therapy, the nurse reinforces that the client should inject the daily dose of insulin into what site?

1 Any site after exercise
2 Only in the arm before exercise
3 A site that will not be exercised
4 Only in the abdomen before exercise

Level of Cognitive Ability: Applying
Client Needs: Health Promotion and Maintenance
Clinical Judgment/Cognitive Skills: Take Action
Integrated Process: Teaching and Learning
Content Area: Adult Health: Endocrine
Health Problem: Adult Health: Endocrine: Diabetes Mellitus

Answer: 3
Rationale: Exercise of a body part increases the rate of absorption of the insulin from that site. For this reason, the client needs to inject insulin into an area that will not be exercised. This will help the client avoid hypoglycemia from rapid insulin absorption. Insulin would be administered at the prescribed time.
Priority Nursing Tip: The underlying mechanism of type 1 diabetes mellitus involves an autoimmune destruction of the insulin-producing beta cells in the pancreas.

Test-Taking Strategy: Focus on the **subject,** insulin injection sites for a client who exercises. Eliminate options 2 and 4 because of the **closed-ended word** "only." From the remaining options, use general knowledge about principles of exercise and diabetes to choose option 3 rather than option 1.

---

137. The nurse is reinforcing home-care instructions regarding skin care to a client receiving external radiation therapy to the chest area for lung cancer. Which statement made by the nurse demonstrates an understanding of this topic?

1 "Use deodorants only once daily."
2 "Limit sun exposure to 3 times a week."
3 "Wear snug-fitting clothing to prevent irritation."
4 "Avoid the use of lotions on the area being treated."

Answer: 4
Rationale: The client is instructed to avoid the use of lotions on the area being treated. The client would be instructed to avoid exposure to the sun. Deodorant would not be used during treatment to the chest area. The client needs to wear loose-fitting clothing over the area to prevent irritation.
Priority Nursing Tip: External radiation therapy uses high-powered x-rays or particles to kill cancer cells. The rays or particles are aimed directly at the tumor from outside the body.

Level of Cognitive Ability: Applying
Client Needs: Health Promotion and Maintenance
Clinical Judgment/Cognitive Skills: Evaluate Outcomes
Integrated Process: Teaching and Learning
Content Area: Adult Health: Oncology
Health Problem: Adult Health: Cancer: Laryngeal/Lung

Test-Taking Strategy: Focus on the **subject,** radiation therapy. Recall that it is important to avoid any substance or material that can irritate the skin in the area receiving the radiation; this will direct you to the correct option.

---

138. A client with chronic kidney disease has been diagnosed with hyperphosphatemia. The nurse reinforces home-care instructions and stresses the need to eliminate which beverage from the diet?

1 Tea
2 Coffee
3 Grape juice
4 Carbonated soda

Answer: 4
Rationale: Foods that are naturally high in phosphates need to be avoided by the client with hyperphosphatemia. These include fish, eggs, milk products, vegetables, whole grains, and carbonated beverages. Coffee, tea, and grape juice are not high in phosphates.
Priority Nursing Tip: Signs and symptoms of acute hyperphosphatemia result from the effects of hypocalcemia, with clients occasionally reporting symptoms such as muscle cramps, tetany, and perioral numbness or tingling.

Level of Cognitive Ability: Applying
Client Needs: Health Promotion and Maintenance
Clinical Judgment/Cognitive Skills: Take Action
Integrated Process: Teaching and Learning
Content Area: Adult Health: Renal and Urinary
Health Problem: Adult Health: Renal and Urinary: Chronic Kidney Disease

Test-Taking Strategy: Focus on the **subject,** hyperphosphatemia and beverages to avoid. Think about the pathophysiology of hyperphosphatemia to assist you in focusing on the client's dietary needs. This will help you eliminate options that are high in phosphates.

---

139. The nurse has conducted dietary teaching with a client diagnosed with iron-deficiency anemia. The nurse determines that the client understands the information if the client states a need to increase the intake of which food?

1 Pineapple
2 Egg whites
3 Kidney beans
4 Refined white bread

Answer: 3
Rationale: The client with iron-deficiency anemia would increase the intake of foods that are naturally high in iron. The best sources of dietary iron are red meat, liver and other organ meats, blackstrap molasses, and oysters. Other good sources of iron are kidney beans, whole-wheat bread, egg yolks, spinach, kale, turnip tops, beet greens, carrots, raisins, and apricots.
Priority Nursing Tip: Signs and symptoms of iron-deficiency anemia may include extreme fatigue and weakness, pale skin, chest pain, fast heartbeat, or shortness of breath.

Level of Cognitive Ability: Evaluating
Client Needs: Health Promotion and Maintenance
Clinical Judgment/Cognitive Skills: Evaluate Outcomes
Integrated Process: Nursing Process/Evaluation
Content Area: Foundations of Care: Therapeutic Diets
Health Problem: Adult Health: Hematological: Anemias

Test-Taking Strategy: Focus on the **subject,** iron-deficiency anemia. Think about the foods that are high in iron, and review each option. Recalling foods that are high in iron will direct you to option 3.

---

140. The nurse is reinforcing home-care instructions with a family whose child is being discharged after a sickle cell crisis. Which intervention would the nurse include in teaching to prevent sickle cell crisis? **Select all that apply.**

❒ 1 Ensure that the child receives a flu shot every year.
❒ 2 Mild discomfort can be treated with a warm bath.
❒ 3 During warm weather make sure the child drinks extra fluids.
❒ 4 Flying in an airplane will have no effect on the disease process.
❒ 5 Contact the primary health care provider immediately if the child becomes short of breath.

Level of Cognitive Ability: Applying
Client Needs: Health Promotion and Maintenance
Clinical Judgment/Cognitive Skills: Take Action
Integrated Process: Teaching and Learning
Content Area: Pediatrics: Hematological
Health Problem: Pediatric-Specific: Sickle Cell

Answer: 1, 2, 3, 5

Rationale: The client with sickle cell disease needs to avoid infections, which can increase metabolic demand and cause dehydration, thereby triggering a sickle cell crisis. The client needs to also avoid dehydration from other causes. Warm weather and mild exercise need not be avoided, but the client needs to take measures to avoid dehydration during these occurrences. Fluid intake is important to prevent dehydration. Warm soaks in a bath can help to relieve some of the discomfort associated with this health problem. If shortness of breath occurs the primary health care provider is contacted because this could be an indication of a sickle cell crisis. Finally, the client needs to avoid high altitudes or flying in nonpressurized aircraft because of the lesser oxygen tension.

Priority Nursing Tip: Measures to prevent sickle cell crisis are those that will increase vasodilation.

Test-Taking Strategy: Focus on the **subject,** sickle cell crisis, and note the word *prevent.* Recalling the causes of sickle cell crisis and that infection increases metabolic demand and can cause dehydration will direct you to the correct options.

---

141. The nurse is reviewing the assignment for the shift. Which client has the lowest risk for acquiring pneumonia during hospitalization?

1 A postoperative client who had local anesthesia
2 A client with a 20-pack-year history of smoking
3 An older adult client with diabetes mellitus admitted from a long-term care facility
4 A postoperative client who developed symptoms of upper respiratory irritation

Level of Cognitive Ability: Analyzing
Client Needs: Health Promotion and Maintenance
Clinical Judgment/Cognitive Skills: Prioritize Hypotheses
Integrated Process: Nursing Process/Data Collection
Content Area: Adult Health: Respiratory
Health Problem: Adult Health: Respiratory: Viral, Bacterial, Fungal Infections

Answer: 1

Rationale: The postoperative client who had local anesthesia for a surgical procedure is at the lowest risk. This client has had no direct insult to the respiratory tract. Clients who have a history of smoking, upper respiratory infection, or chronic disease (e.g., heart, lung, or kidney disease; diabetes mellitus; cancer) are more at risk for developing pneumonia.

Priority Nursing Tip: Air pollution, an insult to the respiratory tree, malnutrition, and dehydration are other miscellaneous risk factors for acquiring pneumonia.

Test-Taking Strategy: Focus on the **subject,** risk factors for pneumonia. Note the words *lowest risk;* these words tell you that the correct option will be the client who does not have a significant risk for developing pneumonia. Apply your knowledge of these factors to the clients presented in each option. Also, noting the words *local anesthesia* will direct you to the correct option.

---

142. The nurse is collecting data from a client with coronary artery disease. The nurse can **best** check for the presence of pallor in which area?
1 The nail beds
2 The fingertips
3 The buccal mucosa
4 Over the palms of the hands

Level of Cognitive Ability: Applying
Client Needs: Health Promotion and Maintenance
Clinical Judgment/Cognitive Skills: Recognize Cues
Integrated Process: Nursing Process/Data Collection
Content Area: Health Assessment: Physical Exam: Heart and Peripheral Vascular
Health Problem: Adult Health: Cardiovascular: Coronary Artery Disease

Answer: 3
Rationale: Pallor is best noted in the buccal mucosa or the conjunctivae, particularly in dark-skinned clients. Cyanosis is best noted in the nail beds, the conjunctivae, and the oral mucosa. Jaundice is best noted in the sclera, at the junction of the hard and soft palates, and over the palms.
Priority Nursing Tip: Pallor is the paleness of the skin and mucous membranes and occurs because of a decreased amount of oxyhemoglobin.

Test-Taking Strategy: Note the **strategic word,** *best.* Focus on the **subject,** checking for pallor. Recalling the definition of pallor and the best techniques to use to check for pallor will direct you to the correct option.

---

143. The nurse reviewing the health record of an infant who was seen in the clinic for a 6-month checkup notes that a developmental assessment was performed. Which assessment finding would indicate that **further follow-up is needed**?
1 Absence of a head lag
2 Interest in environmental stimuli
3 Repetitive performance of a new skill
4 Diminished spontaneous play activity

Level of Cognitive Ability: Analyzing
Client Needs: Health Promotion and Maintenance
Clinical Judgment/Cognitive Skills: Recognize Cues
Integrated Process: Nursing Process/Data Collection
Content Area: Developmental Stages: Infant
Health Problem: N/A

Answer: 4
Rationale: Developmental milestones of the 6-month-old infant include head control with no lag, an interest in environmental stimuli that includes the repetitive performance of learned skills, and motor skills. Early behavioral signs that are suggestive of cognitive impairment include diminished spontaneous activity, irritability, slow feeding, and decreased alertness to voices or movements.
Priority Nursing Tip: Play is an infant's form of communication.

Test-Taking Strategy: Note the **strategic words,** *further follow-up is needed.* These words indicate a **negative event query** and the need to select the abnormal finding. Focus on the **subject,** developmental milestones of an infant. Select the option that indicates an abnormal finding. Noting the word *diminished* in option 4 will direct you to this option.

---

144. Which statement by a school-age child indicates a **need for further teaching** in order to minimize the risk for personal injury while at summer camp?
1 "I need to avoid any bees."
2 "I will apply sunscreen once a day."
3 "I will take swimming lessons while at camp."
4 "I know that I need to shower every day even when camping."

Answer: 2
Rationale: Sunscreen needs to be applied more than once a day. Avoiding bees, taking swimming lessons, and bathing daily are all measures that need to be taught as health promotion measures while camping.
Priority Nursing Tip: Sunscreens are most effective when applied at least 30 minutes before exposure to the sun.

Level of Cognitive Ability: Evaluating
Client Needs: Health Promotion and Maintenance
Clinical Judgment/Cognitive Skills: Evaluate Outcomes
Integrated Process: Teaching and Learning
Content Area: Developmental Stages: Preschool and School Age
Health Problem: N/A

Test-Taking Strategy: Note the **strategic words,** *need for further teaching.* These words indicate a **negative event query** and the need to select the incorrect client statement. Option 2 suggests that the child does not understand that sunscreen would be applied more than once a day to avoid harmful exposure to the sun. The remaining options are statements that present accurate measures to avoid injury.

---

145. A woman is seen in the prenatal clinic and reports experiencing morning sickness. Which self-care measure would the nurse suggest to the client?
1 Eating eggs for breakfast
2 Eating three well-balanced meals every day
3 Eating fatty or spicy foods only at the noontime meal
4 Eating a dry cracker before getting out of bed in the morning

Level of Cognitive Ability: Applying
Client Needs: Health Promotion and Maintenance
Clinical Judgment/Cognitive Skills: Take Action
Integrated Process: Teaching and Learning
Content Area: Maternity: Antepartum
Health Problem: N/A

Answer: 4
Rationale: Morning sickness is associated with increased levels of human chorionic gonadotropin and changes in carbohydrate metabolism. It most often occurs on arising, although a few women experience it throughout the day. Self-care measures include eating a dry cracker or toast before getting out of bed; eating small, frequent meals; and avoiding fatty or spicy foods.
Priority Nursing Tip: Morning sickness is common during the first trimester of pregnancy.

Test-Taking Strategy: Focus on the **subject,** morning sickness. Recall interventions for the management of nausea in general and this complication of pregnancy to direct you to the correct option.

---

146. A client in the third trimester of pregnancy is seen at the clinic and reports urinary frequency. Which self-care measure would the nurse suggest to the client?
1 Restricting fluid intake in the evening
2 Drinking at least 2000 mL of fluid per day
3 Retaining the urine for as long as possible
4 Avoiding large amounts of fluids during the day

Level of Cognitive Ability: Applying
Client Needs: Health Promotion and Maintenance
Clinical Judgment/Cognitive Skills: Take Action
Integrated Process: Teaching and Learning
Content Area: Maternity: Antepartum
Health Problem: N/A

Answer: 2
Rationale: Urinary frequency is present during the first trimester and late in the third trimester of pregnancy. Self-care measures for urinary frequency include emptying the bladder frequently (every 2 hours) and drinking at least 2000 mL of fluid per day. Options 1, 3, and 4 are incorrect and could lead to urinary stasis (option 3) or a fluid volume deficit (options 1 and 4).
Priority Nursing Tip: Increasing fluids in the pregnant woman is necessary to prevent bladder infections due to the pressure from the enlarging uterus on the bladder.

Test-Taking Strategy: Focus on the **subject,** urinary frequency. Eliminate options 1 and 4 first because they are **comparable or alike.** Eliminate option 3 next because it does not make sense to avoid emptying the bladder frequently; this action could lead to urinary stasis and cause discomfort in the woman.

---

147. A pregnant client is seen in the health care clinic with reports of ankle edema. The nurse reinforces self-care measures to prevent the edema. Which statement by the client indicates the **need for further instruction**?

1 "I need to sleep on my left side."
2 "I need to avoid frequent rest periods."
3 "I need to elevate my feet during the day."
4 "I need to avoid standing in one position for long periods."

Level of Cognitive Ability: Applying
Client Needs: Health Promotion and Maintenance
Clinical Judgment/Cognitive Skills: Evaluate Outcomes
Integrated Process: Teaching and Learning
Content Area: Maternity: Antepartum
Health Problem: N/A

Answer: 2
Rationale: Ankle edema is a common occurrence during pregnancy that is caused by decreased venous return from the feet because of gravity. It is a minor discomfort if hypertension and proteinuria are not present. Self-care measures for ankle edema include elevating the feet to hip level during the day, taking frequent rests, sleeping on the left side to avoid pressure on the inferior vena cava, and avoiding standing in one position or place for long periods.
Priority Nursing Tip: Foot and ankle swelling is common in pregnancy; it must be monitored but usually resolves after delivery.

Test-Taking Strategy: Note the **strategic words,** *need for further instruction.* These words indicate a **negative event query** and ask you to select an option that is an incorrect statement. Read each option carefully and visualize its effect in relation to ankle edema; this would direct you to the correct option.

---

148. The nurse is reviewing the records of clients scheduled for prenatal visits today. Which clients are at the **most** risk for an abruptio placentae? **Select all that apply.**

❒ 1 A primipara
❒ 2 A 20-year-old
❒ 3 One who drinks caffeinated beverages
❒ 4 One who smokes half a pack of cigarettes a day
❒ 5 One who works in construction and whose primary job is road drilling

Level of Cognitive Ability: Analyzing
Client Needs: Health Promotion and Maintenance
Clinical Judgment/Cognitive Skills: Prioritize Hypotheses
Integrated Process: Nursing Process/Data Collection
Content Area: Maternity: Antepartum
Health Problem: Maternity: Abruptio Placentae

Answer: 3, 4, 5
Rationale: The highest incidence of abruptio placentae occurs in women who smoke or who use alcohol, cocaine, or caffeine during pregnancy. Other risk factors include having more than five pregnancies, advanced age, and heavy physical labor.
Priority Nursing Tip: Any teratogen that the woman is exposed to could influence fetal development.

Test-Taking Strategy: Note the **strategic word,** *most,* and focus on the **subject,** risk for abruptio placentae. Think about the pathophysiology associated with this complication. Also, recalling general healthy principles will direct you to the correct options.

---

149. The nurse has reinforced instructions to a postpartum client regarding postpartum exercises. Which statement by the client indicates an understanding of the exercises?

1 "The postpartum exercises can result in stress urinary incontinence."
2 "I need to alternately contract and relax the muscles of the perineal area."
3 "Any exercise needs to be delayed for 4 weeks to allow for healing time."
4 "Strenuous exercises will be started while I am in the hospital to evaluate my tolerance."

Level of Cognitive Ability: Evaluating
Client Needs: Health Promotion and Maintenance
Clinical Judgment/Cognitive Skills: Evaluate Outcomes
Integrated Process: Nursing Process/Evaluation
Content Area: Maternity: Postpartum
Health Problem: N/A

Answer: 2
Rationale: Kegel exercises are extremely important to strengthen the muscle tone of the perineal area. Postpartum exercises can begin soon after birth. The initial exercises would be simple, with progression to increasingly strenuous exercises. Postpartum exercises will not result in stress urinary incontinence.
Priority Nursing Tip: Performing Kegel exercises can tighten the pubococcygeal muscle, which will aid in urinary control.

Test-Taking Strategy: Focus on the **subject,** postpartum exercises, and your knowledge of the benefit of exercise to assist you with answering the question. Eliminate options 3 and 4 because of the words *any* and *delayed* and *strenuous.* Next, recalling the benefits of exercise will assist in eliminating option 1.

---

150. The nurse is assigned to care for a hospitalized preschooler who is in traction. The nurse determines that which is the **most appropriate** play activity for the child?

1 Finger painting
2 Listening to music
3 Hand-sewing a picture
4 Reading from a large picture book

Level of Cognitive Ability: Applying
Client Needs: Health Promotion and Maintenance
Clinical Judgment/Cognitive Skills: Take Action
Integrated Process: Nursing Process/Implementation
Content Area: Developmental Stages: Preschool and School Age
Health Problem: Pediatric-Specific: Fractures

Answer: 1
Rationale: A preschooler's play is simple and imaginative. Children of this age like to build and create things. For a bedridden child, the nurse needs to provide an activity that provides stimulation. Option 2 is most appropriate for an adolescent, option 3 is appropriate for a school-age child, and option 4 is appropriate for an infant or a young child.
Priority Nursing Tip: Preschoolers are in the stage of initiative vs. guilt and need to have some control over their activities.

Test-Taking Strategy: Note the **strategic words,** *most appropriate.* Focus on the **subject,** appropriate play activities, and note the age-group of the child. Option 4 can be eliminated because this activity is most appropriate for an infant or a young child. Eliminate option 2 next, knowing that this activity is most appropriate for an adolescent. From the remaining options, recalling that play is simple, imaginative, and creative for the preschooler will direct you to option 1.

---

151. The nurse is reinforcing instructions to the parents of a 10-year-old child diagnosed with hemophilia regarding appropriate activities. Which activity would be safe to suggest for the child?

1 Soccer
2 Football
3 Badminton
4 Skateboarding

Answer: 3
Rationale: Activity guidelines for children with hemophilia are categorized into those that are usually safe, those that are riskier and would be discouraged, and those in which the risks outweigh the benefits and are not recommended. Archery, badminton, fishing, golf, hiking, ping-pong, swimming, and walking are usually considered safe for clients with hemophilia. Options 1, 2, and 4 are riskier and are not recommended for individuals with hemophilia because they present a higher risk for falls or bleeding injuries.

Level of Cognitive Ability: Applying
Client Needs: Health Promotion and Maintenance
Clinical Judgment/Cognitive Skills: Take Action
Integrated Process: Teaching and Learning
Content Area: Pediatrics: Hematological
Health Problem: Pediatric-Specific: Anemias

Priority Nursing Tip: Activities for a child with hemophilia would include only noncontact sports.

Test-Taking Strategy: Focus on the **subject,** safe activities for a child with hemophilia. Understanding the pathology of this disorder will assist you with answering the question. Options 1, 2, and 4 are activities that present a risk of trauma and bleeding.

---

152. Which instruction would the nurse reinforce when discussing the home-care management of multiple sclerosis with a client?

1 Avoid pregnancy.
2 Maintain a low-fiber diet.
3 Avoid taking hot baths or showers.
4 Restrict fluid intake to 1000 mL per day.

Level of Cognitive Ability: Applying
Client Needs: Health Promotion and Maintenance
Clinical Judgment/Cognitive Skills: Take Action
Integrated Process: Teaching and Learning
Content Area: Adult Health: Neurological
Health Problem: Adult Health: Neurological: Multiple Sclerosis

Answer: 3
Rationale: Because fatigue can be precipitated by warm temperatures, the client is instructed to take cool baths and to maintain a cool environmental temperature. A high-fiber diet and an adequate fluid intake of 2000 mL per day are encouraged to prevent alterations in elimination and bowel patterns. The client would not be told to avoid pregnancy, but the nurse would assist the client with making informed decisions regarding pregnancy.
Priority Nursing Tip: Heat, such as hot baths or showers, can cause fatigue and weakness.

Test-Taking Strategy: Focus on the **subject,** home care management for multiple sclerosis. Eliminate option 1 first because it is inappropriate to tell a client to avoid pregnancy. Eliminate options 2 and 4 next because these measures are unhealthy and would promote alterations in elimination patterns for this client.

---

153. A client asks the nurse about the measures that will prevent Lyme disease in children. The nurse would provide which information to the client?

1 A tick needs to be removed by pulling it out of the skin using the fingernails.
2 If a tick falls off a pet, it will die and not be a concern for the family members.
3 Insect repellent needs to be applied to the entire body, except around the eyes and mouth.
4 Children need to wear long pants, long-sleeved shirts, and hats when in wooded or grassy areas.

Level of Cognitive Ability: Applying
Client Needs: Health Promotion and Maintenance
Clinical Judgment/Cognitive Skills: Take Action
Integrated Process: Teaching and Learning
Content Area: Adult Health: Immune
Health Problem: Adult Health: Immune: Lyme Disease

Answer: 4
Rationale: Children need to wear long pants, long-sleeved shirts, and hats when they are in wooded or grassy areas. Ticks need to be removed with tweezers (rather than fingernails) as close to the skin as possible. Insect repellents need to be used with caution and should not be applied to the hands to avoid contact with the child's eyes and mouth. Commercially prepared products should be used on pets to keep them free of ticks. If a tick falls off a pet, it can travel, contact an individual, and attach to the skin.
Priority Nursing Tip: Typical symptoms of Lyme disease include fever, headache, fatigue, and a characteristic skin rash called *erythema migrans.*

Test-Taking Strategy: Focus on the **subject,** measures to prevent Lyme disease. Knowledge of the use of insect repellents will assist you with eliminating option 3. Option 1 can be eliminated next by knowing that direct contact with the tick needs to be avoided. From the remaining options, select option 4 because this intervention will protect children from contact with a tick.

---

154. A clinic nurse reinforces dietary instructions to the parent of a 3-year-old child who was seen in the health care clinic for diarrhea. Which statement by the parent indicates the **need for further instruction**?

1 "It is all right to give my child active-culture yogurt."
2 "I need to encourage my child to drink clear liquids."
3 "I need to avoid giving my child any raw fruits or vegetables."
4 "I need to give my child half a cup of chicken broth every 2 hours."

Level of Cognitive Ability: Evaluation
Client Needs: Health Promotion and Maintenance
Clinical Judgment/Cognitive Skills: Evaluate Outcomes
Integrated Process: Teaching and Learning
Content Area: Pediatrics: Gastrointestinal
Health Problem: Pediatric-Specific: GI and Rectal Problems

Answer: 4
Rationale: When a child has diarrhea, high-sodium broths (e.g., chicken broth) are avoided to prevent electrolyte imbalance. Clear liquids are encouraged. Milk and milk products need to be eliminated, except for active-culture yogurt, which restores the flora of the gastrointestinal tract. Raw fruits and vegetables, beans, spices, and any other foods that cause loose stools would be avoided.
Priority Nursing Tip: Diarrhea is the condition of having at least three loose or liquid bowel movements each day.

Test-Taking Strategy: Focus on the **subject,** diarrhea management, and note the **strategic words,** *need for further instruction.* These words indicate a **negative event query** and ask you to select an option that is an incorrect statement. Think about the food items that promote or control diarrhea. Also, recalling the concern related to electrolyte imbalances will direct you to the correct option.

---

155. A school-age child with type 1 diabetes mellitus is seen in the health care clinic. The nurse reinforces instructions to the child regarding glucose management and the child's interest in playing soccer. Which instruction will the nurse provide to the child?

1 Avoid insulin on the day of soccer practice.
2 Eat lunch 1 hour earlier on the day of soccer practice.
3 The soccer activity needs to be delayed for 1 more year.
4 Eat an extra snack of carbohydrates before the soccer practice starts.

Level of Cognitive Ability: Applying
Client Needs: Health Promotion and Maintenance
Clinical Judgment/Cognitive Skills: Take Action
Integrated Process: Teaching and Learning
Content Area: Pediatrics: Metabolic/Endocrine
Health Problem: Pediatric-Specific: Diabetes Mellitus

Answer: 4
Rationale: Because exercise lowers glucose levels, the child must be taught how to prevent hypoglycemia. The child needs to try to schedule activities to avoid exercising when an insulin dose is peaking and needs to be instructed to eat extra snacks of 15 to 30 g of carbohydrates for each 45 to 60 minutes of exercise. The extra snack before practice will avert the hypoglycemia. Options 1 and 2 are inaccurate management measures for the child with diabetes mellitus. Option 3 is unnecessary.
Priority Nursing Tip: Type 1 diabetes mellitus is a chronic medical condition that occurs when the pancreas produces very little or no insulin. Without insulin, blood glucose levels become higher than normal.

Test-Taking Strategy: Focus on the **subject,** type 1 diabetes mellitus, and your knowledge of the effects of insulin to answer this question. Option 3 can be eliminated because it is unnecessary. From the remaining options, eliminate options 1 and 2 because they are inappropriate choices for the management of diabetes.

---

156. The nurse is reinforcing home-care instructions to the parent of a child with human immunodeficiency virus (HIV) infection. Which statement by the parent indicates the **need for further instruction**?

1 "I need to delay the poliovirus vaccine."
2 "I need to call the pediatrician if my child has a fever."
3 "I need to not allow my child to share toothbrushes with the other children."
4 "If any blood spills occur from a cut on my child, I need to wash the spill with soap and water, rinse it with bleach and water, and allow it to air dry."

Level of Cognitive Ability: Evaluating
Client Needs: Health Promotion and Maintenance
Clinical Judgment/Cognitive Skills: Evaluate Outcomes
Integrated Process: Teaching and Learning
Content Area: Pediatrics: Immune
Health Problem: Pediatric-Specific: Immunodeficiency Disease

Answer: 1
Rationale: The parent would be instructed to keep immunizations up to date and to not delay them. The other options are correct instructions regarding the care of the child with HIV infection.
Priority Nursing Tip: All children with HIV infection need to receive immunizations.

Test-Taking Strategy: Note the **strategic words,** *need for further instruction.* These words indicate a **negative event query** and ask you to select an option that is an incorrect statement. Recalling that immunizations need to always be kept up to date for any child will direct you to option 1.

---

157. Which home-care instruction needs to be included when teaching parents how to prevent infection in their infant after the surgical repair of an inguinal hernia?

1 Restrict all the infant's physical activity.
2 Change the diapers as soon as they become damp.
3 Soak the infant in a tub bath twice a day for the next 5 days.
4 A fever is expected to be present during the postoperative period.

Level of Cognitive Ability: Applying
Client Needs: Health Promotion and Maintenance
Clinical Judgment/Cognitive Skills: Take Action
Integrated Process: Teaching and Learning
Content Area: Pediatrics: Gastrointestinal
Health Problem: Pediatric-Specific: Disorders of Prenatal Development

Answer: 2
Rationale: Changing diapers as soon as they become damp helps reduce the chance of irritation or infection of the incision. Parents are instructed to change diapers more frequently than usual during the day and once or twice during the night. Not all the infant's physical activity is restricted. Parents are instructed to give the child sponge baths instead of tub baths for 2 to 5 days. A fever could indicate the presence of an infection and needs to be reported to the primary health care provider.
Priority Nursing Tip: During surgery to repair the hernia, the bulging tissue is pushed back in. The abdominal wall is strengthened and supported with sutures (stitches), and sometimes mesh.

Test-Taking Strategy: Focus on the **subject**, postsurgical infection control. Eliminate option 1 because of the **closed-ended word** "all." Eliminate option 4 next because a fever indicates infection. From the remaining options, focusing on the subject and recalling the factors that cause infection will direct you to the correct option.

---

158. A client is experiencing difficulty using an incentive spirometer. The nurse reinforces teaching to the client that which action may interfere with the **effective** use of the device?

1 Inhaling slowly
2 Breathing through the nose
3 Removing the mouthpiece to exhale
4 Forming a tight seal around the mouthpiece with the lips

Level of Cognitive Ability: Applying
Client Needs: Health Promotion and Maintenance
Clinical Judgment/Cognitive Skills: Take Action
Integrated Process: Teaching and Learning
Content Area: Adult Health: Respiratory
Health Problem: N/A

Answer: 2
Rationale: Incentive spirometry is ineffective if the client breathes through the nose. The client would exhale, form a tight seal around the mouthpiece, inhale slowly, hold for a count of 3, and then remove the mouthpiece to exhale. The client would repeat the exercise approximately 10 times every hour for best results.
Priority Nursing Tip: In the postsurgical client, the goals of incentive spirometry are to prevent or reduce atelectasis.

Test-Taking Strategy: Focus on the **subject,** effective use of an incentive spirometer, and note the words *may interfere* and the **strategic word,** *effective.* Visualizing the use of the incentive spirometer will direct you to the correct option.

---

159. A client with a respiratory obstructive disorder is unsure of the position to use to breathe more easily. The nurse reinforces the usefulness of which position?

1 Sit upright in bed with the arms crossed over the chest.
2 Lie on the side with the head of the bed at a 45-degree angle.
3 Sit in a reclining chair tilted back slightly and elevate the feet.
4 Sit on the edge of the bed with the arms leaning on an overbed table.

Level of Cognitive Ability: Applying
Client Needs: Health Promotion and Maintenance
Clinical Judgment/Cognitive Skills: Take Action
Integrated Process: Teaching and Learning
Content Area: Adult Health: Respiratory
Health Problem: Adult Health: Respiratory: Obstructive Pulmonary Disease

Answer: 4
Rationale: Proper positioning can decrease episodes of dyspnea in a client. Such positions include sitting upright while leaning on an overbed table, sitting upright in a chair with the arms resting on the knees, and leaning against a wall while standing.
Priority Nursing Tip: A dyspnea scale is a way for a person to describe shortness of breath that he or she feels during exercise. The scale may be used during exercise at pulmonary rehabilitation or at home.

Test-Taking Strategy: Focus on the **subject,** facilitating effective breathing. Option 2 restricts the expansion of the lateral wall of a lung and is eliminated first. From the remaining options, note that options 1 and 3 are **comparable or alike** because they restrict movement of the anterior and posterior walls of the lung.

---

160. A client diagnosed with acquired immunodeficiency syndrome (AIDS) is experiencing fatigue. The nurse reinforces to the client which strategy to conserve energy after discharge to home?

1 Bathe before eating breakfast.
2 Sit for as many activities as possible.
3 Stand in the shower instead of taking a bath.
4 Group all tasks to be performed early in the morning.

Answer: 2
Rationale: The client is taught to conserve energy by sitting for as many activities as possible, including dressing, shaving, preparing food, and ironing. The client would also sit in a shower chair instead of standing while bathing. The client needs to prioritize activities (e.g., eating breakfast before bathing) and would intersperse each major activity with a period of rest. Frequent short rest periods are more effective than fewer longer ones.
Priority Nursing Tip: Fatigue is a common problem involving a physical and mental state of being tired and weak. Physical fatigue and mental fatigue are different, but they often occur together.

Level of Cognitive Ability: Applying
Client Needs: Health Promotion and Maintenance
Clinical Judgment/Cognitive Skills: Take Action
Integrated Process: Teaching and Learning
Content Area: Adult Health: Immune
Health Problem: Adult Health: Immune: Immunodeficiency Syndrome

Test-Taking Strategy: Focus on the **subject,** fatigue, and answer this question by considering the amount of exertion required by the client to perform each of the activities listed in the options. Options 3 and 4 are obviously taxing for the client and are eliminated first. From the remaining options, recall that bathing may take away energy that could be used for eating.

---

161. The nurse has reinforced instructions with a client diagnosed with pleurisy. The nurse determines that the client has understood the instructions about strategies to promote comfort during recuperation when the client states that she or he will do what?

1 Try to take only small, shallow breaths.
2 Take as much pain medication as possible.
3 Lie as much as possible on the unaffected side.
4 Splint the chest wall during coughing and deep breathing.

Level of Cognitive Ability: Evaluating
Client Needs: Health Promotion and Maintenance
Clinical Judgment/Cognitive Skills: Evaluate Outcomes
Integrated Process: Nursing Process/Evaluation
Content Area: Adult Health: Respiratory
Health Problem: Adult Health: Respiratory: Pleurisy

Answer: 4
Rationale: The client with pleurisy needs to splint the chest wall during coughing and deep breathing, which is necessary to prevent atelectasis. The client would also lie on the affected side to minimize movement of the affected chest wall. The client needs to not take only small, shallow breaths because this promotes atelectasis. The client needs to take medication prudently to allow for coughing, deep breathing, and adequate levels of comfort.
Priority Nursing Tip: Pleurisy involves inflammation of the tissue layers (pleura) lining the lungs and inner chest wall. Pleurisy is often associated with the accumulation of fluid between the two layers of pleura, known as *pleural effusion.*

Test-Taking Strategy: Focus on the **subject,** pleurisy-related pain. Option 4 promotes lung expansion while minimizing client discomfort. Option 2 is obviously incorrect because it suggests an unsafe practice. Eliminate option 1 next because taking small, shallow breaths would promote atelectasis. Lying on the unaffected side would stretch the chest wall on the affected side, thereby increasing discomfort, so option 3 can be eliminated.

---

162. A client is to be discharged on warfarin therapy, and the nurse reinforces medication instructions with the client. Which statement by the client would indicate the **need for further teaching**?

1 "I need to have my blood levels checked in 2 weeks."
2 "I need to include more foods high in vitamin K in my diet."
3 "This medicine thins my blood and allows me to clot more slowly."
4 "If I notice any increased bleeding or bruising, I need to call my doctor."

Level of Cognitive Ability: Evaluating
Client Needs: Health Promotion and Maintenance

Answer: 2
Rationale: Warfarin is an oral anticoagulant that is mainly used to prevent thromboembolic events such as thrombophlebitis, pulmonary embolism, and embolism formation caused by atrial fibrillation. Oral anticoagulants prolong the clotting time and are monitored by the prothrombin time and the international normalized ratio. Client education needs to include the signs and symptoms of toxic effects, as well as dietary restrictions related to warfarin therapy, such as limiting foods high in vitamin K because these food items reduce the drug's anticoagulant effect.
Priority Nursing Tip: Vitamin K–containing foods include leafy green vegetables, liver, cheeses, and egg yolks.

Test-Taking Strategy: Note the **strategic words,** *need for further teaching.* These words indicate a **negative event query** and ask you to select an option that is an incorrect statement. Recalling the purpose of warfarin therapy and the role that vitamin K plays in the clotting mechanism will direct you to option 2.

Clinical Judgment/Cognitive Skills: Evaluate Outcomes
Integrated Process: Teaching and Learning
Content Area: Pharmacology: Cardiovascular: Anticoagulants
Health Problem: Adult Health: Hematological: Bleeding/Clotting Disorders

---

163. A teenager returns to the gynecological clinic for a follow-up visit for a sexually transmitted infection (STI). Which statement by the client indicates the **need for further teaching**?

1 "I know you won't tell my parents I'm sick."
2 "I always make sure my boyfriend uses a condom."
3 "I finished all of the antibiotics, just like you said."
4 "My partner doesn't have to come in for treatment."

Level of Cognitive Ability: Evaluating
Client Needs: Health Promotion and Maintenance
Clinical Judgment/Cognitive Skills: Evaluate Outcomes
Integrated Process: Teaching and Learning
Content Area: Adult Health: Reproductive
Health Problem: Adult Health: Reproductive: Inflammatory/Infection Problems

Answer: 4
Rationale: When a client has an STI, all sexual contacts must be notified and treated with medication. Any treatment at a gynecological clinic for teenagers is confidential, and parents will not be contacted, even if the client is younger than 18 years old. Clients need to always finish a medication prescribed by the primary health care provider. Clients need to always use condoms with any sexual contact.
Priority Nursing Tip: STIs are diseases that are passed from one person to another through sexual contact. The infection can be passed through vaginal intercourse, oral sex, and anal sex.

Test-Taking Strategy: Note the **strategic words,** *need for further teaching.* These words indicate a **negative event query** and ask you to select an option that is an incorrect statement. Knowledge of safe sex practices and the treatment of STIs will assist you with answering this question.

---

164. A perinatal client has been instructed about the prevention of genital tract infections. Which statement by the client indicates an understanding of the instructions?

1 "I can douche any time I want."
2 "I can wear my tight-fitting jeans."
3 "I need to avoid the use of condoms."
4 "I need to choose underwear with a cotton panel liner."

Level of Cognitive Ability: Evaluating
Client Needs: Health Promotion and Maintenance
Clinical Judgment/Cognitive Skills: Evaluate Outcomes
Integrated Process: Nursing Process/Evaluation
Content Area: Maternity: Antepartum
Health Problem: Adult Health: Reproductive: Inflammatory/Infection Problems

Answer: 4
Rationale: Wearing items with a cotton panel liner allows for air movement in and around the genital area and assists with the prevention of genital tract infections. Douching needs to be avoided because it places the client at risk for infection. Wearing tight clothes irritates the genital area and does not allow for air circulation. Condoms need to be used to minimize the spread of sexually transmitted infectious diseases.
Priority Nursing Tip: Trichomoniasis is primarily an infection of the urinary and genital tract; it is caused by a parasite.

Test-Taking Strategy: Focus on the **subject,** measures to prevent genital tract infections. Think about the causes of infections. Options 1, 2, and 3 are all incorrect statements regarding client self-care and the prevention of genital tract infections.

---

165. A client who sustained a major burn is resuming an oral diet. The nurse encourages the client to eat a variety of which types of foods to help with continued wound healing and tissue repair?

1. High-protein and high-fat foods
2. High-fat and low-carbohydrate foods
3. High-carbohydrate and low-protein foods
4. High-protein and high-carbohydrate foods

Level of Cognitive Ability: Applying
Client Needs: Health Promotion and Maintenance
Clinical Judgment/Cognitive Skills: Take Action
Integrated Process: Nursing Process/Implementation
Content Area: Adult Health: Integumentary
Health Problem: Adult Health: Integumentary: Burns

Answer: 4
Rationale: To promote adequate healing and to meet continued high metabolic needs, the client with a major burn needs to eat a diet that is high in calories, protein, and carbohydrates. This type of diet also keeps the client in positive nitrogen balance. There is no need to increase the amount of fat in the diet.
Priority Nursing Tip: High-protein foods heal tissues from burns or other skin abnormalities.

Test-Taking Strategy: Focus on the **subject,** a wound-healing diet, and note the words *wound healing and tissue repair.* Use the principles of nutrition as they relate to healing tissues to answer this question; this will direct you to the correct option.

---

166. The nurse has taught the client diagnosed with hypothyroidism about dietary changes to help manage the disorder. The nurse determines that the client understands the information when the client states that it is permissible to continue eating which foods?

1. Shrimp, green beans, and butter
2. Peanut butter, cheese, and red meat
3. Beef liver, carrots, and fried potatoes
4. Apples, whole-grain breads, and low-fat milk

Level of Cognitive Ability: Evaluating
Client Needs: Health Promotion and Maintenance
Clinical Judgment/Cognitive Skills: Evaluate Outcomes
Integrated Process: Nursing Process/Evaluation
Content Area: Adult Health: Endocrine
Health Problem: Adult Health: Endocrine: Thyroid Disorders

Answer: 4
Rationale: Clients with myxedema, or hypothyroidism, have decreased metabolic demands from a reduced metabolic rate. For this reason, they often experience weight gain. The diet needs to be low in calories overall and yet be representative of all food groups. Increased fiber will promote passage of stool through the intestine. This could decrease exposure to any toxic substances. Fiber also contains important vitamins and minerals, which could supplement the low-calorie diet. Option 4 is the only one that contains solely low-calorie foods.
Priority Nursing Tip: Myxedema is a severe form of hypothyroidism. Symptoms of myxedema may include weakness, confusion, low body temperature, swelling of the body, and difficulty breathing.

Test-Taking Strategy: Focus on the **subject,** a diet for hypothyroidism. Remember that when there is more than one part to an option, all of the parts must be correct for the option to be correct. Think about the pathophysiology of hypothyroidism, and analyze each option in terms of dietary content. The correct option is the one that promotes weight reduction by being low in fat and calories.

---

167. The nurse demonstrates to a parent how to correctly take an axillary temperature to determine whether a newborn has a fever. Which action by the parent would indicate the **need for further teaching?**

1 Holding the thermometer securely in place
2 Taking the temperature only after a feeding
3 Recording the actual temperature reading and route
4 Placing the thermometer in the center of the axilla

Level of Cognitive Ability: Evaluating
Client Needs: Health Promotion and Maintenance
Clinical Judgment/Cognitive Skills: Evaluate Outcomes
Integrated Process: Teaching and Learning
Content Area: Skills: Vital Signs
Health Problem: Pediatric-Specific: Fever

Answer: 2
Rationale: It is not necessary to take the newborn's temperature only after a feeding. Options 1, 3, and 4 are correct steps for taking an axillary temperature.
Priority Nursing Tip: Assessment findings associated with the fever provide important indications of the seriousness of the fever.

Test-Taking Strategy: Note the **strategic words,** *need for further teaching.* These words indicate a **negative event query** and ask you to select an option that is an incorrect action. Noting the **closed-ended word** "only" in option 2 will direct you to this option.

---

168. The nurse teaches a client with coronary artery disease about a low-fat diet. The client indicates an understanding of this diet by choosing which foods?

1 Shrimp and bacon salad
2 Liver, potato salad, and sherbet
3 Turkey breast, boiled rice, and angel food cake
4 Lean hamburger steak and macaroni and cheese

Level of Cognitive Ability: Evaluating
Client Needs: Health Promotion and Maintenance
Clinical Judgment/Cognitive Skills: Evaluate Outcomes
Integrated Process: Teaching and Learning
Content Area: Foundations of Care: Therapeutic Diets
Health Problem: Adult Health: Cardiovascular: Coronary Artery Disease

Answer: 3
Rationale: Major sources of fat include organ meats, red meats, salad dressings, eggs, butter, and cheese. All options except option 3 contain high-fat foods.
Priority Nursing Tip: A low-fat diet usually has 30% of calories from fat. Some low-fat diets may be limited to 30 or 50 g per day, which would equal 23% to 38% of a 1200-calorie diet.

Test-Taking Strategy: Focus on the **subject,** low-fat diet options. Eliminate options 1 and 4 first because both a hamburger steak and bacon are high in fat. From the remaining options, look at the foods closely. Option 3 does not contain any high-fat foods. Potato salad will contain mayonnaise, which is high in fat.

---

169. The nurse is reinforcing teaching to a client diagnosed with acquired immunodeficiency syndrome (AIDS) home-care measures for preventing foodborne illnesses. The nurse stresses to the client to avoid which food to prevent a possible illness?

Answer: 2
Rationale: The client is taught to avoid raw or undercooked seafood, meat, poultry, and eggs. Bottled beverages and fruits that the client peels are safe. The client may be taught to avoid syrup, but this is to diminish diarrhea and has nothing to do with foodborne infection.

1 Bananas
2 Raw oysters
3 Bottled water
4 Sugar-free syrup

Level of Cognitive Ability: Applying
Client Needs: Health Promotion and Maintenance
Clinical Judgment/Cognitive Skills: Take Action
Integrated Process: Teaching and Learning
Content Area: Foundations of Care: Infection Control
Health Problem: Adult Health: Immune: Immunodeficiency Syndrome

Priority Nursing Tip: The client with immunodeficiency syndrome needs to avoid unpasteurized milk and dairy products when considering a risk for illness.

Test-Taking Strategy: Focus on the **subject,** the prevention of foodborne illnesses. Sugar-free syrup produces diarrhea but is unrelated to foodborne illness, so option 4 is eliminated first. Bottled water is safe to drink. Eliminate option 1 because the client is taught that fruits that are peeled are safe.

---

170. A client has been prescribed fluconazole for a fungal infection of the skin. The nurse reinforces home-care instructions that include which suggestion when taking this medication?
1 Avoiding exposure to sunlight
2 Limiting alcohol to 2 oz per day
3 Taking the medication with an antacid
4 Taking the medication on an empty stomach

Level of Cognitive Ability: Applying
Client Needs: Health Promotion and Maintenance
Clinical Judgment/Cognitive Skills: Take Action
Integrated Process: Teaching and Learning
Content Area: Pharmacology: Immune: Antifungal
Health Problem: Adult Health: Integumentary: Inflammations/Infections

Answer: 1
Rationale: The client needs to be encouraged avoid exposure to sunlight because the medication increases photosensitivity. The client needs to avoid the concurrent use of any alcohol because the medication is hepatotoxic. It needs to be taken with food or milk, and antacids need to be avoided for 2 hours after it is taken.
Priority Nursing Tip: The client would be taught that fluconazole is an antifungal medication.

Test-Taking Strategy: Focus on the **subject,** client instructions for taking fluconazole. Use general medication guidelines to assist in answering correctly. Begin by eliminating options 2 and 3. Many medications are not well absorbed if an antacid is given concurrently. There are also many medications with which alcohol use is contraindicated for the duration of the therapy. To select between options 1 and 4, you need to know that this medication causes photosensitivity and that it would be taken with food or milk.

---

171. The nurse planning to assist with teaching a teenage client about sexuality would address which topic **first**?
1 Determining the client's knowledge of sexuality
2 Informing the client about the dangers of pregnancy
3 Advising the client to maintain sexual abstinence until marriage
4 Providing written information about sexually transmitted infections

Level of Cognitive Ability: Applying
Client Needs: Health Promotion and Maintenance

Answer: 1
Rationale: The first step in the teaching and learning process is to determine the client's knowledge. The other options may be later steps, depending on the data obtained.
Priority Nursing Tip: When teaching, determine motivation, interest, and level of knowledge before providing information.

Test-Taking Strategy: Note the **strategic word,** *first.* Use the **steps of the nursing process** to answer. Select the option that involves the gathering of data; this will direct you to the correct option.

Clinical Judgment/Cognitive Skills: Generate Solutions
Integrated Process: Teaching and Learning
Content Area: Foundations of Care: Client Teaching
Health Problem: N/A

---

172. The nurse reinforces suggestions to parents about the appropriate actions to take when their toddler has a temper tantrum. Which statement by the parents indicates an understanding of the actions to take?
1 "I will ignore the tantrums as long as there is no physical danger."
2 "I will give frequent reminders that only bad children have tantrums."
3 "I will send my child to a room alone for 10 minutes after every tantrum."
4 "I will reward my child with candy at the end of each day without a tantrum."

Level of Cognitive Ability: Evaluating
Client Needs: Health Promotion and Maintenance
Clinical Judgment/Cognitive Skills: Evaluate Outcomes
Integrated Process: Nursing Process/Evaluation
Content Area: Developmental Stages: Toddler
Health Problem: N/A

Answer: 1
Rationale: Ignoring a negative attention-seeking behavior is the best way to discourage it, provided that the child is safe from injury. Option 2 is untrue and negative. Option 3 gives attention to the tantrum and exceeds the recommended time of 1 minute per year of age for a time-out. Providing candy as a reward is unhealthy and unlikely to ultimately be effective.
Priority Nursing Tip: Tired, hungry, and overstimulated children are more likely to experience tantrums.

Test-Taking Strategy: Use **Maslow's Hierarchy of Needs theory** to answer the question. Recalling that safety is a primary concern will direct you to the correct option.

---

173. The nurse reinforces medication instructions to a client who has been prescribed disulfiram. Which statement by the client indicates the **need for further instruction** regarding the medication?
1 "I'll have to check my aftershave lotion."
2 "I must be careful taking cold medicines."
3 "As long as I don't drink alcohol, I'll be fine."
4 "I'll have to be more careful with the ingredients that I use for cooking."

Level of Cognitive Ability: Evaluating
Client Needs: Health Promotion and Maintenance
Clinical Judgment/Cognitive Skills: Evaluate Outcomes
Integrated Process: Teaching and Learning
Content Area: Pharmacology: Psychotherapeutic: Alcohol Deterrents
Health Problem: Mental Health: Addictions

Answer: 3
Rationale: Clients who are taking disulfiram must be taught that substances that contain alcohol can trigger adverse reactions. Sources of hidden alcohol include foods (e.g., soups, sauces, vinegars), medicines (e.g., cold medicines, mouthwashes), and skin preparations (e.g., alcohol rubs, aftershave lotions).
Priority Nursing Tip: Disulfiram is prescribed for clients who habitually abuse alcohol and need assistance to discontinue alcohol use.

Test-Taking Strategy: Focus on the **subject,** disulfiram, and note the **strategic words,** *need for further instruction.* These words indicate a **negative event query** and ask you to select an option that is an incorrect statement. Recalling that disulfiram is used with clients who have alcoholism and that any form of alcohol needs to be avoided with this medication will direct you to the correct option.

---

174. Which client statement indicates that the client **needs further teaching** about testicular self-examination (TSE)?
1 "I know to report any small lumps."
2 "I examine myself every 2 months."
3 "I examine myself after I take a warm shower."
4 "I feel a cordlike structure in back and going upward."

Level of Cognitive Ability: Evaluating
Client Needs: Health Promotion and Maintenance
Clinical Judgment/Cognitive Skills: Evaluate Outcomes
Integrated Process: Teaching and Learning
Content Area: Adult Health: Oncology
Health Problem: Adult Health: Cancer: Testicular

Answer: 2
Rationale: A TSE needs to be performed every month, and small lumps or abnormalities need to be reported. The spermatic cord finding is normal. After a warm bath or shower, the scrotum is relaxed, thereby making it easier to perform the TSE.
Priority Nursing Tip: If any changes are noticed from one month to the next, the client is instructed to notify his primary health care provider.

Test-Taking Strategy: Focus on the **subject,** testicular self-examination, and note the **strategic words,** *needs further teaching.* These words indicate a **negative event query** and ask you to select an option that is an incorrect statement. Remembering that breast self-examination needs to be performed monthly may assist you with recalling that the TSE is also performed monthly.

---

175. The nurse determines that a client diagnosed with Cushing's syndrome understands the hospital discharge instructions when the client makes which statement?
1 "I need to eat foods low in vitamin D."
2 "I need to check the color of my stools."
3 "I need to check the temperature of my legs at least once a day."
4 "I need to take aspirin rather than acetaminophen for a headache."

Level of Cognitive Ability: Evaluating
Client Needs: Health Promotion and Maintenance
Clinical Judgment/Cognitive Skills: Evaluate Outcomes
Integrated Process: Nursing Process/ Evaluation
Content Area: Adult Health: Endocrine
Health Problem: Adult Health: Endocrine: Adrenal Disorders

Answer: 2
Rationale: Cortisol, which is secreted in clients with Cushing's syndrome, stimulates the secretion of gastric acid; this can result in peptic ulcers and gastrointestinal (GI) bleeding. The client needs to check the stools for signs of GI bleeding. Option 1 is incorrect because Cushing's syndrome causes a thinning of the bones because of the high levels of cortisol in the blood. Adding additional vitamin D to the diet could reduce fractures. Option 3 is incorrect because Cushing's syndrome does not affect temperature changes in the lower extremities. Option 4 is incorrect because aspirin can increase the risk for gastric bleeding and skin bruising.
Priority Nursing Tip: Cushing's syndrome (hypercortisolism) is a hormonal disorder caused by overexposure to the hormone cortisol.

Test-Taking Strategy: Focus on the **subject,** home care instructions for the client with Cushing's syndrome. Knowledge of the pathophysiology related to Cushing's syndrome is necessary to answer this question. Remember that in Cushing's syndrome excessive cortisol is secreted and that cortisol stimulates the secretion of gastric acid, which can result in peptic ulcers and GI bleeding.

---

176. A client with diabetes mellitus is on a diet that has been designed to avoid concentrated sugars. The nurse determines that the client understands the diet plan if which foods are selected?
1 Strawberry yogurt, lettuce salad, and coffee
2 Chicken salad, tomato, Jell-O, tea, and honey

Answer: 4
Rationale: Concentrated sugars are found in fruit yogurt, gelatin desserts, prepared drink mixes, jelly, and sherbet.
Priority Nursing Tip: Most processed foods contain concentrated sugar and sodium.

Test-Taking Strategy: Focus on the **subject,** a low-sugar diet. Read all the food items in each option, noting that options 1, 2, and 3 contain foods that are high in concentrated sugars.

3 Peanut butter and jelly sandwich, sherbet, and cola
4 Tuna sandwich, lettuce salad, watermelon, and herbal tea

Level of Cognitive Ability: Evaluating
Client Needs: Health Promotion and Maintenance
Clinical Judgment/Cognitive Skills: Evaluate Outcomes
Integrated Process: Nursing Process/Evaluation
Content Area: Foundations of Care: Therapeutic Diets
Health Problem: Adult Health: Endocrine: Diabetes Mellitus

---

177. The nurse has reinforced instructions to a client with chronic obstructive pulmonary disease (COPD) regarding home-care measures. Which statement by the client would indicate the **need for further teaching** about nutrition?
1 "I will rest a few minutes before I eat."
2 "I will not eat as much cabbage as I once did."
3 "I will certainly try to drink 3 L of fluid every day."
4 "It's best to eat three large meals a day so that I will get all of my nutrients."

Level of Cognitive Ability: Evaluating
Client Needs: Health Promotion and Maintenance
Clinical Judgment/Cognitive Skills: Evaluate Outcomes
Integrated Process: Teaching and Learning
Content Area: Adult Health: Respiratory
Health Problem: Adult Health: Respiratory: Obstructive Pulmonary Disease

Answer: 4
Rationale: Large meals distend the abdomen and elevate the diaphragm, which may hinder breathing. Resting before eating may decrease the fatigue that is often associated with COPD. Gas-forming foods may cause bloating, which interferes with normal diaphragmatic breathing. Adequate fluid intake helps liquefy pulmonary secretions.
Priority Nursing Tip: Large meals will increase the abdominal diameter and result in pressure on the diaphragm, causing difficulty breathing, particularly in clients with respiratory disorders.

Test-Taking Strategy: Note the **strategic words,** *need for further teaching.* These words indicate a **negative event query** and ask you to select an option that is an incorrect statement. Option 4 suggests that the only way to obtain all of the daily nutrients is by eating three large meals a day; this is a false statement.

---

178. The nurse is reinforcing home-care instructions to a hospitalized client diagnosed with pneumonia. Which statement by the client indicates that the client **requires further discharge teaching**?
1 "I won't need incentive spirometry when I am discharged."
2 "I will take all of my antibiotics even if I do feel 100% better."

Answer: 1
Rationale: Deep breathing and coughing exercises and the use of incentive spirometry need to be practiced for 6 to 8 weeks after the client is discharged from the hospital to keep the alveoli expanded and to promote the removal of lung secretions. If the entire regimen of antibiotics is not taken, the client may experience a relapse. The period of convalescence with pneumonia is often lengthy, and it may be weeks before the client feels a sense of well-being. Adequate rest is needed to maintain progress toward recovery.

3 "I understand that it may be weeks before my usual sense of well-being returns."
4 "It is a good idea for me to take a nap every afternoon for the next couple of weeks."

Level of Cognitive Ability: Evaluating
Client Needs: Health Promotion and Maintenance
Clinical Judgment/Cognitive Skills: Evaluate Outcomes
Integrated Process: Teaching and Learning
Content Area: Adult Health: Respiratory
Health Problem: Adult Health: Respiratory: Viral, Bacterial, Fungal Infections

Priority Nursing Tip: Even after discharge from a hospital for treatment for pneumonia, the respiratory system is still compromised for several weeks after.

Test-Taking Strategy: Focus on the **subject**, home-care instructions after pneumonia, and note the **strategic words,** *requires further discharge teaching.* These words indicate a **negative event query** and ask you to select an option that is an incorrect statement. Think about the pathophysiology of pneumonia and its treatment. The use of an incentive spirometer has a direct relationship to the pneumonia.

---

179. An 18-year-old client is admitted to an inpatient mental health unit with a diagnosis of anorexia nervosa. Health promotion would focus on which goal?
1 Providing a supportive environment
2 Emphasizing social interaction with other clients
3 Examining intrapsychic conflicts and past issues
4 Helping the client identify and examine dysfunctional thoughts and beliefs

Level of Cognitive Ability: Applying
Client Needs: Health Promotion and Maintenance
Clinical Judgment/Cognitive Skills: Generate Solutions
Integrated Process: Nursing Process/Planning
Content Area: Mental Health
Health Problem: Mental Health: Eating Disorders

Answer: 4
Rationale: Health promotion focuses on helping clients recognize and analyze dysfunctional thoughts and on identifying and examining the values and beliefs that maintain these thoughts. Providing a supportive environment is important, but it is not as critical as option 4, and it does not specifically focus on health promotion. Emphasizing social interaction is not appropriate now. Examining intrapsychic conflicts and past issues is not directly related to the client's problem.
Priority Nursing Tip: The main goal for anorexia nervosa treatment is to normalize eating patterns and behaviors to support weight gain. Another goal is to help change distorted beliefs and thoughts that maintain the restrictive eating.

Test-Taking Strategy: Focus on the **subject,** goals for the client with anorexia nervosa. Option 4 is the only option that is specifically client centered. This option also focuses on identifying client issues related to the diagnosis.

---

180. The nurse is assisting with planning home care for a client with a C5 spinal cord injury. During the discharge planning with the client and family, they agree that the **priority** would focus on which facet of care?
1 Maintaining intact skin
2 Regaining bladder and bowel control
3 Performing activities of daily living independently
4 Independently transferring to and from a wheelchair

Answer: 1
Rationale: A C5 spinal cord injury results in quadriplegia with no sensation below the clavicle, including in most of the arms and the hands. The client may maintain partial movement of the shoulders and elbows. Maintaining intact skin is an important outcome for the client with a spinal cord injury. The remaining options are inappropriate for the client with this type of injury because they are unattainable.
Priority Nursing Tip: The skin is the largest system in the body and can be easily traumatized, resulting in breakdown of tissue.

Level of Cognitive Ability: Applying
Client Needs: Health Promotion and Maintenance
Clinical Judgment/Cognitive Skills: Generate Solutions
Integrated Process: Nursing Process/Planning
Content Area: Adult Health: Neurological
Health Problem: Adult Health: Neurological: Spinal Cord Injury

Test-Taking Strategy: Focus on the **subject**, C5 spinal cord injury, and note the **strategic word**, *priority*. Think about the pathophysiology associated with this type of injury. Eliminate options 3 and 4 first because they are **comparable or alike** because they both involve self-care. Knowledge of the effects of a C5 spinal cord injury will assist you with eliminating option 2.

---

181. A client who sustained a thoracic cord injury 1 year ago presents for an office visit with a small reddened area on the coccyx. After reinforcing home-care instructions regarding the relief of pressure on the area with the use of a turning schedule, which action by the nurse is appropriate?

1 Ask a family member to check the skin daily.
2 Teach the client to feel for red and broken areas.
3 Teach the client to use a mirror for skin assessment.
4 Have the client return to the office weekly for a skin check.

Level of Cognitive Ability: Applying
Client Needs: Health Promotion and Maintenance
Clinical Judgment/Cognitive Skills: Take Action
Integrated Process: Nursing Process/Implementation
Content Area: Adult Health: Neurological
Health Problem: Adult Health: Integumentary: Wounds

Answer: 3
Rationale: The client needs to be encouraged to be as independent as possible. The most effective method of skin self-assessment is to use a special mirror to view the skin. Options 1 and 4 involve others in performing a task that the client can perform independently. It is unrealistic to expect the client to return to the office weekly for a skin check. Option 2 is an inaccurate technique because redness cannot be felt. Option 3 is the only option that addresses client self-assessment of redness.
Priority Nursing Tip: T11 and T12 are particularly flexible sections of the spine and are subsequently the most common areas of the thoracic spine that get damaged.

Test-Taking Strategy: Focus on the **subject**, home-care instructions for skin care, and remember that independence is key in the rehabilitation of clients. Recalling this concept will direct you to the correct option.

---

182. The nurse is reinforcing home-care instructions regarding symptom management to a client diagnosed with peptic ulcer disease. Which instruction will the nurse provide the client?

1 Limit the intake of water.
2 Use aspirin to relieve gastric pain.
3 Eat large meals to absorb gastric acid.
4 Eat slowly and chew food thoroughly.

Level of Cognitive Ability: Applying
Client Needs: Health Promotion and Maintenance

Answer: 4
Rationale: The client with a peptic ulcer is taught to eat small, frequent meals to help keep the gastric secretions neutralized. The client needs to eat slowly and chew thoroughly to prevent excess gastric acid secretion. The client needs to drink at least 6 to 8 glasses of water per day to dilute the gastric acid. The use of aspirin is avoided because it is irritating to the gastric mucosa.
Priority Nursing Tip: Two common causes of peptic ulcers are infection with *Helicobacter pylori* bacteria and the use of nonsteroidal antiinflammatory drugs (NSAIDs).

Clinical Judgment/Cognitive Skills: Take Action
Integrated Process: Teaching and Learning
Content Area: Adult Health: Gastrointestinal
Health Problem: Adult Health: Gastrointestinal: Upper GI Disorders

Test-Taking Strategy: Focus on the **subject,** symptom management for peptic ulcer disease. Eliminate option 1 because of the word *limit.* Eliminate option 2, recalling that aspirin is very irritating to the stomach. Eliminate option 3 because of the word *large.* Also, use your knowledge of concepts related to digestion and of substances that are known gastric irritants to direct you to the correct option.

---

183. A client diagnosed with a hiatal hernia asks the nurse about the types of juices that are acceptable to drink. The nurse reinforces that it is acceptable for the client to drink which type of juice?

1 Apple juice
2 Orange juice
3 Tomato juice
4 Grapefruit juice

Level of Cognitive Ability: Applying
Client Needs: Health Promotion and Maintenance
Clinical Judgment/Cognitive Skills: Take Action
Integrated Process: Teaching and Learning
Content Area: Adult Health: Gastrointestinal
Health Problem: Adult Health: Gastrointestinal: Upper GI Disorders

Answer: 1
Rationale: Substances that are irritating to the client with a hiatal hernia include tomato products and citrus fruits, which need to be avoided. Because caffeine stimulates gastric acid secretion, beverages that contain caffeine (e.g., coffee, tea, cola, cocoa) are also eliminated from the diet.
Priority Nursing Tip: Hiatal hernias occur when the muscle tissue surrounding the opening where the esophagus passes into the stomach becomes weak and the upper part of the stomach bulges up through the diaphragm into the chest cavity.

Test-Taking Strategy: Focus on the **subject,** diet for hiatal hernia. Eliminate options 2, 3, and 4 because they are **comparable or alike** in that they are irritating to the gastrointestinal system. Apple juice is the least irritating substance.

---

184. The nurse's teaching plan for the client with seizures includes reinforcing information about the safe use of phenytoin. The nurse reinforces which information to the client?

1 That the anticonvulsant must be taken for life
2 To stop driving a car while taking the medication
3 That seizures can never be completely controlled
4 To avoid skipping a medication dose because it will cause seizures to occur

Level of Cognitive Ability: Applying
Client Needs: Health Promotion and Maintenance
Clinical Judgment/Cognitive Skills: Take Action
Integrated Process: Teaching and Learning
Content Area: Pharmacology: Neurological: Anticonvulsants
Health Problem: Pharmacology: Neurological: Seizure Disorder/Epilepsy

Answer: 4
Rationale: The client needs to be informed about the seriousness of the condition (i.e., skipping a dose of medication places the client at risk for status epilepticus). In some well-controlled cases, the medication can eventually be discontinued. In some states, a client can drive a car if he or she has had no seizures for a year.
Priority Nursing Tip: Neurological medications require consistent use to maintain a blood level at a point whereby seizures are controlled.

Test-Taking Strategy: Focus on the **subject,** phenytoin administration. Eliminate options 1 and 3 because of the **closed-ended words** "must" and "never." Also, general principles related to medication administration will direct you to the correct option.

---

185. A hospitalized client with a spinal cord injury (SCI) experiences bladder spasms and reflex incontinence. When preparing for discharge, the nurse reinforces home-care instructions that include what action?

1 "Avoid caffeine in the diet."
2 "Take your own temperature every day."
3 "Limit fluid intake to 1000 mL every 24 hours."
4 "Catheterize yourself every 2 hours as necessary to prevent spasm."

Level of Cognitive Ability: Applying
Client Needs: Health Promotion and Maintenance
Clinical Judgment/Cognitive Skills: Take Action
Integrated Process: Teaching and Learning
Content Area: Adult Health: Neurological
Health Problem: Adult Health: Neurological: Spinal Cord Injury

Answer: 1
Rationale: Caffeine in the diet can contribute to bladder spasms and reflex incontinence; therefore it needs to be eliminated from the diet of the client with an SCI. Self-monitoring of the temperature would be useful to detect infection but does nothing to alleviate bladder spasms. Limiting fluid intake does not prevent spasm and could place the client at further risk of urinary tract infection. Self-catheterization every 2 hours is too frequent and serves no useful purpose.
Priority Nursing Tip: A risk for reflex incontinence is neurological impairment from multiple sclerosis.

Test-Taking Strategy: Focus on the **subjects,** bladder spasms and reflex incontinence. Eliminate options 3 and 4 first because they are **comparable or alike** in that they increase the client's risk of urinary tract infection and are therefore inappropriate. Choose option 1 rather than option 2 because option 2 would be used to detect infection but does not deal with spasm and incontinence.

---

186. A client diagnosed with atherosclerosis asks the nurse about dietary modifications to lower the risk of heart disease. The nurse encourages the client to eat which food?

1 Fresh cantaloupe
2 Broiled cheeseburger
3 Baked chicken with skin
4 Mashed potatoes with gravy

Level of Cognitive Ability: Applying
Client Needs: Health Promotion and Maintenance
Clinical Judgment/Cognitive Skills: Take Action
Integrated Process: Teaching and Learning
Content Area: Adult Health: Cardiovascular
Health Problem: Adult Health: Cardiovascular: Vascular Disorders

Answer: 1
Rationale: To lower the risk of heart disease, the diet needs to be low in saturated fat and include the appropriate number of total calories. The diet needs to include fewer red meats and more white meat with the skin removed. The dairy products eaten need to be low in fat, and foods with high amounts of empty calories need to be avoided.
Priority Nursing Tip: Atherosclerosis is a disease in which plaque builds up inside the arteries. Plaque is made up of fat, cholesterol, calcium, and other substances found in the blood.

Test-Taking Strategy: Focus on the **subject,** dietary modifications to lower the risk of heart disease. Eliminate options 2 and 3 first because of the fat content of the described meats. Choose option 1 rather than option 4 because fresh fruits and vegetables are naturally low in fat.

---

187. A client with coronary artery disease is being discharged to home after angioplasty that involved the use of the right femoral area as the catheter insertion site. The nurse reinforces home-care instructions to the client and explains that which sign or symptom may be expected after the procedure?

1 A temperature as high as 101 °F
2 Mild discomfort in the right groin

Answer: 2
Rationale: The client may feel some mild discomfort at the catheter insertion site after angioplasty. This is usually relieved by analgesics such as acetaminophen. The client is taught to report to the cardiologist any neurovascular changes to the affected leg, bleeding or bruising at the insertion site, and signs of local infection (e.g., drainage at the site, increased temperature).
Priority Nursing Tip: Angioplasty is also known as *balloon angioplasty* and *percutaneous transluminal angioplasty*. This procedure is minimally invasive and is done to widen narrowed or

3 A large area of bruising in the right groin
4 Coolness or discoloration of the right foot

Level of Cognitive Ability: Applying
Client Needs: Health Promotion and Maintenance
Clinical Judgment/Cognitive Skills: Take Action
Integrated Process: Teaching and Learning
Content Area: Adult Health: Cardiovascular
Health Problem: Adult Health: Cardiovascular: Coronary Artery Disease

obstructed arteries or veins. It is typically used to treat arterial atherosclerosis.

Test-Taking Strategy: Focus on the **subject**, expected occurrences after angioplasty. Knowing that bleeding and infection are complications of the procedure guides you to eliminate options 1 and 3. You would choose option 2 rather than option 4 by knowing that the area may be mildly uncomfortable or that the neurovascular status would not be impaired by the procedure.

---

188. The nurse is reinforcing dietary instructions to a hypertensive client. The nurse encourages which snack food as being acceptable?
1 Frozen pizza
2 Cheese and crackers
3 Canned tomato soup
4 Honeydew melon slices

Level of Cognitive Ability: Applying
Client Needs: Health Promotion and Maintenance
Clinical Judgment/Cognitive Skills: Take Action
Integrated Process: Teaching and Learning
Content Area: Adult Health: Cardiovascular
Health Problem: Adult Health: Cardiovascular: Hypertension

Answer: 4
Rationale: Sodium needs to be avoided by the client with hypertension. Fresh fruits and vegetables are naturally low in sodium. Hypertensive clients are also advised to keep fat intake to less than 30% of the total daily calories. Each of the incorrect options contains high amounts of sodium.
Priority Nursing Tip: Clients with a cardiovascular compromise need to avoid processed foods because most are high in sodium.

Test-Taking Strategy: Focus on the **subject**, a hypertension diet. Recall that the client with hypertension needs to limit sodium intake. Eliminate options 1, 2, and 3 because they are **comparable or alike** and high in sodium. The correct option is a fruit, which is naturally low in sodium.

---

189. The nurse is reinforcing instructions to a client who will be discharged to home with a halo vest. Which instruction would the nurse include in the discussion?
1 Loosen the bolts once a day for bathing.
2 Carry the correct-size wrench to loosen the bolts in an emergency.
3 Have the caregiver use the metal frame to assist the client to sit upright.
4 Perform pin care 3 times a week using hydrogen peroxide or alcohol.

Level of Cognitive Ability: Applying
Client Needs: Health Promotion and Maintenance
Clinical Judgment/Cognitive Skills: Take Action
Integrated Process: Teaching and Learning
Content Area: Adult Health: Musculoskeletal
Health Problem: Adult Health: Musculoskeletal: Skeletal Injury

Answer: 2
Rationale: A halo vest is a device that provides stability and immobility to the cervical area in a client who sustained a cervical fracture. The client is instructed to carry the correct-size wrench in case of an emergency that requires cardiopulmonary resuscitation (CPR). The bolts would never be loosened except in an emergency, and the orthopedic surgeon needs to be notified if the bolts loosen. The metal frame is never used or pulled on for turning or lifting. Pin care needs to be performed at least once a day using soap and water with cotton-tipped swabs or alcohol swabs.
Priority Nursing Tip: Some people who are in a halo vest find it comfortable to sleep in a reclining chair for the first month until they are more used to the halo vest.

Test-Taking Strategy: Focus on the **subject**, a halo vest, and try to visualize its appearance. Eliminate option 3 because pulling on the frame will disrupt the stabilization of the fracture and possibly lead to serious complications. Eliminate option 4 because pin care needs to be performed at least once a day. For the remaining options, remember that the bolts would only be loosened in an emergency.

---

190. What action would the nurse teach the client to avoid while receiving iron therapy to treat iron-deficiency anemia?

1 Eating a low-fiber diet
2 Limiting the intake of fluids
3 Taking the supplement with milk
4 Limiting the intake of animal protein

Level of Cognitive Ability: Applying
Client Needs: Health Promotion and Maintenance
Clinical Judgment/Cognitive Skills: Take Action
Integrated Process: Teaching and Learning
Content Area: Adult Health: Hematological
Health Problem: Adult Health: Hematological: Anemias

Answer: 3
Rationale: The client needs to avoid taking iron with milk or antacids, which decrease the absorption of iron. The client needs to also avoid taking iron with food, if possible. The client needs to increase the intake of natural sources of iron (e.g., meats, fish, poultry). Finally, the client needs to take in sufficient fiber and fluids to prevent constipation, which is a side effect of therapy.
Priority Nursing Tip: Vitamin C increases the absorption of iron.

Test-Taking Strategy: Focus on the **subject,** iron supplement therapy and the action to avoid. Begin to answer this question by eliminating options 1 and 2 by knowing that constipation is a side effect of iron therapy. From the remaining options, recalling the nutritional content of meat products will assist you with eliminating option 4. Remember that milk products or antacids impair the absorption of certain medications.

---

191. A client with a colostomy reports concern over appliance odor. To control the odor, the nurse recommends that the client consume which food?

1 Eggs
2 Yogurt
3 Cucumbers
4 Mushrooms

Level of Cognitive Ability: Applying
Client Needs: Health Promotion and Maintenance
Clinical Judgment/Cognitive Skills: Take Action
Integrated Process: Teaching and Learning
Content Area: Adult Health: Gastrointestinal
Health Problem: Adult Health: Gastrointestinal: Lower GI Disorders

Answer: 2
Rationale: Foods that help eliminate odor from a colostomy include yogurt, buttermilk, spinach, beet greens, and parsley. Foods that cause odor include alcohol, beans, turnips, radishes, asparagus, onions, cucumbers, mushrooms, cabbage, eggs, and fish.
Priority Nursing Tip: The method to eliminate odors from a colostomy is to avoid foods that will normally cause gas production from the gastrointestinal tract.

Test-Taking Strategy: Focus on the **subject,** eliminating colostomy odor. Remember that foods that cause gas in the client with normal gastrointestinal function also cause gas in the gastrointestinal tract of the client with a colostomy. This will assist in eliminating options 1, 3, and 4.

---

192. The nurse is reinforcing instructions about colostomy care to a client. The nurse demonstrates the correct cutting of the appliance by making the circle how much larger than the client's stoma?

1 ½ inch
2 ⅜ inch
3 ¼ inch
4 ⅛ inch

Level of Cognitive Ability: Applying
Client Needs: Health Promotion and Maintenance
Clinical Judgment/Cognitive Skills: Take Action

Answer: 4
Rationale: The size of the opening of the appliance for a client with a colostomy is generally cut ⅛-inch larger than the size of the client's stoma. This minimizes the amount of exposed skin but does not cause pressure on the stoma itself. Options 1, 2, and 3 are incorrect.
Priority Nursing Tip: Cutting the opening of a stoma appliance too large may cause a poor seal, whereas cutting the opening too small can cause abrasions to the stoma site.

Test-Taking Strategy: Focus on the **subject,** colostomy stoma care. Eliminate options 1, 2, and 3 because they are **comparable or alike** and leave too much skin area exposed for possible irritation by gastrointestinal contents.

Integrated Process: Teaching and Learning
Content Area: Adult Health: Gastrointestinal
Health Problem: Adult Health: Gastrointestinal: Lower GI Disorders

---

193. A 10-year-old child is diagnosed with type 1 diabetes mellitus. The nurse prepares to reinforce diabetic teaching to the child and family and plans to provide what instruction?

1 The child needs to monitor insulin requirements and administer his own insulin.
2 The parents need to always be available to monitor the child's insulin requirements.
3 The child's teacher needs to monitor insulin requirements and administer the child's insulin.
4 All the friends and family involved with the child's activities need to monitor the child's insulin requirements.

Level of Cognitive Ability: Applying
Client Needs: Health Promotion and Maintenance
Clinical Judgment/Cognitive Skills: Take Action
Integrated Process: Teaching and Learning
Content Area: Developmental Stages: Preschool and School Age
Health Problem: Pediatric-Specific: Diabetes Mellitus

Answer: 1

Rationale: Most children 9 years old and older can understand the principles of monitoring their own insulin requirements. They are usually responsible enough to determine the appropriate intervention needed to maintain their health. Options 2, 3, and 4 do not support the growth and development level of this child.

Priority Nursing Tip: A 10-year-old child is in the stage of industry vs. inferiority and wants to be responsible and do things correctly.

Test-Taking Strategy: Focus on the **data in the question.** The age of the child indicates that the child can control and be responsible for the health care situation. Eliminate option 4 first because of the **closed-ended word** "all" and because this option is unrealistic. Eliminate option 3 next because the teacher will not take responsibility for health care interventions. Eliminate option 2 because of the **closed-ended word** "always" and because the parents cannot always be available.

---

194. A client has undergone surgery for glaucoma. The nurse reinforces which home-care safety instruction with the client?

1 The sutures are removed after 1 week.
2 Wound healing usually takes 12 weeks.
3 A shield or eye patch needs to be worn to protect the eye.
4 Expect that the vision will be permanently impaired to some degree.

Level of Cognitive Ability: Applying
Client Needs: Health Promotion and Maintenance
Clinical Judgment/Cognitive Skills: Take Action
Integrated Process: Teaching and Learning
Content Area: Adult Health: Eye
Health Problem: Adult Health: Eye: Glaucoma

Answer: 3

Rationale: After ocular surgery, the client needs to wear a shield or eye patch to protect the eye. Healing occurs after approximately 6 weeks. After the postoperative inflammation subsides, the client's vision would return to the preoperative level of acuity. Most sutures used for these operations are absorbable.

Priority Nursing Tip: Glaucoma is a disease that damages the eye's optic nerve.

Test-Taking Strategy: Focus on the **data in the question** and note the word *safety*. Use **Maslow's Hierarchy of Needs theory** to answer this question. Recalling the concepts related to healing after ocular surgery and focusing on safety will direct you to the correct option.

---

195. A client has undergone surgery for cataract removal. Which postoperative occurrence would be reported **immediately** to the surgeon?

1. Eye redness
2. Eye discomfort
3. Decrease in vision
4. Dried matter on the eyelashes

Level of Cognitive Ability: Applying
Client Needs: Health Promotion and Maintenance
Clinical Judgment/Cognitive Skills: Take Action
Integrated Process: Teaching and Learning
Content Area: Adult Health: Eye
Health Problem: Adult Health: Eye: Cataracts

Answer: 3
Rationale: After surgery for cataract removal, the client needs to report a noticeable or sudden decrease in vision to the surgeon. The client is taught to take acetaminophen, which is usually effective for the relief of discomfort. The eye may be slightly reddened postoperatively, but this would gradually resolve. Small amounts of dried material may be present on the eyelashes after sleep; this is expected, and the material would be removed with a warm, damp face cloth.
Priority Nursing Tip: If cataract surgery is needed in both eyes, the surgeon (based on preference) usually will wait at least 2 weeks for the first eye to recover before performing a procedure on the second eye.

Test-Taking Strategy: Focus on the **subject,** the need to call the surgeon, and note the **strategic word,** *immediately.* Note the word *decrease* to direct you to the correct option.

---

196. The nurse reinforces dietary instructions to a client with cirrhosis and ascites. What instruction would the nurse provide?

1. Decrease fat intake.
2. Restrict sodium intake.
3. Decrease carbohydrate intake.
4. Restrict calories to 1500 daily.

Level of Cognitive Ability: Applying
Client Needs: Health Promotion and Maintenance
Clinical Judgment/Cognitive Skills: Take Action
Integrated Process: Teaching and Learning
Content Area: Adult Health: Gastrointestinal
Health Problem: Adult Health: Gastrointestinal: GI Accessory Organs

Answer: 2
Rationale: The client with cirrhosis has ascites and needs to be on a sodium- and possibly fluid-restricted diet because sodium can cause fluid retention. Fat restriction is unnecessary. The diet would supply sufficient carbohydrates to maintain weight and ample protein to rebuild tissue but not enough protein to precipitate hepatic encephalopathy. The total daily calorie intake needs to range between 2000 and 3000.
Priority Nursing Tip: Ascites is a gastroenterological term for an accumulation of fluid in the peritoneal cavity.

Test-Taking Strategy: Focus on the **subject,** cirrhosis and ascites. Recalling the definition of ascites and that it refers to an abnormal accumulation of fluid in the peritoneal cavity will direct you to the correct option.

---

197. Which home-care instruction will the nurse reinforce to the client with a diagnosis of multiple myeloma?

1. Maintain bed rest.
2. Restrict fluid intake to 1000 mL daily.
3. Maintain a high-calorie, low-fiber diet.
4. Notify the primary health care provider if anorexia and nausea persist.

Level of Cognitive Ability: Applying
Client Needs: Health Promotion and Maintenance
Clinical Judgment/Cognitive Skills: Take Action
Integrated Process: Teaching and Learning
Content Area: Adult Health: Oncology

Answer: 4
Rationale: Clients with multiple myeloma need to be taught to watch for signs of hypercalcemia and to report them immediately to the primary health care provider. Anorexia, nausea, vomiting, polyuria, weakness, fatigue, constipation, and dehydration are signs of moderate hypercalcemia. A fluid intake of about 3000 mL daily is necessary to dilute the calcium overload and to prevent protein from precipitating in the renal tubules. Activity is encouraged. Although a high-calorie diet is encouraged, a diet low in fiber will lead to constipation.
Priority Nursing Tip: Multiple myeloma is a malignant neoplasm of the bone marrow.

Test-Taking Strategy: Focus on the **subject,** multiple myeloma. Think about the pathophysiology associated with this disorder and recall that hypercalcemia is a concern in clients with multiple myeloma. Eliminate option 1 first because bed rest

Health Problem: Adult Health: Cancer: Multiple Myeloma

is not indicated. Eliminate option 2 next because this amount of fluid is rather low. Finally, eliminate option 3 because a low-fiber diet is not indicated for this client and can lead to constipation.

---

198. The nurse prepares to reinforce instructions to a postpartum client who is breast-feeding and has developed breast engorgement. Which instruction would the nurse provide to the client?

1 Avoid the use of a bra during engorgement.
2 Apply cool packs to both breasts 20 minutes before a feeding.
3 During feeding, gently massage the breast from the outer areas to the nipple.
4 Feed the infant less frequently, every 4 to 6 hours, using bottle-feeding in between.

Level of Cognitive Ability: Applying
Client Needs: Health Promotion and Maintenance
Clinical Judgment/Cognitive Skills: Take Action
Integrated Process: Teaching and Learning
Content Area: Maternity: Postpartum
Health Problem: Maternity: Infections/Inflammations

Answer: 3
Rationale: The client with breast engorgement needs to be advised to feed frequently, at least every 2½ hours, for 15 to 20 minutes per side. Moist heat would be applied to both breasts for about 20 minutes before a feeding. Between feedings, the parent needs to wear a supportive bra. During a feeding, it is helpful to gently massage the breast from the outer areas to the nipple to stimulate letdown and the flow of milk.
Priority Nursing Tip: Women who are breast-feeding and become engorged need to try home-care measures with heat applications, which will result in vasodilation.

Test-Taking Strategy: Focus on the **subject,** treating breast engorgement. Consider the manifestations that occur with engorgement, and eliminate those options that will not assist with increasing the flow of milk. With this concept in mind, you would be able to eliminate options 2 and 4. From the remaining options, select option 3 because massage would assist with the flow of milk. In addition, a supportive bra would reduce the discomfort that occurs with this condition.

---

199. A client in the third trimester of pregnancy arrives at the obstetrician's office and tells the nurse that she frequently has a backache. Which instruction would the nurse provide to the client to ease the backache?

1 Maintain correct posture.
2 Eat small, frequent meals.
3 Elevate the legs when sitting.
4 Sleep in a supine position on a firm mattress.

Level of Cognitive Ability: Applying
Client Needs: Health Promotion and Maintenance
Clinical Judgment/Cognitive Skills: Take Action
Integrated Process: Teaching and Learning
Content Area: Maternity: Antepartum
Health Problem: Adult Health: Musculoskeletal: Tissue or Ligament Injury

Answer: 1
Rationale: To provide relief from backache, the nurse would advise the client to use good posture and body mechanics; to perform pelvic rock exercises; and to wear flat, supportive shoes. The client would also be instructed to avoid overexertion and to sleep in the lateral position on a firm mattress. Back massage is also helpful. Eating small meals would more specifically help relieve dyspnea. Leg elevation assists the client with varicosities.
Priority Nursing Tip: Backache in the pregnant woman can be relieved by moving the fetus off the spine with correct posture and the pelvic tilt exercise.

Test-Taking Strategy: Focus on the **subject,** measures to relieve a backache. This would assist you with eliminating options 2 and 3. From the remaining options, recalling that the lateral position is most appropriate will direct you to the correct option.

---

200. Which food would the nurse instruct the client with hypertension to avoid while taking spironolactone?

1 Shrimp
2 Popcorn
3 Bananas
4 Crackers

Level of Cognitive Ability: Applying
Client Needs: Health Promotion and Maintenance
Integrated Process: Teaching and Learning
Clinical Judgment/Cognitive Skills: Take Action
Content Area: Pharmacology: Cardiovascular: Diuretics
Health Problem: Adult Health: Cardiovascular: Hypertension

Answer: 3
Rationale: Spironolactone is a potassium-sparing diuretic, and the client needs to avoid foods that are high in potassium, such as whole-grain cereals, legumes, meat, bananas, apricots, orange juice, potatoes, and raisins. Option 3 provides the highest source of potassium and would be avoided.
Priority Nursing Tip: Vomiting, diarrhea, and stomach pain or cramps are side effects of spironolactone.

Test-Taking Strategy: Focus on the **subject,** diet while taking spironolactone, and note the word *avoid.* Begin by eliminating options 2 and 4 because they are food items that are **comparable or alike** in that both are grains. Remembering that fruits, vegetables, and fresh meats are high in potassium will assist with directing you to the correct option.

---

201. The nurse reinforces to the client diagnosed with cystitis to increase intake of which beverage?

1 Tea
2 Water
3 Coffee
4 White wine

Level of Cognitive Ability: Applying
Client Needs: Health Promotion and Maintenance
Clinical Judgment/Cognitive Skills: Take Action
Integrated Process: Teaching and Learning
Content Area: Adult Health: Renal and Urinary
Health Problem: Adult Health: Renal and Urinary: Inflammations/Infections

Answer: 2
Rationale: Cystitis is an inflammatory condition of the urinary bladder and ureters. Water helps flush bacteria out of the bladder, and an intake of 6 to 8 glasses per day is encouraged. Caffeine and alcohol can irritate the bladder, so coffee, tea, and wine are to be avoided.
Priority Nursing Tip: Cystitis is characterized by pain, urgency and frequency of urination, and hematuria.

Test-Taking Strategy: Focus on the **subject,** a measure to treat cystitis. Option 4 needs to be eliminated first because alcohol intake is not encouraged for any disorder. Options 1 and 3 are **comparable or alike** in that both contain caffeine.

---

202. The nurse has reinforced instructions to a female client about measures to prevent recurrence of cystitis. The nurse determines that the client **requires further instruction** when the client verbalizes a need to do what?

1 Take bubble baths for more effective hygiene.
2 Avoid wearing pantyhose while wearing slacks.
3 Drink a glass of water and void after intercourse.
4 Wear underwear made of cotton or with cotton panels.

Answer: 1
Rationale: Cystitis is an inflammatory condition of the urinary bladder and ureters. Measures to prevent cystitis include increasing fluid intake to 3 L per day; eating an acid-ash diet; wiping front to back after urination; taking showers instead of tub baths; drinking water and voiding after intercourse; avoiding bubble baths, feminine hygiene sprays, and perfumed toilet tissue and sanitary pads; and wearing clothes that "breathe" (e.g., cotton pants, no tight jeans, no pantyhose under slacks).
Priority Nursing Tip: To help avoid cystitis, pregnant women would be encouraged to void every 2 hours.

Test-Taking Strategy: Note the **strategic words,** *requires further instruction.* These words indicate a **negative event query** and ask you to select an option that is an incorrect statement. Think about the causes of cystitis to assist in answering the question. This will assist in directing you to the correct option.

Level of Cognitive Ability: Evaluating
Client Needs: Health Promotion and Maintenance
Clinical Judgment/Cognitive Skills: Evaluate Outcomes
Integrated Process: Teaching and Learning
Content Area: Adult Health: Renal and Urinary
Health Problem: Adult Health: Renal and Urinary: Inflammation/Infections

---

203. A client diagnosed with pyelonephritis is being discharged from the hospital, and the nurse reinforces home-care instructions to prevent recurrence. The nurse determines that the client understands the information that was given when the client states an intention to do what?

1 Continue to drink 3 L of fluid each day.
2 Take the prescribed antibiotics until all symptoms subside.
3 Modify fluid intake for the day based on the previous day's output.
4 Report signs and symptoms of urinary tract infection (UTI) if they persist for more than 1 week.

Level of Cognitive Ability: Evaluating
Client Needs: Health Promotion and Maintenance
Clinical Judgment/Cognitive Skills: Evaluate Outcomes
Integrated Process: Nursing Process/Evaluation
Content Area: Adult Health: Renal and Urinary
Health Problem: Adult Health: Renal and Urinary: Inflammation/Infections

Answer: 1
Rationale: Pyelonephritis is an infection of the pelvis and of the parenchyma of the kidney. The client with pyelonephritis needs to take the full course of antibiotic therapy that has been prescribed. The client needs to learn the signs and symptoms of UTI and report them immediately if they occur. The client needs to use all measures recommended to prevent cystitis, which includes drinking 3 L of fluids per day.
Priority Nursing Tip: Pyelonephritis is inflammation of the kidney, typically due to a bacterial infection. Symptoms most often include fever and flank tenderness. This condition can lead to renal scarring.

Test-Taking Strategy: Focus on the **subject,** treatment for pyelonephritis. Begin to answer this question by eliminating option 4, because UTI symptoms would never go unreported for more than a week. Option 2 is eliminated next because antibiotics need to be taken for the full course of treatment to adequately eliminate the infection. From the remaining options, recalling that the client needs to flush the urinary tract well and drink sufficient fluids helps you choose option 1 rather than option 3, which is an inappropriate option.

---

204. A client with nephrotic syndrome needs dietary teaching about how diet can help counteract the effects of altered renal function. The nurse would include which statement in the instructions to the client?

1 "Increase your intake of fish and other high-protein foods."
2 "Increase your intake of fatty foods to prevent protein loss."
3 "Add salt during cooking to replace sodium lost in the urine."
4 "Increase your fluid intake and drink plenty of fluids throughout the day."

Answer: 1
Rationale: Nephrotic syndrome is an abnormal condition of the kidney that is characterized by marked proteinuria, hypoalbuminemia, and edema. Sodium is limited in the nephrotic syndrome diet to help control edema, which is part of the clinical picture. Fluids are not restricted unless hyponatremia is present, but the client is not encouraged to increase fluid intake and/or to drink plenty of fluids throughout the day. Protein is increased unless the glomerular filtration rate is impaired; this helps replace protein lost in the urine and ultimately helps control edema. Hyperlipidemia, which results from the liver's synthesis of lipoproteins in response to hypoalbuminemia, is also part of the clinical picture. Increasing fatty food intake would not be helpful in this circumstance.

Level of Cognitive Ability: Applying
Client Needs: Health Promotion and Maintenance
Clinical Judgment/Cognitive Skills: Take Action
Integrated Process: Teaching and Learning
Content Area: Adult Health: Renal and Urinary
Health Problem: Adult Health: Renal and Urinary: Inflammation/Infections

Priority Nursing Tip: Nephrotic syndrome is usually caused by damage to the small blood vessels in the kidneys that filter waste and excess water from the blood.

Test-Taking Strategy: Focus on the **subject,** nephrotic syndrome, and recall that nephrotic syndrome is characterized by fluid retention and hypoalbuminemia; this would help you eliminate options 3 and 4. To choose between the remaining options, knowing that hyperlipidemia accompanies nephrotic syndrome would help you choose option 1 rather than option 2. You could also choose correctly by recalling that hypoalbuminemia is part of the clinical picture and that protein intake is encouraged.

---

205. The nurse has given dietary instructions to a client to minimize the risk of osteoporosis. The nurse determines that the client understands the instructions if the client verbalizes the need to increase the intake of which food item?

1 Rice
2 Bread
3 Yogurt
4 Chicken

Level of Cognitive Ability: Evaluating
Client Needs: Health Promotion and Maintenance
Clinical Judgment/Cognitive Skills: Evaluate Outcomes
Integrated Process: Nursing Process/Evaluation
Content Area: Adult Health: Musculoskeletal
Health Problem: Adult Health: Musculoskeletal: Osteoporosis

Answer: 3
Rationale: Osteoporosis is a disorder that is characterized by an abnormal loss of bone density and the deterioration of bone tissue. Calcium intake is important to minimize the risk of osteoporosis. The major dietary source of calcium is dairy foods, including milk, yogurt, and a variety of cheeses. Calcium may also be added to certain products (e.g., orange juice), which are then labeled as being "fortified" with calcium. Calcium supplements are available and recommended for those with typically low calcium intake. Rice, bread, and chicken are not high in calcium.
Priority Nursing Tip: A spinal fracture may be caused by osteoporosis, a condition that causes bones to break easily. Height loss can be a warning sign of a spine fracture.

Test-Taking Strategy: Focus on the **subject,** osteoporosis. Think about the pathophysiology of osteoporosis and its causes. Recall that calcium is needed to minimize the risk of osteoporosis, that dairy products are rich in calcium, and that yogurt is a dairy product. None of the incorrect options belong to this food group.

---

206. The nurse is assisting with conducting a health screening for osteoporosis. The nurse would direct health promotion measures to which client with the greatest risk of developing this disorder?

1 A 25-year-old female who jogs
2 A 70-year-old male who consumes excess alcohol
3 A 65-year-old female who smokes cigarettes regularly
4 A 36-year-old male who has been diagnosed with gastroesophageal reflux disease (GERD)

Level of Cognitive Ability: Analyzing
Client Needs: Health Promotion and Maintenance

Answer: 3
Rationale: Osteoporosis is characterized by an abnormal loss of bone density and the deterioration of bone tissue. Risk factors for osteoporosis include being female, postmenopausal, of advanced age, or sedentary; consuming a low-calcium diet; using excessive alcohol; and smoking cigarettes.
Priority Nursing Tip: The long-term use of corticosteroids, anticonvulsants, and furosemide can increase the risk of osteoporosis.

Test-Taking Strategy: Focus on the **subject,** those at greatest risk for osteoporosis. Option 1 is eliminated first, because the 25-year-old female who jogs (thereby using the long bones) has negligible risk. The 36-year-old male with GERD is eliminated next because of no known risk factors. From the remaining options, the 65-year-old female has greater risk (age, gender, postmenopausal, smoking) than the 70-year-old male (age, alcohol consumption).

Clinical Judgment/Cognitive Skills: Recognize Cues
Integrated Process: Nursing Process/Data Collection
Content Area: Adult Health: Musculoskeletal
Health Problem: Adult Health: Musculoskeletal: Osteoporosis

---

207. The nurse is reinforcing dietary home-care instructions to a client diagnosed with pancreatitis. Which food would the nurse instruct the client to avoid?

1 Chili
2 Bagel
3 Spinach
4 Watermelon

Level of Cognitive Ability: Applying
Client Needs: Health Promotion and Maintenance
Clinical Judgment/Cognitive Skills: Take Action
Integrated Process: Nursing Process/Implementation
Content Area: Adult Health: Gastrointestinal
Health Problem: Adult Health: Gastrointestinal: GI Accessory Organs

Answer: 1
Rationale: Pancreatitis is an inflammatory condition of the pancreas that may be acute or chronic. The client needs to avoid alcohol, coffee, tea, spicy foods, and heavy meals, which stimulate pancreatic secretions and produce attacks of pancreatitis. The client is instructed on the benefit of eating small, frequent meals that are high in protein, low in fat, and moderate to high in carbohydrates.
Priority Nursing Tip: Initial treatment for pancreatitis may include fasting. An NPO (nothing by mouth) status provides rest for the pancreas and time for the pancreas to heal.

Test-Taking Strategy: Note the word *avoid.* Focus on the **subject,** pancreatitis, and note that options 2, 3, and 4 are foods that are moderately bland. Option 1 is a spicy food.

---

208. A newborn receives the first dose of hepatitis B vaccine within 12 hours of birth. The nurse reinforces to the parent that the second vaccine is administered when?

1 3 years of age and then during the adolescent years
2 8 months of age and then 1 year after the initial dose
3 6 months of age and then 8 months after the initial dose
4 1 to 2 months of age and then 4 months after the initial dose

Level of Cognitive Ability: Applying
Client Needs: Health Promotion and Maintenance
Clinical Judgment/Cognitive Skills: Take Action
Integrated Process: Nursing Process/Implementation
Content Area: Pharmacology: Immune/Vaccines
Health Problem: Pediatric-Specific: Immunizations

Answer: 4
Rationale: The vaccination schedule for an infant whose parent tests negative for hepatitis B consists of a series of three immunizations given at birth, 1 to 2 months of age, and then again 4 months after the initial dose. An infant whose parent tests positive receives hepatitis B immunoglobulin along with the first dose of the hepatitis B vaccine within 12 hours of birth.
Priority Nursing Tip: Most of the immunizations for infants who require multiple doses are given at 2, 4, and 6 months of age.

Test-Taking Strategy: Focus on the **subject,** administration of the hepatitis B vaccine. Knowledge regarding the immunization schedule for hepatitis B vaccine is necessary to answer this question. Remember that the vaccination schedule for an infant whose parent tests negative consists of a series of three immunizations given at birth, 1 to 2 months of age, and then again 4 months after the initial dose.

---

209. The nurse reinforcing dietary instructions for a child diagnosed with cystic fibrosis tells the parents what type of dietary management is necessary?

1 A low-fat diet
2 A low-protein diet
3 A high-calorie diet
4 A low-sodium diet

Level of Cognitive Ability: Applying
Client Needs: Health Promotion and Maintenance
Clinical Judgment/Cognitive Skills: Take Action
Integrated Process: Teaching and Learning
Content Area: Foundations of Care: Therapeutic Diets
Health Problem: Pediatrics: Cystic Fibrosis

Answer: 3

Rationale: Cystic fibrosis is an inherited autosomal-recessive disorder of the exocrine glands that causes those glands to produce abnormally thick secretions of mucus. It also causes elevation of the sweat electrolytes, increased organic and enzymatic constituents of saliva, and overactivity of the autonomic nervous system. Children with cystic fibrosis are managed with a high-calorie, high-protein diet; pancreatic enzyme replacement therapy; fat-soluble vitamin supplements; and, if nutritional problems are severe, nighttime gastrostomy feedings or total parental nutrition. Fats are not restricted unless steatorrhea cannot be controlled by increased pancreatic enzymes. Sodium intake is unrelated to this disorder.

Priority Nursing Tip: Cystic fibrosis results in muscle wasting, and nutrition therapy is based on increasing muscle mass.

Test-Taking Strategy: Focus on the **subject,** cystic fibrosis. Knowledge of the digestive problems and the dietary management of children with cystic fibrosis is necessary to answer this question. Think about the effect of this disorder on the body. Also note that options 1, 2, and 4 address a diet that is low in a nutritional component.

---

210. The nurse has reinforced instructions with a client who has silicosis about the prevention of self-exposure to silica dust. The nurse determines that the client understands the instructions if the client states a need to wear a mask for which hobby?

1 Painting
2 Gardening
3 Woodworking
4 Pottery making

Level of Cognitive Ability: Evaluating
Client Needs: Health Promotion and Maintenance
Clinical Judgment/Cognitive Skills: Evaluate Outcomes
Integrated Process: Nursing Process/Evaluation
Content Area: Adult Health: Respiratory
Health Problem: Adult Health: Respiratory: Environmental

Answer: 4

Rationale: Silicosis is a lung disorder caused by the continuous long-term inhalation of the dust of the inorganic compound silicon dioxide, which is found in sands, quartzes, flints, and many other stones. Exposure to silica dust occurs with activities such as pottery making and stone masonry. Exposure to finely ground silica, which is found in soaps, polishes, and filters, is also dangerous for these clients. Options 1, 2, and 3 are safe activities because they do not result in exposure to silica sources.

Priority Nursing Tip: A client with silicosis needs to avoid any activities that place a film or dust in the air that can be breathed into the lungs.

Test-Taking Strategy: Focus on the **subject,** activities that lead to silica exposure. It is necessary to have an understanding of the materials that could emit silica dust. Eliminate gardening first, because silica is not a pesticide, and it is not found in average soil. Recall that silica is not inhaled in fumes to help you eliminate woodworking and painting. This information will help direct you to option 4.

---

211. The nurse is reinforcing dietary teaching with a client with hypoparathyroidism who is hypocalcemic. The nurse encourages the client to increase the intake of which food?

1 Apples
2 Yogurt
3 Cooked pasta
4 Chicken breast

Level of Cognitive Ability: Applying
Client Needs: Health Promotion and Maintenance
Clinical Judgment/Cognitive Skills: Take Action
Integrated Process: Teaching and Learning
Content Area: Foundations of Care: Therapeutic Diets
Health Problem: Adult Health: Endocrine: Parathyroid Disorders

Answer: 2
Rationale: Hypocalcemia exists when the blood has too little calcium. Products that are naturally high in calcium are dairy products, including milk, cheese, ice cream, and yogurt. The other options are foods that are low in calcium.
Priority Nursing Tip: High-calcium foods generally have more than 100 mg of calcium per serving.

Test-Taking Strategy: Focus on the **subject,** that the client is experiencing hypocalcemia, and use knowledge of the calcium content of foods. Remember that as a rule, dairy products are naturally high in calcium.

---

212. The nurse reviews the discharge plan of care for a postoperative client who had a cystectomy and a urinary diversion (vesicostomy) created to treat bladder cancer. Teaching to the client would focus on what?

1 Understanding the disease process
2 Understanding how to care for the urinary diversion
3 Accepting the change in body image with the presence of an external pouch
4 Identifying signs of infection of the urinary system and when to call the surgeon

Level of Cognitive Ability: Applying
Client Needs: Health Promotion and Maintenance
Clinical Judgment/Cognitive Skills: Take Action
Integrated Process: Teaching and Learning
Content Area: Adult Health: Oncology
Health Problem: Adult Health: Cancer: Bladder and Kidney

Answer: 2
Rationale: A urinary diversion is a surgical diversion of urinary flow from its usual path through the urinary tract. As a result, the client has impaired urinary elimination. Initial teaching would focus on care of the urinary device. Understanding the disease process would have been completed before surgery. Even though infection can be life threatening if it occurs, this teaching is secondary, as initially the client needs to understand how to care for the device to prevent infection. Accepting a change in body image is a psychosocial need and, according to Maslow's Hierarchy of Needs theory is a later priority.
Priority Nursing Tip: For a client with a urinary diversion, it is important to instruct the client to wash hands and use clean technique when managing the system.

Test-Taking Strategy: Focus on the **subject,** client teaching and urinary diversion. When presented with teaching, it is important to prioritize physiological needs first. Focusing on the **data in the question** will assist in directing you to the correct option. Note the relationship of this data to the correct option.

---

213. The nurse reinforces home-care instructions to the client diagnosed with chronic prostatitis. Which statement by the client would indicate the **need for further instruction**?

1 "There are no restrictions in my diet."
2 "The sitz baths will help my condition."

Answer: 3
Rationale: Prostatitis is an acute or chronic inflammation of the prostate gland that is usually the result of an infection. Interventions include antiinflammatory agents or short-term antimicrobial medication, and the client would be taught about the prescribed regimen. Normal sexual activity is acceptable with chronic prostatitis; with acute conditions, it needs to be avoided

3 "I need to avoid sexual activity for at least 1 month."
4 "I need to take the antiinflammatory medications as prescribed."

Level of Cognitive Ability: Evaluating
Client Needs: Health Promotion and Maintenance
Clinical Judgment/Cognitive Skills: Evaluate Outcomes
Integrated Process: Teaching and Learning
Content Area: Adult Health: Renal and Urinary
Health Problem: Adult Health: Renal and Urinary: Inflammation/Infections

so that the prostate can rest. Sitz baths are recommended. Dietary restrictions are not recommended unless the person finds them to be associated with manifestations.
Priority Nursing Tip: Prostatitis is characterized by urinary problems such as burning or painful urination, the urgent need to urinate, trouble with voiding, difficult or painful ejaculation, and pain in the area between the scrotum and rectum or lower back.

Test-Taking Strategy: Note the **strategic words,** *need for further instruction.* These words indicate a **negative event query** and ask you to select an option that is an incorrect statement. Eliminate option 4 first by using the general principles associated with medication prescriptions. Option 1 can be eliminated next because there is no specific relationship between diet and this disorder. From the remaining options, eliminate option 2 because it would seem reasonable that sitz baths would provide comfort.

---

214. An older adult client diagnosed with iron-deficiency anemia asks the nurse about the food items that are high in iron. The nurse reinforces teaching to the client that which food item is highest in iron?
1 Milk
2 Pork
3 Oranges
4 Broccoli

Level of Cognitive Ability: Applying
Client Needs: Health Promotion and Maintenance
Clinical Judgment/Cognitive Skills: Take Action
Integrated Process: Teaching and Learning
Content Area: Foundations of Care: Therapeutic Diets
Health Problem: Adult Health: Hematological: Anemias

Answer: 4
Rationale: Iron is available in foods of plant and animal origin. Foods that are rich in iron include muscle meats, liver, egg yolks, brewer's yeast, green leafy vegetables, fish, fowl, beans, and cereal grains. Milk is high in calcium, pork is high in thiamine, and oranges are high in vitamin C.
Priority Nursing Tip: A client with mild iron-deficiency anemia may have no signs or symptoms.

Test-Taking Strategy: Focus on the **subject,** the food item that is highest in iron. Remembering that green leafy vegetables are high in iron will direct you to the correct option.

---

215. The nurse reinforces discharge instructions with a client taking ticlopidine to prevent a stroke. Which client statement indicates the **need for further instruction**?
1 "I'll take my medicine as prescribed with meals."
2 "Bloodwork will be done every 2 weeks for the first 3 months."
3 "If I have a cold or run a fever, I will stop taking this medicine."
4 "Side effects with this medicine are different than with my aspirin."

Answer: 3
Rationale: The client is instructed to not discontinue the medication without the primary health care provider's permission. Options 1, 2, and 4 are accurate statements that support appropriate medication therapy.
Priority Nursing Tip: Any change in medication directions needs to be approved by the prescriber.

Test-Taking Strategy: Note the **strategic words,** *need for further instruction.* These words indicate a **negative event query** and ask you to select an option that is an incorrect client statement. Recalling basic principles related to medication administration and that the client would not stop taking the medication without the primary health care provider's approval will direct you to the correct option.

Level of Cognitive Ability: Analyzing
Client Needs: Health Promotion and Maintenance
Clinical Judgment/Cognitive Skills: Evaluate Outcomes
Integrated Process: Teaching and Learning
Content Area: Pharmacology: Cardiovascular: Antiplatelet
Health Problem: Adult Health: Neurological: Stroke

---

216. A client prescribed ticlopidine to prevent clotting in stents asks why bloodwork must be performed so frequently. The nurse reinforces teaching to the client about the importance of bloodwork by making which statement?

1 "I'll have to let your doctor explain that for you."
2 "Don't worry. This bloodwork will only be done 6 times."
3 "I have written information that I will give your family before you leave."
4 "These blood tests are important to check for a reversible side effect called neutropenia."

Level of Cognitive Ability: Applying
Client Needs: Health Promotion and Maintenance
Clinical Judgment/Cognitive Skills: Take Action
Integrated Process: Teaching and Learning
Content Area: Pharmacology: Cardiovascular: Antiplatelets
Health Problem: Adult Health: Hematological: Bleeding/Clotting Disorders

Answer: 4
Rationale: Neutropenia is an abnormally low level of neutrophils that are a common type of white blood cell important to fighting off infections. Option 4 provides the information that the client is requesting and teaches the client. Options 1, 2, and 3 do not address the client's concern or provide education to the client about the medication.
Priority Nursing Tip: Ticlopidine is a medication prescribed to prevent blood clots in stents placed in the heart in an effort to improve long-term patency of the vessel.

Test-Taking Strategy: Focus on the **subject,** the need for regular bloodwork, and use **therapeutic communication techniques.** Option 4 is the only option that addresses the client's question and provides accurate information. The client would not be told not to worry, and options 1 and 3 place the client's question on hold.

---

217. Oral anticoagulant therapy is prescribed for a client with atrial fibrillation. The nurse assists with preparing home-care medication instructions by reinforcing which action?

1 Reporting any signs of bleeding
2 Using a straight razor for shaving
3 Taking aspirin for mild discomfort
4 Using a hard-bristle toothbrush for brushing the teeth

Level of Cognitive Ability: Applying
Client Needs: Health Promotion and Maintenance

Answer: 1
Rationale: Anticoagulant therapy places the client at risk for bleeding, and it is vital that the client know to report bleeding promptly. The client needs to be instructed in the measures that will reduce the likelihood of this adverse effect. An electric razor rather than a straight razor would be used. Acetaminophen would be taken for mild discomfort, because aspirin has antiplatelet properties and will increase the risk of bleeding. A soft toothbrush would be used to prevent bleeding of the gums.
Priority Nursing Tip: Anticoagulants are agents that are used to prevent the formation of blood clots.

Clinical Judgment/Cognitive Skills: Take Action
Integrated Process: Teaching and Learning
Content Area: Pharmacology: Cardiovascular: Anticoagulants
Health Problem: Adult Health: Cardiovascular: Dysrhythmias

Test-Taking Strategy: Focus on the **subject**, home-care instructions for the client on an anticoagulant. Recalling that an anticoagulant medication places the client at risk for bleeding will direct you to option 1.

---

218. A client diagnosed with heart failure (HF) and prescribed furosemide is advised to eat foods that are high in potassium. The nurse reinforces to the client that which food would meet the client's needs?

1 Scalloped potatoes and rice
2 Ham, bacon, and hot dogs
3 Fresh fruits and vegetables
4 Margarine, butter, and cheese

Level of Cognitive Ability: Applying
Client Needs: Health Promotion and Maintenance
Clinical Judgment/Cognitive Skills: Take Action
Integrated Process: Teaching and Learning
Content Area: Foundations of Care: Therapeutic Diets
Health Problem: Adult Health: Cardiovascular: Heart Failure

Answer: 3
Rationale: Heart failure occurs when the heart muscle does not pump blood as well as it should. The body needs a delicate balance of potassium to help the heart and other muscles work properly. Fresh fruits and vegetables are a good source of potassium. Options 1, 2, and 4 identify foods that are either high in sodium or fat and thus would not be consumed by the client with HF.
Priority Nursing Tip: When a client is prescribed a diuretic, it is important to teach the client to avoid foods high in sodium, as they increase fluid retention.

Test-Taking Strategy: Focus on the **subject**, a client with heart failure and the client's need for potassium. Recalling that food items that are high in sodium or fat would not be consumed by the client with HF will assist you with eliminating options 1, 2, and 4.

---

219. A 13-year-old female client is adamantly refusing to take corticosteroid therapy for the treatment of Crohn's disease. What is the **primary** trigger for this behavior?

1 Fear of pain
2 A mental illness
3 Denial of the disease
4 Fear of altered body image

Level of Cognitive Ability: Applying
Client Needs: Health Promotion and Maintenance
Clinical Judgment/Cognitive Skills: Recognize Cues
Integrated Process: Nursing Process/Data Collection
Content Area: Pharmacology: Endocrine/Corticosteroids
Health Problem: Pediatric-specific: Gastrointestinal and Rectal Problems

Answer: 4
Rationale: Corticosteroids can greatly alter the body's appearance by causing weight gain, puffy skin, and a humped back. One of the main concerns in the teenage population is body image. Pain is not a side effect of corticosteroids. There are no data in the question to indicate denial or a mental illness.
Priority Nursing Tip: Body image is the subjective picture or mental image of one's own body.

Test-Taking Strategy: Focus on the **subject**, corticosteroid therapy for an adolescent, and note the **strategic word**, *primary*. Use the concepts of growth and development and your knowledge of the side effects of corticosteroids to answer the question. Recalling that body image is a main concern of the teenager will direct you to the correct option.

---

220. When gathering data about a jaundiced infant, the nurse notes that the serum bilirubin levels have been increasing and that the pediatrician has prescribed phototherapy. After explaining phototherapy to the parents, which statement would indicate the **need for further instruction?**

1 "We understand that home phototherapy is an option."
2 "We will be available for feedings every 2 to 3 hours."
3 "My baby will wear eye patches during this treatment."
4 "We will bring in clean clothes for my baby to wear today."

Level of Cognitive Ability: Evaluating
Client Needs: Health Promotion and Maintenance
Clinical Judgment/Cognitive Skills: Evaluate Outcomes
Integrated Process: Teaching and Learning
Content Area: Maternity: Newborn
Health Problem: Newborn: Hyperbilirubinemia

Answer: 4
Rationale: Hyperbilirubinemia is an elevated level of the pigment bilirubin in the blood. A sufficient elevation of bilirubin produces jaundice. Some degree of hyperbilirubinemia is very common right after birth, especially in premature babies. Clean clothes are not needed because the infant will be wearing only a diaper to facilitate the benefit of the phototherapy. Eye patches will be placed on the infant's eyes. Feedings will be provided every 2 to 3 hours. Phototherapy can be performed at home.
Priority Nursing Tip: Mild infant jaundice often disappears on its own within 2 or 3 weeks.

Test-Taking Strategy: Focus on the **subject,** phototherapy for hyperbilirubinemia, and note the **strategic words,** *need for further instruction.* These words indicate a **negative event query** and ask you to select an option that is an incorrect statement. Recalling that the infant will receive the therapy without clothing other than a diaper will direct you to the correct option.

---

221. As part of the discharge planning for an infant who is to receive home phototherapy, the nurse needs to emphasize what to the parents?

1 Letting the baby sleep through feedings is acceptable.
2 Keeping a list of the number of wet diapers and stools is important.
3 The wearing of eye patches for conventional phototherapy is optional.
4 Taking the baby away from conventional phototherapy lights for hours at a time will not interfere with the goal of the treatment.

Level of Cognitive Ability: Applying
Client Needs: Health Promotion and Maintenance
Clinical Judgment/Cognitive Skills: Take Action
Integrated Process: Teaching and Learning
Content Area: Maternity: Newborn
Health Problem: Newborn: Hyperbilirubinemia

Answer: 2
Rationale: Increasing fluids is encouraged to increase excretion of bilirubin in an infant who is under phototherapy. Keeping a list of the number of wet diapers and stools is important because the infant needs to have 6 to 10 wet diapers a day. The infant needs to be fed every 2 to 3 hours because phototherapy can cause dehydration. The infant would receive phototherapy for 18 hours per day or for the number of hours prescribed by the pediatrician. Patches would be placed over the infant's eyes to protect them from the light.
Priority Nursing Tip: In the standard form of phototherapy, the baby lies in a bassinet or enclosed plastic crib and is exposed to a type of fluorescent light that is absorbed through the baby's skin. Adverse effects from treatment, such as eye damage, dehydration, or sensory deprivation, can occur.

Test-Taking Strategy: Focus on the **subject,** the procedures for phototherapy and client instructions. Use your knowledge of the principles related to phototherapy to answer this question. Recalling that phototherapy can cause dehydration will direct you to the correct option.

---

222. The nurse in a well-baby clinic is providing nutrition instructions to a parent of a 10-month-old infant. Which is the **most** age appropriate?

1 Introduce strained fruits one at a time.
2 Introduce strained vegetables one at a time.
3 Determine whether self-feeding has been initiated.
4 Begin to offer rice cereal mixed with breast milk or formula.

Level of Cognitive Ability: Applying
Client Needs: Health Promotion and Maintenance
Clinical Judgment/Cognitive Skills: Take Action
Integrated Process: Teaching and Learning
Content Area: Developmental Stages: Infant
Health Problem: N/A

Answer: 3
Rationale: Self-feeding can be initiated at the age of approximately 9 months. Rice cereal mixed with breast milk or formula is introduced at the age of 4 months. Strained vegetables, fruits, and meats, introduced one at a time, can begin at the age of 6 months.
Priority Nursing Tip: Fortified infant cereals are an important source of iron, which babies need in their diets around the middle of the first year.

Test-Taking Strategy: Note the **strategic word,** *most.* Focus on the **subject,** infant nutrition. Focusing on the age of the infant will direct you to the correct option. Options 1, 2, and 4 are initiated before the age of 9 months.

---

223. The nurse is collecting physical data from a client and is preparing to auscultate breath sounds on a client with bronchitis. The nurse places the stethoscope in which area to assess bronchovesicular sounds? **Refer to the figure.**

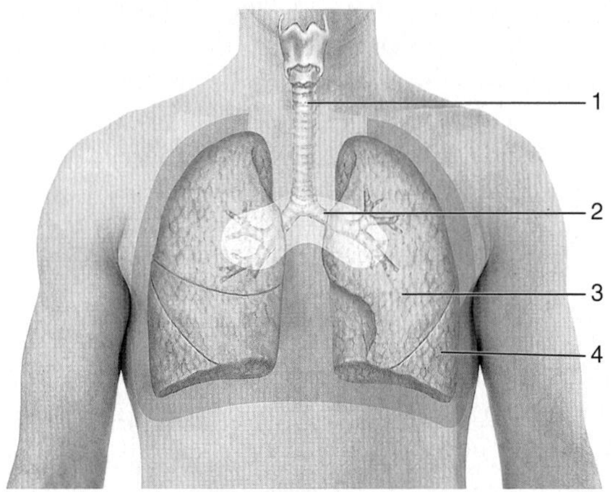

(From Wilson S, Giddens J. *Health assessment for nursing practice*, ed 5. St. Louis, 2016, Mosby.)

Level of Cognitive Ability: Applying
Client Needs: Health Promotion and Maintenance
Clinical Judgment/Cognitive Skills: Recognize Cues
Integrated Process: Nursing Process/Data Collection
Content Area: Health Assessment: Physical Exam: Thorax and Lungs
Health Problem: Adult Health: Respiratory: Upper Airway

Answer: 2
Rationale: Bronchovesicular breath sounds are heard over the main bronchi. Their normal location is specifically between the first and second intercostal spaces at the sternal border anteriorly and at T4 medial to the scapula posteriorly. These sounds are moderate in pitch and medium in intensity, and the duration of inspiration and expiration is equal. Bronchial breath sounds are heard over the trachea. Vesicular breath sounds are heard over the lesser bronchi, the bronchioles, and the lobes.
Priority Nursing Tip: Bronchitis can be acute or chronic and is an inflammation of the lining of the bronchial tubes.

Test-Taking Strategy: Focus on the **subject,** the anatomical location for listening to bronchovesicular sounds. Eliminate options 3 and 4 because they identify similar locations (peripheral lung fields). From the remaining options, recall that bronchial breath sounds are heard over the trachea.

---

224. The nurse teaching a client about the risks of breast cancer identifies which as risk factors? **Select all that apply.**

- ❒ 1 A diet high in fat
- ❒ 2 Age of more than 40 years
- ❒ 3 Menstrual history of late menarche
- ❒ 4 Previous history of cancer in one breast
- ❒ 5 Having the first child after the age of 30
- ❒ 6 Family history of any first-degree relative with breast cancer

Level of Cognitive Ability: Applying
Client Needs: Health Promotion and Maintenance
Clinical Judgment/Cognitive Skills: Take Action
Integrated Process: Teaching and Learning
Content Area: Adult Health: Oncology
Health Problem: Adult Health: Cancer: Breast

Answer: 1, 2, 4, 5, 6
Rationale: Risk factors associated with breast cancer include a menstrual history of early menarche and a birth of the first child after the age of 30. Other risk factors include a previous history of breast cancer; a family history of breast cancer, including any first-degree relative (e.g., mother, sister) with breast cancer; and an age of more than 40 years (incidence increases with age and peaks during the fifth decade). A high-fat diet is associated with an increased risk of cancer.
Priority Nursing Tip: A change in breast size, alongside swelling or redness, may be an early symptom and warning sign of breast cancer.

Test-Taking Strategy: Focus on the **subject,** the risk factors associated with breast cancer. It is necessary to know these risk factors to answer correctly. Use knowledge of the general principles related to cancer to assist in answering correctly.

---

225. The nurse working at a health-screening clinic gathers data from a client to identify the client's risk factors associated with coronary heart disease. The nurse is specifically interested in modifiable risk factors so that a health promotion and maintenance plan of care can be developed for the client. Which factors are considered modifiable? **Select all that apply.**

- ❒ 1 Is physically inactive
- ❒ 2 Is a 45-year-old female
- ❒ 3 Is an African American
- ❒ 4 Has a family history of heart disease
- ❒ 5 Has an elevated serum cholesterol level
- ❒ 6 Has a blood pressure of 158/102 mm Hg

Level of Cognitive Ability: Analyzing
Client Needs: Health Promotion and Maintenance
Clinical Judgment/Cognitive Skills: Recognize Cues
Integrated Process: Nursing Process/Data Collection
Content Area: Adult Health: Cardiovascular
Health Problem: Adult Health: Cardiovascular: Coronary Artery Disease

Answer: 1, 5, 6
Rationale: Modifiable risk factors for coronary artery disease are those that can be modified or reduced with treatment. These include cigarette smoking, hypertension, an elevated serum cholesterol level, physical inactivity, and obesity. Nonmodifiable risk factors are those that cannot be modified or reduced with treatment and include such factors as heredity, race, age, and gender. Clients whose parents had coronary heart disease are at higher risk. Increasing age influences both the risk and severity of the disease. Although men are at higher risk for heart attacks at a younger age, the risk for women increases significantly at menopause. The incidence of coronary heart disease is more prevalent in African American women.
Priority Nursing Tip: Coronary artery disease occurs when a substance called *plaque* builds up inside the coronary arteries.

Test-Taking Strategy: Focus on the **subject,** modifiable risk factors. Recalling that modifiable risk factors are those that can be modified or reduced with treatment will assist you with answering this question. Look at each risk factor listed, and select those that can be changed.

---

226. A client at risk for urinary tract infections is told to drink 3000 mL of fluid every day to decrease the risk. The nurse explains to the client that this equals how many 10-oz glasses of fluid per day to consume the prescribed 3000 mL?

Answer: ______________

Level of Cognitive Ability: Applying
Client Needs: Health Promotion and Maintenance
Clinical Judgment/Cognitive Skills: Take Action
Integrated Process: Teaching and Learning
Content Area: Foundations of Care: Fluids & Electrolytes
Health Problem: Adult Health: Renal and Urinary: Inflammation/Infections

Answer: 10
Rationale: Each 10-oz glass of fluid contains 300 mL (1 oz = 30 mL; therefore 10 oz = 300 mL). The client will need to drink ten 10-oz glasses of fluid daily (3000 mL/300 mL = 10).
Priority Nursing Tip: There are about 3.785 liters in a U.S. gallon of water.

Test-Taking Strategy: Focus on the **subject**, the number of 10-oz glasses of fluid that will equal 3000 mL. First, convert ounces to milliliters to determine the number of milliliters in each 10-oz glass of fluid. Next, divide the amount of fluid prescribed by the number of milliliters in each 10-oz glass of fluid.

---

227. The nurse is providing home-care instructions to a client who has had vascular bypass surgery on a lower limb. To prevent the complications associated with the surgical procedure, the nurse reinforces to the client to do what? **Select all that apply.**
- ❒ 1 Initiate a daily walking regimen.
- ❒ 2 Avoid lifting anything heavier than 30 pounds.
- ❒ 3 Take a tub bath daily to keep the incision clean.
- ❒ 4 Eat a high-fiber diet and drink plenty of liquids.
- ❒ 5 Promptly report signs of incisional infection to the surgeon.
- ❒ 6 Expect to feel fatigued and plan for rest periods throughout the day.

Level of Cognitive Ability: Applying
Client Needs: Health Promotion and Maintenance
Clinical Judgment/Cognitive Skills: Take Action
Integrated Process: Teaching and Learning
Content Area: Adult Health: Cardiovascular
Health Problem: Adult Health: Cardiovascular: Vascular Disorders

Answer: 1, 4, 5, 6
Rationale: Vascular bypass surgery is performed to restore blood flow when a life- or limb-threatening arterial occlusion is present. To prevent complications postoperatively, the nurse teaches the client to avoid lifting anything heavier than 10 pounds until approved by the surgeon. Items that weigh more than 10 pounds will cause pressure and stress on the incision. To prevent complications associated with incisional healing, the client is also taught to avoid tub baths and instead to shower daily until the incision is healed. The client needs to advance activity gradually as tolerated and initiate a daily walk. Fatigue is expected, and the client needs to plan for rest periods throughout the day. A high-fiber diet and liquids will prevent constipation.
Priority Nursing Tip: A vascular bypass is a surgical procedure that is done to redirect blood flow from one area to another.

Test-Taking Strategy: Focus on the **subject**, vascular bypass surgery postoperative care and teaching, and note the words *lower limb.* Use general postoperative teaching guidelines to assist you with selecting the correct option. Eliminate option 2 because of the words *30 pounds.* Eliminate option 3 by focusing on the principles related to infection and healing.

CHAPTER

8

Psychosocial Integrity Practice Questions

1. When collecting data from a client with a history of hypertension, the nurse determines that the client would benefit from biofeedback as an adjunctive therapy. Which client statement supports this determination?
   1 "I have such a stressful job, you wouldn't believe it."
   2 "It is so hard giving up all the salty foods that I enjoy."
   3 "I don't have the money to pay for the pills that I take every day."
   4 "It is hard for me to get to the bus to come in to the clinic for my blood pressure checks."

Level of Cognitive Ability: Analyzing
Client Needs: Psychosocial Integrity
Clinical Judgment/Cognitive Skills: Analyze Cues
Integrated Process: Nursing Process/Data Collection
Content Area: Mental Health
Health Problem: Mental Health: Coping

Answer: 1
Rationale: Biofeedback is one of several stress management techniques that may be useful for clients whose hypertension is aggravated by stress. Option 2 indicates the need for further dietary management. Options 3 and 4 relate to financial and environmental issues that are interfering with treatment.
Priority Nursing Tip: Hypertension can strain the heart, damage blood vessels, and increase the risk of heart attack, stroke, kidney problems, and death.

Test-Taking Strategy: Focus on the **subject,** the purpose of biofeedback training. Knowing that biofeedback is a stress management technique enables you to eliminate each of the incorrect options.

---

2. A 10-month-old infant is hospitalized for respiratory syncytial virus. Which interventions would the nurse stress to the parents to promote the infant's development?
   1 The need to routinely contain the infant in order to prevent tubes from being dislodged
   2 The importance of washing hands, wearing a mask, and keeping the infant as quiet as possible
   3 The benefit of following the home feeding schedule and encouraging the infant to be held only by the parents
   4 The appropriateness of providing a consistent routine that includes touching, rocking, and cuddling throughout the hospitalization

Answer: 4
Rationale: Hospitalization may have an adverse psychological effect on an infant. A consistent routine that is accompanied by touching, rocking, and cuddling helps the infant develop trust and provides sensory stimulation. Option 2 identifies good infection control methods, but these measures will not help meet the developmental task. It is important to follow the home routine, if possible, but touching and holding only by the parents is not enough. A contained infant may regress.
Priority Nursing Tip: Infants require human contact to develop appropriately psychologically, and this is especially important during times of childhood stress.

Level of Cognitive Ability: Applying
Client Needs: Psychosocial Integrity
Clinical Judgment/Cognitive Skills: Take Action
Integrated Process: Nursing Process/Implementation
Content Area: Developmental Stages: Infant
Health Problem: Pediatric-Specific: Bronchitis/Bronchiolitis/Respiratory Syncytial Virus

Test-Taking Strategy: Focus on the **data in the question,** age of the child, and the **subject,** developmental needs. Eliminate option 2 because it does not address psychosocial development. Eliminate options 1 and 3 because of the words *routinely* and *only,* respectively. Focusing on the subject will direct you to the correct option.

---

3. A client with a prescription for a 12-lead electrocardiogram (ECG) has never had this procedure done before. The nurse **most effectively** reduces the client's anxiety when making which statement?

1 "It would take only about 5 minutes to complete the ECG"
2 "Would you be less anxious if a family member remains with you?"
3 "The test is noninvasive, so it will not cause you any type of pain."
4 "Are you anxious because of the possibility you have a heart problem?"

Level of Cognitive Ability: Evaluating
Client Needs: Psychosocial Integrity
Clinical Judgment/Cognitive Skills: Evaluate Outcomes
Integrated Process: Caring
Content Area: Mental Health
Health Problem: Mental Health: Coping

Answer: 3

Rationale: A common concern about diagnostic tests that are unfamiliar is whether they will be painful. Reinforcing that the ECG does not require any type of action that would cause the client discomfort, but rather uses painless electrodes that are applied to the chest and limbs, will best minimize the client's anxiety level. To ask a question regarding the client's concern about heart disease is appropriate but does not address the common concern regarding pain. Although it is true that an ECG takes less than 5 minutes to complete, this information is unlikely to address the client's concerns. Having family present may minimize the client's concern, but it does not adequately address the common concern of whether the test will be painful.

Priority Nursing Tip: The 12-lead ECG is made up of the three standard limb leads (I, II, and III), the augmented limb leads (aVR, aVL, and aVF), and the six precordial leads (V1, V2, V3, V4, V5, and V6).

Test-Taking Strategy: Focus on the **subject,** reducing the client's anxiety, and the **strategic words,** *most effectively*. Options 1, 2, and 4 are factual statements but are not stated to reduce anxiety. Option 3 is the only reassuring statement, which addresses the focus of the question.

---

4. The nurse would identify which statements made by a client diagnosed with anorexia nervosa as having a **need for follow-up**?

1 "I check my weight every day without fail."
2 "I exercise 4 to 5 hours every day to keep my figure."
3 "I've been told that I am 5% below my ideal body weight."
4 "All my friends are interested in being thin and looking good."

Level of Cognitive Ability: Evaluating
Client Needs: Psychosocial Integrity
Clinical Judgment/Cognitive Skills: Evaluate Outcomes
Integrated Process: Nursing Process/Data Collection
Content Area: Mental Health
Health Problem: Mental Health: Eating Disorders

Answer: 2

Rationale: Exercising 4 to 5 hours every day is excessive physical activity and unrealistic for a 16-year-old client. The nurse would explore this statement to find out why the client feels that she needs to exercise this much to maintain her figure. Concern about physical attractiveness is a common issue for teenagers; this is not considered a major threat to the client's physical well-being unless it becomes an obsession. A weight of 15% or more below the ideal body weight is characteristic of anorexia nervosa. It is not considered abnormal to check the weight every day; however, many anorexics check their weight up to 20 times a day.

Priority Nursing Tip: Teenagers, especially girls, are susceptible to internal and external pressures to be "thin." The most common means of achieving this goal is through diet and exercise. Abusive behavior with diet and exercise can lead to anorexia nervosa.

Test-Taking Strategy: Focus on the **subject,** anorexia nervosa, and note the **strategic words,** *need for follow-up.* Knowledge of the characteristics associated with anorexia nervosa directs you to the correct option.

---

5. A mental health home health nurse is caring for a depressed child with suicidal tendencies. Which statement made by the client's parent requires **immediate** intervention?

1 "I'm concerned, as all he seems to do is cry for long periods."
2 "I've noticed that my child gave one of his friends his signed baseball."
3 "I'm concerned because all he seems to do is spend time alone in his room."
4 "I would like to know if a sleeping pill can be prescribed, as he is always tired."

Level of Cognitive Ability: Analyzing
Client Needs: Psychosocial Integrity
Clinical Judgment/Cognitive Skills: Evaluate Outcomes
Integrated Process: Nursing Process/Data Collection
Content Area: Mental Health
Health Problem: Mental Health: Suicide

Answer: 2
Rationale: Suicide precautions would be implemented if a depressed client begins to give away belongings because this may be an indication that the client feels the belongings are no longer needed. Options 1, 3, and 4 are indicative of depression but are not as definitive as option 2 with regard to the client contemplating suicide.
Priority Nursing Tip: Depression is a risk factor for suicide. Depressed individuals must be frequently assessed for indications that they are planning their death.

Test-Taking Strategy: Focus on the **subject**, depression and suicide, and note the **strategic word**, *immediate*. Note that option 2 identifies the possible formulation of a suicidal plan, meaning there is no longer any need for personal belongings.

---

6. The nurse is collecting data from a client who survived a fire 2 months ago that killed two roommates. The client is reporting insomnia, difficulty concentrating, nervousness, and hypervigilance. Which problem has **priority** and would be included in the client's plan of care?

1 Fear
2 Anxiety
3 Ineffective coping
4 Complicated grieving

Level of Cognitive Ability: Analyzing
Client Needs: Psychosocial Integrity
Clinical Judgment/Cognitive Skills: Analyze Cues
Integrated Process: Nursing Process/Planning
Content Area: Mental Health
Health Problem: Mental Health: Post-Traumatic Stress Disorder

Answer: 2
Rationale: Anxiety is the client problem most evidenced by the symptoms. Post-traumatic stress disorder is precipitated by events that are overwhelming, unpredictable, and sometimes life threatening. Typical symptoms of post-traumatic stress disorder include difficulty concentrating, sleep disturbances, intrusive recollections of the traumatic event, hypervigilance, and anxiety. A phobia is an irrational fear of something or someone that interferes with daily living; this client is not exhibiting fear. Ineffective coping is defined as an inability to form an understanding of the stressors. This client may have ineffective coping, but it is not defined by the symptoms of nervousness and hypervigilance. Complicated grieving occurs from the distress of death and manifests in functional impairment. This individual is not functionally impaired.
Priority Nursing Tip: Experiencing a traumatic event can lead to extreme stress that results in recurring flashbacks and anxiety regarding the event.

Test-Taking Strategy: Focus on the **data in the question** and note the **strategic word**, *priority*. Recalling that hypervigilance is a common symptom of post-traumatic stress disorder directs you to option 2.

---

7. A 16-year-old client is hospitalized with pneumonia. Which statement represents a potential developmental problem and indicates the **need for follow-up**?

1 "Do I need to worry about giving my friends pneumonia?"
2 "I think I'm still too tired to have my friends visit me."
3 "Is it okay if I have a couple of friends in to visit me this evening?"
4 "I had my mom tell my friends I couldn't have visitors while I'm in the hospital."

Level of Cognitive Ability: Analyzing
Client Needs: Psychosocial Integrity
Clinical Judgment/Cognitive Skills: Analyze Cues
Integrated Process: Nursing Process/Data Collection
Content Area: Developmental Stages: Adolescent
Health Problem: Pediatric-Specific: Pneumonia

Answer: 4

Rationale: Adolescents who withdraw from peers into isolation struggle with developing identity; therefore option 4 would cause the nurse to be concerned. Option 1 demonstrates that the client is concerned for the safety of his or her friends. Option 2 is an expression of a realistic situation related to the disease process. Option 3 demonstrates a healthy interest in companionship.

Priority Nursing Tip: According to Erickson's stages of psychosocial development, an adolescent faces the task of identity vs. role confusion.

Test-Taking Strategy: Note the **strategic words,** *need for follow-up.* These words indicate a **negative event query** and the need to select the concerning statement by the adolescent. Options 1, 2, and 3 indicate reactions within normal behavior for a teenager hospitalized for an illness. Option 4 indicates that the client may be withdrawing from suitable relationships.

---

8. During an obstetrician office visit, a prenatal client is told that she tested positive for human immunodeficiency virus (HIV). The client cries and is significantly distressed about this news. Which statement by the nurse is appropriate?

1 "Your life won't change at this time."
2 "Your baby will not be susceptible to HIV."
3 "Have you considered notifying the baby's father?"
4 "It appears that you are upset. I will sit with you for a while."

Level of Cognitive Ability: Applying
Client Needs: Psychosocial Integrity
Clinical Judgment/Cognitive Skills: Take Action
Integrated Process: Nursing Process/Implementation
Content Area: Mental Health
Health Problem: Mental Health: Grief/Loss

Answer: 4

Rationale: A potential life-threatening diagnosis such as HIV can stimulate fear in the client. The best response is to support the client. Sitting with the client, holding a hand, offering support, and acknowledging the client's grief is most helpful at this time. There are no data in the question to support the responses for option 1 or 2. These options are providing false hope. Option 3 is helpful but does not address the response that the client is exhibiting.

Priority Nursing Tip: Being informed of a serious health problem will cause fear in the client. The nurse needs to recognize this possibility and provide a caring and supportive response.

Test-Taking Strategy: Focus on the **data in the question**. A client who is distressed and crying supports the client problem of fear. Options 1 and 2 are inappropriate responses to this situation. Option 3 is a concern for the client with HIV, but there are no **data in the question** to support this action.

---

9. The nurse is caring for a client recovering from a myocardial infarction. The nurse determines that the client is exhibiting signs of depression when the client demonstrates what behavior?

1 Reports inability to play web-based games and engage in social networking
2 Ignores activity restrictions and does not report the experience of chest pain with activity
3 Expresses apprehension about leaving the hospital and requests someone to stay with him at night
4 Consumes only 25% of meals and shows little interest when client education is reinforced

Level of Cognitive Ability: Applying
Client Needs: Psychosocial Integrity
Clinical Judgment/Cognitive Skills: Analyze Cues
Integrated Process: Nursing Process/Data Collection
Content Area: Mental Health
Health Problem: Mental Health: Mood Disorders

Answer: 4
Rationale: Signs of depression include withdrawal, crying, anorexia, and apathy. The inability to engage in activities suggests a lack of physical or cognitive ability. Ignoring symptoms and activity restrictions is a sign of denial. Apprehension is a sign of anxiety.
Priority Nursing Tip: Experiencing a myocardial infarction is both physically and emotionally trying. Depression is a common outcome of such an event and generally results in a decrease in interest in areas of importance.

Test-Taking Strategy: Focus on the **subject,** signs of depression. Think about the characteristics of depression to assist in answering correctly. Option 4 is the only option that identifies depression.

---

10. A client who has a new gastrostomy feeding tube refuses to participate in the plan of care, will not make eye contact, and does not speak to family or visitors. The nurse recognizes that this client is using which coping mechanism?

1 Denial
2 Distancing
3 Self-control
4 Problem solving

Level of Cognitive Ability: Applying
Client Needs: Psychosocial Integrity
Clinical Judgment/Cognitive Skills: Recognize Cues
Integrated Process: Nursing Process/Data Collection
Content Area: Mental Health
Health Problem: Mental Health: Coping

Answer: 2
Rationale: Distancing is an unwillingness or inability to discuss events. Self-control is demonstrated by stoicism and hiding feelings. Problem solving involves making plans and verbalizing what will be done. Denial is the rejection of reality as being too painful to face.
Priority Nursing Tip: Coping skills are methods a person uses to deal with stressful situations. Obtaining and maintaining good coping skills does take practice. However, utilizing these skills becomes easier over time.

Test-Taking Strategy: Focus on the **data in the question** to identify the coping mechanism that the client uses. The words *refuses, will not,* and *does not* are all indicative of ineffective coping.

---

11. The nurse is caring for a client diagnosed with esophageal varices. The client says, "I deserve this. I brought it on myself by drinking too much alcohol." Which is the **best** response from the nurse?

1 "Would you like to talk to the hospital chaplain?"
2 "Is there some reason you feel you deserve this?"
3 "That is something to think about when you leave the hospital."
4 "It's true that esophageal varices can result from alcohol abuse."

Level of Cognitive Ability: Applying
Client Needs: Psychosocial Integrity
Clinical Judgment/Cognitive Skills: Take Action
Integrated Process: Communication and Documentation
Content Area: Mental Health
Health Problem: Mental Health: Therapeutic Communication

Answer: 2
Rationale: Esophageal varices are often a complication of cirrhosis of the liver, and the most common type of cirrhosis is caused by chronic alcohol abuse. Option 1 blocks communication. Options 3 and 4 are judgmental. Option 2 allows the client to discuss feelings.
Priority Nursing Tip: Open-ended questioning is the most therapeutic means of encouraging the client to discuss situations that appear to be stress producing.

Test-Taking Strategy: Note the **strategic word,** *best.* Use **therapeutic communication techniques** to answer the question. Option 1 could block the nurse–client communication process. Options 3 and 4 are judgmental. The open-ended question in option 2 promotes the expression of feelings. Remember that the client's feelings and concerns would be addressed first.

---

12. An older client is admitted to the hospital after falling and hitting his head at home. The client wakes up at night and states, "I'm so scared. Where am I? What's happening?" The nurse would make which response?

1 "Hold my hand. Try to concentrate and tell me your name."
2 "You fell and hit your head. Your family brought you here."
3 "You're in the hospital after a fall. It's normal to feel scared."
4 "There's no reason to be scared. You're safe here in the hospital."

Level of Cognitive Ability: Applying
Client Needs: Psychosocial Integrity
Clinical Judgment/Cognitive Skills: Take Action
Integrated Process: Communication and Documentation
Content Area: Mental Health
Health Problem: Mental Health: Therapeutic Communication

Answer: 3
Rationale: Reflecting is using the client's own words or feelings when responding. In option 3, the nurse gives information to the client in addition to reflecting the client's feelings. In option 2, the nurse gives information but does not deal with the client's emotional needs. In option 1, the nurse attempts to calm the client but blocks communication by changing the subject. In option 4, the nurse does not provide the client with an opportunity to express feelings, thereby blocking communication.
Priority Nursing Tip: Being in a strange environment, especially after a head injury, can result in temporary disorientation. The nurse would calmly reorient the client to person, place, and time while acknowledging his or her concerns.

Test-Taking Strategy: Use **therapeutic communication techniques** to answer the question. Remember to respond to the client's emotional needs. Avoid blocks to communication, and focus on the client's feelings and concerns.

---

13. The parent of a toddler who is hospitalized for pneumonia must leave their child alone. Which **initial** behavior will the nurse **most likely** observe in this child?

1 Playing quietly with a favorite toy
2 Crying loudly and kicking both legs
3 Silently curled in bed with a blanket
4 Sucking the thumb and rocking back and forth

Level of Cognitive Ability: Applying
Client Needs: Psychosocial Integrity
Clinical Judgment/Cognitive Skills: Analyze Cues
Integrated Process: Nursing Process/Data Collection
Content Area: Developmental Stages: Toddler
Health Problem: Pediatric-Specific: Pneumonia

Answer: 2
Rationale: The stages of separation anxiety include protest, despair, and detachment. Crying loudly and kicking both legs is a protest behavior that is seen during the first stage of separation. Option 1 is incorrect because the behavior reflects detachment, which is the third stage of separation. Options 3 and 4 are incorrect and are unlikely to be noted in this situation.
Priority Nursing Tip: Toddlers are especially sensitive to being separated from familiar family members. This is a normal developmental stage and would be expected and appropriately dealt with.

Test-Taking Strategy: Note the **strategic words,** *initial* and *most likely,* after the parent's departure. This directs you to look for the toddler's immediate behavioral response to separation. Think about the developmental stages of children and separation anxiety to answer correctly.

---

14. A preschool-age child placed in traction for the treatment of a femur fracture begins wetting the bed. Which response by the nurse is **most appropriate** in handling this regressive behavior?

1 "We need to put a diaper on you."
2 "You are too old to be doing this."
3 "Stop this nonsense; you need a time-out."
4 "Let's get you cleaned up and see if there's a book you like."

Level of Cognitive Ability: Applying
Client Needs: Psychosocial Integrity
Clinical Judgment/Cognitive Skills: Take Action
Integrated Process: Nursing Process/Implementation
Content Area: Mental Health
Health Problem: Mental Health: Coping

Answer: 4
Rationale: The monotony of immobilization can lead to sluggish intellectual and psychomotor responses. Although option 2 may seem like an appropriate response, option 4 is a more accurate description of the intervention to the behavior. Regressive behaviors are not uncommon in immobilized children and usually do not require professional intervention. Options 1, 2, and 3 are more negative responses and can lead to other maladaptive behaviors in the child.
Priority Nursing Tip: Extreme stress can result in regression of developmental behaviors at any age.

Test-Taking Strategy: Focus on the **subject,** managing regressive behavior in a preschooler, and note the **strategic words,** *most appropriate.* Eliminate options 1 and 3, as they may cause more harm to the child's development. Eliminate option 2 next because bedwetting by an immobilized child is not unusual. Also, recall that regression is a normal psychological response to immobilization. The nurse would not focus on the behavior and instead would offer alternative options for the child.

---

15. The nurse is collecting data on the client with a diagnosis of mania. Which findings assist the nurse in evaluating the client's status? **Select all that apply.**

❒ 1 Weight gain
❒ 2 Flattened affect
❒ 3 Inflated self-esteem
❒ 4 Inability to concentrate
❒ 5 Rapid speech patterns

Level of Cognitive Ability: Evaluating
Client Needs: Psychosocial Integrity
Clinical Judgment/Cognitive Skills: Evaluate Outcomes
Integrated Process: Nursing Process/Data Collection
Content Area: Mental Health
Health Problem: Mental Health: Mood Disorder

Answer: 3, 4, 5
Rationale: The manic client typically forgets to eat and therefore demonstrates a weight loss and is likely to be excited and animated rather than depressed with flattened affect. The manic client also demonstrates rapid speech, inflated self-esteem, and an inability to concentrate.
Priority Nursing Tip: In extreme cases, mania can induce hallucinations and other psychotic symptoms.

Test-Taking Strategy: Note the **subject,** characteristics associated with mania. Think about this condition and what occurs to answer correctly. Also note the relationship of the description of mania and the characteristics in the correct options.

---

16. The husband of a client who has a Sengstaken–Blakemore tube states, "I really hoped that having that tube down her nose the first time would convince my wife to quit drinking." Based on this statement, which response by the nurse is appropriate?

1 "Alcoholism is a disease that affects the whole family."
2 "Please discuss your feelings with your support group."
3 "I think you are a very good and loving person to stay with your wife."
4 "You sound frustrated with dealing with your wife's drinking problem."

Level of Cognitive Ability: Applying
Client Needs: Psychosocial Integrity
Clinical Judgment/Cognitive Skills: Take Action
Integrated Process: Communication and Documentation
Content Area: Mental Health
Health Problem: Mental Health: Therapeutic Communication

Answer: 4
Rationale: The nurse would use therapeutic communication techniques to assist the client (in this case, the client's spouse) with expressing his feelings about his wife's chronic illness. The nurse focuses on the spouse's feelings in option 4. Stereotyping (option 1), avoiding the subject (option 2), and expressing an opinion (option 3) are examples of communication blocks.
Priority Nursing Tip: Indications for placement of a Sengstaken–Blakemore tube include acute, life-threatening bleeding from esophageal or gastric varices that does not respond to medical therapy.

Test-Taking Strategy: Use **therapeutic communication techniques.** With communication questions, identify the use of therapeutic tools (option 4) and blocks to communication (options 1, 2, and 3). Remember to always focus on the client's feelings and concerns first.

---

17. The nurse is caring for a client on suicide precautions. Which statement made by the client suggests to the nurse that the client has developed a potentially credible suicide plan?

1 "Hanging yourself seems easy enough."
2 "I could end it by driving my car into a tree."
3 "I'm thinking about getting some medications to take."
4 "I will use my gun and go into the woods behind my house."

Level of Cognitive Ability: Analyzing
Client Needs: Psychosocial Integrity
Clinical Judgment/Cognitive Skills: Analyze Cues
Integrated Process: Nursing Process/Data Collection
Content Area: Mental Health
Health Problem: Mental Health: Suicide

Answer: 4
Rationale: The more specific the plan, the greater the likelihood of a successful suicide. Option 4 designates thought and planning with a deadly weapon. Options 1, 2, and 3 are vague statements for a suicidal plan.
Priority Nursing Tip: When a depressed individual has the ability to concentrate sufficiently to formulate a lethal, realistic plan, the risk for a successful suicide is significant.

Test-Taking Strategy: Focus on the **subject,** a credible suicide plan. Recognizing the attention to details on a plan in option 4 will help you select the correct option.

---

18. A client is admitted to the hospital for a partial thyroidectomy. While preparing the client for surgery, the nurse gathers information about psychosocial problems that may cause preoperative anxiety. Which issue would be a **priority** concern?

1 Changes in body image
2 Sexual dysfunction and infertility
3 Imposed dietary restrictions postoperatively
4 Developing gynecomastia and hirsutism postoperatively

Level of Cognitive Ability: Analyzing
Client Needs: Psychosocial Integrity
Clinical Judgment/Cognitive Skills: Recognize Cues
Integrated Process: Nursing Process/Data Collection
Content Area: Adult Health: Endocrine
Health Problem: Adult Health: Endocrine: Thyroid Disorders

Answer: 1
Rationale: Because the incision is in the neck area, clients often worry about thyroid surgery out of fear of having a large postoperative scar. Having all or part of the thyroid gland removed does not cause the client to experience gynecomastia or hirsutism. Sexual dysfunction and infertility would occur only if the entire thyroid is removed and the client is not placed on thyroid replacement medications. Dietary restrictions are not prescribed.
Priority Nursing Tip: Surgeries that result in physical changes to the exterior of the body often produce anxiety.

Test-Taking Strategy: Note the **strategic word,** *priority*. Focusing on the **subject,** the potential for postoperative anxiety, and recalling the anatomical location of this surgical procedure will direct you to the correct option.

---

19. The nurse is caring for a client diagnosed with type 2 diabetes mellitus who has been hospitalized for hyperosmolar hyperglycemic syndrome. The client expresses concern about this syndrome recurring. Based on the client's expressed concern, which statement by the nurse is appropriate?

1 "This isn't likely to happen again."
2 "Don't worry; your family will know how to help you."
3 "Let's talk about your concerns with this complication."
4 "Perhaps you need to consider talking with your doctor."

Level of Cognitive Ability: Applying
Client Needs: Psychosocial Integrity
Clinical Judgment/Cognitive Skills: Take Action
Integrated Process: Communication and Documentation
Content Area: Adult Health: Endocrine
Health Problem: Mental Health: Therapeutic Communication

Answer: 3
Rationale: Because the client has expressed a concern, the nurse would focus on the client's feelings that are the basis of the concern. Option 3 is the only option that addresses the client's feelings. Options 1 and 2 are inappropriate and provide false reassurance. Option 4 is inappropriate and a premature statement.
Priority Nursing Tip: Nurses use therapeutic communication techniques to provide support and information to clients.

Test-Taking Strategy: Use **therapeutic communication techniques** to answer the question. Focus on the information in the question that stresses the client's concern; this will direct you to the correct option.

---

20. The nurse is explaining necessary lifestyle changes to a client with angina. Which client statement identifies a maladaptive response to coping?
1 "How many children did you say you had?"
2 "It's work's fault that this happened to me."
3 "Are you sure that the pain is from my heart?"
4 "I'm afraid to go to sleep; what if this happens at night?"

Level of Cognitive Ability: Analyzing
Client Needs: Psychosocial Integrity
Clinical Judgment/Cognitive Skills: Evaluate Outcomes
Integrated Process: Nursing Process/Data Collection
Content Area: Adult Health: Cardiovascular
Health Problem: Mental Health: Coping

Answer: 1
Rationale: Denial is a defense mechanism that allows the client to minimize a threat; it manifests by a refusal to discuss what has happened and a redirection of the discussion to an unrelated topic. Denial is a common early reaction associated with chest discomfort, angina, or myocardial infarction. Anger is often manifested by "acting out" behaviors and blaming. Depression manifests through passive behaviors. Fear and anxiety are usually manifested as a result of symptoms of sympathetic nervous system arousal.
Priority Nursing Tip: A defense mechanism is a mental process (e.g., repression or projection) initiated, typically unconsciously, to avoid conscious conflict or anxiety.

Test-Taking Strategy: Focus on the **subject**, maladaptive response to coping. Select the option that best fits this description. Note that in option 1, the correct option, the client redirects the discussion to an unrelated topic.

---

21. The nurse is caring for a client who has verbalized suicidal ideation. Which statement indicates that the client is at **highest** risk for suicide?
1 "I'm just useless. I want someone to take me out and shoot me!"
2 "There is nothing left for me in this life. I just wish I could die!"
3 "God has commanded me to jump off the city bridge tomorrow."
4 "I tried to kill myself last year, but nothing about my life improved."

Level of Cognitive Ability: Analyzing
Client Needs: Psychosocial Integrity
Clinical Judgment/Cognitive Skills: Analyze Cues
Integrated Process: Nursing Process/Data Collection
Content Area: Mental Health
Health Problem: Mental Health: Suicide

Answer: 3
Rationale: The formulation of a suicide plan indicates the client's serious intent. The likelihood of suicide increases when manifestations of auditory command hallucinations (voices telling the client to commit suicide) are present. In option 3, the client identifies an auditory command hallucination and a suicide plan. The nature of the psychosis is highly lethal, and the suicide plan includes an active lethal method, a time, and a place.
Priority Nursing Tip: Any statement made by a client that reflects hopelessness or interest in dying must be taken seriously.

Test-Taking Strategy: Note the **strategic word,** *highest,* and focus on the **subject,** suicidal statements. Note that option 3 identifies a suicide plan that includes an active lethal method, a time, and a place.

---

22. The care plan of a client diagnosed with cancer of the bladder includes the client problem of experiencing fear. Which client statement **best** supports the inclusion of this problem into the client's care plan?

1 "I wish I'd never gone to the doctor at all."
2 "I'm so concerned that I won't live through all this."
3 "I'll never feel like myself once I can't go to the bathroom normally."
4 "I will have no help at home after going through this awful surgery."

Level of Cognitive Ability: Analyzing
Client Needs: Psychosocial Integrity
Clinical Judgment/Cognitive Skills: Analyze Cues
Integrated Process: Nursing Process/Data Collection
Content Area: Mental Health
Health Problem: Mental Health: Crisis

Answer: 2
Rationale: The client must be able to identify the object of fear for *fear* to be an actual client problem. This client is expressing a fear of death related to cancer in option 2. Option 1 is vague and nonspecific; further exploration is necessary to associate this statement with a client problem. Option 3 reflects a problem with body image. The statement in option 4 reflects a problem with the inability to care for self at home.
Priority Nursing Tip: The description of fear is explained by a variety of terms, such as *concern, anxiety,* and *apprehension.*

Test-Taking Strategy: Focus on the **subject**, supporting the existence of client fear, and note the **strategic word,** *best.* Note that the client problem includes wording about the uncertain outcome of surgery that is supported by option 2. Eliminate option 1 because it is a general statement. Options 3 and 4 focus on the self after surgery but do not contain statements about an uncertain outcome.

---

23. The nurse suspects that a client is depressed after experiencing an acute myocardial infarction (MI). What behavior by the client helps the nurse verify this suspicion?

1 Ignoring prescribed activity restrictions
2 Frequently observed crying during the day
3 Expresses concern about being transferred from the telemetry unit
4 States being apprehensive about engaging in a rehabilitation program

Level of Cognitive Ability: Analyzing
Client Needs: Psychosocial Integrity
Clinical Judgment/Cognitive Skills: Analyze Cues
Integrated Process: Nursing Process/Data Collection
Content Area: Mental Health
Health Problem: Mental Health: Coping

Answer: 2
Rationale: The emotional and behavioral reactions of a client after MI are varied. Depression manifests by withdrawal, crying, or apathy. Option 1 is more indicative of denial. Option 3 indicates common post-MI concerns. Option 4 is more indicative of dependence and fear.
Priority Nursing Tip: Demonstrated behaviors of depression include those that represent sadness, despair, and hopelessness.

Test-Taking Strategy: Focus on the **subject,** a client who is depressed. All options are behaviors that manifest in the client after an MI; however, the question is asking about depression. Note that the incorrect options indicate behavioral responses other than those associated with depression. Also, note the relationship of the word *depressed* to the word *crying* in the correct option.

---

24. An older adult client shares with the nurse that his son, daughter-in-law, and their three children have unexpectedly moved into the house "to care for" him. Which statement made by the client causes the nurse to suspect that the client is being exploited?
1 "The children are too noisy, but overall it's helped me get over my wife's death."
2 "Since my wife died, I've been lonely, so having them around is okay."
3 "As long as my son keeps contributing to the household expenses, they can stay."
4 "My son asked me to deed the house to him but promises it will still be my home."

Answer: 4
Rationale: The exploitation of older adults can include taking over the client's bank accounts, deeds, stock portfolios, or wills. Option 1 addresses some adjustment to the expansion of the family, but that is expected. In option 2, the client is stating positive reasons that extended families can be helpful. Option 3 states the client's complete satisfaction with the expansion of the family.
Priority Nursing Tip: Family dynamics can be very complicated. Autonomy and independence are generally vigorously protected. Loss of such rights can indicate exploitation.

Test-Taking Strategy: Focus on the **subject,** older adult exploitation. Recalling the definition and examples of this form of abuse will assist you with eliminating options 1, 2, and 3.

Level of Cognitive Ability: Analyzing
Client Needs: Psychosocial Integrity
Clinical Judgment/Cognitive Skills: Analyze Cues
Integrated Process: Nursing Process/Data Collection
Content Area: Mental Health
Health Problem: Mental Health: Abusive Behaviors

---

25. The nurse is gathering information from members of a family who share a history of both physical and verbal abuse directed toward each other. Which characteristic will the nurse **initially** focus on?
1 The coping style of individual family members
2 The use of community resources by family members
3 The possible existence of family anger directed toward the nurse
4 The use of denial regarding the violent nature of the family's behavior

Answer: 1
Rationale: The nurse would initially collect data about each family member. Although some family members may regard the nurse's interventions as intrusive, this is not the focus of an initial assessment of a violent family. Denial may be one of the coping styles of the family, but it is not specific to a family experiencing violence. Although the use of community resources is important, the coping style of each family member would be determined first.
Priority Nursing Tip: Assessment of a dysfunctional family initially involves data collection regarding individual family members.

Test-Taking Strategy: Note the **strategic word,** *initially.* Eliminate options 2, 3, and 4 because they are **comparable or alike** and relate to data collection about the family as a unit. Option 1 is the only option that addresses the individual family members.

Level of Cognitive Ability: Applying
Client Needs: Psychosocial Integrity
Clinical Judgment/Cognitive Skills: Recognize Cues
Integrated Process: Nursing Process/Data Collection
Content Area: Mental Health
Health Problem: Mental Health: Abusive Behaviors

---

26. The nurse is assisting with the care of a client on a mechanical ventilator. Which symptomatology supports that the client is experiencing difficulty adapting to treatment? **Select all that apply.**

❒ 1 Hypotension
❒ 2 Bradycardia
❒ 3 Hand clenching
❒ 4 Pupillary dilation
❒ 5 Heightened awareness

Level of Cognitive Ability: Analyzing
Client Needs: Psychosocial Integrity
Clinical Judgment/Cognitive Skills: Analyze Cues
Integrated Process: Nursing Process/Data Collection
Content Area: Mental Health
Health Problem: Mental Health: Coping

Answer: 3, 4, 5

Rationale: Signs of anxiety include behaviors such as clenched hands, heightened awareness, wide eyes, pupil dilation, startle response, furrowed brow, clinging to the family or staff, or physical lashing out. Because anxiety stimulates the sympathetic nervous system, the client may also exhibit palpitations, chest pain, tachycardia, an increased respiratory rate, an elevated blood glucose level, and hand tremors. In anxious states, tachycardia is present rather than bradycardia and hypertension rather than hypotension.

Priority Nursing Tip: Anxiety can result in both physical and psychological symptoms.

Test-Taking Strategy: Focus on the **subject,** experiencing difficulty adapting to treatment. Recalling that anxiety stimulates the sympathetic nervous system and knowing the effects of sympathetic stimulation will direct you to options 3, 4, and 5.

---

27. An exercise stress test is prescribed for a client who has experienced recent episodes of severe chest pain. As the nurse is preparing the client for the test, the client states, "Maybe I shouldn't bother going. I wonder if I need to just take more medication instead." The nurse would make which response to the client?

1 "Can you tell me more about how you're feeling?"
2 "Don't you really want to control your heart disease?"
3 "Most people tolerate the procedure well without any complications."
4 "Don't worry. Emergency equipment is available if it would be needed."

Level of Cognitive Ability: Applying
Client Needs: Psychosocial Integrity
Clinical Judgment/Cognitive Skills: Recognize Cues
Integrated Process: Communication and Documentation
Content Area: Adult Health: Cardiovascular
Health Problem: Mental Health: Therapeutic Communication

Answer: 1

Rationale: Anxiety and fear are often present before stress testing. The nurse uses questioning as a communication method to explore a client's feelings and concerns. Only option 1 is an open-ended question that is phrased to encourage the sharing of concerns by the client. Options 2, 3, and 4 are nontherapeutic and do not focus on the client's feelings.

Priority Nursing Tip: A stress test usually involves walking on a treadmill or riding a stationary bike while the client's heart rhythm, blood pressure, and breathing are monitored.

Test-Taking Strategy: Use **therapeutic communication techniques** to answer the question. Only option 1 focuses on the client's feelings. Remember to focus on client feelings and concerns first.

---

28. A term newborn diagnosed with Hirschsprung's disease is crying. The nurse observes that the parents are hesitant to hold their newborn. Based on this observation, what would be the nurse's **initial** focus?

1. How to safely support an infant's head and neck
2. How to manage this congenital disorder
3. How to help the parents bond with their newborn
4. How to comfort a crying baby

Level of Cognitive Ability: Applying
Client Needs: Psychosocial Integrity
Clinical Judgment/Cognitive Skills: Take Action
Integrated Process: Nursing Process/Implementation
Content Area: Maternity/Newborn
Health Problem: Mental Health: Coping

Answer: 3
Rationale: One of the main objectives is to help parents adjust to the congenital disorder in their child and to foster infant–parent bonding. All the other options assume the cause of the hesitation. Once bonding is established, the other options can be addressed.
Priority Nursing Tip: The parent–child bond can be seriously impaired when the child is born with a congenital disorder because such an event will cause a large amount of parental stress. Education about the unknown disorder is an important positive intervention in fostering parent–child bonding.

Test-Taking Strategy: Focus on the **subject,** the parents' hesitance to hold their newborn, and the **strategic word,** *initial.* This may indicate a need to help the parents accept their child even though the newborn has a serious medical condition. Only option 3 addresses this concern.

---

29. The nurse is caring for a client diagnosed with chronic depression. Which finding will the nurse identify as requiring **immediate** attention?

1. Sleeping for 12 to 18 hours every night
2. Verbalizing feelings of being "hopeless"
3. Requesting to call a member of his support team
4. Describing self as "never feeling better than right now"

Level of Cognitive Ability: Analyzing
Client Needs: Psychosocial Integrity
Clinical Judgment/Cognitive Skills: Analyze Cues
Integrated Process: Nursing Process/Data Collection
Content Area: Mental Health
Health Problem: Mental Health: Suicide

Answer: 4
Rationale: The depressed individual who has a sudden mood elevation after a period of being depressed is identified as being at risk to carry out suicidal intent. Options 1, 2, and 3 would require documentation and reporting but are not the most significant findings.
Priority Nursing Tip: Once a depressed individual has decided to end their life, the depression the individual feels is often lifted.

Test-Taking Strategy: Note the **strategic word,** *immediate.* Recalling that the depressed individual who has a sudden mood elevation is at risk to carry out a suicide intent will direct you to the correct option.

---

30. The nurse is preparing a client for electroconvulsive therapy (ECT). The client is pacing and says to the nurse, "How do I know this will work? I really don't understand how it can help me now. It may kill me." How does the nurse **best** respond to the client's expressed concern?

1 Assisting the client with resolving ambivalence about the decision to receive ECT
2 Planning with the client how ECT will help the client's return to daily functioning
3 Asking the client to recall what the client remembers about ECT from discussions
4 Exploring the meaning of the client's comment about ECT in a calm, supportive manner

Level of Cognitive Ability: Applying
Client Needs: Psychosocial Integrity
Clinical Judgment/Cognitive Skills: Take Action
Integrated Process: Nursing Process/Implementation
Content Area: Mental Health
Health Problem: Mental Health: Therapeutic Communication

Answer: 4
Rationale: In this situation, the client presents with anxiety before ECT. Only option 4 addresses the client's feelings and concerns. Although options 1, 2, and 3 may be components of caring for the client, these options do not address the subject of the question.
Priority Nursing Tip: ECT seems to cause changes in brain chemistry that can reverse symptoms of certain mental illnesses.

Test-Taking Strategy: Note the **strategic word,** *best.* Use **therapeutic communication techniques,** and note that only option 4 addresses the client's concerns. Remember to address the client's feelings and concerns first.

---

31. A parent refuses to have their child immunized because of fear that a serious injury will result. To identify the basis of the parent's concern, the nurse would make which statement to the parent?

1 "Are you afraid that the child is going to die from the injection?"
2 "There will be slight discomfort at the time of the injection, and that is all."
3 "Children are immunized every day without ever experiencing a problem."
4 "May we talk about the concerns you have about immunizing your child?"

Level of Cognitive Ability: Applying
Client Needs: Psychosocial Integrity
Clinical Judgment/Cognitive Skills: Take Action
Integrated Process: Communication and Documentation
Content Area: Pediatrics: Infectious and Communicable Diseases
Health Problem: Mental Health: Therapeutic Communication

Answer: 4
Rationale: Option 4 acknowledges the parent's concern, which provides an opportunity for the parent to respond to the nurse's open-ended question. Option 1 is an attempt to verify an assumption that is not supported by the question. Options 2 and 3 block communication.
Priority Nursing Tip: Vaccines are important to prevent infectious disease.

Test-Taking Strategy: Use **therapeutic communication techniques** to answer the question. The correct option demonstrates empathy and helps the parent focus on specific fears so that the nurse can clarify information. Options 1, 2, and 3 use blocking strategies by assuming what the parent fears, giving false reassurances, and devaluing the parent's feelings, respectively.

---

32. The nurse is caring for a client with a diagnosis of terminal ovarian cancer. While providing care, the nurse identifies that the client is in the bargaining phase of coping when hearing the client make which statement?

1. "There's nothing I can do to make this better for myself or my family."
2. "I need to make a will and spend quality time with my family and friends."
3. "If I just stay away from my family, it will be easier for them when I am gone."
4. "If I can just live long enough to attend my daughter's graduation, I'll be ready to die."

Level of Cognitive Ability: Analyzing
Client Needs: Psychosocial Integrity
Clinical Judgment/Cognitive Skills: Analyze Cues
Integrated Process: Nursing Process/Data Collection
Content Area: Adult Health: Oncology
Health Problem: Mental Health: Coping

Answer: 4
Rationale: Bargaining is the phase of coping in which dying persons try to negotiate by making deals with their God or fate. Option 1, 2, and 3 indicate depression, acceptance, and isolation, respectively.
Priority Nursing Tip: A grieving individual generally processes through a series of stages that help the individual accept impending death.

Test-Taking Strategy: Focus on the **subject,** the bargaining phase of coping. Read each client statement, and use your understanding of the grieving process. This will direct you to the correct option.

---

33. A neonate is experiencing withdrawal symptoms related to maternal medication abuse during pregnancy. Which neonate characteristic is **most likely** to affect the parent–baby bond **initially**?

1. Sleeps only when swaddled
2. Feedings require an orogastric tube
3. Hyperextends their body and avoids eye contact
4. Becomes irritable in response to noise and light

Level of Cognitive Ability: Analyzing
Client Needs: Psychosocial Integrity
Clinical Judgment/Cognitive Skills: Recognize Cues
Integrated Process: Nursing Process/Data Collection
Content Area: Maternity/Newborn
Health Problem: Newborn: Addicted Newborn

Answer: 3
Rationale: A hyperextended posture and gaze aversion make the parent–baby relationship and bond most difficult to establish. The neonate is showing its disinterest by not looking at the parent's face. Parents often feel that they do not know a child until they are able to look into the baby's eyes. In addition, the hyperextended posture makes the neonate difficult to hold and cuddle. Swaddling does not interfere with the typical bonding behaviors. There is ample time to engage in bonding techniques other than at feeding times. The irritability can be managed by minimizing the triggering stimuli.
Priority Nursing Tip: Parent–child bonding is affected by any situation that interferes with normal holding, cuddling, and mutual interest.

Test-Taking Strategy: Focus on the **subject**, identifying the neonate behavior that will make the parent–baby bond difficult to establish. Also note the **strategic words,** *most likely* and *initially.* Recall that gaze aversion and hyperextension are viewed as rejection of the parent by the neonate. All the other options provide only minimal barriers to the bonding process.

---

34. A client will be self-administering an anticoagulant subcutaneously at home and confides to the nurse that "I'm not sure I will be able to give myself these shots." How does the nurse **best** address the client's concern?

1 "Maybe your wife can give you your shot."
2 "Don't worry. Your doctor knows what's best for you."
3 "You'll be fine after you get used to giving your own shots."
4 "What is it about taking this medication at home that worries you?"

Level of Cognitive Ability: Applying
Client Needs: Psychosocial Integrity
Clinical Judgment/Cognitive Skills: Take Action
Integrated Process: Communication and Documentation
Content Area: Skills: Medication Administration
Health Problem: Mental Health: Therapeutic Communication

Answer: 4
Rationale: Option 4 restates the client's concern and provides the opportunity to verbalize feelings. Option 1 offers advice without knowing what the client's concerns really are. Options 2 and 3 identify false reassurance, which invalidates the client's concern.
Priority Nursing Tip: Heparin is an anticoagulant and can be administered subcutaneously. It is used to decrease the clotting ability of the blood and help prevent harmful clots from forming in blood vessels.

Test-Taking Strategy: Use **therapeutic communication techniques** to answer this question. Also note the **strategic word,** *best.* Remember to focus on the client's feelings and concerns; this will direct you to the correct option.

---

35. A pregnant client with mild anemia reports that her prescribed iron supplement is causing nausea, constipation, and heartburn and that she plans to stop the medication. What is the nurse's **best** response?

1 "In time you will get used to the side effects."
2 "Your baby needs that iron, so you shouldn't stop taking it."
3 "Do not stop taking your medication without talking to the doctor."
4 "These discomforts will become less bothersome with continued use."

Level of Cognitive Ability: Applying
Client Needs: Psychosocial Integrity
Clinical Judgment/Cognitive Skills: Take Action
Integrated Process: Communication and Documentation
Content Area: Pharmacology: Hematological Medications/Medications for Anemia
Health Problem: Adult Health: Hematological: Anemias

Answer: 4
Rationale: Pregnant clients need iron supplements because the fetus places extra demands on the maternal circulation. The correct option addresses the issues that are bothersome to the client. Option 1 places the client's issue of the side effects on hold. Options 2 and 3 show the nurse's disapproval of the client's feelings.
Priority Nursing Tip: Therapeutic communication between nurse and client is the most effective technique to encourage a client to discuss his or her feelings and concerns.

Test-Taking Strategy: Note the **strategic word,** *best,* and focus on the **subject,** side effects of iron supplementation. Your knowledge of the side effects of iron supplements will help direct you to the correct option. Additionally, the use of **therapeutic communication techniques** will direct you to the correct option.

---

36. The nurse is reinforcing a dietary regimen with a pregnant client who has mild anemia when the client states, "My iron pills will have to do; I can't afford to buy any of that fancy food." The nurse responds to the client **best** when making what statement?

1 "Ask your family for financial help."
2 "Ground beef is cheap and rich in iron."
3 "Let's look into food options you can afford."
4 "Iron is very important to the health of both you and the baby."

Level of Cognitive Ability: Applying
Client Needs: Psychosocial Integrity
Clinical Judgment/Cognitive Skills: Take Action
Integrated Process: Communication and Documentation
Content Area: Pharmacology: Hematological Medications: Medications for Anemia
Health Problem: Adult Health: Hematological: Anemias

Answer: 3
Rationale: Option 3 validates the concern that the client has with income and attempts to provide a workable solution. The nurse offers help in a nonthreatening manner that will allow the client to accept being involved in solving the problem. The remaining options either postpone or minimize the problem.
Priority Nursing Tip: Anemia is a condition marked by a deficiency of red blood cells or of hemoglobin in the blood, resulting in pallor and weariness.

Test-Taking Strategy: Use **therapeutic communication techniques** and note the **strategic word,** *best.* Note that the correct option is the only one that addresses the client's concern. Remember to always focus on the client's concerns.

---

37. The nurse is caring for a client undergoing radiation therapy. Which client statement indicates the **most** common concern of clients receiving this therapy?

1 "I'm not certain that this is the best intervention."
2 "This treatment is very expensive and time consuming."
3 "I'm worried that I will be radioactive after the treatments."
4 "This is just one of several options that I have for treatment."

Level of Cognitive Ability: Analyzing
Client Needs: Psychosocial Integrity
Clinical Judgment/Cognitive Skills: Analyze Cues
Integrated Process: Nursing Process/Data Collection
Content Area: Adult Health: Oncology
Health Problem: Mental Health: Coping

Answer: 3
Rationale: Radiation therapy is often a source of fear and misconceptions for clients and their families. Some of the most common fears and misconceptions include fear of being burned, fear of being radioactive, fear of treatment failure, and concern about adverse effects. Options 1, 2, and 4 identify concerns, but they do not identify the most common client concern of radiation therapy.
Priority Nursing Tip: Radiation therapy (also called *radiotherapy*) is a cancer treatment that uses high doses of radiation to kill cancer cells and shrink tumors. At low doses, radiation is used in x-rays to see inside your body, as with x-rays of your teeth or broken bones.

Test-Taking Strategy: Focus on the **subject,** the common concerns, and note the **strategic word,** *most.* Note the relationship between the words *radiation* in the question and *radioactive* in the correct option.

---

38. The nurse implements what intervention to facilitate positive outcomes during pregnancy?

1 Discussion of reproductive issues with a woman and her sexual partner
2 Education of all males as to the issues and spread of sexually transmitted infections
3 Encouragement of safe-sex practices among couples 18 years old and older in all cultures
4 Promoting the discussion of sexual practices of all women with their health care providers

Level of Cognitive Ability: Applying
Client Needs: Psychosocial Integrity
Clinical Judgment/Cognitive Skills: Take Action
Integrated Process: Nursing Process/Implementation
Content Area: Maternity: Antepartum
Health Problem: N/A

Answer: 1
Rationale: The nurse providing care to women in their childbearing years must be familiar with the framework within which the client lives and operates. After this is achieved, appropriate communication techniques can be used to facilitate client care and to identify health promotion educational strategies. Options 2, 3, and 4 generalize clients.
Priority Nursing Tip: Consistent exposure to positive role models is an excellent way to emphasize respect and admiration for diversity.

Test-Taking Strategy: Focus on the **subject,** facilitating positive outcomes. Eliminate options 2, 3, and 4 because these options identify situations that generalize childbearing clients. Also, note the **closed-ended word** "all" in these incorrect options.

---

39. While discussing a pregnant client's dietary and drinking habits with the client, the nurse observes that the client has difficulty concentrating and appears agitated. The nurse would proceed with data collection using which guideline?

1 A nonjudgmental approach may help gain maternal trust when discussing sensitive issues.
2 Provoking maternal guilt may help the woman recognize her problem and seek support services.
3 A discussion of the possible consequences of drinking during pregnancy would be postponed until the client is better prepared cognitively.
4 Women respond negatively to a hopeful message regarding the potential benefits of drinking cessation during pregnancy.

Level of Cognitive Ability: Applying
Client Needs: Psychosocial Integrity
Clinical Judgment/Cognitive Skills: Recognize Cues
Integrated Process: Caring
Content Area: Maternity: Antepartum
Health Problem: Mental Health: Addictions

Answer: 1
Rationale: The potential effects of alcohol abuse during pregnancy for both the parent and fetus have been well documented. The nurse using therapeutic communication techniques would express genuine concern with suspected abusers to motivate positive behavioral changes during the antenatal period. Options 2, 3, and 4 are inappropriate and inaccurate guidelines because they do not facilitate therapeutic communication or address the issues of abuse.
Priority Nursing Tip: Offspring of parents abusing alcohol during pregnancy are known to suffer from developmental delays and/or a variety of behavioral changes.

Test-Taking Strategy: Use **therapeutic communication techniques** to answer the question. Remember to display a nonjudgmental attitude and to focus on the client's feelings.

---

40. During report the nurse received information that a client with hypertension is refusing to take the prescribed medication spironolactone. The nurse suspects that this refusal results from which adverse effect?

1 Edema
2 Weight loss
3 Muscle atrophy
4 Decreased libido

Level of Cognitive Ability: Analyzing
Client Needs: Psychosocial Integrity
Clinical Judgment/Cognitive Skills: Analyze Cues
Integrated Process: Nursing Process/Data Collection
Content Area: Pharmacology: Cardiovascular/Diuretic
Health Problem: Adult Health: Cardiovascular/Hypertension

Answer: 4

Rationale: Spironolactone is a potassium-sparing diuretic. The nurse would be alert to the fact that the client taking spironolactone may experience body image changes as a result of threatened sexual identity. These body image changes are related to decreased libido, gynecomastia in males, and hirsutism in females. Muscle atrophy is unrelated to this medication. Weight loss is an expected outcome of taking the medication. Edema is a reason for taking the medication.

Priority Nursing Tip: Potassium-sparing diuretics are used as adjunctive therapy, together with other medications, in the treatment of hypertension and management of heart failure.

Test-Taking Strategy: Focus on the **subject**, spironolactone and the client's refusal. Also note the client's diagnosis. Recalling the adverse effects of spironolactone and that medication compliance is a problem with antihypertensive medications will direct you to the correct option.

---

41. The nurse is caring for a client who is experiencing psychomotor agitation. Which activity is **most appropriate** for the nurse to plan for the client?

1 A chess game with staff
2 Playing volleyball with other clients
3 Reading magazines quietly in the dayroom
4 Working crossword puzzles from the newspaper

Level of Cognitive Ability: Applying
Client Needs: Psychosocial Integrity
Clinical Judgment/Cognitive Skills: Generate Solutions
Integrated Process: Nursing Process/Planning
Content Area: Mental Health
Health Problem: Mental Health: Coping

Answer: 2

Rationale: With psychomotor agitation, it is best to provide activities that involve the use of the hands and gross motor movements. These activities include table tennis, volleyball, finger painting, drawing, and working with clay. These activities give the client an appropriate way of discharging motor tension. Options 3 and 4 are sedentary activities that will not address discharging psychomotor agitation. Option 1 requires concentrating and a more intensive use of the thought processes.

Priority Nursing Tip: People with psychomotor agitation engage in movements such as pacing, tapping with toes or fingers, or rapid talking; these movements serve no purpose.

Test-Taking Strategy: Note the **strategic words,** *most appropriate*. Focus on the **subject**, psychomotor agitation. Note the diagnosis of the client, and recall that activities that involve the use of the hands and gross motor movements are best for this client.

42. Which intervention is appropriate for a depressed client whose plan of care is based in part on the client problem of poor nutrition? **Select all that apply.**

❒ 1 Remaining with the client during meals to assist with eating

❒ 2 Completing the food menu for the client during the depressed period

❒ 3 Encouraging the client to consume high-protein, high-calorie fluids frequently

❒ 4 Providing a variety of high-protein snacks frequently throughout the day and evening

❒ 5 Allowing the client to earn privileges by consuming appropriate amounts of food daily

Level of Cognitive Ability: Applying
Client Needs: Psychosocial Integrity
Clinical Judgment/Cognitive Skills: Generate Solutions
Integrated Process: Nursing Process/Planning
Content Area: Skills: Nutrition
Health Problem: Mental Health: Mood Disorder

Answer: 1, 3, 4
Rationale: It is inappropriate for the nurse to complete the food menu for the client. Instead, the client would be offered dietary choices and asked which foods or drinks he or she likes. The client is more likely to eat the foods provided if he or she has selected the foods and may have foods that he or she likes. It is nontherapeutic to bribe the client with privileges for eating. Options 1, 3, and 4 are appropriate interventions for the client with depression with this client problem.
Priority Nursing Tip: The depressed individual is likely to lack both interest and energy to eat sufficient amounts of nutritious food and fluids. It is a nursing responsibility to provide the client with easily eaten, nutritious food and beverages.

Test-Taking Strategy: Focus on the **subject,** depression and poor nutrition. Think about the characteristics of a depressed client and nursing considerations, then focus on interventions that may further nutritional intake.

---

43. The nurse is assigned to care for a client demonstrating manic characteristics. The plan of care addresses the client's problem with interacting socially related to altered thought processes. Which activity would the nurse **initially** provide for the client related to this client problem?

1 Writing in a personal journal
2 Playing checkers with another client
3 Attending a movie in the auditorium
4 Going on a supervised trip to a local mall

Level of Cognitive Ability: Applying
Client Needs: Psychosocial Integrity
Clinical Judgment/Cognitive Skills: Take Action
Integrated Process: Nursing Process/Implementation
Content Area: Mental Health
Health Problem: Mental Health: Mood Disorders

Answer: 1
Rationale: When the client is manic, solitary activities that require a short attention span or mild physical exertion are best initially, such as writing, painting, finger painting, woodworking, or walking with the staff. Solitary activities minimize stimuli, and mild physical activities release tension constructively. When less manic, the client may join one or two other clients in quiet, nonstimulating activities. Competitive games would be avoided because they can stimulate aggression and cause increased psychomotor activity.
Priority Nursing Tip: Bipolar disorder is associated with episodes of mood swings ranging from depressive lows to manic highs.

Test-Taking Strategy: Note the **strategic word,** *initially.* Focus on the **data in the question.** Note that options 2, 3, and 4 are **comparable or alike** in that they are all activities that involve another individual. Option 1 is the only solitary activity that will minimize stimuli.

44. The nurse documents that a client diagnosed with schizophrenia presents an inappropriate affect. Which behavior describes this type of behavioral response as observed by the nurse?

1 Crying most of the day
2 Blank staring for hours
3 Mumbling loudly to himself or herself
4 Laughing when another client is crying

Level of Cognitive Ability: Applying
Client Needs: Psychosocial Integrity
Clinical Judgment/Cognitive Skills: Recognize Cues
Integrated Process: Nursing Process/Data Collection
Content Area: Mental Health
Health Problem: Mental Health: Schizophrenia

Answer: 4
Rationale: An inappropriate affect refers to an emotional response to a situation that is not congruent with the tone of the situation. A bizarre affect such as grimacing, giggling, or mumbling to oneself is marked when the client is unable to relate logically to the environment. A blunted affect is a minimal emotional response and expresses the client's outward affect; it may not coincide with the client's inner emotions. A flat affect is an immobile facial expression or a blank look.
Priority Nursing Tip: Affect is related to the expression of emotions.

Test-Taking Strategy: Focus on the **subject,** inappropriate affect. A knowledge of affect and how it is reflective of emotional well-being will help direct you to the correct option.

---

45. The nurse is gathering data from a client admitted to the hospital with a diagnosis of coronary artery disease. During the interviewing process, the client tells the nurse that life has been quite stressful. The nurse would take which therapeutic action **initially**?

1 Arranging a psychiatric consult for the client
2 Sharing with the client that stress is common these days
3 Assisting the client in writing down the sources of daily stress
4 Encouraging the client to talk about the sources of personal stress

Level of Cognitive Ability: Applying
Client Needs: Psychosocial Integrity
Clinical Judgment/Cognitive Skills: Take Action
Integrated Process: Nursing Process/Implementation
Content Area: Mental Health
Health Problem: Mental Health: Coping

Answer: 4
Rationale: The nurse encourages the client to verbalize personal stressors so that strategies for coping with unavoidable stress can be explored. Option 1 is a premature action. Option 2 does not address the client's concerns. Option 3 may be appropriate but is not the first action.
Priority Nursing Tip: Verbalization of the sources of a problem is the first step in managing the problem.

Test-Taking Strategy: Note the **strategic word,** *initially,* and focus on the **subject,** managing stress. An understanding of how to best manage stress will assist with directing you to the correct option. Remember to focus on the client's feelings first.

---

46. The nurse is caring for a client admitted to the hospital with a diagnosis of coronary artery disease. While gathering data from the client during the interviewing process, the client tells the nurse about the occasional use of cocaine. What is the nurse's **priority** action to **best** ensure appropriate care?

1. Report the client to the police for illegal medication use.
2. Explain to the client what effect the medication has on the heart.
3. Inform the client that medication abuse is physically dangerous.
4. Notify the client's primary health care provider of the cocaine use.

Level of Cognitive Ability: Applying
Client Needs: Psychosocial Integrity
Clinical Judgment/Cognitive Skills: Take Action
Integrated Process: Nursing Process/Implementation
Content Area: Mental Health
Health Problem: Mental Health: Addictions

Answer: 4
Rationale: Notifying the client's primary health care provider will best ensure that the client will receive appropriate care. The remaining options do not address the immediate physical threat cocaine use presents for this client.
Priority Nursing Tip: Client safety has priority when considering client care interventions.

Test-Taking Strategy: Focus on the **subject**, cocaine use, and the **strategic words**, *priority* and *best*. Understanding that treatment is initiated by the primary health care provider will help direct you to the correct option.

---

47. A client presents with "bad indigestion" and tells the nurse that the pain is "probably related to the greasy cheeseburger I ate a few hours ago." The nurse's care will be based on what **primary** understanding of a myocardial infarction (MI)?

1. A diet high in fat can cause an MI.
2. MI symptomatology can mimic gastrointestinal distress.
3. An MI is a major cardiological event that can cause death.
4. Denial is a major factor in not seeking immediate MI treatment.

Level of Cognitive Ability: Applying
Client Needs: Psychosocial Integrity
Clinical Judgment/Cognitive Skills: Analyze Cues
Integrated Process: Nursing Process/Analysis
Content Area: Adult Health: Cardiovascular
Health Problem: Mental Health: Coping

Answer: 4
Rationale: An individual's first response to the pain that he or she is experiencing is denial because the individual cannot believe that he or she is really having an MI; this in turn keeps the individual from seeking immediate medical treatment. Knowing that this is a common response, the nurse will be better able to help the client face the reality of the situation. Options 1, 2, and 3 may be true but are not the foundational principle upon which nursing care would be provided.
Priority Nursing Tip: Women are more likely to have atypical symptoms of an MI than men.

Test-Taking Strategy: Focus on the **subject**, response to a possible MI, and your knowledge of the psychological effects that an individual experiences during an MI. Noting the **strategic word**, *primary*, will direct you to the correct option.

---

48. The nurse assigned to care for a postpartum client will promote maternal–infant bonding after discharge when reinforcing which intervention?

1 Avoid using a high-pitched voice when speaking to their infant.
2 Allow the infant to sleep in the parental bed between the parents.
3 Hold and cuddle the infant closely to comfort the infant when crying.
4 Let grandparents assume a portion of the infant's care so that the parents may rest.

Level of Cognitive Ability: Applying
Client Needs: Psychosocial Integrity
Clinical Judgment/Cognitive Skills: Take Action
Integrated Process: Nursing Process/Implementation
Content Area: Maternity: Postpartum
Health Problem: N/A

Answer: 3

Rationale: Holding and cuddling the infant closely initiates a positive experience for the parents. It is self-quieting and consoles the infant. The use of a high-pitched voice and participating in infant care are other methods of promoting maternal–infant attachment. An infant would not be allowed to sleep in the parental bed between parents because of the danger of suffocation and because the couple will require meaningful rest and time to be alone as a couple.

Priority Nursing Tip: Parent–child bonding is best achieved when there is ample opportunity to connect both physically and emotionally.

Test-Taking Strategy: Focus on the **subject,** parental bonding. Note the relationship of the subject and the words *hold and cuddle the infant closely.* The correct option is the only one that addresses the issue of bonding accurately.

---

49. The nurse is assigned to care for a postpartum client. When collecting data regarding the new parent's anxieties, which client statement indicates the strongest potential for a problem with parental–infant attachment?

1 "I just feel so weepy all the time."
2 "His toothless grin reminds me of Granddaddy's smile."
3 "I'm tired; can someone in the nursery feed the baby so I can sleep?"
4 "Why did this baby have to inherit my mother-in-law's ugly big nose?"

Level of Cognitive Ability: Analyzing
Client Needs: Psychosocial Integrity
Clinical Judgment/Cognitive Skills: Analyze Cues
Integrated Process: Nursing Process/Data Collection
Content Area: Maternity: Postpartum
Health Problem: N/A

Answer: 4

Rationale: Negativity about the baby's features may interfere with the parent's ability to bond with and care for the infant. Positive statements and identification with family members help the parent identify with the infant, thus promoting attachment. Fatigue and mild postpartum depression are expected responses and may cause the parent to feel weepy and to request the staff to assume care of the infant temporarily; however, after a period of rest, the parent needs to begin to assume the care of the infant.

Priority Nursing Tip: Parent–child bonding is in most danger when the child is connected to unpleasant events or situations in a parent's mind.

Test-Taking Strategy: Focus on the **subject,** barriers to maternal–infant attachment. Note that in option 4, the client expresses negativity about the baby's features.

---

50. A client with a spinal cord injury (SCI) tells the nurse, "It's so depressing that I'll never get to have sex again." How would the nurse address the client's concerns?

1 "It must feel horrible to know you can never have sex again."
2 "It is still possible to have a sexual relationship, but it will be different."
3 "You're young, so you'll adapt to this more easily than if you were older."
4 "Because of body reflexes, sexual functioning will be no different than before."

Level of Cognitive Ability: Applying
Client Needs: Psychosocial Integrity
Clinical Judgment/Cognitive Skills: Take Action
Integrated Process: Communication and Documentation
Content Area: Adult Health: Neurological
Health Problem: Adult Health: Neurological: Spinal Cord Injury

Answer: 2
Rationale: It is possible to have a sexual relationship after an SCI, but it will be different from what the client experienced before the injury. Males may experience reflex erections, although they may not ejaculate. Females can have adductor spasm. Option 1 does not promote continued discussion of the client's concerns. Options 3 and 4 are incorrect statements.
Priority Nursing Tip: Sexual counseling may help the client adapt to changes in sexuality after an SCI.

Test-Taking Strategy: Focus on the **subject,** sexual function after an SCI. Knowledge regarding the altered physiology after SCI and **therapeutic communication techniques** will assist you with answering the question. Eliminate option 1 because it is a communication block. Eliminate options 3 and 4 next because they are incorrect statements.

---

51. A family member of a client who was just diagnosed with a brain tumor is distraught and feeling guilty for not encouraging the client to seek medical evaluation earlier. The nurse plans to incorporate a response to this family member's concern based on what fact?

1 There are few early symptoms of brain tumors.
2 It is true that brain tumors are easily recognizable.
3 Brain tumors are seldom detected until very late in their course.
4 The symptoms of brain tumor may be easily attributed to other causes.

Level of Cognitive Ability: Applying
Client Needs: Psychosocial Integrity
Clinical Judgment/Cognitive Skills: Generate Solutions
Integrated Process: Nursing Process/Planning
Content Area: Adult Health: Neurological
Health Problem: Adult Health: Cancer/Brain Tumors

Answer: 4
Rationale: The signs and symptoms of a brain tumor vary depending on the location of the tumor, and they may easily be attributed to another cause. Options 1, 2, and 3 are incorrect statements.
Priority Nursing Tip: Guilt is often assumed inappropriately, and the nurse can help relieve unwarranted negative emotions by providing appropriate education on the cause of the illness.

Test-Taking Strategy: Focus on the **data in the question.** Eliminate options 1 and 3 first because they contain the **closed-ended words** "few" and "seldom," respectively. From the remaining options, it is necessary to know that the symptoms of brain tumor can be vague and that they may easily be attributed to another cause.

---

52. A client who has experienced extensive surgery on the gastrointestinal tract has been prescribed total parenteral nutrition (TPN). The client tells the nurse, "I think I'm going crazy. I feel as if I'm starving, yet that bag is supposed to be feeding me." What is the **best** response by the nurse to address the client's concern?

1 "Don't worry; the sensations will soon go away."
2 "I'll be sure to mention those sensations to your doctor."
3 "I'll check to be sure the solution is being mixed correctly."
4 "TPN can't stop your stomach from sending hunger signals to your brain."

Level of Cognitive Ability: Applying
Client Needs: Psychosocial Integrity
Clinical Judgment/Cognitive Skills: Take Action
Integrated Process: Nursing Process/Implementation
Content Area: Foundations of Care: Communication
Health Problem: Adult Health: Gastrointestinal/Nutrition Problems

Answer: 4
Rationale: When it is empty, the stomach does send signals to the brain to stimulate hunger. The client would be told that this is normal. Some clients also experience food cravings for the same reason. Options 1 and 2 will block the communication process. Option 3 will produce fear.
Priority Nursing Tip: Communication that provides the client with an explanation for the client's concern is generally the most therapeutic intervention.

Test-Taking Strategy: Note the **strategic word,** *best.* Use **therapeutic communication techniques** and an understanding of TPN to answer the question. Begin to answer this question by eliminating option 3 first; this statement could frighten the client and lessen the client's trust in the health care team. Eliminate options 1 and 2 because they do not respond to the client's concerns. The correct option is the only response that acknowledges the client's concern and addresses it.

---

53. A licensed practical nurse (LPN) observes assistive personnel (AP) talking in an unusually loud voice to a client with delirium. Which of these actions would the LPN take to address the AP's behavior?

1 Ask the AP immediately why it is necessary to speak so loudly.
2 Inform the client in a calm, normal voice that everything is all right.
3 Explain to the AP that yelling in the client's room is tolerated only if the client is talking loudly.
4 Ask the AP to step outside of the client's room and discuss appropriate communication techniques.

Level of Cognitive Ability: Applying
Client Needs: Psychosocial Integrity
Clinical Judgment/Cognitive Skills: Take Action
Integrated Process: Nursing Process/Implementation
Content Area: Leadership/Management: Delegating/Supervising
Health Problem: N/A

Answer: 4
Rationale: The nurse must determine that the client is safe and then discuss the matter with the AP in an area in which the conversation cannot be heard by the client. If the client hears the conversation, the client may become more confused or agitated. In addition, option 1 could unnecessarily embarrass the AP.
Priority Nursing Tip: Constructive criticism regarding the delivery of care needs to be addressed immediately and in private.

Test-Taking Strategy: Use **therapeutic communication techniques** and effective management practices. An understanding of effective communication techniques will direct you to the correct option.

---

54. An adolescent diagnosed with chronic inflammatory bowel disease presents with profuse watery diarrhea after eating pizza at a party earlier in the day. The client states, "I don't want to be different from my friends." Based on the statement, the nurse determines that the client is at **most** risk for which problem?

1 Depression
2 Dehydration
3 Celiac crisis
4 Altered self-esteem

Level of Cognitive Ability: Analyzing
Client Needs: Psychosocial Integrity
Clinical Judgment/Cognitive Skills: Analyze Cues
Integrated Process: Nursing Process/Data Collection
Content Area: Mental Health
Health Problem: Mental Health: Coping

Answer: 4
Rationale: The client expresses concern about being different. This statement is associated with a self-esteem issue. Data provided in the question do not support a diagnosis of depression. Dehydration and celiac crisis are physiological problems.
Priority Nursing Tip: Psychosocial problems involve dysfunctions that include both emotional and cognitive issues.

Test-Taking Strategy: Note the **strategic word,** *most.* Focus on the **data in the question,** noting the client's feelings of being different; this would direct you to the correct option.

---

55. The nurse is assisting with developing a plan of care for a 1-month-old infant hospitalized for intussusception. Which measure provides psychosocial support for the parent–child relationship?

1 Provide educational materials on the disorder.
2 Encourage the parents to room-in with the infant.
3 Initiate home nutritional support as early as possible.
4 Encourage the parents to go home and get some sleep.

Level of Cognitive Ability: Applying
Client Needs: Psychosocial Integrity
Clinical Judgment/Cognitive Skills: Generate Solutions
Integrated Process: Nursing Process/Planning
Content Area: Developmental Stages: Infant
Health Problem: Pediatric-Specific: Gastrointestinal and Rectal Problems

Answer: 2
Rationale: Rooming-in is effective for reducing separation anxiety and preserving the parent–child relationship. It is stressful for the parents when a child is ill and hospitalized. Telling a parent to go home and sleep will not relieve this stress. Although educational materials are beneficial, they will not provide psychosocial support for the parent–child relationship. Home nutritional support is not directed at the psychosocial concerns of this situation.
Priority Nursing Tip: Rooming-in is the practice followed in hospitals in which the baby's crib is kept by the side of the parent's bed.

Test-Taking Strategy: Focus on the **subject,** providing psychosocial support to the parents and the child. Note that the correct option is the only one that provides an interaction between the child and the parents.

---

56. Which comment made by the parents of an infant who is scheduled for inguinal hernia repair surgery **requires follow-up** by the nurse?

1. "I wonder if he will be able to have children."
2. "We will need to change his diaper more frequently now."
3. "I understand that surgery will repair the hernia completely."
4. "We were told not to put him into water for a few days after surgery."

Level of Cognitive Ability: Evaluating
Client Needs: Psychosocial Integrity
Clinical Judgment/Cognitive Skills: Evaluate Outcomes
Integrated Process: Nursing Process/Evaluation
Content Area: Pediatrics: Gastrointestinal
Health Problem: Pediatric-Specific: Disorders of Prenatal Development

Answer: 1
Rationale: The anatomical location of hernias frequently causes more psychological concern to the parents than does the actual condition or treatment; the parents may think that the disorder affects future reproductive ability. Options 2, 3, and 4 all indicate the parents' accurate understanding.
Priority Nursing Tip: An inguinal hernia is a protrusion of abdominal cavity contents through the inguinal canal.

Test-Taking Strategy: Focus on the **strategic words,** *requires follow-up.* These words indicate a **negative event query** and the need to select the comment that is a concern. The correct option reflects parental fear and identifies a need for follow-up.

---

57. A licensed practical nurse is assisting a school nurse with conducting a crisis intervention group. The clients are high school students whose classmate recently committed suicide at the school. The students experiencing disbelief are reviewing details about finding the student dead in a bathroom. Based on this information, what would be the nurse's **first** intervention?

1. Reinforce the students' sense of growth through this death.
2. Inquire how the students coped with death events in the past.
3. Reinforce the students' ability to work through this death event.
4. Inquire about the students' perception of their classmate's suicide.

Level of Cognitive Ability: Applying
Client Needs: Psychosocial Integrity
Clinical Judgment/Cognitive Skills: Take Action
Integrated Process: Nursing Process/Implementation
Content Area: Mental Health
Health Problem: Mental Health: Grief/Loss

Answer: 4
Rationale: It is essential to first determine the students' perception of the suicide. Inquiring about the students' perception of the death will specifically identify the appraisal of the suicide and the meaning of the perception. Although option 2 is exploratory, it does not address the "here and now" appraisal in terms of the classmate's suicide. Although the nurse is interested in how clients have coped in the past, this inquiry would not be the most immediate.
Priority Nursing Tip: Communication that provides the client with support to explore the cause of their concern is generally the most therapeutic intervention; this can only be accomplished when the client's perception of events is understood.

Test-Taking Strategy: Note the **strategic word,** *first.* Focus on the **subject,** reacting to a suicide, and select the option that deals with the here and now. Options 1 and 3 are **comparable or alike** in that they attempt to foster clients' self-esteem; such an approach is premature at this point.

58. Which action will **most likely** calm a client who experiences periodic agitation while recovering from a traumatic head injury?

1 Giving the client a soft object to hold
2 Assigning the client a new task to master
3 Turning the television on to a musical program
4 Making the client aware that the behavior is undesirable

Level of Cognitive Ability: Applying
Client Needs: Psychosocial Integrity
Clinical Judgment/Cognitive Skills: Take Action
Integrated Process: Nursing Process/Implementation
Content Area: Adult Health: Neurological
Health Problem: Mental Health: Neurocognitive Impairment

Answer: 1

Rationale: Decreasing environmental stimuli aids in reducing agitation for the head-injured client. Introducing a new task may be frustrating. The television increases stimuli. Option 4 identifies a nontherapeutic approach. The correct option helps distract the client with a motor activity—holding a soft object.

Priority Nursing Tip: The damaged brain cannot process information as it normally does, which may lead to increased intracranial pressure and, in later stages of recovery, agitation and restlessness.

Test-Taking Strategy: Focus on the **subject**, calming an agitated, brain-injured client. Note the **strategic words,** *most likely.* Eliminating options that may increase stimuli, agitation, and frustration would direct you to the correct option.

---

59. A client recovering from a stroke (brain attack) has become irritable and angry about the associated limitations. The nurse would take which approach to help the client regain motivation to succeed?

1 Use supportive statements to correct behavior.
2 Ignore the behavior, knowing that the client is grieving.
3 Encourage longer and more frequent visitation with the spouse.
4 State that nursing experience lets the nurse know how the client feels.

Level of Cognitive Ability: Applying
Client Needs: Psychosocial Integrity
Clinical Judgment/Cognitive Skills: Take Action
Integrated Process: Nursing Process/Implementation
Content Area: Adult Health: Neurological
Health Problem: Mental Health: Coping

Answer: 1

Rationale: Clients who have had strokes have many and varied needs. The client may need negative behaviors pointed out so that correction can take place, as well as support and praise for accomplishments. The client may be grieving or may have damage to cerebral inhibitory centers; however, the behavior should not be ignored. Spouses of stroke clients are often grieving, so more visits may not be helpful; short visits are often encouraged. Stating that you know how someone feels is inappropriate.

Priority Nursing Tip: Whereas a healthy relationship depends on the emotional space provided by personal boundaries, codependent personalities have difficulties in setting such limits; defining and protecting boundaries efficiently may be for them a vital part of regaining mental health.

Test-Taking Strategy: Use **therapeutic communication techniques.** The correct option is the only one that addresses client feelings and supportive care.

---

60. A client admitted to the hospital with a broken hip is experiencing periods of confusion. The nurse assists with developing a plan of care related to disturbed thought processes. The nurse understands that which psychosocial outcome has the **highest priority** for this client?

1 Improved sleep patterns
2 Reducing family fears and anxiety
3 Independently meeting self-care needs
4 Increased ability to concentrate and make decisions

Level of Cognitive Ability: Analyzing
Client Needs: Psychosocial Integrity
Clinical Judgment/Cognitive Skills: Generate Solutions
Integrated Process: Nursing Process/Planning
Content Area: Mental Health
Health Problem: Mental Health: Neurocognitive Impairment

Answer: 4

Rationale: The client needs to be able to concentrate and make decisions. When the client is able to do that, the nurse can work with the client to achieve the other outcomes. All remaining options are goals that are secondary to increased concentration and decision making.

Priority Nursing Tip: Acute confusion is often called *delirium,* or an acute confusional state.

Test-Taking Strategy: Note the **strategic words,** *highest priority,* and focus on the **subject,** confusion. Look for the option that will have the greatest impact on the client's ability to function. This will assist in eliminating options 1 and 2. Next eliminate option 3 because it is unrealistic at this time, considering that the word *independently* is in this option. The correct option will make the greatest difference in the client's ability to achieve the remaining goals.

---

61. A young terminally ill client with breast cancer talks privately with the nurse. The nurse identifies the client problem of anticipatory grief in which client behavior?

1 The client expresses prolonged emotional reactions and outbursts.
2 The client discusses what her family will go through when she dies.
3 The client ignores untreated medical conditions that require treatment.
4 The client cries every time the nurse comes into the room.

Level of Cognitive Ability: Analyzing
Client Needs: Psychosocial Integrity
Clinical Judgment/Cognitive Skills: Analyze Cues
Integrated Process: Nursing Process/Data Collection
Content Area: Mental Health
Health Problem: Mental Health: Grief/Loss

Answer: 2

Rationale: The nurse can determine the client's stage of grief by observing behavior. This is extremely important so that an appropriate plan of care can be developed. The correct option identifies anticipatory grief in the form of the client's concern of events once she dies. The remaining options are examples of dysfunctional grieving.

Priority Nursing Tip: Anticipatory grief involves dealing with issues related to the loss that is expected to occur through effective communication concerning the loss.

Test-Taking Strategy: Focus on the **subject,** anticipatory grief. Note that the incorrect options are **comparable or alike** in that they deal with the here and now rather than events in the future.

---

62. A licensed practical nurse notes that a client in labor begins to saturate the bed with sanguineous fluid; upon assessment the nurse finds pallor, light-headedness, and blood pressure of 89/42 mm Hg. The client asks, "What is happening to me? I feel so funny. Is the baby okay? I'm so scared." The nurse bases the response on the fact that the client is experiencing what emotional response?
   1 Panic secondary to shock
   2 Anticipatory grieving related to the fear of dying
   3 Altered tissue perfusion related to intranatal hemorrhage
   4 Anxiety related to unexpected and ambiguous sensations

Level of Cognitive Ability: Analyzing
Client Needs: Psychosocial Integrity
Clinical Judgment/Cognitive Skills: Analyze Cues
Integrated Process: Nursing Process/Data Collection
Content Area: Maternity/Intrapartum
Health Problem: Mental Health: Crisis

Answer: 4
Rationale: Feelings of loss of control because of the unknown are common causes of anxiety especially if the client is feeling unexpected and ambiguous sensations. Apprehension and feelings of impending doom are also associated with shock, but the case situation does not suggest panic at this point. Anticipatory grieving occurs when there is knowledge of an impending loss, but it is not operative in a sudden situational crisis such as this one. There is no supportive data indicating that the intranatal hemorrhage is occurring.
Priority Nursing Tip: When an individual experiences a loss of control, real or imagined, a common response is a sense of anxiety.

Test-Taking Strategy: Focus on the **data in the question.** Note the relationship between the words *I feel so funny* in the question and *unexpected and ambiguous sensations* in the correct option.

---

63. The nurse has just assessed a client at 20 weeks' gestation. The client is experiencing new bleeding and reports less fetal movement. The client begins to cry quietly while holding her abdomen with her hands and murmurs, "No, no, you can't go, my little man." Which response by the nurse is **most appropriate**?
   1 "There is no need to be upset. Everything will be fine."
   2 "I have notified the primary health care provider to come."
   3 "You seem to be upset; I will stay with you if you would like."
   4 "So, you are having a boy. What are you going to name him?"

Level of Cognitive Ability: Applying
Client Needs: Psychosocial Integrity
Clinical Judgment/Cognitive Skills: Take Action
Integrated Process: Nursing Process/Implementation
Content Area: Maternity: Antepartum
Health Problem: Mental Health: Grief and Loss

Answer: 3
Rationale: Anticipatory grieving occurs when a client has knowledge of an impending loss. Anticipatory grieving is appropriate when any signs of fetal distress accelerate. The nurse would listen attentively to the client and use clarifying and focusing to assist the client with expressing his or her feelings. "There is no need to be upset..." provides false reassurance. "So, you are having a boy..." is a distraction technique that does not acknowledge the client's feelings. "I have notified the primary health care provider ..." informs the client of what interventions the nurse has done; however, this can make the client more upset. "You seem to be upset; I will stay with you if you would like" acknowledges the client's concerns, and staying with the client provides support and reassurance during a difficult time.
Priority Nursing Tip: According to the American Congress of Obstetricians and Gynecologists, when doing kick counts, the parent ideally would feel at least 10 fetal movements within 2 hours.

Test-Taking Strategy: Focus on the **data in the question.** Note the **strategic words,** *most appropriate.* Option 1 provides false reassurance, and option 4 distracts the client. These can be eliminated as they do not provide support. Option 2 increases anxiety and worsens the sense of loss. The correct option provides the most support and acknowledges the client's feelings.

---

64. A postoperative client diagnosed with an ileus has a nasogastric tube inserted. After being provided with an explanation of its purpose and insertion procedure, the client says to the nurse, "I'm not sure I can tolerate this procedure." How does the nurse address the client's concern?

1 "Are you afraid of having the tube inserted?"
2 "If you don't have this tube put down, you will just continue to vomit."
3 "Are you feeling tired and frustrated with your recovery from surgery?"
4 "It is your right to refuse any procedure. I'll notify the primary health care provider."

Level of Cognitive Ability: Applying
Client Needs: Psychosocial Integrity
Clinical Judgment/Cognitive Skills: Take Action
Integrated Process: Communication and Documentation
Content Area: Adult Health: Gastrointestinal
Health Problem: Mental Health: Therapeutic Communication

Answer: 3
Rationale: The correct option assists the client with expressing and exploring feelings, which can lead to effective problem solving. Options 2 and 4 are examples of barriers to effective communication in that the nurse does not address the client's concerns. Option 1 states a true fact but does not address the nursing responsibility to identify why the client is refusing the treatment.
Priority Nursing Tip: A nasogastric tube enables the drainage of gastric contents, decompressing the stomach.

Test-Taking Strategy: Use **therapeutic communication techniques.** The correct option is an open-ended question and a communication tool that focuses on the client's feelings.

---

65. A client is admitted to the hospital with a bowel obstruction secondary to a recurrent malignancy. After the primary health care provider inserts a Miller–Abbott tube, the client asks the nurse, "Do you think this is worth all this trouble?" What is the appropriate nursing response?

1 Stating, "Let's give this tube a chance."
2 Staying with the client and being silent.
3 Asking, "Are you wondering whether you are going to get better?"
4 Sharing, "I remember a case similar to yours, and the tube relieved the obstruction."

Level of Cognitive Ability: Applying
Client Needs: Psychosocial Integrity
Clinical Judgment/Cognitive Skills: Take Action
Integrated Process: Communication and Documentation
Content Area: Adult Health: Oncology
Health Problem: Mental Health: Therapeutic Communication

Answer: 3
Rationale: The nurse needs to use therapeutic communication tools when assisting a client with a chronic terminal illness to express feelings. The nurse would listen attentively to the client and use clarifying and focusing to assist the client with expressing his or her feelings. Changing the subject (option 1), responding with inappropriate silence (option 2), and offering false reassurance (option 4) are examples of barriers to communication.
Priority Nursing Tip: A Miller–Abbott tube is used to treat obstructions in the small intestine through intubation of a device that is around 3 meters long and has a distal balloon at one end.

Test-Taking Strategy: Use **therapeutic communication techniques** when responding to the client and focus on the **subject,** the client's concern. The correct option encourages the client to verbalize, whereas the remaining options are blocks to communication.

---

66. A client receiving total parenteral nutrition (TPN) and intralipids says to the nurse, "I was always overweight until I had this illness. I'm not sure I want to get that fat again. The other intravenous fluids are probably enough." The nurse would make which **initial** response to the client?

1 "I understand what you mean. I've dieted most of my life."
2 "Tell me how being ill has affected the way you think of yourself."
3 "Fatty acids are essential for life. You'll develop deficiencies without the fats."
4 "I think you need to discuss this decision with the primary health care provider."

Level of Cognitive Ability: Applying
Client Needs: Psychosocial Integrity
Clinical Judgment/Cognitive Skills: Take Action
Integrated Process: Communication and Documentation
Content Area: Foundations of Care: Communication
Health Problem: Mental Health: Therapeutic Communication

Answer: 2
Rationale: Clients receiving long-term TPN are at risk for the development of essential fatty acid deficiency. However, the client's response requires more than an informational response initially. The nurse uses tools of therapeutic communication to assist the client with expressing feelings and dealing with the aspects of illness and treatment. Blocks to communication, such as giving opinions (option 1), placing the client's feelings on hold (option 4), and giving information too soon (option 3), will not assist the client with coping effectively.
Priority Nursing Tip: Lipid emulsion or fat emulsion refers to an emulsion of lipids for human intravenous use.

Test-Taking Strategy: Note the **strategic word,** *initial.* Use **therapeutic communication techniques.** The correct option is the only one that encourages the client to express feelings.

---

67. A client diagnosed with terminal cancer is using opioid analgesics for pain relief. The client expresses concern about becoming addicted to the pain medication. How can the nurse allay this anxiety?

1 Encouraging the client to hold off as long as possible between doses of pain medication
2 Telling the client an option is to take lower doses of medications even though the pain may not be as well controlled
3 Explaining to the client that his or her fears are justified but would be of no concern during the final stages of illness
4 Explaining to the client that addiction rarely occurs when the medication is taken appropriately to relieve pain

Level of Cognitive Ability: Applying
Client Needs: Psychosocial Integrity
Clinical Judgment/Cognitive Skills: Take Action
Integrated Process: Caring
Content Area: Adult Health: Oncology
Health Problem: Mental Health: Addictions

Answer: 4
Rationale: Clients who are prescribed opioid analgesics often have well-founded fears about addiction, even in the face of pain. The nurse has a responsibility to give correct information about the likelihood of addiction while still maintaining adequate pain control. Addiction is rare for individuals who are taking medication to relieve pain. Allowing the client to be in pain is not acceptable nursing practice. The remaining option is correct only in that it acknowledges the client's fear, but addressing the final stages of illness is inappropriate at this time.
Priority Nursing Tip: Most cancer pain is caused by the tumor pressing on bones, nerves, or other organs in the body.

Test-Taking Strategy: Focus on the **subject,** a client's concern about opioid addiction. Eliminate options 1 and 2, which are unacceptable nursing practices. Eliminate option 3 because it is only partially correct. An understanding of effective opioid therapy for pain management will direct you to the correct option.

---

68. A client is highly anxious about receiving chest physical therapy (CPT) for the first time. When planning the client's care, the nurse provides the client with what reassurance?

1 CPT has relatively few associated risks.
2 CPT can resolve all of the client's respiratory symptoms.
3 CPT always assists the client with coughing more effectively.
4 CPT will assist with mobilizing secretions to help breathing.

Level of Cognitive Ability: Applying
Client Needs: Psychosocial Integrity
Clinical Judgment/Cognitive Skills: Generate Solutions
Integrated Process: Nursing Process/Planning
Content Area: Adult Health: Respiratory
Health Problem: Mental Health: Coping

Answer: 4
Rationale: CPT is a respiratory treatment that will mobilize secretions to enhance more effective breathing. Risks are associated with CPT, including cardiac, gastrointestinal, neurological, and pulmonary complications. CPT will indirectly assist the client with coughing if the secretions have been mobilized and the cough stimulus is present. CPT is an intervention to assist with clearing secretions, but it will not resolve all respiratory symptoms.
Priority Nursing Tip: Problems related to respiratory secretions can be caused by infection or aspiration, or by pooling of normal oropharyngeal secretions in a client who is weak or unable to swallow or cough effectively.

Test-Taking Strategy: Focus on the **subject,** the purpose of CPT. Eliminate options 2 and 3 because of the **closed-ended words** "all" and "always." An understanding of CPT will help direct you to the correct option.

---

69. A client diagnosed with cardiomyopathy is demonstrating behaviors that are often associated with depression. Which assessment finding supports this diagnosis? **Select all that apply.**

❐ 1 Consumes only 10% to 15% of each meal
❐ 2 Remains awake for long periods during the night
❐ 3 Repeatedly tells family that "I will never get better"
❐ 4 Reports shortness of breath when walking to the bathroom
❐ 5 States, "I'm not interested in watching sports on TV anymore"

Level of Cognitive Ability: Analyzing
Client Needs: Psychosocial Integrity
Clinical Judgment/Cognitive Skills: Analyze Cues
Integrated Process: Nursing Process/Data Collection
Content Area: Adult Health: Cardiovascular
Health Problem: Mental Health: Mood Disorders

Answer: 1, 2, 3, 5
Rationale: Depression is a common problem among clients who have long-term and debilitating illnesses. Poor appetite, feelings of hopelessness, a loss of interest in pleasurable activities, and dysfunctional sleeping patterns are all symptoms associated with depression. Option 4 is not related to depression and is probably a result of the cardiac problem.
Priority Nursing Tip: Depression is generally associated with behaviors that demonstrate a lack of interest and joy in life, as well as problems with attending to basic physiological needs.

Test-Taking Strategy: Focus on the **data in the question,** and use your related knowledge to identify the classic signs of depression. This will assist in eliminating option 4.

---

70. Which psychosocial intervention is **most important** for a pregnant client hospitalized for diabetes mellitus?

1 Evaluate the client's fears related to pregnancy and diabetes.
2 Teach the client about the risks of preterm labor and the signs to watch for.
3 Teach the client and her family about diabetes mellitus and its implications.
4 Provide support about interrupted family processes related to hospitalization.

Level of Cognitive Ability: Analyzing
Client Needs: Psychosocial Integrity
Clinical Judgment/Cognitive Skills: Generate Solutions
Integrated Process: Nursing Process/Planning
Content Area: Maternity: Antepartum
Health Problem: Mental Health: Coping

Answer: 4

Rationale: The most important psychosocial risk is to the well-being of the family because of the hospitalization of the parent. Options 1 and 2 are psychosocial problems, but the client's risks are not directly associated with hospitalization. The client may experience fears related to pregnancy and diabetes; however, evaluating these fears is a long-term goal and not related to the current hospitalization.

Priority Nursing Tip: The client's psychosocial well-being involves the minimization of anxiety related to hospitalization.

Test-Taking Strategy: Focus on the **subject**, a psychosocial intervention associated with hospitalization, and note the **strategic words,** *most important.* Eliminate options that are not directly associated with the client's hospitalization.

---

71. A new parent is trying to decide whether to have their baby boy circumcised. The nurse makes which statement to the parent to assist with making this decision?

1 "I had my son circumcised, and I am so glad."
2 "Circumcision is a difficult decision. Let's discuss the questions that you have."
3 "You know, they say it prevents cancer and sexually transmitted infections, so I would definitely have my son circumcised."
4 "Circumcision is a personal decision, but your pediatrician is the best, and you know it's better to get it done now rather than later."

Level of Cognitive Ability: Applying
Client Needs: Psychosocial Integrity
Clinical Judgment/Cognitive Skills: Take Action
Integrated Process: Communication and Documentation
Content Area: Maternity/Newborn
Health Problem: Newborn: Circumcision

Answer: 2

Rationale: Circumcision can be a difficult decision for parents, and the nurse would provide the client with the opportunity to discuss feelings and concerns and to ask questions. Options 1, 3, and 4 identify nontherapeutic communication techniques in that they offer personal opinion and advice to the client. The nurse's personal thoughts and feelings would not be part of the educational process.

Priority Nursing Tip: For some families, circumcision is a religious ritual. Circumcision can also be a matter of family tradition, personal hygiene, or preventive health care.

Test-Taking Strategy: Focus on the **subject,** concern about circumcision. Eliminate options 1 and 3 because they are **comparable or alike** in that the nurse is referring to his or her son. In addition, options 1, 3, and 4 are communication blocks because the nurse is providing a personal opinion to the client. Informed decision making is the key point to consider when selecting the correct option in this question.

---

72. The nurse is assisting with the planning of care for a client who is experiencing anxiety after a myocardial infarction. Which nursing intervention would be included in the plan of care to address the cause of the anxiety?

1 Answer questions with factual information.
2 Provide detailed explanations of all procedures.
3 Administer the antianxiety medication as prescribed.
4 Encourage family involvement during the acute phase.

Level of Cognitive Ability: Applying
Client Needs: Psychosocial Integrity
Clinical Judgment/Cognitive Skills: Generate Solutions
Integrated Process: Nursing Process/Planning
Content Area: Adult Health: Cardiovascular
Health Problem: Mental Health: Anxiety Disorder

Answer: 1
Rationale: Accurate information reduces fear, strengthens the nurse–client relationship, and assists the client with dealing realistically with the situation. Providing detailed information may increase the client's anxiety; the information provided should be simple and clear. Encouraging family involvement may be helpful, but it does not address the cause of the anxiety. Although antianxiety medication may be helpful, administering it will not address the root of the client's concern.
Priority Nursing Tip: Providing the client with accurate information will assist the client in the management of anxiety by eliminating the unknown and giving the client power over the situation.

Test-Taking Strategy: Focus on the **subject,** managing anxiety. Eliminate option 3 because medication would not be the first intervention used to alleviate anxiety. Eliminate option 2 next because of the word *detailed.* From the remaining options, eliminate option 4 because family involvement does not reduce anxiety in all situations.

---

73. A client recovering from an acute myocardial infarction is scheduled for discharge in 12 hours. Which action suggests that the client is in the denial phase of grieving?

1 Requests a sedative for sleep at 10:00 PM
2 Expresses hesitancy about leaving the hospital
3 Consumes only 25% of the foods and fluids given for supper
4 Walks up and down three flights of stairs without supervision

Level of Cognitive Ability: Analyzing
Client Needs: Psychosocial Integrity
Clinical Judgment/Cognitive Skills: Analyze Cues
Integrated Process: Nursing Process/Data Collection
Content Area: Adult Health: Cardiovascular
Health Problem: Mental Health: Coping

Answer: 4
Rationale: Ignoring activity limitations and avoiding lifestyle changes are signs of denial during the process of grieving. Walking up and down three flights of stairs would be a supervised activity during the rehabilitation process. Option 1 is an appropriate client action on the evening before discharge. Option 2 may be a manifestation of anxiety or fear rather than denial. Option 3 is a manifestation of depression rather than denial.
Priority Nursing Tip: The term *myocardial infarction* focuses on the myocardium (the heart muscle) and the changes that occur in it due to the sudden deprivation of circulating blood.

Test-Taking Strategy: Focus on the **subject,** the denial phase. Option 1 is an appropriate client action. Option 2 identifies anxiety or fear. Option 3 identifies depression. Option 4 is the only option that suggests denial in the client.

---

74. Which statement by a client indicates the use of a positive coping mechanism during treatment for Hodgkin's disease?

1 "I will not leave the house bald."
2 "I don't want to see anyone if I lose my hair."
3 "I will be one of the few who don't lose their hair."
4 "I have always wanted red hair, so that's the color wig I got."

Level of Cognitive Ability: Evaluating
Client Needs: Psychosocial Integrity
Clinical Judgment/Cognitive Skills: Evaluate Outcomes
Integrated Process: Nursing Process/Evaluation
Content Area: Adult Health: Oncology
Health Problem: Mental Health: Coping

Answer: 4
Rationale: A combination of radiation and chemotherapy often causes alopecia in clients with Hodgkin's disease. To use positive coping mechanisms, the client must identify personal feelings and use problem-solving positive interventions to deal with the side effects of treatment. Option 4 is the only option that indicates a positive coping mechanism. Options 1 and 2 involve avoidance, and option 3 indicates denial.
Priority Nursing Tip: A positive coping mechanism is one that recognizes and accepts the painful truth while allowing the individual to deal with it in a healthy manner.

Test-Taking Strategy: Focus on the **subject,** a positive coping mechanism, and use your understanding of positive coping. Option 4 is the only option that is a positive statement.

---

75. A client is admitted to the hospital with a diagnosis of diabetic ketoacidosis (DKA). The client's daughter shares, "My mother died last month, and now this. We've been following all of the instructions from the doctor, but he is still sick. What am I doing wrong?" What response would the nurse make?

1 "It may get very difficult to manage diabetic care as your father gets older."
2 "Maybe we can keep your father in the hospital for a while longer to give you a rest."
3 "You should consider having a home health nurse manage your father's diabetic care."
4 "Emotional stress can trigger DKA even when appropriate diabetic care is being given."

Level of Cognitive Ability: Applying
Client Needs: Psychosocial Integrity
Clinical Judgment/Cognitive Skills: Take Action
Integrated Process: Communication and Documentation
Content Area: Mental Health
Health Problem: Mental Health: Therapeutic Communication

Answer: 4
Rationale: Environment, infection, or an emotional stressor can initiate the pathophysiological mechanism of DKA. Options 1 and 3 inappropriately substantiate the daughter's feelings of guilt. Option 2 is neither necessary nor cost-effective.
Priority Nursing Tip: A trigger for DKA is stress, which would be aggressively addressed in the diabetic client.

Test-Taking Strategy: Focus on the **client of the question** (the client's daughter) and the **data in the question.** Eliminate options 1, 2, and 3 because they do not directly address the daughter's expressed feelings of guilt.

---

76. The nurse is assisting with planning goals for a victim of rape. Which short-term goals are appropriate for inclusion in the client's plan of care? **Select all that apply.**

- ❒ 1 The client will verbalize feelings about the rape event.
- ❒ 2 The client will resolve feelings of fear and anxiety related to the rape trauma.
- ❒ 3 The client will experience physical healing of the wounds that were incurred at the time of the rape.
- ❒ 4 The client will participate in the treatment plan by keeping appointments and following through with treatment options.
- ❒ 5 The client will demonstrate control over the event by talking about it only when asked to by mental health professionals.

Level of Cognitive Ability: Applying
Client Needs: Psychosocial Integrity
Clinical Judgment/Cognitive Skills: Generate Solutions
Integrated Process: Nursing Process/Planning
Content Area: Mental Health
Health Problem: Mental Health: Coping

Answer: 1, 3, 4
Rationale: Short-term goals will include those appropriate for the beginning stages of dealing with the rape trauma. Clients will initially be expected to keep appointments, participate in care, begin to explore feelings, and begin to heal the physical wounds that were inflicted at the time of the rape. Option 2, the resolution of feelings, is a long-term goal, whereas option 5 is inappropriate and nontherapeutic because expressing feelings is critical to the recovery of a traumatized client.
Priority Nursing Tip: A short-term goal is something you want to accomplish in the near future. The near future can mean today, this week, this month, or in some situations even this year.

Test-Taking Strategy: Focus on the **subject,** appropriate short-term goals related to rape recovery. Note the words *short-term goals* and *appropriate.* The word *resolve* in option 2 indicates that this is a long-term goal. Also note the **closed-ended word** "only" in option 5, an incorrect option.

---

77. A client with a diagnosis of cancer is scheduled for surgery in the morning. The nurse recognizes that the client is exhibiting denial when the client is heard making which statement?

1. "Oh my Lord, I'm not ready for you to take me home."
2. "I'm not having surgery; there's nothing wrong with me."
3. "If you can't take me to the operating room, I don't want to go."
4. "If anyone tries to take me out of this room, I'll hurt them badly."

Level of Cognitive Ability: Analysis
Client Needs: Psychosocial Integrity
Clinical Judgment/Cognitive Skills: Recognize Cues
Integrated Process: Nursing Process/Data Collection
Content Area: Adult Health: Mental Health
Health Problem: Mental Health: Coping

Answer: 2
Rationale: Defense mechanisms protect against anxiety. Denial (option 2) is the defense mechanism that blocks out painful or anxiety-inducing events or feelings. In this case, the client cannot deal with the upcoming surgery for cancer and therefore denies that he or she is ill. Hopelessness (option 1) is a client problem of anticipated loss. Option 3 is a bargaining technique and not a coping technique. Option 4 is a maladaptive coping mechanism of acting out.
Priority Nursing Tip: Anxiety is a feeling of worry, nervousness, or unease, typically about an imminent event or something with an uncertain outcome.

Test-Taking Strategy: Focus on the **subject,** an indication of denial. Eliminate options 1 and 3 first because these are not defense mechanisms. From the remaining options, focus on the **subject** to direct you to the correct option.

78. The nurse who works in an industrial setting is given a memo that indicates that a large number of employees will be laid off during the next 2 weeks. A review of previous layoffs suggested that workers experienced role crises, indecision, and depression. Using these data, the nurse assists with planning for the layoff by suggesting the need for which intervention?

1 Helping the workers acquire unemployment benefits to avoid a gap in income
2 Reducing the staff in the occupational health department of the industrial setting
3 Notifying insurance carriers of the upcoming event to assist with potential health alterations
4 Identifying referral, counseling, and vocational retraining services for the employees being laid off

Level of Cognitive Ability: Applying
Client Needs: Psychosocial Integrity
Clinical Judgment/Cognitive Skills: Generate Solutions
Integrated Process: Nursing Process/Planning
Content Area: Mental Health
Health Problem: Mental Health: Crisis

Answer: 4
Rationale: In this case, option 4 is the only intervention; the other options may or may not need to occur. The nurse would need to know more about the industry to determine whether options 1, 2, or 3 would be necessary or possible.
Priority Nursing Tip: Adjustment to psychosocial stressors, such as a loss of employment, is often facilitated by the availability of mental health services.

Test-Taking Strategy: Focus on the **data in the question.** Options 1, 2, and 3 are more industry specific, and one would need to know more about the industrial setting than is presented in the question. In addition, the correct option is the **umbrella option,** which includes several options.

---

79. During the discharge planning of a small-for-gestational-age (SGA) infant, the nurse makes an appointment for an evaluation by a developmental specialist. The parent says to the nurse, "I am not sure that going to a specialist is necessary just because the baby is small." Which statement is the appropriate response by the nurse?

1 "Your baby is very small and needs to be evaluated by the developmental specialist."
2 "A lot of parents need to have their babies evaluated by the developmental specialist."
3 "I feel that it is the best thing for you to have the baby evaluated by the developmental specialist."
4 "Let's discuss the purpose and the benefits of such a referral, and I'll try to answer any questions."

Level of Cognitive Ability: Applying
Client Needs: Psychosocial Integrity
Clinical Judgment/Cognitive Skills: Take Action
Integrated Process: Communication and Documentation
Content Area: Maternity: Newborn
Health Problem: Newborn: Gestational Age Problems

Answer: 4
Rationale: SGA infants are at risk for poor postnatal growth and for neurological and developmental handicaps. By providing the parent with an opportunity to discuss the appointment, the nurse uses a therapeutic communication technique and addresses the parent's need for understanding. Options 1, 2, and 3 are nontherapeutic responses that do not address the parent's concerns.
Priority Nursing Tip: *Gestational age* is the common term used during pregnancy to describe how far along the pregnancy is. It is measured in weeks, from the first day of the woman's last menstrual cycle to the current date. Although the gestational age may be calculated from the parent's last menstrual period and by ultrasonography during pregnancy, the date of the last menstrual period is not always accurate, and ultrasonography is not always performed.

Test-Taking Strategy: Use **therapeutic communication techniques** to answer the question. Only the correct option addresses the parent's concern. Options 1 and 3 provide advice from the nurse's viewpoint and opinion. Option 2 is a generalized statement that does not address the parent's individual concern.

---

80. A toddler is admitted to the hospital with a fever of unknown origin. The mother has three other children she cares for, and the father is out of town on business. The mother's time at the hospital is limited to the hours that the other children are in school. The nurse demonstrates an understanding of the toddler's psychosocial development by making which statement to the mother?

1 "Your child is egocentric, which allows a child to self-comfort."
2 "It is better to leave without saying goodbye so that your child will not be upset."
3 "Games such as peekaboo and hide-and-seek will help your child understand that you will return."
4 "Your child is too old to be having separation anxiety. Crying is just a way children have of controlling their parents."

Level of Cognitive Ability: Applying
Client Needs: Psychosocial Integrity
Clinical Judgment/Cognitive Skills: Take Action
Integrated Process: Communication and Documentation
Content Area: Developmental Stages: Toddler
Health Problem: N/A

Answer: 3
Rationale: In the correct option, the nurse suggests ways in which the child can be helped to develop object permanence. Options 1, 2, and 4 do not meet the psychosocial needs of a toddler who is being separated from a caregiver.
Priority Nursing Tip: Before 8 months, a baby will think that an object has disappeared if it is covered or hidden from view. The concept that objects exist even when they cannot be seen is called object permanence.

Test-Taking Strategy: Focus on the **data in the question,** including the age of the child and the psychosocial development that occurs during this time. This knowledge will assist in directing you to the correct option.

---

81. The nurse is caring for a client diagnosed with coronary artery disease. When entering the client's room, which observation requires a **priority** intervention?

1 The client's lunch tray has not been touched.
2 The client is working on his laptop computer.
3 The client is quietly praying using rosary beads.
4 The client is laughing loudly at a television program.

Level of Cognitive Ability: Analyzing
Client Needs: Psychosocial Integrity
Clinical Judgment/Cognitive Skills: Take Action
Integrated Process: Nursing Process/Data Collection
Content Area: Adult Health: Cardiovascular
Health Problem: Adult Health: Cardiovascular: Coronary Artery Disease

Answer: 2
Rationale: Rest and relaxation are crucial for clients with angina because stress and emotional tension can trigger episodes of pain. The volume of client laughter is not related to triggering episodes of pain. Praying is a positive coping mechanism. Although nutrition is important, the nurse is most concerned with the finding related to stress.
Priority Nursing Tip: Stress, both physical and emotional, is a trigger for cardiac-focused pain.

Test-Taking Strategy: Note the **strategic word,** *priority.* Focus on the **data in the question** and note the client's diagnosis. Think about the factors that can trigger anginal pain, and remember that a common reaction is denial; this will direct you to the correct option.

---

82. A stillborn infant delivered a few hours ago remains in the room with the family. Which statement by the nurse will further assist the family during their initial period of grief?

1 "What did you name your baby?"
2 "You seem upset. Do you need a tranquilizer?"
3 "I feel so bad. I don't understand why this happened either."
4 "You can continue holding your baby for another 15 minutes."

Level of Cognitive Ability: Applying
Client Needs: Psychosocial Integrity
Clinical Judgment/Cognitive Skills: Take Action
Integrated Process: Caring
Content Area: Maternity/Postpartum
Health Problem: Mental Health: Grief/Loss

Answer: 1
Rationale: Nurses would explore measures that assist the family with creating memories of a stillborn infant so that the existence of the child is confirmed and the parents can complete the grieving process. The correct option identifies this measure and demonstrates a caring and empathetic response. Option 2 devalues the parents' feelings and is inappropriate. Option 3 is inappropriate and reflects a lack of knowledge on the nurse's part. Option 4 is uncaring.
Priority Nursing Tip: The loss of a child is traumatic for families. The most therapeutic initial intervention will focus on providing acknowledgment of their loss.

Test-Taking Strategy: Use **therapeutic communication techniques.** Choose the option that demonstrates a caring and empathetic nursing response and that meets the psychosocial needs of the client and family.

---

83. A primigravida client diagnosed with a urinary tract infection repeatedly verbalizes concern. The nurse determines that which statement made by the client is the **priority** concern?

1 "I'm worried that my infant will be born deaf."
2 "I cannot deal with the pain of this pregnancy."
3 "I'm so tired of having accidents because of this pregnancy."
4 "I know that I will need to drink more water and eat fewer veggies."

Level of Cognitive Ability: Analyzing
Client Needs: Psychosocial Integrity
Clinical Judgment/Cognitive Skills: Generate Solutions
Integrated Process: Nursing Process/Data Collection
Content Area: Maternity/Antepartum
Health Problem: Maternity: Infections/Inflammations

Answer: 1
Rationale: The primary concern for this client is fear for the safety of her fetus (rather than for her own safety). There is no information in the question to support options 2 and 3. Option 4 is true; however, it does not address issues regarding fetal safety.
Priority Nursing Tip: The uterus sits directly on top of the bladder. As the uterus grows, its increased weight can block the drainage of urine from the bladder, causing an infection.

Test-Taking Strategy: Note the **strategic word,** ***priority.*** Focus on the **subject,** the client's concerns, and the **data in the question.** There is no information in the question to support options 2, 3, and 4.

---

84. A pregnant client is diagnosed with sickle cell anemia. Which is the **most important** psychosocial intervention at this time to foster mental health wellness?

1 Providing her with all available information about the disease
2 Providing emotional support by encouraging her to talk about her concerns
3 Avoiding further stress to the client by not discussing the topic of the disease
4 Allowing the client to be alone if she is observed crying as a coping mechanism

Level of Cognitive Ability: Applying
Client Needs: Psychosocial Integrity
Clinical Judgment/Cognitive Skills: Take Action
Integrated Process: Nursing Process/Implementation
Content Area: Maternity: Antepartum
Health Problem: Mental Health: Coping

Answer: 2
Rationale: The most important psychosocial intervention is to provide emotional support to the client and family. Option 1 overwhelms the client with information while the client is trying to cope with the news of the disease. Option 3 is nontherapeutic. Option 4 is only appropriate if the client asks to be alone.
Priority Nursing Tip: Supportive therapy allows the client to express feelings, explore alternatives, and make decisions in a safe, caring environment.

Test-Taking Strategy: Focus on the **subject**, psychosocial intervention, and note the **strategic words**, *most important*. Eliminate options 1 and 3 because of the words *all* and *avoiding*, respectively. In addition, these actions are nontherapeutic. From the remaining options, remember that the client's feelings are the priority and that an important role of the nurse is to provide emotional support.

---

85. The nurse is assisting with the immediate postdelivery care of a newborn with a suspected diagnosis of erythroblastosis fetalis. The nurse makes which therapeutic statement to the parents at this time to address their **immediate** stress?

1 "Your newborn is very sick but is receiving excellent care."
2 "This is a common neonatal problem; you need not be overly concerned."
3 "There is no need to worry. We have the most updated equipment in this hospital."
4 "You must have many concerns. Please allow me to answer any questions you have."

Level of Cognitive Ability: Applying
Client Needs: Psychosocial Integrity
Clinical Judgment/Cognitive Skills: Take Action
Integrated Process: Communication and Documentation
Content Area: Maternity/Newborn
Health Problem: Newborn: Erythroblastosis Fetalis

Answer: 4
Rationale: Parental concern and anxiety are expected and are related to the care of the newborn with erythroblastosis fetalis. This anxiety results from a lack of knowledge about the disease process, treatment, and expected outcomes. Parents need to be encouraged to verbalize their concerns and to participate in care as appropriate. Their concerns will not be addressed by providing false assurance or by avoiding the concerns.
Priority Nursing Tip: Erythroblastosis fetalis is a type of hemolytic anemia that results from maternal–fetal blood group incompatibility involving the Rh factor and the ABO blood groups.

Test-Taking Strategy: Focus on the **subject**, providing parental support, and note the **strategic word** *immediate*. Eliminate options 2 and 3 because they are **comparable or alike** in that they both provide false assurance. In addition, they are blocks to communication. The wording in option 1 would frighten the parents. Remember to address clients' feelings and concerns.

---

86. A licensed practical nurse (LPN) is assisting a school nurse with weighing all the high school students. One of the teenagers who has type 1 diabetes mellitus has gained 15 pounds since last year with no gain in height. This teenager tells the nurse that she eats alone in the cafeteria at lunchtime and is very concerned about not looking attractive. Based on this data, the LPN would suggest what screening for the teenager?

1 Depression
2 Bulimia nervosa
3 An insulin deficiency
4 An alcohol abuse problem

Level of Cognitive Ability: Applying
Client Needs: Psychosocial Integrity
Clinical Judgment/Cognitive Skills: Generate Solutions
Integrated Process: Nursing Process/Planning
Content Area: Mental Health
Health Problem: Mental Health: Mood Disorder

Answer: 1
Rationale: Diabetic teenagers are at risk for depression and suicide, which is frequently manifested by changing insulin and eating patterns. Social isolation is another clue. Remember that weight loss is a symptom of type 1 diabetes and that an insulin deficiency would have the same effect. Bulimic clients may be of normal weight, but they control weight gain by purging. Alcohol abuse is more likely to be related to weight loss.
Priority Nursing Tip: Teenagers are at risk for a variety of psychosocial disorders, with depression being observed often among this age group.

Test-Taking Strategy: Focus on the **data in the question** and associate these data with the characteristics of each condition in the options. This will direct you to the correct option.

---

87. The nurse is conducting an information session with a class of high school students about the risk of sexually transmitted infections (STIs). What opening statement will **best** encourage participation within the group?

1 "Please feel free to share your personal experiences with the group."
2 "Anything shared with the group today will remain strictly confidential."
3 "At the end of the class, condoms will be distributed to everyone in the class."
4 "Our goal today is to describe ways to prevent acquiring an STI."

Level of Cognitive Ability: Applying
Client Needs: Safe and Effective Care Environment
Clinical Judgment/Cognitive Skills: Take Action
Integrated Process: Nursing Process/Implementation
Content Area: Leadership/Management: Ethical/Legal
Health Problem: Adult Health: Reproductive: Inflammatory/Infection Problems

Answer: 2
Rationale: The correct option states the rules for confidentiality, which will help the high school students develop trust when sharing sensitive issues with the group. Option 1 offers the opportunity to share personal experiences but with no promise of confidentiality. Option 3 may be an incentive for those attending to stay but implies that participation during the class is not required to get the reward. Option 4 is a good introduction to the topic but does not foster trust, especially among those who may already have an STI.
Priority Nursing Tip: Confidentiality is a client right and strictly adhered to by all health care providers.

Test-Taking Strategy: Focus on the **subject,** an opening statement to encourage participation, and note the **strategic word,** *best.* Think about confidentiality, trust building, and sharing. Eliminate option 4, which focuses on content, and option 1, which addresses format. From the remaining options, note that the correct option addresses the subject of confidentiality.

---

88. A client tells the nurse, "My doctor says I can have the breast biopsy and go home the same day, but I'm afraid. My husband's dead and my son lives so far away, so I'm alone. What happens if something goes wrong?" What response would the nurse provide to address the client's concern?

1 "Don't worry. This procedure is done all the time without any recovery problems."
2 "Is it possible for you to get an alarm system so that if you fall it will alert someone to come?"
3 "You seem very concerned about going home without help. Have you discussed your concerns with your doctor?"
4 "Your concern is well voiced. I advise you to call your son and request that he come home immediately. You can't be too careful."

Level of Cognitive Ability: Applying
Client Needs: Psychosocial Integrity
Clinical Judgment/Cognitive Skills: Take Action
Integrated Process: Communication and Documentation
Content Area: Mental Health
Health Problem: Mental Health: Coping

Answer: 3

Rationale: The response would address the client's concerns. In option 3, the correct option, the nurse uses reflection to direct the client's feelings and concerns. In option 1, the nurse provides false reassurance and minimizes the client's concerns. In option 2, the nurse is projecting the client's own fears, and the problem solving suggested by the nurse is histrionic and provokes fear and anxiety. In option 4, the nurse is trying to solve problems for the client but is overly controlling and takes the decision making out of the client's hands.

Priority Nursing Tip: A breast biopsy is an example of a same-day procedure. In most health care facilities, core biopsies can be performed and the pathology known the following day, providing the woman with rapid results.

Test-Taking Strategy: Use **therapeutic communication techniques** to address the **subject,** the client's concern about being discharged. Eliminate options 1, 2, and 4 because they are nontherapeutic and do not address the client's feelings. Remember that the priority is to address the client's feelings.

---

89. A pregnant client diagnosed with preeclampsia is admitted to the hospital. The nurse notes that the client continues to review work-related papers several hours a day between numerous visits from fellow students, family, and friends. Which nursing intervention would **initially** be implemented to ensure appropriate nursing care?

1 Developing a routine with the client to balance work and rest needs
2 Asking the client why she is not complying with the prescription of rest
3 Including a significant other in helping the client understand the need for rest
4 Instructing the client that the health of the baby is more important than work

Level of Cognitive Ability: Applying
Client Needs: Psychosocial Integrity
Clinical Judgment/Cognitive Skills: Take Action
Integrated Process: Nursing Process/Implementation
Content Area: Maternity: Antepartum
Health Problem: Maternity: Gestational Hypertension/Preeclampsia and Eclampsia

Answer: 1

Rationale: Rest is vital to the health of both client and child when dealing with the diagnosis of preeclampsia. The correct option involves the client in the decision making. In options 2 and 4, the nurse is judging the client's decisions and asking probing questions; this will cause a breakdown in communication. Option 3 persuades the client's significant others to disagree with the client's actions; this could cause problems with the client's self-esteem and also affect the nurse–client relationship.

Priority Nursing Tip: Preeclampsia is a condition in pregnancy characterized by high blood pressure and possibly proteinuria.

Test-Taking Strategy: Note the **strategic word,** ***initially.*** Use **therapeutic communication techniques** to address the problem. Eliminate options 2, 3, and 4 because these are blocks to communication. The correct option is therapeutic and the most thorough nursing action because it addresses rest and work and involves the client in the decision-making process.

---

90. A pregnant client is newly diagnosed with gestational diabetes. She is crying, and she keeps repeating, "What have I done to cause this? If I could only live my life over." The nurse identifies the client as experiencing what emotional conflict?

1 A risk for injury to the fetus related to maternal distress
2 A disturbance in body image related to complications of pregnancy
3 A disturbance in self-concept related to complications of pregnancy
4 A lack of understanding regarding diabetic self-care during pregnancy

Level of Cognitive Ability: Analyzing
Client Needs: Psychosocial Integrity
Clinical Judgment/Cognitive Skills: Analyze Cues
Integrated Process: Nursing Process/Data Collection
Content Area: Maternity: Antepartum
Health Problem: Maternity: Diabetes

Answer: 3
Rationale: The client is putting the blame for the diabetes on herself, thus lowering her self-concept or image. She is expressing fear and grief. There is no information in the question to support options 1, 2, and 4.
Priority Nursing Tip: Guilt is often assumed inappropriately, and the nurse can help relieve unwarranted negative emotions by providing appropriate education on the cause of the illness the client is experiencing.

Test-Taking Strategy: Use the **data in the question** and focus on the **subject,** the client's feelings of guilt. This will assist you with selecting the correct option.

---

91. A client says to the nurse, "I'm going to die, and I wish my family would stop hoping for a cure! I get so angry when they carry on like this! After all, I'm the one who's dying." The nurse would make which therapeutic response to the client to further discuss the client's comment?

1 "Have you shared your feelings with your family?"
2 "Well, it sounds as if you're being pretty pessimistic."
3 "I think we need to talk more about your anger with your family."
4 "You're feeling angry that your family continues to hope for you to be cured?"

Level of Cognitive Ability: Applying
Client Needs: Psychosocial Integrity
Clinical Judgment/Cognitive Skills: Take Action
Integrated Process: Communication and Documentation
Content Area: Mental Health
Health Problem: Mental Health: Therapeutic Communication

Answer: 4
Rationale: The nurse's initial intervention is to fully understand the client's feelings. Reflection is the therapeutic communication technique that redirects the client's feelings back to validate what the client is saying. In option 1, the nurse is attempting to assess the client's ability to openly discuss feelings with family members. In option 2, the nurse makes a judgment and is nontherapeutic. In option 3, the nurse attempts to use focusing, but the attempt addresses a premature statement.
Priority Nursing Tip: Therapeutic communication is defined as the face-to-face process of interacting that focuses on advancing the physical and emotional well-being of a client.

Test-Taking Strategy: Use **therapeutic communication techniques** to eliminate options 1, 2, and 3. The correct option is the only one that address a therapeutic communication technique and that redirects the client's feelings back to validate what the client is saying.

---

92. The nurse is caring for an older adult client who says, "I don't want to talk with you. You're only the nurse. I'll wait for my doctor." Which nursing response is therapeutic in this situation?

1 "I'll leave you now and call your doctor."
2 "Are you saying that you need to talk to your doctor?"
3 "I'm assigned to work with you. Your doctor placed you in my hands."
4 "I'm angry with the way you've dismissed me. I am your nurse, not your servant."

Level of Cognitive Ability: Applying
Client Needs: Psychosocial Integrity
Clinical Judgment/Cognitive Skills: Take Action
Integrated Process: Communication and Documentation
Content Area: Foundations of Care: Communication
Health Problem: Mental Health: Therapeutic Communication

Answer: 2
Rationale: The nurse's initial intervention is to fully understand the client's feelings. In the correct option, the nurse uses the therapeutic communication of reflection to redirect the client's feelings back for validation. Note that the nurse does not reflect a negative option but instead focuses on the client's desire to talk with the primary health care provider. Options 1, 3, and 4 are nontherapeutic. Remember that the nurse places the client's well-being first and foremost while engaged in nursing care.
Priority Nursing Tip: Validation as a therapeutic communication technique between nurse and client is an effective technique to encourage clients to discuss their feelings, concerns, and needs.

Test-Taking Strategy: Focus on the **subject,** therapeutic communication for clients who are using defensive statements to drive others away. Use **therapeutic communication techniques.** You can easily eliminate options 3 and 4 because these are nontherapeutic responses. Option 1 is a social response and intervention that reinforces the continuation of this behavior.

---

93. A client and their newborn infant have undergone human immunodeficiency virus (HIV) testing, and the test results for both clients are positive. The news is devastating, and the client is crying. The nurse demonstrates an understanding of client support by implementing what intervention **immediately**?

1 Leaving the client to grieve privately
2 Listening quietly while the client talks and cries
3 Describing the progressive stages and treatments of HIV to the client
4 Calling an HIV counselor to make an appointment for the client and baby

Level of Cognitive Ability: Applying
Client Needs: Psychosocial Integrity
Clinical Judgment/Cognitive Skills: Take Action
Integrated Process: Nursing Process/Implementation
Content Area: Maternity/Postpartum
Health Problem: Mental Health: Therapeutic Communication

Answer: 2
Rationale: This client has just received devastating news and needs to have someone present with them as they begin to cope with this issue. The nurse needs to sit and actively listen while the client talks and cries to best encourage the expression of maternal feelings and needs. Calling an HIV counselor may be helpful but is not what the client needs at this time. The other options are inappropriate for this stage of coping with the news that both the client and the infant are HIV positive.
Priority Nursing Tip: The therapeutic use of silence allows clients to determine the flow of the conversation.

Test-Taking Strategy: Noting the **strategic word,** *immediately,* and focusing on the **subject,** supporting the client, will assist you with eliminating options 3 and 4. From the remaining options, remember to address the client's feelings and to support the client.

---

94. The nurse employed in a home-care agency is assigned to provide care to a recently widowed man who is estranged from his only son. When the nurse arrives at the client's home, the ordinarily immaculate house is in chaos, and the client is disheveled, with alcohol on his breath. Which statement by the nurse is **effective** in addressing the client's current situation?

1 "This probably isn't a good time to visit."
2 "You seem to be having a very troubling time."
3 "How much have you been drinking and for how long?"
4 "Do you think your wife would want you to behave like this?"

Level of Cognitive Ability: Applying
Client Needs: Psychosocial Integrity
Clinical Judgment/Cognitive Skills: Take Action
Integrated Process: Communication and Documentation
Content Area: Mental Health
Health Problem: Mental Health: Therapeutic Communication

Answer: 2
Rationale: The nurse's initial intervention is to fully understand the client's feelings. The therapeutic statement is the one that helps the client explore his situation and express his feelings. Option 2 identifies the use of reflection and will assist the client with beginning to express his feelings. As this happens, the nurse can assist the client with discussing the reasons behind his alienation from his only child. In option 1, the nurse uses humor to avoid therapeutic intimacy and effective problem solving. In option 3, the nurse uses admonishment and tries to shame the client, which is nontherapeutic; this belittles the client, causes anger, and may evoke acting out by the client. In option 4, the nurse uses social communication.
Priority Nursing Tip: Therapeutic communication is supported best when the communication is focused on the client's feelings and based on the observations of potentially unhealthy behaviors.

Test-Taking Strategy: Note the **strategic word,** *effective.* Use **therapeutic communication techniques**. Option 2 is the only option that addresses the client's feelings.

---

95. A client says to the nurse, "I don't do anything right. I'm such a loser." To encourage further discussion, the nurse would make which statement?

1 "Everything will get better."
2 "You are not a loser; you are sick."
3 "You don't think you do anything right?"
4 "I'm sure you do things right some of the time."

Level of Cognitive Ability: Applying
Client Needs: Psychosocial Integrity
Clinical Judgment/Cognitive Skills: Take Action
Integrated Process: Communication and Documentation
Content Area: Mental Health
Health Problem: Mental Health: Therapeutic Communication

Answer: 3
Rationale: The nurse's initial intervention is to fully understand the client's feelings. The correct option encourages the client to verbalize feelings. With this question, the nurse can learn more about what the client really means. This option repeats the client's statement and allows the communication to stay open. The remaining options are closed statements and do not encourage the client to further explore feelings.
Priority Nursing Tip: Therapeutic communication includes the use of restatement of the client's verbal statements.

Test-Taking Strategy: Use **therapeutic communication techniques.** The correct option is the only one that restates and identifies a therapeutic response and that allows the client to verbalize feelings.

---

96. A client who is experiencing suicidal thoughts says to the nurse, "It just doesn't seem worth it anymore. Why not just end it all?" The nurse would gather data from the client by using which response?

1 "Did you sleep at all last night?"
2 "Tell me what you mean by that."
3 "I know you have had a stressful night."
4 "I'm sure your family is worried about you."

Level of Cognitive Ability: Applying
Client Needs: Psychosocial Integrity
Clinical Judgment/Cognitive Skills: Analyze Cues
Integrated Process: Communication and Documentation
Content Area: Mental Health
Health Problem: Mental Health: Suicide

Answer: 2

Rationale: The nurse's initial intervention is to fully understand the client's feelings. The correct option encourages the client to tell the nurse more about his or her current thoughts. Options 1 and 3 change the subject and block communication. Option 4 is false reassurance and may also block communication.

Priority Nursing Tip: Any statement that suggests suicidal ideations must be clarified and discussed with the client in order to ensure his or her safety.

Test-Taking Strategy: Use **therapeutic communication techniques.** Options 3 and 4 can be eliminated because they do not reflect data collection. Although option 1 is involved in data collection, the data are not directed to the focus of the **subject**, suicide. The correct option is directly related to the subject.

---

97. A parent confides to the nurse, "I am afraid that my child may have another febrile seizure." What response by the nurse addresses the parent's concerns **best**?

1 "Tell me what frightens you the most about seizures."
2 "Don't worry about something that you cannot control."
3 "Most children will never experience a second seizure."
4 "Acetaminophen can prevent another seizure from occurring."

Level of Cognitive Ability: Applying
Client Needs: Psychosocial Integrity
Clinical Judgment/Cognitive Skills: Take Action
Integrated Process: Communication and Documentation
Content Area: Foundations of Care: Communication
Health Problem: Pediatric-Specific: Seizures

Answer: 1

Rationale: The nurse's initial intervention is to fully understand the client's feelings. The correct option is the one response that is an open-ended statement and that provides the parent with an opportunity to express her feelings. Option 2 is incorrect because it blocks communication by giving a flippant response to an expressed fear. Options 3 and 4 are incorrect because the nurse is giving false assurance that a seizure will not recur or that it can be prevented in this woman's child.

Priority Nursing Tip: A febrile seizure is associated with a high body temperature but without any serious underlying health issue. Febrile seizures most commonly occur in children between the ages of 6 months and 5 years.

Test-Taking Strategy: Note the **strategic word,** *best.* Use **therapeutic communication techniques** to determine which option encourages the client to express her feelings. Options 2, 3, and 4 are nontherapeutic and block communication. Option 1 focuses on feelings and concerns.

---

98. A client has just given birth to a baby who has a cleft lip and palate. Which nursing intervention will address the **most immediate** parent–child need?

1 Arranging for a family counseling consult to address family concerns
2 Assuring the client that the disfigurements can be surgically corrected
3 Supporting bonding by encouraging rooming-in rather than the nursery for the baby
4 Assisting the client in learning to meet the child's long-term unique feeding needs

Answer: 3

Rationale: Often, the client who has given birth to a child with a facial disfigurement will stress the parent–child relationship. The parent–child bonding process can be affected negatively. The correct option helps support parent–child bonding. The remaining options are interventions that can be addressed after bonding issues are considered.

Priority Nursing Tip: The birth of a child with physical anomalies represents a loss of the perfect child to the parent(s) and will be mourned as would any loss.

Test-Taking Strategy: Focus on the **subject,** parent–child need. Note the **strategic words,** *most immediate.* The correct option deals with the immediate need for effective bonding. The remaining options are issues that can be addressed later.

Level of Cognitive Ability: Applying
Client Needs: Psychosocial Integrity
Clinical Judgment/Cognitive Skills: Take Action
Integrated Process: Nursing Process/Implementation
Content Area: Maternity/Postpartum
Health Problem: Mental Health: Coping

---

99. A client scheduled for cardiac stress testing initially expresses a fear that his or her heart will "give out" during the procedure. Which current client behavior **requires further follow-up**?

1 The client verbally expresses fear about his or her own mortality.
2 The client appears distracted when the procedure is discussed.
3 The client asks numerous, detailed questions about the stress test.
4 The client expresses frustration that the test needs to be performed.

Answer: 2

Rationale: Demonstrating disinterest in discussing the procedure indicates possible denial on the part of the client. Expressions of fear, anxiety, and frustration are examples of expected client behaviors.

Priority Nursing Tip: A cardiac stress test may require medication changes before the test. For example, the cardiologist may prescribe that the client stop taking prescribed beta blockers for 48 hours and calcium channel blockers for 24 hours before the test.

Test-Taking Strategy: Note the **strategic words,** *requires further follow-up.* These words indicate a **negative event query** and the need to select the client behavior that identifies a concern. Options 1, 3, and 4 contain evidence of communication on the client's part. Not talking indicates a barrier and would require additional interventions.

Level of Cognitive Ability: Analyzing
Client Needs: Psychosocial Integrity
Clinical Judgment/Cognitive Skills: Analyze Cues
Integrated Process: Nursing Process/Data Collection
Content Area: Adult Health: Cardiovascular
Health Problem: Mental Health: Coping

---

100. After the vaginal delivery of a large-for-gestational-age (LGA) male infant, the nurse wraps the infant in a warm blanket and hands the newborn to the parent. The parent demonstrates reluctance to touch the baby and verbalizes concern about the infant's facial bruising. To enhance parental–infant attachment, how would the nurse respond?

1 "Bruising is common in large babies and nothing to be concerned about."
2 "The bruising is temporary, and it is important to interact with your infant."
3 "The bruising is caused by polycythemia, which usually leads to jaundice."
4 "The bruising on your baby's face seems to be causing you some concern."

Level of Cognitive Ability: Applying
Client Needs: Psychosocial Integrity
Clinical Judgment/Cognitive Skills: Take Action
Integrated Process: Nursing Process/Implementation
Content Area: Maternity/Postpartum
Health Problem: Mental Health: Coping

Answer: 4

Rationale: The parent of an LGA infant with facial bruising may be reluctant to interact with the infant because of concern surrounding birth-related bruising. The nurse's initial intervention is to fully understand the client's feelings. Acknowledging the concern is the priority action. The concern would not be minimized with false assurances. The remaining options may contain factual information but fail to address the parent's concerns.

Priority Nursing Tip: LGA is often defined as a weight, length, or head circumference that lies above the 90th percentile for that gestational age.

Test-Taking Strategy: Focus on the **data in the question** and the need to enhance bonding. Use **therapeutic communication techniques** to lead you to the correct option, which addresses the parent's concerns.

---

101. A client diagnosed with myasthenia gravis confides that she is concerned that her husband will no longer find her physically attractive. The nurse would plan to encourage what intervention **initially**?

1 Tell the client to not dwell on the negative.
2 Encourage the client to start a support group.
3 Insist that the client reach out and face this diagnosis.
4 Encourage the client to share her feelings with her husband.

Level of Cognitive Ability: Applying
Client Needs: Psychosocial Integrity
Clinical Judgment/Cognitive Skills: Generate Solutions
Integrated Process: Nursing Process/Planning
Content Area: Adult Health: Neurological
Health Problem: Mental Health: Coping

Answer: 4

Rationale: Encouraging the client to share her feelings with her husband directly addresses the client's concern. Encouraging the client to start a support group will not address the client's immediate and individual concern. Options 1 and 3 are blocks to communication and avoid the client's concern.

Priority Nursing Tip: Myasthenia gravis is caused by a breakdown in the normal communication between nerves and muscles. More specifically, there is a defect in the action of acetylcholine at neuromuscular junctions.

Test-Taking Strategy: Focus on the **subject,** concern related to attractiveness, and note the **strategic word,** *initially*. The correct option is the only one that addresses the client's immediate concern. Remember to address the client's feelings first.

---

102. A 9-year-old child is hospitalized long-term in traction after a car accident. What intervention **best** promotes the psychosocial development of this child?

1 Access to a telephone to call family and friends
2 Encouraging the use of an iPod with headphones
3 Providing computer games, television, and videos at the bedside
4 Arranging for tutoring to keep the child up-to-date with schoolwork

Level of Cognitive Ability: Applying
Client Needs: Psychosocial Integrity
Clinical Judgment/Cognitive Skills: Take Action
Integrated Process: Nursing Process/Implementation
Content Area: Developmental Stages: Preschool and School Age
Health Problem: Pediatric-Specific: Fractures

Answer: 4
Rationale: The developmental task of the school-age child is industry versus inferiority. The child achieves success by mastering skills and knowledge. Maintaining schoolwork provides for accomplishment and prevents feelings of inferiority that may result from lagging behind the class. The other options provide diversion and are of lesser importance for a child of this age.
Priority Nursing Tip: Industry versus inferiority is the fourth stage of Erik Erikson's theory of psychosocial development. Children are at the stage where they will be learning to read and write, to do sums, and to do things on their own.

Test-Taking Strategy: Note the **strategic word,** *best,* and note the age of the child. Options 1, 2, and 3 are **comparable or alike** in that they address social and diversional issues. Option 4 best addresses the psychosocial development.

---

103. A client who is in halo traction says to the nurse, "I can't get used to this contraption. I can't see properly on the side, and I keep misjudging where everything is." How would the nurse respond?

1 "Few people ever get used to that thing."
2 "If I were you, I would consider the surgery."
3 "Practice scanning with your eyes after standing up and before you move."
4 "Your peripheral vision will soon adapt to the restrictions caused by the halo."

Level of Cognitive Ability: Applying
Client Needs: Psychosocial Integrity
Clinical Judgment/Cognitive Skills: Take Action
Integrated Process: Communication and Documentation
Content Area: Adult Health: Neurological
Health Problem: Adult Health: Neurological: Spinal Cord Injury

Answer: 3
Rationale: The response the nurse provides in the correct option offers a problem-solving strategy that helps increase the client's peripheral vision. In option 1, the nurse provides a social response that contains emotionally charged language and that could increase the client's anxiety. In option 2, the nurse undermines the client's faith in the medical treatment being used by giving advice that is insensitive and unprofessional. Option 4 is inaccurate information.
Priority Nursing Tip: The halo is a ring that surrounds the head and is attached by pins to the outer portion of the skull. It is used to stabilize the cervical spine or to correct its alignment.

Test-Taking Strategy: Focus on the **data in the question.** Use **therapeutic communication techniques,** and note that the correct option relates to the data.

104. An older adult client was admitted to the acute care facility with a hip fracture. Which client statement supports a psychologically adaptive response to the situation?

1 "Hurry up and go away. I want to be alone."
2 "What took you so long? I called for you 30 minutes ago."
3 "I wish you nurses would leave me alone! You're always telling me what to do!"
4 "It's so hard to concentrate since the doctor talked with me about the surgery tomorrow."

Level of Cognitive Ability: Evaluating
Client Needs: Psychosocial Integrity
Clinical Judgment/Cognitive Skills: Evaluate Outcomes
Integrated Process: Nursing Process/Evaluation
Content Area: Adult Health: Musculoskeletal
Health Problem: Mental Health: Coping

Answer: 4
Rationale: Stress is likely to bring about anxiety. The correct option is reflective of a person with moderate anxiety and supports a psychologically adaptive response to the situation. Option 1 demonstrates withdrawal behavior. Option 2 is a demanding response. Option 3 demonstrates acting out by the client. Demanding, acting-out, and withdrawn clients have not coped with or adjusted to injury or disease.
Priority Nursing Tip: Anxiety can cause alterations in a person's cognitive abilities.

Test-Taking Strategy: Focus on the **subject,** a psychologically adaptive response. Remember that age, limited mobility, and medications often contribute to anxiety and confusion; this would direct you to the correct option. Also note that options 1, 2, and 3 are **comparable or alike** and identify negative behaviors.

---

105. What is the **most effective** way for the nurse to help the parents of a preterm newborn develop appropriate attachment behaviors?

1 Placing family pictures in the infant's view
2 Encouraging the parents to touch and speak to their infant often
3 Reporting only the infant's positive qualities and progress to the parents
4 Providing information about infant development and stimulation guidelines

Level of Cognitive Ability: Applying
Client Needs: Psychosocial Integrity
Clinical Judgment/Cognitive Skills: Take Action
Integrated Process: Nursing Process/Implementation
Content Area: Maternity/Postpartum
Health Problem: Newborn: Preterm and Postterm Newborn

Answer: 2
Rationale: The parents' involvement through touch and voice establishes and initiates the attachment process in the relationship. Their active participation builds confidence and supports the parenting role. Family pictures are ineffective for an infant with limited distance vision. Providing information and emphasizing only positives do not relate to the attachment process, nor are these actions helpful.
Priority Nursing Tip: A preterm birth is a birth that takes place more than 3 weeks before the baby's estimated due date.

Test-Taking Strategy: Note the **strategic words,** *most effective.* Focusing on the **subject,** attachment behaviors, will assist in directing you to the correct option. Also note that the incorrect options are not directly associated with attachment.

---

106. A client angrily tells the nurse that the doctor purposefully provided wrong information. Which nursing responses encourage therapeutic communication? **Select all that apply.**

❒ 1 "I'm certain the doctor would not lie to you."
❒ 2 "I'm not sure what information you are referring to."
❒ 3 "Are you comfortable talking to your doctor about this?"
❒ 4 "Can you describe the information that you are talking about?"
❒ 5 "I think you will feel differently when you have time to think about this."

Level of Cognitive Ability: Applying
Client Needs: Psychosocial Integrity
Clinical Judgment/Cognitive Skills: Take Action
Integrated Process: Communication and Documentation
Content Area: Foundations of Care: Communication
Health Problem: Mental Health: Therapeutic Communication

Answer: 2, 3, 4
Rationale: Therapeutic communication addresses client concerns, seeks clarification, acknowledges feelings, or encourages open and direct communication. Options 1 and 5 hinder communication by disagreeing with the client; this technique could make the client defensive and block further communication. Options 2 and 4 attempt to clarify what the client is referring to. Option 3 attempts to explore whether the client is comfortable talking to the doctor about this issue and encourages direct confrontation.
Priority Nursing Tip: The goals of therapeutic communication are to help a client feel cared for and understood and to establish a relationship in which the client feels free to express any concerns.

Test-Taking Strategy: Focus on the **subject,** responses that encourage therapeutic communication. Using **therapeutic communication techniques** will direct you to the correct options.

---

107. A client diagnosed with major depression says to the nurse, "I ought to have died. I've always been a failure." What response by the nurse would be **most appropriate** to support the needed discussion?

1 "I see a lot of positive things in you."
2 "Don't you still have a great deal to live for?"
3 "Feeling like a failure is part of your illness."
4 "You've been feeling like a failure for some time now?"

Level of Cognitive Ability: Applying
Client Needs: Psychosocial Integrity
Clinical Judgment/Cognitive Skills: Take Action
Integrated Process: Communication and Documentation
Content Area: Mental Health
Health Problem: Mental Health: Mood Disorders

Answer: 4
Rationale: The nurse must initially explore the meaning and the feelings associated with the client's statement. The correct option demonstrates an attempt to respond to the feelings expressed by a client, which is an effective therapeutic communication technique called *restating*. The remaining options block communication because they minimize the client's experience and do not facilitate the exploration of the client's expressed feelings.
Priority Nursing Tip: Depression can be a result of an individual's poor sense of self-esteem.

Test-Taking Strategy: Note the **strategic words,** *most appropriate.* Use **therapeutic communication techniques.** Select the option that directly addresses client feelings and concerns. The correct option is the only one that is stated in the form of an open-ended question that will encourage the verbalization of feelings.

---

108. Two months after a right mastectomy for breast cancer, a client comes to the primary health care provider's office for a scheduled follow-up. Which primary prevention measure would the nurse implement at this time?

1 Teach breast self-examination (BSE) to the client.
2 Assist the client in choosing an appropriate supportive bra.
3 Educate the client regarding chemotherapy and radiation.
4 Reinforce teaching regarding reconstructive breast therapy.

Level of Cognitive Ability: Applying
Client Needs: Psychosocial Integrity
Clinical Judgment/Cognitive Skills: Take Action
Integrated Process: Nursing Process/Implementation
Content Area: Adult Health: Oncology
Health Problem: Adult Health: Cancer: Breast

Answer: 1
Rationale: Primary prevention measures are those that assist in preventing the illness or future events. Breast self-care measures such as the BSE need to be taught. Options 2, 3, and 4 are not primary prevention measures.
Priority Nursing Tip: The loss of a breast can be extremely impactful to a woman's sense of self-esteem. Primary prevention education assists the client in gaining control and evaluating future issues.

Test-Taking Strategy: Focus on the **subject,** primary prevention measures associated with breast cancer. Recall that primary prevention measures are those that assist in preventing the illness or future events. Thus, eliminate options 2, 3, and 4 because they are not primary prevention measures.

---

109. When planning the care of a client diagnosed with terminal cancer, one of the goals is for the client to verbalize acceptance of impending death. Which client statement indicates that this goal is met?

1 "I'd like to have my family here when I die."
2 "It would be easier to die if I'd had an unhappy life."
3 "I just want to live until I've accomplished my life goals."
4 "I want to go to my daughter's wedding. Then I'll be ready to die."

Level of Cognitive Ability: Evaluating
Client Needs: Psychosocial Integrity
Clinical Judgment/Cognitive Skills: Evaluate Outcomes
Integrated Process: Nursing Process/Evaluation
Content Area: Adult Health: Oncology
Health Problem: Mental Health: Grief and Loss

Answer: 1
Rationale: Acceptance of impending death is characterized by peaceful plans; often the client wants loved ones near. None of the other options demonstrates acceptance.
Priority Nursing Tip: The Kübler-Ross model, or the five stages of grief, postulates a series of emotions experienced by terminally ill clients before death, or people who have lost a loved one, wherein the five stages are denial, anger, bargaining, depression, and acceptance.

Test-Taking Strategy: Focus on the **subject,** acceptance of impending death. Note that options 2, 3, and 4 are **comparable or alike** in that they all demonstrate negotiating for something else to happen before death occurs. Only the correct option reflects acceptance.

---

110. Which intervention would the nurse implement for the client with breast cancer who has a body image disturbance related to chemotherapy-induced alopecia?

1 Educating the client that wigs are often paid for by health insurance
2 Teaching the client the importance of rinsing the mouth after eating
3 Suggesting that the client use cosmetics to hide medication-induced rashes
4 Teaching the client proper dental hygiene with the use of a foam toothbrush

Level of Cognitive Ability: Applying
Client Needs: Psychosocial Integrity
Clinical Judgment/Cognitive Skills: Take Action
Integrated Process: Nursing Process/Implementation
Content Area: Adult Health: Oncology
Health Problem: Adult Health: Cancer: Breast

Answer: 1
Rationale: The temporary or permanent thinning or loss of hair known as *alopecia* is common among oncology clients receiving chemotherapy. This often causes a body image disturbance that can be addressed with the use of wigs, hats, or scarves. Options 2, 3, and 4 are unrelated to alopecia.
Priority Nursing Tip: Self-perception of appearance has a great impact on an individual's ability to recover from any physical loss.

Test-Taking Strategy: Focus on the **subject,** alopecia. Remember that alopecia means loss of hair. Eliminate options 2, 3, and 4 because they are **comparable or alike** in that they are addressing a subject other than alopecia.

---

111. A client diagnosed with hyperparathyroidism says to the nurse, "I can't stay on this diet. It is too difficult for me." How would the nurse respond to facilitate a discussion about the client's concerns?

1 "Most people do find this diet plan difficult to adhere to."
2 "It really isn't difficult to stick to this diet. Just avoid milk products."
3 "You are having a difficult time staying on this plan. Let's discuss this."
4 "It is very important that you stay on this diet to avoid forming renal calculi."

Level of Cognitive Ability: Applying
Client Needs: Psychosocial Integrity
Clinical Judgment/Cognitive Skills: Take Action
Integrated Process: Communication and Documentation
Content Area: Foundations of Care: Therapeutic Communication
Health Problem: Adult Health: Endocrine: Parathyroid Disorders

Answer: 3
Rationale: The nurse must initially explore the meaning and the feelings associated with the client's statement. By paraphrasing the client's statement, the nurse can encourage the client to express feelings. The nurse also sends feedback to the client that the message was understood. Option 1 agrees with the client but offers no support. Option 2 is giving advice, which blocks communication. Option 4 devalues the client's feelings.
Priority Nursing Tip: Paraphrasing is a communication technique that allows for both clarification and broader discussion of a client's concerns.

Test-Taking Strategy: Focus on the **subject,** the client's concerns. Use **therapeutic communication techniques.** The correct option is the only one that supports further discussion, allowing the nurse to address the client's feelings.

---

112. The nurse is caring for a client who recently had a bilateral adrenalectomy. Which goal will the nurse include in the client's plan of care to meet the expected needs of the client?

1 Preventing social isolation
2 Managing stressful situations
3 Receiving occupational therapy
4 Accepting changes in body image

Level of Cognitive Ability: Applying
Client Needs: Psychosocial Integrity
Clinical Judgment/Cognitive Skills: Generate Solutions
Integrated Process: Nursing Process/Planning
Content Area: Adult Health: Endocrine
Health Problem: Adult Health: Endocrine: Adrenal Disorders

Answer: 2
Rationale: Adrenalectomy can lead to adrenal insufficiency. Adrenal hormones are essential for maintaining homeostasis in response to stressors. Options 1, 3, and 4 are not directly related to the client's diagnosis.
Priority Nursing Tip: Laparoscopic adrenalectomy for symptomatic Cushing's disease may be a treatment option for some clients.

Test-Taking Strategy: Focus on the **data in the question,** noting the client's diagnosis. Recalling that an adrenalectomy can lead to adrenal insufficiency and recalling the relationship of an adrenalectomy to the stress response will direct you to the correct option.

---

113. Which statement made by a client diagnosed with anorexia nervosa indicates that treatment has been **effective**?

1 "I'll eat until I don't feel hungry."
2 "I no longer have a weight problem."
3 "I don't want to starve myself anymore."
4 "My friends and I went out and ate lunch today."

Level of Cognitive Ability: Evaluating
Client Needs: Psychosocial Integrity
Clinical Judgment/Cognitive Skills: Evaluate Outcomes
Integrated Process: Nursing Process/Evaluation
Content Area: Mental Health
Health Problem: Mental Health: Eating Disorders

Answer: 4
Rationale: Anorexia nervosa is usually seen in adolescent girls who try to establish identity and control by self-imposed starvation. Options 1, 2, and 3 are verbalizations of the client's intentions. The correct option is a measurable action that can be verified.
Priority Nursing Tip: The exact causes of anorexia nervosa are unknown.

Test-Taking Strategy: Focus on the **subject,** anorexia nervosa, and note the **strategic word,** *effective.* Understanding of the disease process will help you in selecting the option that is measurable and that can be verified.

---

114. The nurse is reinforcing home-care instructions to a client diagnosed with heart failure. The client interrupts by saying, "What's the use? I'll never remember all of this, and I'll probably die anyway!" The nurse makes which interpretation about the client's response?

1 Anger about the new medical regimen
2 Concern over the teaching strategies used by the nurse
3 Insufficient financial resources to pay for the medications
4 Anxiety and the fear of an uncertain death continue to persist

Answer: 4
Rationale: Anxiety often develops after heart failure as the fear of death persists, and there is often a long and difficult period of adjustment. The client's statement does not appear to be associated with issues identified by options 1, 2, and 3.
Priority Nursing Tip: Anxiety and fear can place strain on a failing heart.

Level of Cognitive Ability: Analyzing
Client Needs: Psychosocial Integrity
Clinical Judgment/Cognitive Skills: Analyze Cues
Integrated Process: Nursing Process/Data Collection
Content Area: Adult Health: Cardiovascular
Health Problem: Mental Health: Coping

Test-Taking Strategy: Focus on the **data in the question.** Note the relationship between the client's statement and option 4. There is no evidence in the question to support options 1, 2, or 3.

---

115. A client who is to be discharged with a temporary colostomy tells the nurse, "I'm still uncomfortable caring for this bag." The client asks, "Can't I stay here until the doctor puts things back the way they were?" What response would the nurse provide to address the client's concerns?

1 "Because this is only temporary, you could hire a nurse companion until your reversal surgery is scheduled."
2 "So you're saying that you don't feel comfortable on your own yet even though you've practiced changing your colostomy?"
3 "Well, I doubt your insurance will pay for extended hospitalization just so you can get comfortable with caring for the colostomy, but we can ask."
4 "So going home still feels pretty overwhelming. Would you like me to arrange for home health nursing assistance until you're feeling more comfortable?"

Level of Cognitive Ability: Applying
Client Needs: Psychosocial Integrity
Clinical Judgment/Cognitive Skills: Take Action
Integrated Process: Communication and Documentation
Content Area: Foundations of Care: Communication
Health Problem: Mental Health: Therapeutic Communication

Answer: 4
Rationale: The client is expressing feelings of helplessness and abandonment. The correct option assists with meeting these needs by acknowledging the concern and suggesting a possible solution. Option 1 provides a solution that would probably overwhelm the client. Option 2 restates but focuses on the subject, helplessness, without addressing the expressed concern. Option 3 provides what is probably accurate information but the words *just to* can be interpreted by the client as belittling.
Priority Nursing Tip: Reversing a loop colostomy involves a cut (incision) being made around the stoma so that the surgeon can access the inside of the abdomen. The upper section of the colon is then reattached to the remaining section of the colon.

Test-Taking Strategy: Focus on the **subject,** fear and dependency. Eliminate options 1 and 3 first because they are impractical solutions. From the remaining options, look for the one that addresses the client's feelings and concerns. Option 2 involves restating but focuses on the subject of helplessness. The correct option addresses both fear and dependency needs.

---

116. A client diagnosed with schizophrenia is demonstrating mutism. What response would the nurse provide when the family wants diagnostic tests done to determine the cause of the speechlessness?

1 "The client can control this and will begin to speak when ready to do so."
2 "The client will speak again when there is a strong enough need to do so."
3 "This is a common problem with schizophrenia; it will resolve in a few days."
4 "The problem does not stem from a physiological problem with the organs of communication."

Level of Cognitive Ability: Applying
Client Needs: Psychosocial Integrity
Clinical Judgment/Cognitive Skills: Take Action
Integrated Process: Nursing Process/ Implementation
Content Area: Mental Health
Health Problem: Mental Health: Schizophrenia

Answer: 4

Rationale: Mutism is the absence of verbal speech. The client diagnosed with schizophrenia does not communicate verbally despite an intact physical structural ability to speak, but rather for reasons rooted in the mental condition. The mutism may resolve on its own, persist for long periods, or may be permanent. The condition is not one the client can necessarily control.

Priority Nursing Tip: A trauma may produce such overwhelming stress that the individual becomes mute. Assist the client to use alternative means to express feelings, such as through music, art therapy, or writing.

Test-Taking Strategy: Focus on the **subject,** the inability to speak. Use knowledge of mutism and of its relationship to schizophrenia to assist in directing you to the correct option.

---

117. A client diagnosed with schizophrenia exhibits clang associations. The nurse recognizes this distorted speech behavior when the client makes which statement?

1 "You asked about my home. I've gone to the laundromat."
2 "Polly wants a cracker. Polly wants a cracker. Polly wants a cracker."
3 "I am a spy for the FBI. I am an eye, an eye in the sky. The sky is like a big lie."
4 "Yes, I have been a very bad boy. I've been mentally abusing my neighbor's boy."

Level of Cognitive Ability: Analyzing
Client Needs: Psychosocial Integrity
Clinical Judgment/Cognitive Skills: Analyze Cues
Integrated Process: Nursing Process/Data Collection
Content Area: Mental Health
Health Problem: Mental Health: Schizophrenia

Answer: 3

Rationale: Clang associations often take the form of rhyming. Echolalia is an involuntary parrot-like repetition of words spoken by others. Tangential speech is characterized by a tendency to digress from an original topic of discussion using a common word that connects two unrelated thoughts. Loosened associations are a sign of disordered thought processes in which the person speaks with frequent changes of subject; the content is related only obliquely (if at all) to the subject matter.

Priority Nursing Tip: Repetition of words or phrases that are similar in sound and in no other way (rhyming) is one of the patterns of altered thought and language noted in clients with schizophrenia.

Test-Taking Strategy: Focus on the **subject,** clang speech and associations. Think about the description of this type of speech. Recalling that rhyming occurs in clang associations will direct you to the correct option.

118. The nurse is assisting with planning the hospital discharge of an adolescent who has been newly diagnosed with type 1 diabetes mellitus. The client expresses concern to the nurse about self-administering insulin while in school with other students around. Which statement by the nurse supports the client's need at this time?

1 "Oh, don't worry about that! We'll figure something out."
2 "You could leave school early and take your insulin at home."
3 "The school nurse could provide a private area for you to take your insulin."
4 "There is no need to be embarrassed by your diabetes. Lots of people have this disease."

Level of Cognitive Ability: Applying
Client Needs: Psychosocial Integrity
Clinical Judgment/Cognitive Skills: Take Action
Integrated Process: Communication and Documentation
Content Area: Developmental Stages: Adolescent
Health Problem: Pediatric-Specific: Diabetes Mellitus

Answer: 3
Rationale: In the therapeutic caring relationship, the nurse offers information that will promote or assist the client to reach a decision that optimizes a sense of well-being, such as in the correct option. Option 2 requires a change in lifestyle. Options 1 and 4 are inappropriate statements and blocks to communication.
Priority Nursing Tip: If a child is age 10 years or older, he or she may be able to give insulin with supervision.

Test-Taking Strategy: Focus on the **subject,** concern about self-administering insulin while in school. Eliminate options 1 and 4 because they are nontherapeutic responses and nonsupportive to the client. Select option 3 because it promotes the client's ability to stay at school, whereas option 2 requires a change in school attendance hours.

---

119. A client who was admitted to the hospital for recurrent thyroid storm is preparing for discharge. The client is anxious about the illness and at times emotionally labile. Which approach does the nurse include in the care plan to address these emotional symptoms?

1 Assist the client with identifying coping skills, support systems, and potential stressors.
2 Avoid teaching the client anything about the disease until he or she is emotionally stable.
3 Confront the client and explain that he or she must control the anxiety if he or she wants to go home.
4 Reassure the client that everything will be fine when he or she is able to avoid or minimize personal stressors.

Level of Cognitive Ability: Applying
Client Needs: Psychosocial Integrity
Clinical Judgment/Cognitive Skills: Generate Solutions
Integrated Process: Nursing Process/Planning
Content Area: Adult Health: Endocrine
Health Problem: Mental Health: Coping

Answer: 1
Rationale: It is normal for clients who experience thyroid storm to continue to be anxious and emotionally labile at the time of discharge. The best intervention is to help the client cope with these changes in behavior and perhaps anticipate potential stressors so that symptoms will not be as severe. Confrontation in option 3 will only heighten the client's anxiety. Option 2 avoids the subject, and option 4 provides false reassurance.
Priority Nursing Tip: During thyroid storm, an individual's heart rate, blood pressure, and body temperature can rise to dangerously high levels.

Test-Taking Strategy: Focus on the **subject,** that the client is anxious. Use **therapeutic communication techniques** to answer. This will direct you to the correct option.

120. A client newly diagnosed with tuberculosis (TB) will be on respiratory isolation in the hospital for at least 2 weeks. Which intervention is vital to prevent social isolation in the client?

1 Using the delivery of care time as opportunities to socialize
2 Educating the family on the importance of touch as a means of socializing
3 Providing the client with a roommate who also is diagnosed with TB
4 Removing the room's clock so that the client will not obsess about time

Level of Cognitive Ability: Applying
Client Needs: Psychosocial Integrity
Clinical Judgment/Cognitive Skills: Take Action
Integrated Process: Nursing Process/Implementation
Content Area: Adult Health: Respiratory
Health Problem: Adult Health: Respiratory/Tuberculosis

Answer: 1

Rationale: The nurse would encourage social contact with staff because the presence of others can offer positive stimulation. Although touch is important to help the client feel socially acceptable, it is not in this case a substitute for regular and consistent human contact. A roommate with TB is inappropriate because such clients would be provided a private room. The clock is needed to facilitate the client's orientation to time.

Priority Nursing Tip: Social isolation is a state of complete or near-complete lack of contact between an individual and society. It differs from loneliness, which reflects a temporary lack of contact with other humans.

Test-Taking Strategy: Focus on the **subject,** preventing social isolation in the client, and focus on the **data in the question.** Recalling that TB is contagious will assist in eliminating option 2. Next eliminate option 4 because a clock provides orientation. To select from the remaining options, remembering the basic principles related to sensory deprivation will direct you to the correct one.

---

121. During report, the nurse is told that a client has signed a consent form for the amputation of a limb severely burned in an accident that occurred while the client was intoxicated. The nurse notes that the client is tearful and socially withdrawn. Which intervention is therapeutic at this time?

1 Reflecting back to the client, "You seem sad and troubled"
2 Requesting medication to assist the client in the management of depression
3 Allowing the client to have some time alone to grieve over the future loss of the limb
4 Suggesting to the client a need for counseling and treatment for alcohol abuse issues

Level of Cognitive Ability: Applying
Client Needs: Psychosocial Integrity
Clinical Judgment/Cognitive Skills: Take Action
Integrated Process: Nursing Process/Implementation
Content Area: Mental Health
Health Problem: Mental Health: Grief/Loss

Answer: 1

Rationale: It is the nurse's responsibility to initiate a discussion about the client's apparent sadness and social withdrawal. Reflection statements tend to elicit a deeper awareness of feelings. In addition, the correct option validates the perception that the client is upset. Option 4 is inappropriate and a block to communication. Options 2 and 3 initiate interventions prematurely.

Priority Nursing Tip: Loss of a body part has a great potential for initiating depression.

Test-Taking Strategy: Focus on the **subject,** the client's concerning behavior. Use **therapeutic communication techniques.** Select the option that encourages the client to express feelings; this will direct you to the correct option.

---

122. Which statement made by a client diagnosed with left-sided Bell's palsy **requires follow-up** by the nurse?

1. "My left eye is tearing a lot."
2. "I have trouble closing my left eyelid."
3. "I can't taste anything on the left side."
4. "Living like this forever just isn't fair."

Level of Cognitive Ability: Evaluating
Client Needs: Psychosocial Integrity
Clinical Judgment/Cognitive Skills: Evaluate Outcomes
Integrated Process: Nursing Process/Evaluation
Content Area: Adult Health: Neurological
Health Problem: Adult Health: Neurological: Bell's Palsy

Answer: 4
Rationale: Bell's palsy is a temporary inflammatory condition that involves the facial nerve (cranial nerve VII). It is important for the nurse to identify the client's fears and to formulate a plan for helping clients deal with them. Options 1, 2, and 3 are expected findings in a client with Bell's palsy.
Priority Nursing Tip: Bell's palsy is usually temporary, with symptoms resolving after several weeks to months. Many clients fear that they have had a stroke when the symptoms appear, and they commonly believe that the paralysis is permanent.

Test-Taking Strategy: Focus on the **subject,** the client's fears related to Bell's palsy. Note the **strategic words,** *requires follow-up.* These words indicate a **negative event query** and the need to select the statement of concern. Options 1, 2, and 3 identify expected findings in clients with this condition. The correct option identifies an inaccurate understanding of the disorder and requires further exploration.

---

123. The nurse is assisting with caring for a client newly diagnosed with diabetes mellitus who is anxious about the self-administration of insulin. The nurse would **initially** implement what intervention to help manage the client's fear?

1. Teach a family member to give the client the insulin.
2. Help the client identify the root cause of their expressed fears.
3. Have the client practice giving injections to an orange until the anxiety is gone.
4. Administer the insulin until the client feels confident enough to assume responsibility.

Level of Cognitive Ability: Applying
Client Needs: Psychosocial Integrity
Clinical Judgment/Cognitive Skills: Take Action
Integrated Process: Nursing Process/Implementation
Content Area: Adult Health: Endocrine
Health Problem: Mental Health: Coping

Answer: 2
Rationale: Therapeutic communication between the nurse and client will assist in identifying what the client is fearful of regarding the administration of the insulin and will allow for interventions to help minimize the fears. Options 1 and 4 place the client in a dependent role. Option 3 is unrealistic in view of the subject of the question.
Priority Nursing Tip: Fear is a barrier to effective client self-care.

Test-Taking Strategy: Focus on the **subject,** the fear of self-administration of insulin. Next, note the **strategic word,** *initially.* The correct option focuses directly on the client and the client's fear.

---

124. An adolescent is admitted to the hospital diagnosed with hyperglycemia resulting from a failure to adhere to the prescribed plan of care. The client states, "I'm fed up with having my life ruled by doctors and machines!" The nurse identifies that the client is experiencing what emotional conflict?

1 Distress related to loss of autonomy
2 Anxiety related to the personal crisis
3 Confusion related to the chronic illness
4 Agitation as a result of elevated blood glucose levels

Level of Cognitive Ability: Analyzing
Client Needs: Psychosocial Integrity
Clinical Judgment/Cognitive Skills: Analyze Cues
Integrated Process: Nursing Process/Data Collection
Content Area: Developmental Stages: Adolescent
Health Problem: Mental Health: Coping

Answer: 1
Rationale: Adolescents strive for identity and independence, and this question describes a common fear of loss of autonomy. The correct option relates to the subject, failure to follow the prescribed regimen and feelings of powerlessness. There is no indication of either confusion or anxiety. The cause of the agitation is emotional, not physical.
Priority Nursing Tip: Chronic illness can result in a loss of autonomy and independence; this can be especially frustrating to a teenager.

Test-Taking Strategy: Focus on the **data in the question.** Eliminate option 2 because, although the client may be experiencing a personal crisis, there is no evidence of anxiety. Eliminate option 3 because there are no data to support confusion. Eliminate option 4 because there are no data to support that the agitation is a result of a physical dysfunction.

---

125. The parents of a newborn with cleft lip and tetralogy of Fallot discuss how their life plans for the child will need to be altered. Based on this conversation, the nurse would **initially** focus on which client issues?

1 Impaired adjustment
2 Anticipatory grieving
3 Dysfunctional grieving
4 Disabled family coping

Level of Cognitive Ability: Applying
Client Needs: Psychosocial Integrity
Clinical Judgment/Cognitive Skills: Generate Solutions
Integrated Process: Nursing Process/Planning
Content Area: Maternity: Newborn
Health Problem: Mental Health: Grief and Loss

Answer: 2
Rationale: Anticipatory grieving involves the intellectual and emotional responses and behaviors that individuals and families use to work through the process of modifying their self-concept with the perception of potential loss. There is no supporting evidence that any of the other options exist.
Priority Nursing Tip: The birth of a child with a disability is a trigger for parental loss and potentially poor parent bonding.

Test-Taking Strategy: Focus on the **data in the question.** Also note the **strategic word,** *initially.* Noting the word *altered* in the question would immediately lead you to one of the options related to grieving. From this point, eliminate options 3 and 4 because there are no data to indicate that the grieving is dysfunctional.

---

126. A client being prepared for a parathyroidectomy states, "I guess I'll have to learn to love wearing a scarf after this surgery!" The nurse identifies which as a psychosocial concern?

1 Acute pain from surgery
2 Avoidance of public places
3 Altered physical appearance
4 Decreased physical mobility

Level of Cognitive Ability: Analyzing
Client Needs: Psychosocial Integrity
Clinical Judgment/Cognitive Skills: Analyze Cues
Integrated Process: Nursing Process/Data Collection
Content Area: Adult Health: Endocrine
Health Problem: Mental Health: Coping

Answer: 3
Rationale: The client's statement reflects a psychosocial concern about appearance after surgery; thus altered physical appearance would be a potential problem. Option 2 is inappropriate because the client is addressing the concern rather than avoiding or denying it. Options 1 and 4 identify physiological problems.
Priority Nursing Tip: A common psychosocial stressor to a body-altering surgery is that the resulting change to the body will be unacceptable.

Test-Taking Strategy: Focus on the **data in the question.** The client is expressing a concern, not avoidance of the perceived problem, so eliminate option 2. Because the client is expressing a psychosocial concern, eliminate options 1 and 4.

---

127. The husband of a client diagnosed with Graves' disease expresses concern that the client has been nervous, unable to concentrate on even trivial tasks, and often demonstrates outbursts of temper. Based on this information, the nurse asks the client what assessment question?

1 "How do you handle grief over a loss?"
2 "How often do you spend time with old friends?"
3 "Can you tell me about how you are coping with the disease?"
4 "Are you experiencing any problems with your medication?"

Level of Cognitive Ability: Applying
Client Needs: Psychosocial Integrity
Clinical Judgment/Cognitive Skills: Analyze Cues
Integrated Process: Nursing Process/Data Collection
Content Area: Adult Health: Endocrine
Health Problem: Mental Health: Coping

Answer: 3
Rationale: Family and friends may report that the client with Graves' disease has become more irritable or depressed, especially after discharge from the hospital. The signs and symptoms in the question support data for the problem of ineffective coping and are unrelated to grief, social isolation, or adherence to therapies.
Priority Nursing Tip: Chronic illnesses often require adjustments to autonomy, independence, well-being, and wellness. These adjustments require effective coping mechanisms if the individual is to experience fullness of life.

Test-Taking Strategy: Focus on the **data in the question.** Your understanding of the psychological effects of chronic illness will help you identify the correct option. There is no information in the question that supports options 1, 2, and 4.

---

128. The nurse is caring for a client diagnosed with hypoparathyroidism. When assisting with planning for the client's discharge, the nurse identifies which data as a potential psychosocial problem related to the condition?

1 Reluctance to retire because of economic concerns
2 Anxiety related to the need for lifelong interventions
3 Acute pain related to cold intolerance secondary to decreased metabolic rate
4 Constipation related to decreased peristaltic action secondary to decreased metabolic rate

Level of Cognitive Ability: Applying
Client Needs: Psychosocial Integrity
Clinical Judgment/Cognitive Skills: Analyze Cues
Integrated Process: Nursing Process/Data Collection
Content Area: Adult Health: Endocrine
Health Problem: Mental Health: Coping

Answer: 2

Rationale: The medical management of hypoparathyroidism is aimed at continuous monitoring correcting the hypocalcemia. Knowing that the interventions are lifelong can create some anxiety for the client, and this problem needs to be addressed before discharge. Retirement is an economic concern for many individuals and not necessarily associated with the diagnosis. The other options are unrelated to this disorder and are physiological problems rather than psychosocial concerns.

Priority Nursing Tip: Chronic illness can result in both physical and psychosocial stressors.

Test-Taking Strategy: Focus on the **data in the question** and the words *psychosocial problem.* This will assist in eliminating options 3 and 4. Next think about the pathophysiology of this disorder to answer correctly.

---

129. A client diagnosed with human immunodeficiency virus (HIV) is in early labor. The woman confides to the nurse, "I know I will have a very sick baby." The nurse would make which therapeutic response to begin to address the client's concerns?

1 "It's a real possibility, but don't focus on that right now."
2 "You have concerns about how HIV will affect your baby?"
3 "Our neonatal unit will provide your baby with quality care."
4 "You are very sick, and we'll know immediately whether your baby is sick as well."

Level of Cognitive Ability: Applying
Client Needs: Psychosocial Integrity
Clinical Judgment/Cognitive Skills: Take Action
Integrated Process: Communication and Documentation
Content Area: Maternity: Intrapartum
Health Problem: Mental Health: Coping

Answer: 2

Rationale: The nurse's initial intervention would be to encourage the client to further discuss concerns. The correct option is a therapeutic response that will elicit additional information from the client. It addresses the therapeutic communication technique of paraphrasing. The client needs to know that her baby will not look sick at birth and that there will be a period of uncertainty before it is known whether the baby has acquired HIV. The client's concern would not be dismissed, nor would she be given false reassurances.

Priority Nursing Tip: HIV has a strong potential to be transmitted to the unborn child from an infected parent.

Test-Taking Strategy: Focus on the **subject,** the client's concerns. Use **therapeutic communication techniques.** The correct option is an open-ended question that will provide an opportunity for the client to verbalize her concerns. None of the other options provide that opportunity.

---

130. A client who is scheduled for an abdominal peritoneoscopy says to the nurse, "Do people ever have problems with this procedure?" Which response **best** addresses the client's concern?

1 "It sounds as if you may be having concerns about actually having the procedure."
2 "Any invasive procedure brings risk with it. You need to report any shoulder pain immediately."
3 "There is seldom any trouble with this procedure. Have you heard stories of people experiencing problems?"
4 "There are relatively few problems, especially if you are having local anesthesia, but vaginal bleeding should be reported immediately."

Level of Cognitive Ability: Applying
Client Needs: Psychosocial Integrity
Clinical Judgment/Cognitive Skills: Take Action
Integrated Process: Communication and Documentation
Content Area: Adult Health: Gastrointestinal
Health Problem: Mental Health: Coping

Answer: 1
Rationale: The nurse's initial intervention would be to encourage the client to further discuss concerns. A therapeutic response, such as option 1, is one that facilitates the client's expression of feelings and directly addresses the client's concerns. Initially discussing potential complications is likely to cause anxiety about the procedure. The topic of risks would not be minimized because the procedure does present risks.
Priority Nursing Tip: Laparoscopy, also called *peritoneoscopy,* is a procedure that permits visual examination of the abdominal cavity with an optical instrument called a *laparoscope,* which is inserted through a small incision made in the abdominal wall.

Test-Taking Strategy: Note the **strategic word,** *best.* Use **therapeutic communication techniques.** The correct option is the therapeutic response because it supports the information provided in the question and provides an opportunity for the client to verbalize concerns.

---

131. When planning to meet the client's emotional needs during a precipitous labor, the nurse can anticipate that the client will demonstrate which needs? **Select all that apply.**

❒ 1 More severe pain than with a normal labor
❒ 2 Increased fears regarding the effect on the infant
❒ 3 A sense of satisfaction regarding the quick labor
❒ 4 A need for support in maintaining a sense of control
❒ 5 A decreased desire for pain medication due to the shortness of the labor

Level of Cognitive Ability: Applying
Client Needs: Psychosocial Integrity
Clinical Judgment/Cognitive Skills: Recognize Cues
Integrated Process: Nursing Process/Planning
Content Area: Maternity: Intrapartum
Health Problem: Maternity: Precipitous Labor and Delivery

Answer: 1, 2, 4
Rationale: The client experiencing a precipitous labor may have more difficulty maintaining control because of the abrupt onset of labor and its quick progression. This may be very different from previous labor experiences; therefore the client needs support from the nurse to understand and adapt to the rapid progression. The contractions often increase in intensity quickly, thus adding to the client's pain, anxiety, and lack of control. The client may also have an increased amount of concern about the effect of labor on the baby. Lack of control over the situation in combination with increased pain and anxiety can result in a decreased level of satisfaction with the labor and delivery experience. The nature of such a labor generally does not create a sense of satisfaction or a lesser need/desire for pain medication.
Priority Nursing Tip: Labor often causes the client to feel a loss of control over her body.

Test-Taking Strategy: Focus on the **data in the question.** Remembering the various characteristics of a precipitous labor, such as an abrupt onset and a quick progression, will help direct you to the correct options.

---

132. The nurse is assisting with care for a client who presents in active labor with a history of a previous cesarean delivery. She is upset and expresses concern for the safety of her baby and for herself. What is the appropriate response from the nurse to **best** address the woman's concerns?

1. "I'll notify your doctor about the concerns you are having."
2. "Don't worry. This is not an unusual situation for us to handle."
3. "We'll talk about your concerns as soon as I check your baby."
4. "I can understand that you are fearful. Tell me what you need from me."

Level of Cognitive Ability: Applying
Client Needs: Psychosocial Integrity
Clinical Judgment/Cognitive Skills: Take Action
Integrated Process: Communication and Documentation
Content Area: Maternity/Intrapartum
Health Problem: Mental Health: Therapeutic Communication

Answer: 4
Rationale: Pregnant clients have concern for the safety of their babies during labor and delivery. A calm attitude with realistic reassurances is an important aspect of client care. Dismissing or ignoring the client's concerns as described in the other options can lead to increased fear and lack of cooperation.
Priority Nursing Tip: The maternal fear of one's body not being able to tolerate a vaginal birth after experiencing a cesarean delivery is common and would be effectively addressed through education.

Test-Taking Strategy: Note the **strategic word,** *best.* Use **therapeutic communication techniques,** and eliminate option 2, which blocks therapeutic communication using a cliché and false reassurance. Eliminate option 3, which places the client's feelings on hold. Look for the option that reflects acceptance of the client's feelings and provides realistic reassurances; this will direct you to option 4.

---

133. During an initial physical examination of a newborn, the neonatologist discovers cryptorchidism. When teaching the family, the nurse identifies understanding of the condition through which statement?

1. "Our son is at risk for atrophy of his penis and scrotum."
2. "Our son is at risk for becoming sterile if this is not corrected."
3. "Our son is diagnosed with testicular cancer and will need treatment."
4. "Our son's testicles are twisted and painful; we will need to apply heat."

Level of Cognitive Ability: Evaluating
Client Needs: Psychosocial Integrity
Clinical Judgment/Cognitive Skills: Evaluate Outcomes
Integrated Process: Nursing Process/Evaluation
Content Area: Pediatrics: Renal and Urinary
Health Problem: Pediatric-Specific: Urological Structural Abnormalities

Answer: 2
Rationale: Cryptorchidism is a condition in which one or both of the testes fail to descend from the abdomen into the scrotum. Infertility could occur with this disorder because sperm production is decreased in the undescended testes. None of the remaining options are associated with this condition.
Priority Nursing Tip: The psychological effects of an "empty scrotum" (cryptorchidism) could affect self-perception, as well as the client's ability to reproduce.

Test-Taking Strategy: Focus on the **subject,** an understanding of cryptorchidism. Knowledge of the characteristics of this disorder will direct you to the correct option.

---

134. Cranial surgery is performed on a 15-year-old client who sustained a head injury. Which psychosocial issue would the nurse prepare the client to experience that is **most** related to self-esteem?

1 Anxiety
2 Fear of crowds
3 Temporary alopecia
4 Short-term memory loss

Level of Cognitive Ability: Applying
Client Needs: Psychosocial Integrity
Clinical Judgment/Cognitive Skills: Generate Solutions
Integrated Process: Nursing Process/Planning
Content Area: Developmental Stages: Adolescent
Health Problem: Pediatric-Specific: Head Injury

Answer: 3
Rationale: Body image is a main focus for an adolescent; appearance is very important and is linked with peer acceptance in this age group. A loss of hair in the head area alters the adolescent's appearance. None of the remaining options are directly associated with a self-esteem–related problem.
Priority Nursing Tip: Alopecia is the partial or complete absence of hair from areas of the body where it normally grows.

Test-Taking Strategy: Note the **strategic word,** *most,* and focus on the **subject,** self-esteem issues related to cranial surgery. Remember that adolescents' focus at this stage of growth and development is body image and how peers perceive them. Based on this focus, you can eliminate unrelated options.

---

135. A client of an infant diagnosed with hydrocephalus is concerned about the complication of developmental disabilities. The client states, "I'm not sure if I can care for my baby at home." What nursing response **best** addresses the client's concern?

1 "Are you aware that all babies have individual needs?"
2 "Parents instinctively know what is best for their babies."
3 "You have concerns about your baby's condition and care?"
4 "There is no reason to worry. You have a good pediatrician."

Level of Cognitive Ability: Applying
Client Needs: Psychosocial Integrity
Clinical Judgment/Cognitive Skills: Take Action
Integrated Process: Communication and Documentation
Content Area: Maternity: Newborn
Health Problem: Mental Health: Therapeutic Communication

Answer: 3
Rationale: The nurse's initial intervention would be to encourage the client to further discuss concerns. The correct option involves the therapeutic technique of paraphrasing or restating the client's concerns. In option 1, the nurse is minimizing the social needs involved with the baby's diagnosis, which is harmful for the nurse–parent relationship. In options 2 and 4, the nurse is offering false reassurance; these types of responses will block communication.
Priority Nursing Tip: Hydrocephalus and its long-term effects can be a parental stressor and must be effectively addressed to minimize unrealistic expectations and poor parent–infant bonding.

Test-Taking Strategy: Note the **strategic word,** *best,* and use **therapeutic communication techniques.** The correct option is the only therapeutic technique that will provide the client with an opportunity to verbalize her concerns.

---

136. A child in day care has been diagnosed with impetigo. The parent of another child who attends the day care tells the nurse, "My child takes a bath every day, so that's okay, right?" What response would the nurse provide to address the parent's concerns?

1 "You sound worried about your child developing impetigo."
2 "The problem is easy to manage if you bring it to your pediatrician's attention."
3 "Does everyone in the family know the importance of proper hand-washing technique?"
4 "There is no need to worry; just keep your child out of day care until the problem is resolved."

Level of Cognitive Ability: Applying
Client Needs: Psychosocial Integrity
Clinical Judgment/Cognitive Skills: Take Action
Integrated Process: Communication and Documentation
Content Area: Pediatrics: Infectious and Communicable Diseases
Health Problem: Mental Health: Therapeutic Communication

Answer: 1
Rationale: The nurse's initial intervention would be to encourage the client to further discuss concerns. By paraphrasing what the parent tells the nurse, the nurse is addressing the parent's thoughts, as in the correct option. All of the other options are blocks to communication because they tend to minimize the parent's concerns.
Priority Nursing Tip: Impetigo is a common and highly contagious skin infection that mainly affects infants and children. Impetigo usually appears as red sores on the face, especially around a child's nose and mouth, and on hands and feet.

Test-Taking Strategy: Focus on the **subject,** the client's concerns. Use **therapeutic communication techniques.** The correct option is the therapeutic option, and it includes the technique of paraphrasing; this is the only option that will provide the client with an opportunity to verbalize her concerns.

---

137. A school-aged child is hospitalized for a compound fracture. What nursing intervention **best** addresses the family's needs?

1 Giving priority to those issues that affect the care of the child
2 Prioritizing the needs that are affecting the child's separation from family
3 Sharing with the family that identifying and meeting their needs is a priority
4 Explaining to the family that the child's physical care will take priority over family needs

Level of Cognitive Ability: Applying
Client Needs: Psychosocial Integrity
Clinical Judgment/Cognitive Skills: Take Action
Integrated Process: Caring
Content Area: Foundations of Care: Communication
Health Problem: Mental Health: Therapeutic Communication

Answer: 3
Rationale: When caring for individuals and families, it is important to ask questions about specific needs and means of treatment. An understanding of the family's beliefs and health practices is essential to successful interventions for that particular family. None of the remaining options attend to exploring family needs.
Priority Nursing Tip: Family-centered care is an approach involving a partnership between the family as a unit and their health care providers.

Test-Taking Strategy: Note the **strategic word,** *best,* and focus on the **subject,** child and family needs. Options 1, 2, and 4 are **comparable or alike** in that they ignore the family practices and values of the client. The correct option addresses the needs of the family and the child.

---

138. A client with a thoracic vertebra (T1) spinal cord injury has just learned that the cord was completely severed. The client says, "I'm no good to anyone. I might as well be dead." What response **best** demonstrates the nurse's therapeutic communication skills?

1. "Don't say that; you're not a useless person at all."
2. "It makes me uncomfortable when you talk this way."
3. "I'll ask the psychologist to see you about these feelings."
4. "I sense you are feeling pretty bad about things right now."

Level of Cognitive Ability: Applying
Client Needs: Psychosocial Integrity
Clinical Judgment/Cognitive Skills: Take Action
Integrated Process: Communication and Documentation
Content Area: Adult Health: Neurological
Health Problem: Mental Health: Therapeutic Communication

Answer: 4
Rationale: The nurse's initial intervention would be to encourage the client to further discuss concerns. Restating and reflecting keep the communication open and show interest that will encourage the client to expand on the current feelings of unworthiness and loss that require exploration. The nurse blocks communication by showing disapproval (option 1) or discomfort (option 2) or by postponing a discussion of issues (option 3).
Priority Nursing Tip: The chronic nature of the effects of a spinal cord injury can have massive impact on the individual's self-esteem.

Test-Taking Strategy: Note the **strategic word,** *best.* Use **therapeutic communication techniques.** Review the options and consider the effect that they may have on the client's ability to further discuss his or her concerns. The correct option identifies the therapeutic communication technique of restating and reflecting and thus encourages discussion.

---

139. The nurse enters the room of a client diagnosed with coronary artery disease and finds her quietly crying. After determining that there is no physiological reason for the client's distress, what response would the nurse provide to further gather data about the client?

1. "I will telephone a family member for you to talk to."
2. "Please tell me a little about what has you so upset."
3. "Try not to be so upset. Psychological stress is bad for your heart."
4. "I understand how you feel. I'd cry too if I had a major heart attack."

Level of Cognitive Ability: Applying
Client Needs: Psychosocial Integrity
Clinical Judgment/Cognitive Skills: Take Action
Integrated Process: Communication and Documentation
Content Area: Adult Health: Cardiovascular
Health Problem: Mental Health: Therapeutic Communication

Answer: 2
Rationale: The nurse's initial intervention would be to encourage the client to further discuss concerns. Clients with heart disease often experience anxiety or fear. The nurse encourages the client to express concerns by showing genuine interest and by facilitating communication using therapeutic communication techniques like those in the correct option. None of the other options address the client's feelings or promote client verbalization.
Priority Nursing Tip: The physiological results of chronic disorders can have a massive impact on the development of depression.

Test-Taking Strategy: Focus on the **subject,** the client's concerns. Use **therapeutic communication techniques.** Select the option that has an exploratory approach to identify why the client is upset. This will direct you to option 2 as the response that addresses the client's feelings and promotes client verbalization.

---

140. A client with a recent complete thoracic (T4) spinal cord transection tells the nurse that he will walk as soon as spinal shock subsides. The most accurate basis for planning the nurse's response is an understanding of what characteristic behavior associated with the grief process?

1 The client is bargaining by insisting that walking is possible when the shock subsides.
2 Acceptance that walking is dependent on the improvement of the basic trauma results.
3 The client's anger has created a delusion of possible recovery when the shock lessens.
4 Denial can be protective while the client deals with the anxiety created by the new disability.

Level of Cognitive Ability: Applying
Client Needs: Psychosocial Integrity
Clinical Judgment/Cognitive Skills: Recognize Cues
Integrated Process: Nursing Process/Planning
Content Area: Adult Health: Neurological
Health Problem: Mental Health: Coping

Answer: 4

Rationale: During the adjustment period that occurs for the first few weeks after a spinal cord injury, clients may use denial as a defense mechanism. Denial may temporarily decrease anxiety, and it is a normal part of grieving. After spinal shock abates, denial may impair rehabilitation if its use is prolonged or excessive. However, rehabilitation programs include psychological counseling to deal with grief. Options 1, 2, and 3 are inaccurate explanations of the described behaviors.

Priority Nursing Tip: Defense mechanisms can be helpful when appropriately used to assist the client in adjusting to a traumatic event, especially for the short term.

Test-Taking Strategy: Focus on the **data in the question** and the **subject,** grieving process. Select the option that describes the mechanism most used in the short term during the grieving process. Also, note the client's statement, which is an indication of denial.

---

141. Maladaptive coping behavior can occur in response to a loss or change in the body associated with surgery. In this situation, the nurse would include which action in the nursing care plan?

1 Explaining to the client that open grieving is abnormal
2 Encouraging the client to express feelings about body changes
3 Advising the client to seek psychological treatment immediately
4 Delaying interaction with individuals who have experienced similar losses is not appropriate at this time

Level of Cognitive Ability: Applying
Client Needs: Psychosocial Integrity
Clinical Judgment/Cognitive Skills: Generate Solutions
Integrated Process: Nursing Process/Planning
Content Area: Mental Health
Health Problem: Mental Health: Coping

Answer: 2

Rationale: Surgery can alter a client's body image. The onset of problems with coping with these changes may occur during the immediate or extended postoperative stage. Nursing interventions primarily involve providing psychological support, and the nurse would encourage the client to express feelings. Options 1, 3, and 4 are inaccurate interventions because they are barriers to the sharing of feeling and needs.

Priority Nursing Tip: In psychology, coping means to invest a conscious effort to solve personal and interpersonal problems in order to try to master, minimize, or tolerate stress and conflict.

Test-Taking Strategy: Focus on the **subject,** coping with body changes. Use **therapeutic communication techniques.** Remember that options that block communication (e.g., giving advice, option 3) and showing disapproval (options 1 and 4) are incorrect. Always focus on the client's feelings first.

---

142. A client experiencing pulmonary edema exhibits severe anxiety as the nurse prepares to leave the room to get a change of bed linen. Which intervention will meet the needs of the client in a holistic manner?

1 Encourage the client to watch television as a distraction.
2 Stay with the client until the client is capable of managing the anxiety.
3 Instruct the client to use the call bell if anything is needed while the nurse is out of the room.
4 Promise that the client will be alone only long enough for the nurse to get the bed linen.

Level of Cognitive Ability: Applying
Client Needs: Psychosocial Integrity
Clinical Judgment/Cognitive Skills: Take Action
Integrated Process: Nursing Process/Implementation
Content Area: Mental Health
Health Problem: Mental Health: Anxiety Disorder

Answer: 2
Rationale: Pulmonary edema is accompanied by extreme fear and anxiety. Because the client typically experiences a sense of impending doom, the nurse would remain with the client as much as possible. None of the other options provide for the psychological needs of the client in distress.
Priority Nursing Tip: A person experiencing emotional distress would not be left alone unless absolutely necessary because doing so can result in an escalation of the anxiety and cause an emotional crisis.

Test-Taking Strategy: Focus on the **subject**, care of the client experiencing severe anxiety. The word *holistic* in the question guides you to consider both the physical and emotional needs of the client; this will direct you to the correct option.

---

143. The family of a client who is hospitalized for a myocardial infarction is visibly anxious and distressed about the client's condition. How can the nurse provide support for the family?

1 Offering them food and beverages on a regular basis
2 Allowing visiting times to meet the client's condition and family needs
3 Promising to provide frequent telephone updates if they go home and rest
4 Arranging for the hospital chaplain to sit with them until the crisis passes

Level of Cognitive Ability: Applying
Client Needs: Psychosocial Integrity
Clinical Judgment/Cognitive Skills: Take Action
Integrated Process: Nursing Process/Implementation
Content Area: Adult Health: Cardiovascular
Health Problem: Mental Health: Coping

Answer: 2
Rationale: The use of flexible visiting hours meets the needs of the client and family by reducing the anxiety levels of both. Offering the family food and beverages does not provide emotional support. Although the chaplain may provide support, it is unrealistic for the chaplain to stay until the client stabilizes; in addition, the religious preference of the family may be incompatible with this option. Encouraging the family to go home is nontherapeutic.
Priority Nursing Tip: Emotional support is generally best provided when allowing flexibility in the ways the client/family needs are met.

Test-Taking Strategy: Focus on the **subject**, emotional support for a family in stress. Options 1 and 3 may or may not be helpful, depending on the client and family situation. Coffee and beverages, although probably helpful for many visitors, do not provide support and can also be obtained in the hospital cafeteria. This leaves the correct option as the intervention with the most value because it presents flexibility.

---

144. A client diagnosed with unstable angina says to the nurse, "I'm so afraid; I can't stop thinking that something bad will happen when I'm alone." How can the nurse meet the client's **most immediate** need?

1 Telephoning family to come to the hospital
2 Staying with the client while discussing the client's fear
3 Using television to distract the client
4 Giving reassurance that the client is being monitored closely by staff

Level of Cognitive Ability: Applying
Client Needs: Psychosocial Integrity
Clinical Judgment/Cognitive Skills: Take Action
Integrated Process: Nursing Process/Implementation
Content Area: Adult Health: Cardiovascular
Health Problem: Mental Health: Coping

Answer: 2
Rationale: When a client experiences fear, the nurse can provide a calm, safe environment by offering appropriate reassurance with the therapeutic use of touch and by remaining with the client as much as possible. Discussing the fear will also help the client begin to manage it effectively. The actions in the remaining options fail to provide immediate support to the client.
Priority Nursing Tip: Unstable angina is a condition in which the heart does not get enough blood flow and oxygen.

Test-Taking Strategy: Focus on the **subject,** managing a client's fear. Options 1 and 3 can be eliminated first because they do not provide direct support to the client. From the remaining options, focus on the **strategic words,** *most immediate;* this will direct you to the correct option.

---

145. A client who experiences vasospasm associated with Raynaud's disease tells the nurse that "all I do is think about the stressful nature of my job." What **initial** intervention would the nurse urge to help the client address the expressed concern?

1 Seek a less stressful form of employment.
2 Consider attending a local stress management program.
3 Accept a referral to a psychologist who specializes in stress management.
4 Avoid stressful situations because they can trigger an increase in vasospasms.

Level of Cognitive Ability: Applying
Client Needs: Psychosocial Integrity
Clinical Judgment/Cognitive Skills: Take Action
Integrated Process: Nursing Process/Implementation
Content Area: Adult Health: Cardiovascular
Health Problem: Mental Health: Coping

Answer: 2
Rationale: Stress can trigger the vasospasm that occurs with Raynaud's disease, so referral to a stress management program or the use of biofeedback training may be helpful. These measures teach clients a variety of techniques to reduce or minimize stress. Options 1 and 4 are unrealistic. Option 3 is not necessarily required at this time.
Priority Nursing Tip: Raynaud's disease is characterized by spasm of the arteries in the extremities, especially the fingers. The spasm is typically brought on by constant cold or stress and leads to pallor, pain, numbness, and, in severe cases, gangrene.

Test-Taking Strategy: Note the **strategic word,** *initial,* and focus on the **subject,** managing stress. Note the word *consider* in the correct option. This option provides the client with both assistance and the opportunity to make an independent decision.

---

146. A client with an oral endotracheal tube attached to a mechanical ventilator is being weaned. The nurse caring for the client determines that which strategies are recommended to help manage the client's anxiety during this process? **Select all that apply.**

❒ 1 Evaluating pulse oximetry on a continual basis
❒ 2 Talking to the client during the delivery of care
❒ 3 Encouraging supportive family and friends to visit
❒ 4 Turning the television on to watch favorite programs
❒ 5 Providing antianxiety medications on a regular basis

Level of Cognitive Ability: Applying
Client Needs: Psychosocial Integrity
Clinical Judgment/Cognitive Skills: Take Action
Integrated Process: Nursing Process/Implementation
Content Area: Adult Health: Respiratory
Health Problem: Mental Health: Coping

Answer: 2, 3, 4
Rationale: The client may exhibit anxiety during the weaning process for a variety of reasons; therefore distractions such as radio, television, and visitors are still very useful. Talking to the client is also a positive distraction. Pulse oximetry is a beneficial assessment component to evaluate weaning but has little distraction value. Antianxiety medications and opioid analgesics are used cautiously in the client being weaned from a mechanical ventilator. These medications may interfere with the weaning process by suppressing the respiratory drive.
Priority Nursing Tip: Antianxiety medication can have an effect on respiratory function.

Test-Taking Strategy: Focus on the **subject,** managing anxiety. To answer this question accurately, you would identify the activities that could distract the client and so help minimize feelings of anxiety and fear. This understanding will help you select the correct options.

---

147. A client suspected of having a pulmonary embolism who is scheduled for pulmonary angiography expresses fear regarding pain and the exposure to radiation. The nurse would provide which response to help provide the client with a sense of control and understanding of what to expect?

1 "The procedure is somewhat painful, but there is minimal exposure to radiation."
2 "Discomfort may occur with needle insertion, and there is minimal exposure to radiation."
3 "There is very mild pain throughout the procedure, and the exposure to radiation is negligible."
4 "There is no pain, although a moderate amount of radiation must be used to obtain accurate results."

Level of Cognitive Ability: Applying
Client Needs: Psychosocial Integrity
Clinical Judgment/Cognitive Skills: Take Action
Integrated Process: Nursing Process/Implementation
Content Area: Adult Health: Respiratory
Health Problem: Adult Health: Respiratory: Pulmonary Embolism

Answer: 2
Rationale: Pulmonary angiography involves minimal exposure to radiation. The procedure is painless, although the client may feel discomfort with the insertion of the needle for the catheter that is used for dye injection. All the remaining options inaccurately describe the experience, especially in the areas concerning the client.
Priority Nursing Tip: A pulmonary angiogram is an angiogram of the blood vessels of the lungs. The procedure is done with a special contrast dye injected into the body's blood vessels; x-rays are taken.

Test-Taking Strategy: Focus on the **subject,** fear related to a pulmonary angiogram. An understanding of the pain and radiation danger involved is needed to select the correct option.

---

148. A client has an initial positive result of an enzyme-linked immunosorbent assay (ELISA) test and asks the nurse for an explanation of the results. The nurse's response is based on what understanding of this diagnostic test associated with HIV?

1 The ELISA is definitive for HIV, so a diagnosis will be made and treatment begun.
2 There are occasional false-positive readings with this test, so a Western blot test will be done.
3 There is a high rate of false-positive results with this test, so the test will be repeated for accuracy.
4 The combination of positive results for both the ELISA and the Western blot tests is needed to confirm a diagnosis.

Level of Cognitive Ability: Applying
Client Needs: Psychosocial Integrity
Clinical Judgment/Cognitive Skills: Take Action
Integrated Process: Nursing Process/Implementation
Content Area: Adult Health: Immune
Health Problem: Adult Health: Immune: Immunodeficiency Syndrome

Answer: 3
Rationale: If the ELISA test results are positive, the test is repeated. If the test is positive a second time, then a Western blot test, which is more specific, is performed to confirm the finding. The client is not considered HIV positive unless the Western blot test is positive. The ELISA is a fast and relatively inexpensive test, but it carries a high false-positive rate.
Priority Nursing Tip: Diagnosis of any disorder, whether physical or emotional, is rarely made based on one criterion.

Test-Taking Strategy: Focus on the **data in the question** and an understanding of the ELISA test. Recall that HIV infection is not diagnosed with a single laboratory test and that this test has a high rate of false-positive results. With this in mind, eliminate options 1 and 4 first. To choose correctly between the remaining options, it is necessary to understand that the ELISA would be repeated and that a Western blot test would be done to confirm these results.

---

149. A client hospitalized during an acute period of mania is restless and slaps another client. How will the nurse respond in order to provide safety to all clients and staff?

1 "You cannot hit other people. Come with me to your room now."
2 "You're lucky that you didn't get hit right back; don't do that again."
3 "I understand that you are not feeling well, but hurting others doesn't help."
4 "If you are having difficulty controlling yourself right now, I will help you."

Level of Cognitive Ability: Applying
Client Needs: Psychosocial Integrity
Clinical Judgment/Cognitive Skills: Take Action
Integrated Process: Communication and Documentation
Content Area: Foundations of Care: Safety
Health Problem: Mental Health: Violence

Answer: 4
Rationale: The client with mania may exhibit aggression. The nurse would respond using therapeutic communication techniques and would set limits on the client's behavior. The statement in the correct option conveys understanding and sets limits on the client's behavior. The statement in option 1 sets limits on the client's behavior but is lacking in understanding. The remaining options fail to either display understanding or to provide limits.
Priority Nursing Tip: A client experiencing difficulty controlling his or her behavior needs an outside source of control.

Test-Taking Strategy: Focus on the **data in the question** and note the **subject,** client violence and providing milieu safety. The client is in need of both understanding and behavioral limits. The correct option is the only one that provides both.

---

150. A client diagnosed with renal cell carcinoma of the left kidney is scheduled for a nephrectomy. When told that the right kidney appears normal at this time, the client expresses concern that dialysis will ultimately be needed. The nurse would respond to the client's concern based on what fact?

1 Dialysis could be unlikely as long as the client adheres to treatment.
2 Dialysis will be necessary since a kidney was removed.
3 There is a strong likelihood that the client will need dialysis within 5 to 10 years.
4 One kidney is adequate to meet the needs of the body as long as it has normal function.

Level of Cognitive Ability: Applying
Client Needs: Psychosocial Integrity
Clinical Judgment/Cognitive Skills: Take Action
Integrated Process: Nursing Process/Implementation
Content Area: Adult Health: Renal and Urinary
Health Problem: Adult Health: Cancer: Bladder and Kidney

Answer: 4
Rationale: Fear about having only one functioning kidney is common among clients who must undergo nephrectomy for renal cancer. These clients need emotional support and reassurance that the remaining kidney will be able to fully meet the body's metabolic needs as long as it has normal function. Options 1, 2, and 3 are incorrect statements.
Priority Nursing Tip: Adherence to treatment has a positive effect on prognosis.

Test-Taking Strategy: Focus on the **data in the question** and the client's concern. Recalling the level of function of a single kidney and that one remaining kidney would be able to fully meet the body's metabolic needs as long as it has normal function will direct you to the correct option.

---

151. A psychosocial plan of care for a client with a diagnosis of acute pulmonary edema would include strategies for what potential complication?

1 Reducing anxiety
2 Increasing fluid volume
3 Decreasing cardiac output
4 Promoting a positive body image

Level of Cognitive Ability: Applying
Client Needs: Psychosocial Integrity
Clinical Judgment/Cognitive Skills: Generate Solutions
Integrated Process: Nursing Process/Planning
Content Area: Adult Health: Cardiovascular
Health Problem: Adult Health: Cardiovascular: Pulmonary Edema

Answer: 1
Rationale: When cardiac output falls as a result of acute pulmonary edema, the sympathetic nervous system is stimulated. Stimulation of the sympathetic nervous system results in the fight-or-flight reaction, which further impairs cardiac function. The goal of treatment is to increase cardiac output. Fluid volume would be decreased. Disturbed body image is not a common problem among clients with acute pulmonary edema.
Priority Nursing Tip: Psychosocial planning focuses on mood, cognitive, and affect disorders.

Test-Taking Strategy: Focus on the **subject,** the potential complications of acute pulmonary edema. Considering the physiological manifestations of this condition will assist you with eliminating options 2 and 3. Recalling that anxiety is often a result of the associated severe dyspnea that occurs will direct you to the correct option.

152. A client diagnosed with acute kidney injury (AKI) is experiencing difficulty remembering and understanding instructions because of an elevated blood urea nitrogen (BUN) level. Which interventions will the nurse implement when communicating with this client? **Select all that apply.**

- ❒ 1 Provide directions using simple but clear language.
- ❒ 2 Include the family in discussions related to care whenever possible.
- ❒ 3 Educate the client at the end of the day to help maximize concentration.
- ❒ 4 Give thorough and complete explanations when discussing treatment options.
- ❒ 5 Substitute verbal instructions with written ones to allow for revisiting the instructions.

Answer: 1, 2

Rationale: The client with AKI may have difficulty remembering information and instructions because of the effects of an increased BUN level and anxiety. Communication would be clear, simple, and understandable. The family is included whenever possible. It is the primary health care provider's responsibility to explain treatment options. Educating at the end of the day will have little impact on the problem. Providing only written instructions does not adequately address the client's cognitive issues.

Priority Nursing Tip: Communication problems can be minimized by using applicable communication techniques and including family in discussions.

Test-Taking Strategy: Focus on the **data in the question.** Note that the client is having difficulty remembering and understanding instructions because of an elevated BUN level. Recalling the basic principles of effective communication will help you recognize that options 1 and 2 are helpful for maintaining effective communication about appropriate subjects.

Level of Cognitive Ability: Applying
Client Needs: Psychosocial Integrity
Clinical Judgment/Cognitive Skills: Take Action
Integrated Process: Nursing Process: Implementation
Content Area: Foundations of Care/ Communication
Health Problem: Adult Health: Renal and Urinary: Acute Kidney Injury

---

153. The nurse is assisting with planning care for a client who has been newly diagnosed with active tuberculosis (TB). When addressing the psychosocial needs of the client, what would be identified as the **primary** goal?

1 The client will list all instructions for care and explain when to use each.
2 The client will verbalize ways to lessen the risk of transmitting the infection.
3 The client will share with the nursing staff fears about the disease and prognosis.
4 The client will ask questions and actively seek information about the disease and care.

Answer: 3

Rationale: Addressing psychosocial needs relates to helping the client deal with his or her feelings. Goals for the client focus on the open expression of feelings and fears and the development of coping skills for dealing with the illness and the care required. Options 1, 2, and 4 do not address psychosocial needs.

Priority Nursing Tip: TB is an infectious disease that primarily affects the lungs and is usually caused by the bacterium *Mycobacterium tuberculosis.*

Test-Taking Strategy: Focus on the **subject,** psychosocial needs of the client, and note the **strategic word,** *primary.* Recall that addressing the client's fears and concerns is a primary nursing goal.

Level of Cognitive Ability: Applying
Client Needs: Psychosocial Integrity
Clinical Judgment/Cognitive Skills: Generate Solutions
Integrated Process: Nursing Process/Planning
Content Area: Adult Health: Respiratory
Health Problem: Adult Health: Respiratory: Tuberculosis

154. What would be the nurse's **primary** focus when collecting data during the psychosocial assessment of a client diagnosed with human immunodeficiency virus (HIV)?

1 The presence of any concerns or fears
2 What type of emotional support the client is in need of
3 How the client perceives the illness has affected his or her life
4 Which family member will assume the client's care upon discharge

Level of Cognitive Ability: Applying
Client Needs: Psychosocial Integrity
Clinical Judgment/Cognitive Skills: Recognize Cues
Integrated Process: Nursing Process/Data Collection
Content Area: Adult Health: Immune
Health Problem: Mental Health: Coping

Answer: 1
Rationale: When collecting data about the psychosocial needs of a client with HIV, the nurse would address the issue of client concerns or fears. Asking how the illness has affected life and the support the client needs are important assessment questions, but neither has the priority of a fears assessment. Asking about care at home is an important discharge planning issue, but it is not the primary concern among the options provided.
Priority Nursing Tip: HIV is a chronic disease process that affects every aspect of an individual's life.

Test-Taking Strategy: Note the **strategic word,** *primary.* Focus on the **subject,** psychosocial assessment, and use **therapeutic communication techniques.** Recalling that the primary intervention when addressing psychosocial needs is addressing the client's feelings will direct you to the correct option.

---

155. A client diagnosed with hyperparathyroidism talks to the nurse about the dietary changes prescribed by the endocrinologist. What response would the nurse provide when the client states, "I guess I'll never be able to eat ice cream and yogurt again"?

1 "Why do you say that?"
2 "There are lots of other foods you can eat."
3 "Ice cream has too much fat content, anyway."
4 "You don't think you will be able to eat ice cream at all?"

Level of Cognitive Ability: Applying
Client Needs: Psychosocial Integrity
Clinical Judgment/Cognitive Skills: Take Action
Integrated Process: Communication and Documentation
Content Area: Adult Health: Endocrine
Health Problem: Mental Health: Therapeutic Communication

Answer: 4
Rationale: Treatment for clients with hyperparathyroidism includes a low-calcium diet. Ice cream and yogurt are high in calcium and need to be restricted. The nurse would respond by rephrasing the client's statement. Options 1, 2, and 3 are examples of communication blocks (e.g., giving advice, requesting an explanation).
Priority Nursing Tip: Dietary restrictions are generally very difficult for an individual to effectively adjust to.

Test-Taking Strategy: Focus on the **subject,** the client's concerns. Use **therapeutic communication techniques** to answer the question. The correct option seeks to validate what the nurse heard to determine whether additional instruction is needed.

---

156. A client scheduled for chorionic villus sampling tells the nurse, "I'm not sure I want to have this test." Which response by the nurse will **best** encourage the client to discuss her statement further?

1 "It's your decision to make."
2 "Tell me what concerns you have."
3 "What negative things have you heard?"
4 "Why don't you want to have this test?"

Level of Cognitive Ability: Applying
Client Needs: Psychosocial Integrity
Clinical Judgment/Cognitive Skills: Take Action
Integrated Process: Communication and Documentation
Content Area: Foundations of Care: Communication
Health Problem: Mental Health: Therapeutic Communication

Answer: 2
Rationale: The nurse needs to gather more data and assist the client with exploring her feelings about the test. None of the other options provide this opportunity for further discussion.
Priority Nursing Tip: Concerns about a diagnostic procedure, especially one that involves an unborn fetus, make consenting to the procedure often very stressful.

Test-Taking Strategy: Note the **strategic word,** ***best.*** Use **therapeutic communication techniques** to answer the question. The correct option addresses the client's concern by encouraging further discussion.

---

157. How would the nurse respond when a client states, "It will be so hard to wait for the results of this amniocentesis. I don't know what I will do if something goes wrong"?

1 "You sound concerned about having this test done."
2 "You are in good hands; your doctor is very competent."
3 "It's not good for your baby when you become upset or worry."
4 "This test has been done for many years with few reported complications."

Level of Cognitive Ability: Applying
Client Needs: Psychosocial Integrity
Clinical Judgment/Cognitive Skills: Take Action
Integrated Process: Communication and Documentation
Content Area: Foundations of Care: Communication
Health Problem: Mental Health: Therapeutic Communication

Answer: 1
Rationale: The nurse needs to gather more data and assist the client with exploring her feelings about the test. Therefore option 1 is correct. None of the remaining options focus on the client's feelings and concerns.
Priority Nursing Tip: An amniocentesis presents some risks to the fetus.

Test-Taking Strategy: Focus on the **subject,** the client's concerns. Use **therapeutic communication techniques** to answer the question. The correct option addresses the client's concern, whereas the remaining options block further communication.

---

158. A hospitalized client is being prepared for discharge to home in 2 days. The client has been eating a regular diet for a week but is still receiving intermittent enteral tube feedings. How would the nurse respond when the client expresses concern that he or she will not be able to do the tube feedings at home?

1 "Have you discussed your feelings with your doctor?"
2 "Do you want to stay in the hospital for a few more days?"
3 "Tell me more about your concerns with your diet after going home."
4 "Your tube feedings will no longer be necessary after your discharge."

Level of Cognitive Ability: Applying
Client Needs: Psychosocial Integrity
Clinical Judgment/Cognitive Skills: Take Action
Integrated Process: Communication and Documentation
Content Area: Foundations of Care: Communication
Health Problem: Mental Health: Therapeutic Communication

Answer: 3

Rationale: A client often has fears about leaving the secure, cared-for environment of the hospital. The correct option provides the client with an opportunity to further discuss those fears. Option 1 places the client's concern on hold. Option 2 is not related to the client's concern. There are no data to indicate that the tube feedings will be discontinued.

Priority Nursing Tip: Fear can have a large negative impact on the individual's perceived ability to manage self-care procedures such as enteral tube feedings.

Test-Taking Strategy: Focus on the **subject,** the client's concerns. Use **therapeutic communication techniques** to answer the question. Remember to always focus on the client's concerns. The correct option is the only one that addresses the client's concerns.

---

159. A client will be receiving continuous parenteral nutrition at home for long-term nutritional therapy. Which potential problem is a **priority** concern?

1 Hopelessness
2 Social isolation
3 Low self-esteem
4 Fluid volume deficit

Level of Cognitive Ability: Applying
Client Needs: Psychosocial Integrity
Clinical Judgment/Cognitive Skills: Recognize Cues
Integrated Process: Nursing Process/Data Collection
Content Area: Mental Health
Health Problem: Mental Health: Coping

Answer: 2

Rationale: This client will be receiving continuous parenteral nutrition for the long term and thus isolated from psychological and physical stimuli outside the home. Fluid volume excess (rather than deficit) is most likely to occur. There are no data in the question to support option 1 or 3.

Priority Nursing Tip: Social isolation leads to depression, poor healing, and decreased adherence to medical regimens.

Test-Taking Strategy: Focus on the **data in the question** and note the **strategic word,** *priority.* Think about the potential impact of needing to receive continuous parenteral nutrition at home. This will assist in directing you to the correct option.

---

160. The nurse is collecting data about a client's psychosocial adjustment to a newly applied body cast. The nurse would give **priority** to the data concerning what area of the assessment?

1 Home environment
2 Usual coping techniques
3 Presence of at-home care support
4 Ability to perform activities of daily living

Level of Cognitive Ability: Applying
Client Needs: Psychosocial Integrity
Clinical Judgment/Cognitive Skills: Recognize Cues
Integrated Process: Nursing Process/Data Collection
Content Area: Mental Health
Health Problem: Mental Health: Coping

Answer: 2
Rationale: When collecting data about the client's psychosocial adjustment, the nurse would first address the client's usual coping techniques because adjusting to this situation will require a healthy set of skills. Options 1, 3, and 4 do not address psychosocial issues.
Priority Nursing Tip: The presence of healthy coping mechanisms is a primary factor in the adjustment to stress.

Test-Taking Strategy: Focus on the **subject,** psychosocial adjustment, and focus on the **strategic word,** *priority.* The correct option is the only one that addresses the client's psychosocial needs.

---

161. A client who has been on bed rest in a private room for 1 week is now allowed up as tolerated. The client has been exhibiting periods of confusion for 2 days before this change in activity prescription. Which intervention would the nurse implement to **best** decrease the confusion?

1 Range-of-motion exercises three times a day to increase strength
2 Ambulation to the client's bathroom at least three times a day
3 Increasing the distance the client walks by 5 feet each day
4 Progressive ambulation in the hall three times a day

Level of Cognitive Ability: Applying
Client Needs: Psychosocial Integrity
Clinical Judgment/Cognitive Skills: Take Action
Integrated Process: Nursing Process/Implementation
Content Area: Mental Health
Health Problem: Mental Health: Neurocognitive Impairment

Answer: 4
Rationale: Confusion in this situation is probably due to decreased sensory stimulation as a result of being in a private room. Ambulating the client in the hall will increase sensory stimulation and may decrease confusion. Options 2 and 3 do not provide the best methods for increasing sensory stimulation. The question addresses ambulation rather than range-of-motion exercises.
Priority Nursing Tip: Sensory stimulation uses everyday objects to arouse one or more of the five senses (hearing, sight, smell, taste, and touch), with the goal of evoking positive feelings.

Test-Taking Strategy: Note the **strategic word,** *best,* and focus on the **subject,** increased sensory stimulation and decreasing confusion. Understanding activities related to increased stimulation will help eliminate options 2 and 3 while directing you to the correct option.

---

162. A client with a history of pulmonary emboli is scheduled for the insertion of an inferior vena cava (IVC) filter. The nurse checks on the client 1 hour after the primary health care provider has explained the procedure and obtained informed consent. The client is lying in bed, wringing her hands, and says to the nurse, "I'm not sure about this. What if it doesn't work and I'm just as bad off as before?" Which concern is the likely reason for the client's statement?

1 Anxiety related to the possibility of death
2 Ineffective coping related to the treatment regimen
3 Lack of knowledge related to the surgical procedure
4 Fear related to the potential risks and outcome of surgery

Level of Cognitive Ability: Analyzing
Client Needs: Psychosocial Integrity
Clinical Judgment/Cognitive Skills: Analyze Cues
Integrated Process: Nursing Process/Data Collection
Content Area: Mental Health
Health Problem: Mental Health: Crisis

Answer: 4
Rationale: This client has indicated fear regarding the surgical procedure and its outcome. Anxiety is present when the client cannot identify the source of the uneasy feelings. Deficient knowledge is characterized by a lack of appropriate information. Ineffective coping is appropriate when the client is not making necessary adaptations to deal with daily life.
Priority Nursing Tip: IVC filter placement is most commonly indicated for deep venous thrombosis (DVT) or pulmonary embolism (PE) when anticoagulation therapy is contraindicated.

Test-Taking Strategy: Focus on the **data in the question** and the client's statement to assist with directing you to the correct option. Note the relationship of the client's statement to option 4. The client's statement supports fear related to the potential risks and outcome of surgery.

---

163. A client who experienced a myocardial infarction (MI) 4 days ago refuses to dangle at the bedside and says, "If my doctor tells me to do it, I will." How would the nurse respond to the client's statement?

1 "Well, it's your choice to do what you want to do."
2 "I'm confident your doctor wants you to do this."
3 "If you don't do this, you'll likely take longer to recover."
4 "This is part of your treatment plan to help with recovering safely."

Level of Cognitive Ability: Applying
Client Needs: Psychosocial Integrity
Clinical Judgment/Cognitive Skills: Take Action
Integrated Process: Communication and Documentation
Content Area: Adult Health: Cardiovascular
Health Problem: Mental Health: Coping

Answer: 4
Rationale: Clients may experience numerous emotional and behavioral responses after an MI. Dependency is one response that may be manifested by the client's refusal to perform any tasks or activities unless they have been approved by the primary health care provider. Performing or refusing to perform activities that may seem harmful is indicative of denial, which is commonly noted after MI. The nurse needs to acknowledge the client's concerns and explain what care is recommended by standard protocols. Options 2 and 3 do not attempt to provide an explanation for the treatment. Option 1 is true; however, the client needs to have an explanation as to how refusal of treatment can affect the client's health.
Priority Nursing Tip: An individual faced with a major health threat may develop a dependency on others to make decisions. The individual needs the support and reassurance of protocols to make informed choices.

Test-Taking Strategy: Focus on the **data in the question.** Use **therapeutic communication techniques** to answer correctly. Eliminate options that fail to provide the client with support and understanding of the prescribed treatment.

---

164. The nurse is collecting data from a client admitted to the hospital with a diagnosis of renal calculi. The client states to the nurse, "I'm scared to death that it'll come back. That was the worst pain I ever had." Based on this conversation, the nurse suggests including which client problem into the plan of care?

1 Fear related to anticipation of recurrent severe pain
2 Pain related to presence of calculus in the right ureter
3 Urinary retention related to obstruction of the urinary tract by calculi
4 Lack of knowledge related to lack of information about the disease process

Level of Cognitive Ability: Applying
Client Needs: Psychosocial Integrity
Clinical Judgment/Cognitive Skills: Generate Solutions
Integrated Process: Nursing Process/Planning
Content Area: Adult Health: Renal and Urinary
Health Problem: Adult Health: Renal and Urinary: Obstructive Problems

Answer: 1
Rationale: The anticipation of the recurring pain is the client's concern. There is no evidence that the client has a calculus in the right ureter or that urinary retention or a knowledge deficit exists.
Priority Nursing Tip: Fear of pain is a strong emotion, especially once severe pain has been experienced.

Test-Taking Strategy: Focus on the **data in the question** and the client's statement to assist with directing you to the correct option. Note the relationship of the words in the client's statement to the word *fear* in the correct option.

---

165. A neonatal intensive care nurse observes parents at the bedside of their infant and hears the parent state, "She is so tiny and fragile. I'll never be able to hold her with all those tubes." Based on this statement, the nurse plans to add what problem to the plan of care?

1 Caregiver role strain
2 Inadequate problem-solving skills
3 Compromised family coping
4 Risk for altered parenting abilities

Level of Cognitive Ability: Applying
Client Needs: Psychosocial Integrity
Clinical Judgment/Cognitive Skills: Analyze Cues
Integrated Process: Nursing Process/Planning
Content Area: Maternity/Newborn
Health Problem: Mental Health: Coping

Answer: 4
Rationale: One of the problems for the parents of a high-risk neonate is the risk for altered parenting abilities. The initial focus of intervention for the parents of a preterm small-for-gestational-age (SGA) infant is to assist parent–infant bonding. Option 1 addresses the strain of a caregiver, which, during the initial hospitalization, is too early to apply. Option 2 addresses nonacceptance of a health status change or an inability to solve problems or set goals. Option 3 involves the identification of a lack of coping mechanisms. At this time, there are inadequate data to accurately identify these problems, although they may become relevant at a later time.
Priority Nursing Tip: A neonatal intensive care unit (NICU) is an intensive care unit specializing in the care of ill or premature newborn infants.

Test-Taking Strategy: Focus on the **data in the question.** Eliminate options 2 and 3 first because these options identify actual problems that do not exist. When selecting from the remaining options, note the words *I'll never be able to hold her.* Note the relationship between these words and the words *altered parenting abilities* in the correct option.

---

166. The nurse is caring for a client who will be wearing a cast for several weeks. The nurse determines that the client is expressing difficulty coping when the client makes what statement?

1 "I'm so upset I won't be able to work while I'm in this cast."
2 "I feel so helpless, and I don't want to be a burden to anyone."
3 "If I get a shower chair and place my leg in plastic, I can bathe."
4 "My wife is going to have to help me until I can get around on my own."

Level of Cognitive Ability: Analyzing
Client Needs: Psychosocial Integrity
Clinical Judgment/Cognitive Skills: Analyze Cues
Integrated Process: Nursing Process/Data Collection
Content Area: Adult Health: Musculoskeletal
Health Problem: Mental Health: Coping

Answer: 2
Rationale: Illness can present a unique experience and often frustrate and challenge the client into feeling powerless. There is no evidence in the question that anxiety (option 1) exists or that there is compromised family coping (option 4). Although there may be a self-care deficiency (option 3), it does not demonstrate the client's inability to cope.
Priority Nursing Tip: Situations that result in a loss of independence can lead to a sense of powerlessness.

Test-Taking Strategy: Focus on the **subject,** a client having difficulty coping. Select the client statement that demonstrates a sense of powerlessness. Noting the words *helpless* and *burden* in option 2 will direct you to this option.

---

167. The nurse working in a rehabilitation center witnesses a postoperative coronary artery bypass graft client and his spouse arguing after a rehabilitation session. To identify the client's concern, the nurse would make which statement?

1 "Let's talk about what upset you."
2 "Oh, don't let this get you down."
3 "It will seem better tomorrow. Smile."
4 "You need not get upset. It will affect your heart."

Level of Cognitive Ability: Applying
Client Needs: Psychosocial Integrity
Clinical Judgment/Cognitive Skills: Recognize Cues
Integrated Process: Communication and Documentation
Content Area: Adult Health: Cardiovascular
Health Problem: Mental Health: Therapeutic Communication

Answer: 1
Rationale: Therapeutic communication techniques assist with the flow of communication and always focus on the client. Open-ended statements allow the client to verbalize, thus giving the nurse some direction for clarifying the client's true feelings. In addition, acknowledging the client's feelings without inserting personal values or judgments is a method of therapeutic communication. Options 2, 3, and 4 do not encourage verbalization by the client.
Priority Nursing Tip: Stress can have a negative effect on health and wellness.

Test-Taking Strategy: Focus on the **subject,** the client's concerns. Use **therapeutic communication techniques.** Remember to always focus on the client's feelings; this will direct you to the correct option.

---

168. As the nurse approaches a client with schizophrenia who was recently admitted to the inpatient unit of a psychiatric hospital, the client says, "Quit following me. You're with the FBI; I can tell by the way you're walking." The nurse documents this statement as what type of dysfunctional thinking?

1 Delusionary
2 Hallucinatory
3 Circumstantial
4 Loose association

Level of Cognitive Ability: Applying
Client Needs: Psychosocial Integrity
Clinical Judgment/Cognitive Skills: Recognize Cues
Integrated Process: Communication and Documentation
Content Area: Mental Health
Health Problem: Mental Health: Schizophrenia

Answer: 1

Rationale: Delusions are false fixed beliefs that cannot be corrected with reasoning. Most commonly, delusional thinking involves themes of reference, persecution, grandiosity, jealousy, and control. Hallucinations are defined as sensory perceptions for which there is no external stimulus. The most common types of hallucinations are auditory, visual, olfactory, and tactile. Circumstantiality is a pattern of speech characterized by indirectness and delay before a person gets to the point or answers a question; the client gets caught up in countless details and explanations. Associative looseness is an alteration in speech that consists of threads (associations) that tie one thought or concept to another.

Priority Nursing Tip: Possible symptoms of psychosis include delusions, hallucinations, incoherent speech, and agitation.

Test-Taking Strategy: Focus on the **subject,** a client who is exhibiting disturbed thought processes. Next, focus on the client's statement and determine what type of altered thought process the client is expressing. Recalling the definitions of each item in the options will direct you to the correct option.

---

169. A client with schizophrenia hospitalized on the mental health unit is displaying manipulative behavior. Which action by a health care provider demonstrates a **need for further teaching** in managing such behavior?

1 Communicating to the client the behaviors that are expected
2 Identifying the manipulative behaviors that the client exhibits
3 Arguing with the client to ensure that views of a situation are shared
4 Describing clearly the consequences of not staying within identified limits

Level of Cognitive Ability: Evaluating
Client Needs: Psychosocial Integrity
Clinical Judgment/Cognitive Skills: Evaluate Outcomes
Integrated Process: Teaching and Learning
Content Area: Mental Health
Health Problem: Mental Health: Schizophrenia

Answer: 3

Rationale: The nurse would avoid getting into arguments with the manipulative client. The other options listed are helpful interventions that will eventually assist the client with setting limits on his or her own behavior.

Priority Nursing Tip: Attempting to get the manipulative individual to accept alternative points of view will only serve to escalate the behavior.

Test-Taking Strategy: Focus on the **subject,** managing the manipulative client. Note the **strategic words,** *need for further teaching.* These words indicate a **negative event query** requiring you to select an inappropriate action. Use your knowledge of management techniques effective in caring for this behavior to direct you to the correct option. Also, note the word *arguing* in the correct option. This is an inappropriate behavior.

---

170. A client with mobility problems due to a fracture is having trouble initiating the stream of urine when using the bedside commode. It is determined that the reason for the problem is psychosocial. The nurse demonstrates an understanding of the likely cause when encouraging what intervention?

1 Encouraging the client to increase fluid intake by 500 mL daily
2 Running water in the bathroom sink as a cue to assist to begin urinating
3 Reviewing medications for the presence of any that can cause such a side effect
4 Asking the client to use the bathroom call bell so that staff can be alerted to the need to return to bed

Level of Cognitive Ability: Applying
Client Needs: Psychosocial Integrity
Clinical Judgment/Cognitive Skills: Take Action
Integrated Process: Nursing Process/Implementation
Content Area: Skills: Elimination
Health Problem: Adult Health: Musculoskeletal: Skeletal Injury

Answer: 4
Rationale: A lack of privacy may inhibit the ability of the client to void. Using a commode behind a curtain may inhibit voiding in some people. Providing privacy and the use of a bathroom is an appropriate intervention when staff can assist in ambulating. The remaining options focus on physiological issues.
Priority Nursing Tip: Paruresis is a condition in which the person is unable to urinate in the presence of others.

Test-Taking Strategy: Focus on the **data in the question** and note the words *that the reason for the problem is psychosocial.* The correct option is the only one that addresses a psychosocial issue rather than a physiological one.

---

171. While the nurse is providing care, the client says, "My doctor just told me that my cancer has spread and that I have less than 6 months to live." How would the nurse respond to **best** meet the client's psychosocial needs?

1 "Would it be helpful for you to discuss this with me more?"
2 "There are no easy answers in times like this, are there?"
3 "Let's focus on how you'd like to live your final days."
4 "Do you believe that miracle cures occur almost daily?"

Level of Cognitive Ability: Applying
Client Needs: Psychosocial Integrity
Clinical Judgment/Cognitive Skills: Take Action
Integrated Process: Communication and Documentation
Content Area: Adult Health: Oncology
Health Problem: Mental Health: Crisis

Answer: 1
Rationale: The client has just received very distressing news. In the correct option, the nurse encourages the client to discuss feelings. Option 2 expresses the nurse's feelings rather than facilitating the client's feelings. Option 3 is patronizing and stereotypical. Option 4 provides a social communication and false hope.
Priority Nursing Tip: Terminal illness means that the individual has an incurable disease that cannot be adequately treated and is reasonably expected to result in death.

Test-Taking Strategy: Note the **strategic word,** *best.* Use **therapeutic communication techniques.** Note that option 1 is the only option that provides the opportunity for the client to express feelings.

---

172. A client with a temporary endotracheal tube gets frustrated easily when trying to communicate with the nurse. The nurse encourages the client to implement what intervention?

1 Use pictures or the word board
2 Have his family interpret for him
3 Practice stress management techniques
4 Remember that this is a temporary situation

Level of Cognitive Ability: Applying
Client Needs: Psychosocial Integrity
Clinical Judgment/Cognitive Skills: Take Action
Integrated Process: Communication and Documentation
Content Area: Foundations of Care: Communication
Health Problem: Mental Health: Coping

Answer: 1
Rationale: The client with an endotracheal tube in place cannot speak, and the nurse needs to devise an alternative communication system with the client. The use of a picture or word board is the simplest method of communication because it only requires the client to point at a word or object. Options 3 and 4 will not address the client's need to communicate effectively. Option 2 is not a reliable method for communication.
Priority Nursing Tip: Being able to communicate effectively is a basic need and must be addressed whenever possible.

Test-Taking Strategy: Focus on the **subject,** impaired communication. Options 3 and 4 do not address the client's need to communicate. Because the family may not necessarily know what the client is trying to communicate, option 2 could add to the client's frustration. Thus the picture or word board is the easiest and least frustrating method of communication for the client.

---

173. A client has been receiving the antidepressant protriptyline. The client demonstrates an understanding of the medication's expected effects when making what statements? **Select all that apply.**

❒ 1 "I expect that my appetite will improve."
❒ 2 "I will need to be careful because I may be drowsy."
❒ 3 "I'm looking forward to my memory improving."
❒ 4 "This medication is supposed to decrease anxiety as well."
❒ 5 "I'm told I'll have fewer delusional thoughts on the medication."

Level of Cognitive Ability: Evaluating
Client Needs: Psychosocial Integrity
Clinical Judgment/Cognitive Skills: Evaluate Outcomes
Integrated Process: Nursing Process/Evaluating
Content Area: Pharmacology/Psychotherapeutic: Tricyclic Antidepressants
Health Problem: Mental Health: Mood Disorders

Answer: 1, 4
Rationale: Protriptyline is an antidepressant used to treat various forms of depression and anxiety. Expected effects of the medication include improved appetite and a reduced level of anxiety. Drowsiness is a side effect, but the medication will not affect cognition or delusions.
Priority Nursing Tip: Antidepressants focus on the reduction of the symptoms of depression.

Test-Taking Strategy: Note the **data in the question** and focus on the **subject,** the expected effects of the medication. Eliminate option 2 because this is a side effect. Next, use knowledge about the medication and eliminate options 3 and 5 because the medication will not affect cognition or delusions.

---

174. A client with heart failure who develops a pleural effusion and is to undergo thoracentesis is afraid of not being able to tolerate the procedure. The nurse provides support and reassurance when making which response?

1 "I'll be right by your side, but the procedure will be painless as long as you don't move and stay still."
2 "The procedure takes only 1 to 2 minutes, so you might try to get through it by mentally counting up to 120."
3 "The insertion of the needle may be painful, but you need to remain still. I'll stay with you throughout the entire procedure to help you any way I can."
4 "The needle is uncomfortable going in, but the pain can be controlled by rhythmically breathing in and out. I'll be with you to coach your breathing."

Level of Cognitive Ability: Applying
Client Needs: Psychosocial Integrity
Clinical Judgment/Cognitive Skills: Take Action
Integrated Process: Communication and Documentation
Content Area: Adult Health: Cardiovascular
Health Problem: Adult Health: Cardiovascular: Heart Failure

Answer: 3
Rationale: The needle insertion for thoracentesis is painful for the client. The nurse tells the client how important it is to remain still during the procedure so that the needle does not injure visceral pleura or lung tissue. The procedure takes longer than 1 to 2 minutes and may take up to 1 hour, depending on the client's condition. The client may also need to hold his or her breath at certain points during the procedure. The nurse reassures the client during the procedure and helps the client hold the proper position.
Priority Nursing Tip: Thoracentesis is an invasive procedure to remove fluid or air from the pleural space for diagnostic or therapeutic purposes.

Test-Taking Strategy: Focus on the **subject,** thoracentesis. Specific knowledge of the procedure is needed to answer correctly. Recalling that thoracentesis is an invasive procedure may help to direct you to the correct option.

---

175. A client diagnosed with chronic respiratory failure responds to the resulting dyspnea with anxiety, which worsens the condition. The nurse teaches the client to **best** interrupt the dyspnea–anxiety–dyspnea cycle by encouraging what interventions? **Select all that apply.**

❒ 1 Relaxation
❒ 2 Distraction
❒ 3 Biofeedback
❒ 4 Guided imagery
❒ 5 Thought interruption

Level of Cognitive Ability: Applying
Client Needs: Psychosocial Integrity
Clinical Judgment/Cognitive Skills: Take Action
Integrated Process: Teaching and Learning
Content Area: Adult Health: Respiratory
Health Problem: Mental Health: Coping

Answer: 1, 2, 3, 4
Rationale: The anxious client with dyspnea would be taught interventions to decrease anxiety. These methods include relaxation, biofeedback, guided imagery, and distraction, and they will stop the escalation of feelings of dyspnea. Thought interruption is used to disrupt dysfunctional sensory perceptions such as command hallucinations.
Priority Nursing Tip: Fear and anxiety can be managed by using stress reduction techniques.

Test-Taking Strategy: Note the **strategic word,** *best.* Focus on the **subject,** interrupting the dyspnea–anxiety–dyspnea cycle. Select the techniques listed that are reliable methods of reducing stress and anxiety.

---

176. A client who has undergone the drainage of a pleural effusion is in pain. The nurse addresses this client's needs when implementing what interventions? **Select all that apply.**

- ❒ 1 Providing pain medication for the client
- ❒ 2 Offering verbal support and reassurance
- ❒ 3 Leaving the client alone to encourage rest
- ❒ 4 Assisting the client with finding positions of comfort
- ❒ 5 Reinforcing that the pain is only a temporary problem

Level of Cognitive Ability: Applying
Client Needs: Psychosocial Integrity
Clinical Judgment/Cognitive Skills: Take Action
Integrated Process: Caring
Content Area: Adult Health: Respiratory
Health Problem: Adult Health: Neurological: Pain

Answer: 1, 2, 4
Rationale: The pain associated with the drainage of a pleural effusion is minimized by positioning the client for comfort and administering analgesics for pain relief. The nurse also addresses the client's emotional pain by offering verbal support and understanding. It is not helpful to leave the client alone for extended periods, because the pain may be augmented by isolation. Stressing the temporary nature of the pain will not help the client manage the pain currently.
Priority Nursing Tip: Pleural effusion is excess fluid that accumulates in the pleural cavity, the fluid-filled space that surrounds the lungs. This excess can impair breathing by limiting the expansion of the lungs.

Test-Taking Strategy: Focus on the **subject,** interventions for pain management. Basic knowledge of pain management techniques and of the principles of nursing care will direct you to the correct options.

---

177. The nurse is caring for a client who has experienced a pulmonary embolism and is currently restless and anxious. The nurse uses which approach when communicating with this client?

1 Explaining each treatment in great detail
2 Giving simple, clear directions and explanations
3 Having the family reinforce the nurse's directions
4 Limiting communication until the client's emotions have stabilized

Level of Cognitive Ability: Applying
Client Needs: Psychosocial Integrity
Clinical Judgment/Cognitive Skills: Take Action
Integrated Process: Communication and Documentation
Content Area: Foundations of Care: Communication
Health Problem: Adult Health: Respiratory: Pulmonary Embolism

Answer: 2
Rationale: The client who has experienced a pulmonary embolism is fearful and apprehensive. The nurse effectively communicates with this client by staying with the client; providing simple, clear, and accurate information; and acting in a calm, efficient manner. Options 1, 3, and 4 will produce more anxiety for the client and the client's family.
Priority Nursing Tip: A pulmonary embolism (embolus) is a serious, potentially life-threatening condition. It is due to a blockage in a blood vessel in the lungs.

Test-Taking Strategy: Note the **data in the question** and focus on the subject, the client's response. Use **therapeutic communication techniques** to answer this question. Options 1 and 4 represent the least effective communication strategies and may be eliminated first. Having the family reinforce the directions may place stress on the family. The nurse gives simple, clear information to the client who is in distress.

---

178. The nurse is collecting data from an older widowed client admitted to the hospital with a hip fracture. Which data obtained by the nurse supports that the client is at risk for disturbed thought processes? **Select all that apply.**

- ❒ 1 Eyeglasses left at home
- ❒ 2 Hearing aid currently needs new batteries
- ❒ 3 Diagnosed with type 2 diabetes 2 years ago
- ❒ 4 Only child is out of the country on a business trip
- ❒ 5 Takes aspirin daily since experiencing a myocardial infarction last year

Level of Cognitive Ability: Analyzing
Client Needs: Psychosocial Integrity
Clinical Judgment/Cognitive Skills: Analyze Cues
Integrated Process: Nursing Process/Data Collection
Content Area: Mental Health
Health Problem: Mental Health: Neurocognitive Impairment

Answer: 1, 2, 4
Rationale: This client is at risk for confusion and disorientation as a result of dysfunctional hearing and vision. The lack of family contact may also contribute to the problem. The other options would present little risk for disturbed thought processes.
Priority Nursing Tip: Acute injuries and immobility issues can stress an older adult, causing episodes of confusion.

Test-Taking Strategy: Note the **data in the question.** The wording of the question asks you to look for the options that will increase the potential for confusion and disorientation. Keeping this in mind will assist in directing you to the correct options.

---

179. A client is admitted to the hospital after experiencing a traumatic below-the-knee amputation of the left foot. The client tells the nurse, "I think I'm going crazy. I can feel my left foot itching." What response demonstrates the nurse's understanding of the condition?

1. "This is a normal response; it's called phantom limb pain."
2. "These sensations are a response to the nerves that were damaged."
3. "It is normal to be in denial about traumatically losing a limb as you did."
4. "The trauma of your amputation will certainly require psychological support."

Level of Cognitive Ability: Applying
Client Needs: Psychosocial Integrity
Clinical Judgment/Cognitive Skills: Take Action
Integrated Process: Nursing Process/Implementation
Content Area: Adult Health: Musculoskeletal
Health Problem: Adult Health: Musculoskeletal: Amputation

Answer: 2
Rationale: Phantom limb sensations are felt in the area of the amputated limb and can include itching, warmth, and cold. The sensations are caused by intact peripheral nerves in the area that has been amputated. Whenever possible, clients would be prepared for these normal sensations. The client may also feel painful sensations in the amputated limb, which is called *phantom limb pain.* The origin of the pain is less understood, but, whenever possible, the client would also be prepared for this occurrence. These sensations do not present an abnormal or psychological problem.
Priority Nursing Tip: Many individuals with an amputation experience phantom sensations in their amputated limb, and the majority of the sensations are painful.

Test-Taking Strategy: Note the **data in the question.** Knowing that sensation and pain may be felt in the amputated limb helps you eliminate options 3 and 4 first because the sensations are not abnormal responses. Next note that the client is experiencing sensations, not pain. This will direct you to option 2. The correct option provides an explanation for the sensations the client is experiencing.

---

180. A client who has had a spinal fusion and the insertion of hardware is extremely concerned about the perceived lengthy rehabilitation period. The client expresses concerns about finances and the ability to return to prior employment. The nurse demonstrates an understanding of the client's needs when making which statement?

1 "Your surgeon should be made aware of your financial concerns."
2 "Let's consider requesting a social services consult to discuss these concerns."
3 "The physical therapist should be aware of ways to help speed up your recovery."
4 "The unit's clinical nurse specialist is prepared to help clients deal with these problems."

Level of Cognitive Ability: Applying
Client Needs: Psychosocial Integrity
Clinical Judgment/Cognitive Skills: Take Action
Integrated Process: Nursing Process/Implementation
Content Area: Adult Health: Musculoskeletal
Health Problem: Mental Health: Coping

Answer: 2

Rationale: After spinal surgery, concerns about finances and employment are best handled by referral to a social worker; this health care member is aware of the best information about resources available to the client. The physical therapist has knowledge of techniques for increasing mobility and endurance. An occupational therapist would have knowledge of techniques for activities of daily living and items related to occupation, but this is not one of the options. The clinical nurse specialist and surgeon are not the best resources for providing specific information related to financial resources.

Priority Nursing Tip: Spinal fusion is surgery to permanently connect two or more vertebrae in the spine, eliminating motion between them.

Test-Taking Strategy: Note the **data in the question.** An understanding of the roles of the various members of the health care team helps you answer this question. Focus on the **subject,** concern about finances; this will direct you to the social worker as the optimal resource in this situation.

---

181. A client is fearful about having an arm cast removed. The nurse supports the client by implementing which intervention?

1 Showing the client the cast cutter and explaining how it works
2 Educating the client to the fact that the saw makes a loud noise
3 Offering to stay with the client while the cast is being removed
4 Reassuring the client that the risk of being cut is minimal

Level of Cognitive Ability: Applying
Client Needs: Psychosocial Integrity
Clinical Judgment/Cognitive Skills: Take Action
Integrated Process: Nursing Process/Implementation
Content Area: Adult Health: Musculoskeletal
Health Problem: Mental Health: Coping

Answer: 1

Rationale: Because of misconceptions about the cast-cutting blade, clients may be fearful about having a cast removed. The nurse would show the cast cutter to the client before it is used and explain that the client may feel heat, vibration, and pressure. The remaining options do not fully address the client's concerns.

Priority Nursing Tip: Allowing an individual to have hands-on experience with procedural equipment often has an anxiety-reducing effect.

Test-Taking Strategy: Focus on the **subject,** client fears about cast removal. Option 3 provides no information to the client. Options 2 and 4 give accurate information but are not reassuring. The correct option gives the client the most reassurance because it best prepares the client for what will occur when the cast is removed.

---

182. A client admitted to the mental health unit with a diagnosis of panic disorder is prescribed a medication to depress the central nervous system and relax the client. The nurse will prepare educational information about which classification of medications?

1 A benzodiazepine
2 A tricyclic antidepressant
3 A monoamine oxidase inhibitor (MAOI)
4 A selective serotonin reuptake inhibitor (SSRI)

Level of Cognitive Ability: Applying
Client Needs: Psychosocial Integrity
Clinical Judgment/Cognitive Skills: Generate Solutions
Integrated Process: Nursing Process/Planning
Content Area: Pharmacology/Psychotherapeutics: Antianxiety/Anxiolytics
Health Problem: Mental Health: Anxiety Disorder

Answer: 1

Rationale: A benzodiazepine antianxiety agent depresses the central nervous system (CNS) and induces relaxation in clients with panic disorders. Options 2, 3, and 4 are classified as antidepressants and act by stimulating the CNS to elevate mood.

Priority Nursing Tip: A panic attack is the abrupt onset of intense fear or discomfort that reaches a peak within minutes and includes at least four of the following symptoms: palpitations, pounding heart, or accelerated heart rate; sweating; trembling or shaking; and sensations of shortness of breath or smothering.

Test-Taking Strategy: Focus on the **subject,** a medication that will depress the central nervous system and relax the client. Eliminate options 2, 3, and 4 because they are **comparable or alike** in that they are antidepressants.

---

183. A client scheduled for an implanted port for intermittent chemotherapy treatments says, "I'm not sure if I can handle having a tube coming out of me all the time. What will my friends think?" What intervention would the nurse implement to address the client's concern?

1 Notifies the oncologist of the client's concerns
2 Shows the client various central line tubes and catheters
3 Explains that an implanted port is not visible because it is under the skin
4 Reminds the client that his or her friends will not react negatively to the port

Level of Cognitive Ability: Applying
Client Needs: Psychosocial Integrity
Clinical Judgment/Cognitive Skills: Take Action
Integrated Process: Nursing Process/Implementation
Content Area: Foundations of Care: Communication
Health Problem: Mental Health: Therapeutic Communication

Answer: 3

Rationale: What the client says in this situation indicates that the client would be educated about the implanted port. An implanted port is placed under the skin and is not visible, and there is no visible tubing. Tubing is used only when the port is accessed intermittently and the intravenous line is connected. Showing the client various other tubes will not be beneficial because the client will not be using them. It is premature to notify the oncologist. It is inappropriate to make assurances that are not guaranteed.

Priority Nursing Tip: Chemotherapy can produce many fears for the person who needs to receive this treatment.

Test-Taking Strategy: Focus on the **data in the question** and on the **subject,** the client's concerns. Use knowledge about the physiology of an implanted port. Recalling that a port is placed under the skin will direct you to the correct option.

---

184. A client displays signs of anxiety because of pain resulting from an infiltration at an intravenous (IV) site. When preparing the client for required removal and reinsertion of the IV catheter, the nurse would make what statement?

1. "I'm sure you want this IV out."
2. "This will be a relatively painless experience. Just look out the window and relax. Don't worry."
3. "Just relax and take a deep breath. I'll stay with you while the RN inserts the new IV."
4. "I can see that you're anxious. The removal of the IV shouldn't be painful, but there will be some discomfort when the new catheter is inserted."

Level of Cognitive Ability: Applying
Client Needs: Psychosocial Integrity
Clinical Judgment/Cognitive Skills: Take Action
Integrated Process: Communication and Documentation
Content Area: Foundations of Care: Communication
Health Problem: Mental Health/Therapeutic Communication

Answer: 4

Rationale: Although discontinuing an IV line is a painless experience, it is not therapeutic to tell a client not to worry. Option 1 does not acknowledge the client's feelings and does not let the client know that an infiltrated IV line will need to be restarted. Option 3 does not address the client's feelings. The correct option addresses the client's anxiety and honestly informs the client that the IV line will need to be restarted. This option uses the therapeutic technique of giving information, and it also acknowledges the client's feelings.

Priority Nursing Tip: Signs and symptoms of infiltration include swelling, discomfort, burning, tightness, cool skin, and blanching.

Test-Taking Strategy: Note the **data in the question.** When answering communication questions, remember to use **therapeutic communication techniques.** The correct option is the only one that addresses the client's feelings.

---

185. A toddler with suspected conjunctivitis is crying and refuses to sit still during the eye examination. The nurse minimizes the child's resistance by making what statement?

1. "Would you like to see the flashlight?"
2. "Don't be scared. The light won't hurt you."
3. "If you will sit still, the exam will be over soon."
4. "I know you are upset. Will you let me do this exam later?"

Level of Cognitive Ability: Applying
Client Needs: Psychosocial Integrity
Clinical Judgment/Cognitive Skills: Take Action
Integrated Process: Developmental Stages: Toddler
Health Problem: Pediatric-Specific: Conjunctivitis

Answer: 1

Rationale: Fears in this age-group can be decreased by getting the child actively involved in the examination. Option 2 tells the child how to feel. Option 3 gives advice and ignores the child's feelings. Although option 4 acknowledges feelings, it puts off the inevitable.

Priority Nursing Tip: Distraction may be helpful in managing anxiety.

Test-Taking Strategy: Note the **data in the question** and that the child is a toddler. Using the child's developmental level and **therapeutic communication techniques** will direct you to the correct option.

186. A shy and timid client with acute pyelonephritis is scheduled for a voiding cystourethrogram. The nurse interprets that this client could **most likely** benefit from increased psychosocial support and teaching about what aspect of the procedure?

1 Radioactive contrast is injected into the bladder.
2 Radiopaque contrast is injected into the bloodstream.
3 The client must void while the micturition process is filmed.
4 The procedure requires lying on an x-ray table in a cold room.

Level of Cognitive Ability: Applying
Client Needs: Psychosocial Integrity
Clinical Judgment/Cognitive Skills: Recognize Cues
Integrated Process: Nursing Process/Planning
Content Area: Adult Health: Renal and Urinary
Health Problem: Adult Health: Renal and Urinary: Inflammation/Infections

Answer: 3
Rationale: Having to void in the presence of others can be very embarrassing for clients and may actually interfere with the client's ability to void. The other options are not as likely to embarrass the client.
Priority Nursing Tip: A voiding cystourethrogram is a test done to examine the bladder and urethra while the bladder fills and empties.

Test-Taking Strategy: Note the **strategic words,** *most likely.* Note the **data in the question.** Begin to answer this question by eliminating options 1 and 2, because the contrast material is inserted into the bladder with a catheter. From the remaining options, it is necessary to know that the client has to void to allow for the filming of the movement of urine through the lower urinary tract.

---

187. A client in a manic state exits her room topless and begins making sexual remarks and gestures toward the staff and her peers. What is the **initial** nursing action to manage this situation?

1 Quietly approach the client, escort her to her room, and assist her with getting dressed.
2 Confront the client about the inappropriateness of her behavior and offer her a time-out in seclusion.
3 Approach the client, cover her with a blanket, and insist that she go to her room immediately.
4 Ask the other clients to go to their rooms while calmly discussing her behavior after providing her with a shirt.

Level of Cognitive Ability: Applying
Client Needs: Psychosocial Integrity
Clinical Judgment/Cognitive Skills: Take Action
Integrated Process: Nursing Process/Implementation
Content Area: Mental Health
Health Problem: Mental Health/Mood Disorders

Answer: 1
Rationale: A person who is experiencing mania lacks insight and judgment, has poor impulse control, and is highly excitable. The nurse must take control without creating increased stress or anxiety in the client. A quiet, firm approach while distracting the client (i.e., walking her to her room and assisting her with dressing) achieves the goals of having the client dressed appropriately and preserving her psychosocial integrity. Options 2, 3, and 4 are inappropriate actions because the client's needs are not focused upon.
Priority Nursing Tip: The immediate needs for which the nurse is responsible are milieu management and client safety.

Test-Taking Strategy: Note the **strategic word,** *initial,* and the **data in the question.** The goal of the interaction is to provide the milieu and the client with a safe environment. Insisting that the client go to her room may be met with a great deal of resistance. Confronting the client and offering her a consequence of a time-out may be meaningless to her.

---

188. A client who had cardiac surgery and his family express anxiety regarding how to cope with the recuperative process after discharge and without the support of the staff. The nurse provides information regarding which available resource?

1 The United Way
2 The local library
3 The local caregivers support group
4 The American Heart Association Mended Hearts Club

Level of Cognitive Ability: Applying
Client Needs: Psychosocial Integrity
Clinical Judgment/Cognitive Skills: Take Action
Integrated Process: Nursing Process/Planning
Content Area: Adult Health: Cardiovascular
Health Problem: Mental Health: Coping

Answer: 4

Rationale: Most clients and families benefit from knowing that there are available resources to help them cope with the stress of self-care management at home. These can include telephone contact with the surgeon, the cardiologist, and the nurse; cardiac rehabilitation programs; and community support groups such as the American Heart Association Mended Hearts Club, which is a nationwide program with local chapters. The United Way provides resources for clients with various disorders and is not specific to the client with a cardiac problem. The local caregivers support group is not focused on client care, but rather the needs of the caregivers. The local library provides resources but does not provide support via an interactive process.

Priority Nursing Tip: Providing information on appropriate care resources is a nursing responsibility.

Test-Taking Strategy: Focus on the **data in the question.** Of the four options, three list organizations and one lists a library. Eliminate the library first because the client and family need resources for coping, which implies the need for an interactive process. From the remaining options, focusing on the type of surgery addressed in the question will direct you to the correct option.

---

189. A client diagnosed with obsessive-compulsive disorder is upset and agitated and repeatedly paces the unit for hours each night, following the same route each time. When the client asks, "Will you walk with me?" how would the nurse respond to **best** meet the client's needs?

1 "I will walk with you, and we can talk if you want."
2 "No, it is bedtime. Let me walk you back to your room."
3 "Go to sleep now. We can talk together tomorrow afternoon."
4 "I'm sorry, I can't. But I will get someone else to walk with you."

Level of Cognitive Ability: Applying
Client Needs: Psychosocial Integrity
Clinical Judgment/Cognitive Skills: Take Action
Integrated Process: Communication and Documentation
Content Area: Mental Health
Health Problem: Mental Health: OCD

Answer: 1

Rationale: The response in the correct option acknowledges the client's feelings and provides an avenue for a release of the client's anxieties. Each of the incorrect options represents a block to communication. The wording in each of these responses does not indicate that the client is valued, nor does it acknowledge the client's feelings.

Priority Nursing Tip: Joining in client-initiated activities if asked is a useful communication technique.

Test-Taking Strategy: Note the **strategic word,** ***best.*** Use **therapeutic communication techniques.** Eliminate each of the incorrect options because they do not deal with the client's concerns or promote further communication. Remember that the client's feelings need to be addressed first.

---

190. A client with superficial varicose veins says to the nurse, "I hate these things. They're so ugly. I wish I could get them to go away." To **best** meet the client's concerns, how would the nurse respond?

1 "You need to try sclerotherapy. It's really helpful."
2 "There's not much you can do after you get them."
3 "I understand how you feel, but they really don't look too bad."
4 "What have you been told about varicose veins and their management?"

Level of Cognitive Ability: Applying
Client Needs: Psychosocial Integrity
Clinical Judgment/Cognitive Skills: Take Action
Integrated Process: Communication and Documentation
Content Area: Adult Health: Cardiovascular
Health Problem: Mental Health: Therapeutic Communication

Answer: 4

Rationale: The client is expressing distress about their physical appearance and has a risk for body image disturbance. The nurse collects data regarding what the client has been told. Options 1, 2, and 3 are nontherapeutic responses because they tend to minimize the client's concerns or to offer advice.

Priority Nursing Tip: Determining the extent of an individual's knowledge on a particular subject is an appropriate initial intervention.

Test-Taking Strategy: Note the **strategic word,** *best.* Use the **steps of the nursing process** and **therapeutic communication techniques** to answer the question; this will direct you to the correct option. Remember that data collection is the first step of the nursing process.

---

191. A client who has been diagnosed with chronic kidney disease has been told that hemodialysis will be required. The client becomes angry and states, "I'll never be the same now." The nurse bases further care on the fact that the client is demonstrating what emotional response?

1 Fear
2 Anxiety
3 Depression
4 Disturbed body image

Level of Cognitive Ability: Analyzing
Client Needs: Psychosocial Integrity
Clinical Judgment/Cognitive Skills: Recognize Cues
Integrated Process: Nursing Process/Planning
Content Area: Adult Health: Renal and Urinary
Health Problem: Adult Health: Renal and Urinary: Chronic Kidney Disease

Answer: 4

Rationale: The client with renal failure may become angry because of the need for dialysis and the permanence of the alteration. Because of the physical change and the change in lifestyle that may be required to manage a severe renal condition, the client may experience body image disturbance. Although options 1, 2, and 3 may occur, these problems are not associated with the data in the question.

Priority Nursing Tip: Changes to one's body can result in a disturbance in one's perception of body image.

Test-Taking Strategy: Note the **data in the question,** especially the client's statement, *I'll never be the same now.* Note that the client's statement focuses on the self, which is consistent with a disturbance in body image; this will direct you to the correct option.

---

192. The nurse observes that a client who is recovering from a myocardial infarction (MI) is crying silently. The nurse explores the client's feelings by implementing what intervention?

1 Spending time merely sitting quietly by the client
2 Assuring the client that the condition will improve
3 Distracting the client by discussing the news of the day
4 Encouraging family members to visit the client frequently

Answer: 1

Rationale: Sitting quietly by the client conveys caring and acceptance. The remaining options do not address the client's feelings and instead ignore the client's behavior.

Priority Nursing Tip: Spending time with the client, even when verbal communication does not occur, can be beneficial to the client.

Test-Taking Strategy: Focus on the **subject,** the client's behaviors. Use **therapeutic communication techniques** to answer this question. Options 2, 3, and 4 can be easily eliminated because they ignore the client's feelings. The correct option conveys caring and acceptance.

Level of Cognitive Ability: Applying
Client Needs: Psychosocial Integrity
Clinical Judgment/Cognitive Skills: Take Action
Integrated Process: Caring
Content Area: Adult Health: Cardiovascular
Health Problem: Mental Health: Therapeutic Communication

---

193. The nurse caring for a client with newly diagnosed diabetes mellitus is assisting with developing a teaching plan. The nurse addresses which client situation **initially**?

1 Fear of administering insulin
2 Knowledge of the diabetic diet
3 Denial regarding having diabetes
4 Depression regarding lifestyle changes

Answer: 3

Rationale: When diabetes mellitus is diagnosed, the client will usually go through the phases of grief, including denial, fear, anger, bargaining, depression, and acceptance. Denial is the phase that is the most detrimental to the teaching and learning process. If the client is denying the fact that he or she has diabetes mellitus, then he or she probably will not listen to discussions about the disease or how to manage it. Denial must be identified before the nurse can develop a teaching plan.

Priority Nursing Tip: Acceptance of a situation is the initial step in managing the situation.

Test-Taking Strategy: Note the **strategic word,** *initially.* All of the options may be appropriate; however, note that options 1, 2, and 4 are related to very specific components of teaching. The correct option is the **umbrella option,** and, considering the principles of teaching and learning, this aspect needs to be determined before teaching begins.

Level of Cognitive Ability: Analyzing
Client Needs: Psychosocial Integrity
Clinical Judgment/Cognitive Skills: Generate Solutions
Integrated Process: Nursing Process/Planning
Content Area: Adult Health: Endocrine
Health Problem: Adult Health: Endocrine: Diabetes Mellitus

---

194. The nurse reinforcing teaching with a client taking conjugated estrogen would plan to address which psychosocial issue related to the medication?

1 The client needs to notify the primary health care provider if migraine headaches occur.
2 Estrogen should be used with caution by individuals with a family history of breast or reproductive cancer.

Answer: 3

Rationale: Conjugated estrogen can cause changes in client affect, mood, and behavior. Aggression, depression, or both can also occur. All the remaining options are correct but address physiological needs. Option 3 is the only psychosocial need noted.

Priority Nursing Tip: Medication therapy can result in both physical and/or psychosocial side effects.

3 The medication may cause mood and affect changes, and may need to be discontinued if depression occurs.
4 Hyperglycemia is a possible side effect, and the client would be informed about signs and symptoms to report to the primary health care provider.

Level of Cognitive Ability: Applying
Client Needs: Psychosocial Integrity
Clinical Judgment/Cognitive Skills:
Integrated Process: Nursing Process/Implementation
Content Area: Pharmacology: Endocrine: Androgens, Estrogens, Progestins
Health Problem: Mental Health: Mood Disorders

Test-Taking Strategy: Note the **data in the question** while also noting the word *psychosocial.* Eliminate options 1, 2, and 4 because they are **comparable or alike** and address physiological issues.

---

195. A client with newly diagnosed diabetes mellitus has been seen in the clinic for 3 consecutive days with the symptomatology of hyperglycemia. The client says to the nurse, "I'm sorry to keep bothering you every day, but I just can't give myself those awful shots." What response will address the client's needs?

1 "I would find it hard to give myself a shot, too."
2 "You must learn to give yourself the insulin shots."
3 "Let me see if the doctor can change your medication."
4 "I'm sorry you are having trouble, so let's discuss the problem."

Level of Cognitive Ability: Applying
Client Needs: Psychosocial Integrity
Clinical Judgment/Cognitive Skills: Take Action
Integrated Process: Communication and Documentation
Content Area: Adult Health: Endocrine
Health Problem: Adult Health: Endocrine: Diabetes Mellitus

Answer: 4
Rationale: It is important to determine and deal with a client's underlying fear of self-injection. The nurse would determine whether a client needs additional instructions. Positive reinforcement is necessary instead of focusing on negative behaviors (option 1). Scare tactics (option 2) would not be used. The nurse would not offer a change in regimen that cannot be accomplished (option 3).
Priority Nursing Tip: Fear can be the unconscious cause of an individual's inability to perform necessary self-care.

Test-Taking Strategy: Use **therapeutic communication techniques,** and focus on the **subject,** needed adherence to insulin therapy. Options 1 and 2 are nontherapeutic because they fail to address the concern, and option 3 may give false reassurance about a change in medication. The correct option focuses on the subject and is the therapeutic response.

---

196. The nurse asks a client diagnosed with diabetes mellitus to have a family member attend an educational conference about the self-administration of insulin. When asked why that is necessary, how would the nurse respond to **best** describe the role of family in client care?

1 "Family members are at a high risk of developing diabetes."
2 "Family members can take over giving you your shots when necessary."
3 "Families often work together to develop strategies for the management of diabetes."
4 "Nurses need someone familiar with your condition to call to check on your progress."

Level of Cognitive Ability: Applying
Client Needs: Psychosocial Integrity
Clinical Judgment/Cognitive Skills: Take Action
Integrated Process: Nursing Process/Implementation
Content Area: Skills: Client Teaching
Health Problem: Adult Health: Endocrine: Diabetes Mellitus

Answer: 3
Rationale: Families or significant others may be included in diabetes education to assist with adjustment to the diabetic regimen. Although options 1 and 2 may be accurate, they are not the most appropriate response in relation to the subject of the question. Option 4 devalues the client, disregards the subject of independence, and promotes powerlessness.
Priority Nursing Tip: Clients benefit when their support system includes caring family members.

Test-Taking Strategy: Note the **strategic word,** *best.* Use **therapeutic communication techniques.** The correct option involves a collaborative response and addresses the client's question.

---

197. A young adult client has recently been diagnosed with polycystic kidney disease (PKD). The nurse assists in planning a series of discussions with the client that are intended to help with adjustment to the disorder. The nurse plans to include information on which psychosocial issue?

1 Ongoing fluid restriction
2 Need for genetic counseling
3 Risk for hypotensive episodes
4 Depression regarding massive edema

Level of Cognitive Ability: Applying
Client Needs: Psychosocial Integrity
Clinical Judgment/Cognitive Skills: Generate Solutions
Integrated Process: Nursing Process/Planning
Content Area: Adult Health: Renal and Urinary
Health Problem: Adult Health: Renal and Urinary: Hereditary Diseases

Answer: 2
Rationale: Adult PKD is a hereditary disorder that is inherited as an autosomal-dominant trait. Because of this, the client and the extended family would have genetic counseling. The remaining issues are not psychosocial in nature.
Priority Nursing Tip: PKD is an inherited disorder in which clusters of cysts develop primarily within the kidneys, causing the kidneys to enlarge and lose function over time.

Test-Taking Strategy: Focus on the **subject,** psychosocial issues related to PKD. Because massive edema and the need for fluid restriction are not part of the clinical picture of the client with PKD, options 1 and 4 are eliminated first. From the remaining options, you would need to know either that this disorder is hereditary in nature or that the client would exhibit hypertension rather than hypotension. Also note that options 1, 3, and 4 are **comparable or alike** and are physiological issues.

---

198. The nurse is caring for an older adult client diagnosed with mild depression. The client asks, "What do you think I need to do about my home? My son thinks I need to sell it and move into something smaller now that I'm alone." How would the nurse respond to **best** support the client in the decision-making process?

1 "That is a decision only you can make."
2 "I agree with your son. As you age, you will find that smaller, one-floor living is best."
3 "What would you like to do? As your depression lifts, you'll be more able to decide what's best for you."
4 "Why not wait until you're feeling less depressed to make such an important decision? You've only been taking your medication for a few months."

Level of Cognitive Ability: Applying
Client Needs: Psychosocial Integrity
Clinical Judgment/Cognitive Skills: Take Action
Integrated Process: Communication and Documentation
Content Area: Mental Health
Health Problem: Mental Health: Therapeutic Communication

Answer: 3
Rationale: The therapeutic response is the one that encourages the client to make his or her own decisions. This approach provides the client with a sense of personal empowerment that will relieve his or her powerlessness. If the client is moderately or severely depressed, decision making is difficult. Option 1 is incorrect because the nurse provides a social response rather than a therapeutic one, which may undermine the client's confidence, sense of support, and mutuality. Option 2 is incorrect because the nurse agrees with the client's son and makes a judgment, which is unprofessional and nontherapeutic. Option 4 is incorrect because the nurse provides procrastination and avoidance as models for problem solving.
Priority Nursing Tip: The older adult experiencing acute or chronic illness is faced with many difficult decisions that can be overwhelming.

Test-Taking Strategy: Note the **strategic word,** ***best.*** Note the **data in the question,** and use **therapeutic communication techniques** that focus on the client's feelings and concerns. The correct option addresses the client's concerns directly.

---

199. A terminally ill client's spouse says to the nurse, "I don't think I can come anymore and watch her die. It's chewing me up too much!" How would the nurse respond to address the spouse's needs?

1 "I know it's hard for you, but she would know if you're not there, and you'd feel guilty all the rest of your days."
2 "I think you're making the right decision. Your wife knows you love her. You don't have to come. I'll take care of her."
3 "It's hard to watch someone you love die. You've been here with your wife every day. Are you taking any time for yourself?"
4 "I wish you'd focus on your wife's pain rather than yours. I know it's hard, but this isn't about what's happening to you, you know."

Level of Cognitive Ability: Applying
Client Needs: Psychosocial Integrity
Clinical Judgment/Cognitive Skills: Take Action
Integrated Process: Caring
Content Area: Foundations of Care: Communication
Health Problem: Mental Health: Therapeutic Communication

Answer: 3
Rationale: The husband is the subject of this question. The therapeutic response is the one that reflects the nurse's understanding of the husband's stress and emotional pain. Option 1 makes a statement that the nurse cannot know is true (the wife may in fact not know whether the husband visits), and predicting feelings of guilt is inappropriate. Option 2 is inappropriate because it fosters dependency and gives advice, which is nontherapeutic. Option 4 is an example of a nontherapeutic and judgmental attitude.
Priority Nursing Tip: Those experiencing the loss of loved ones generally experience many stressors that benefit from the caring attention of others.

Test-Taking Strategy: Note the **client of the question,** the spouse, and use **therapeutic communication techniques** to address the spouse. The correct option is the only one that addresses the spouse's feelings.

---

200. An older client at a retirement center spits out food and throws it on the floor during a Thanksgiving dinner in the community dining room. The client yells, "This turkey is dry and cold! I can't stand the food here!" How would the nurse respond to **best** address the client's behavior?

1. "Please don't ruin this celebration for yourself and everyone else."
2. "Holidays can be hard. Let's go to the kitchen and get food that is more to your liking."
3. "I think you had better return to your apartment, where a new meal will be served to you."
4. "One of the things that the residents of this group agreed on was that anyone who did not use appropriate behavior would be asked to leave the dining room."

Level of Cognitive Ability: Applying
Client Needs: Psychosocial Integrity
Clinical Judgment/Cognitive Skills: Take Action
Integrated Process: Communication and Documentation
Content Area: Foundations of Care/Communication
Health Problem: Mental Health: Therapeutic Communication

Answer: 2
Rationale: The therapeutic response identifies that the client's behavior stems from some troubled feelings with which the client is struggling. Option 1 is an angry, aggressive, nontherapeutic response, and it is humiliating to the client. Option 3 could provoke a regressive struggle between the nurse and client and cause more explosive behavior on the client's part. In option 4, the nurse is authoritative, but trying to expel the client would be inappropriate, and it might set up an aggressive struggle between the nurse and the client. Asking the client to accompany the nurse to the kitchen respects the client's need for control, removes the angry client from the dining room, and may offer the nurse an opportunity to identify what is happening to the client.
Priority Nursing Tip: Respect shown to and by the nurse is a critical element of therapeutic communication.

Test-Taking Strategy: Note the **strategic word,** *best.* Use **therapeutic communication techniques.** The correct option is the only one that focuses on the client's feelings.

---

201. An older adult client diagnosed with emphysema is at a primary health care provider's office for a follow-up visit. When the client is found smoking at the front door of the office complex, how would the nurse respond to **best** meet the client's needs?

1. "Well, I can see you never got to the stop-smoking clinic."
2. "I'm glad I caught you smoking. Now let's decide what you are going to do to stop."
3. "Do you realize that you are making your respiratory problems even more severe by smoking?"
4. "I notice that you are smoking. Did you explore the stop-smoking program at the senior citizens' center?"

Level of Cognitive Ability: Applying
Client Needs: Psychosocial Integrity
Clinical Judgment/Cognitive Skills: Take Action
Integrated Process: Communication and Documentation
Content Area: Adult Health: Respiratory
Health Problem: Adult Health: Respiratory: Obstructive Pulmonary Disease

Answer: 4
Rationale: The correct option places the decision making in the client's hands and provides an avenue for the client to share what may be expressions of frustration at an inability to stop what is essentially a physiological addiction. Option 1 is a disciplinary and sarcastic remark that places a barrier between the nurse and client within the therapeutic relationship. Option 2 is preachy and judgmental, and it is an example of a countertransference issue for the nurse. Option 3 is a preachy statement that demeans the client.
Priority Nursing Tip: Even if emphysema is at an incurable point, quitting smoking can still improve one's quality of life.

Test-Taking Strategy: Note the **strategic word,** *best.* Use your knowledge of **therapeutic communication techniques** and how they can help a client make adaptive decisions about health. The correct option encourages the client to discuss the problem further and explore ways to manage the smoking. All the remaining options are accusatory and unlikely to encourage discussions.

---

202. A client is to have blood drawn to test arterial blood gas levels. While the respiratory therapist is performing an Allen's test, the client says to the nurse, "What is he doing? No one else has done that!" On the basis of the understanding of this test, the nurse would make which appropriate response to the client?

1 "I assure you that this is the correct procedure. I cannot account for what others do."
2 "This step is crucial to safe blood withdrawal. I would not let anyone take my blood until they did this."
3 "This is a routine precautionary step that makes sure that your circulation is intact before a blood sample is obtained."
4 "Oh, you have questions about this? You should insist that everyone do this procedure before drawing your blood."

Answer: 3

Rationale: Allen's test is performed to assess collateral circulation in the hand before blood is drawn from an artery. The nurse's most therapeutic response gives information. Option 1 is defensive and nontherapeutic in that it offers false reassurance. Option 2 demonstrates client advocacy that is overly controlling, quite aggressive, and undermining of treatment. Option 4 is aggressive, controlling, and nontherapeutic with its disapproving stance.

Priority Nursing Tip: A positive Allen's test shows that the client does not have a dual blood supply to the hand, which is a negative indication for using the radial arteries.

Test-Taking Strategy: Focus on the **data in the question** and use **therapeutic communication techniques** to address the client's concerns. The correct option is the only therapeutic response, and it provides information to the client.

Level of Cognitive Ability: Applying
Client Needs: Psychosocial Integrity
Clinical Judgment/Cognitive Skills: Take Action
Integrated Process: Communication and Documentation
Content Area: Foundations of Care: Diagnostic Tests
Health Problem: Mental Health: Therapeutic Communication

---

203. A client reports difficulty in concentrating, outbursts of anger, inability to sleep, and constantly feeling "keyed up." The nurse obtaining data from the client discovers that the symptoms started about 6 months ago after the client was involved in a serious auto accident. The nurse would institute which intervention **initially** to address the client's needs?

1 Isolate the client to his or her room until a psychiatric evaluation is obtained.
2 Educate the client in various adaptive coping mechanisms to deal with anxiety.
3 Evaluate the client's precipitating event(s) and gradually introduce the client to the event(s).
4 Distract the client when he feels "keyed up" to avoid outbursts of anger.

Answer: 2

Rationale: The client's history and symptomatology suggest the presence of post-traumatic stress disorder (PTSD). The client would be educated on various adaptive coping mechanisms to deal with the anxiety effectively. None of the remaining options address the client's immediate needs for anxiety management.

Priority Nursing Tip: The term *adaptive coping mechanism* generally refers to constructive (helpful) coping strategies that tend to reduce stress. In contrast, other coping strategies may be known as maladaptive if they increase stress.

Level of Cognitive Ability: Applying
Client Needs: Psychosocial Integrity
Clinical Judgment/Cognitive Skills: Take Action
Integrated Process: Nursing Process/Implementation
Content Area: Mental Health
Health Problem: Mental Health: Post-Traumatic Stress Disorder

Test-Taking Strategy: Note the **strategic word,** *initially.* Focus on the **data in the question** to determine that the client is experiencing PTSD, and use your knowledge of PTSD to identify the appropriate intervention to manage the client's signs and symptoms.

---

204. A client who is very demanding says to the nurse, "I can't get any help with my care! I call and call, but the nurses never answer my light. Last night one of them told me their were other clients besides me! I'm very sick, but the nurses don't care!" To **best** meet the client's needs, how would the nurse respond?

1 "I'm so sorry this happened to you. Do you want to report the nurse?"
2 "The nurses work very hard and usually come as quickly as they can."
3 "Is it hard for you to be unable to get out of bed and have to ask for help?"
4 "I can hear your anger. That nurse had no right to speak to you that way. It won't happen again."

Level of Cognitive Ability: Applying
Client Needs: Psychosocial Integrity
Clinical Judgment/Cognitive Skills: Take Action
Integrated Process: Communication and Documentation
Content Area: Foundations of Care: Communication
Health Problem: Mental Health: Therapeutic Communication

Answer: 3
Rationale: In the correct option, the nurse displays empathy as she shares her perceptions. Sharing perceptions asks the client to validate the nurse's understanding of what the client is feeling and thinking. It opens the door for the client to share concerns, fears, and anxieties. Option 1 is sympathetic but inappropriate because of the negative comment about another nurse. In option 2, the nurse is assertive and defends the nursing staff without validating the client. In option 4, the nurse expresses the client's frustration by labeling the client's feelings as angry and disapproving of the nursing staff.
Priority Nursing Tip: Feeling helpless is a very stressful emotion for most individuals.

Test-Taking Strategy: Note the **strategic word,** *best.* Use **therapeutic communication techniques** and note the **data in the question.** The correct option is the only one that encourages the client to express feelings.

---

205. The nurse caring for a hospitalized client with an alcohol abuse disorder is reviewing the client's discharge outcomes. Which statement made by the client indicates the **most** positive outcome regarding the client's prognosis?

1 "I'll start an exercise program."
2 "I'm going to take a biofeedback class."
3 "I'll stop drinking with friends after work."
4 "I'll continue to attend Alcoholics Anonymous meetings."

Level of Cognitive Ability: Evaluating
Client Needs: Psychosocial Integrity
Clinical Judgment/Cognitive Skills: Evaluate Outcomes
Integrated Process: Nursing Process/Evaluation
Content Area: Mental Health
Health Problem: Mental Health: Addictions

Answer: 4
Rationale: All of the outcomes deserve support by the nurse, but the correct option, which will help the client abstain from alcohol and provide the client with a support group, is the most positive outcome.
Priority Nursing Tip: The most positive outcome is one that supports behaviors that the client needs to adopt.

Test-Taking Strategy: Note the strategic word, *most.* Focus on the subject, the most positive outcome. From the options presented, the correct option directly addresses the client's disorder. Alcoholics Anonymous has the greatest potential to provide impulse control.

206. A client has a long leg cast applied after fracturing his right proximal tibia. During rounds that night, the nurse finds the client restless, withdrawn, and quiet. Which **initial** statement by the nurse is appropriate when considering therapeutic communication techniques?

1 "Are you uncomfortable?"
2 "Tell me what you are feeling."
3 "Do you need pain medication?"
4 "You'll feel better in the morning."

Level of Cognitive Ability: Applying
Client Needs: Psychosocial Integrity
Clinical Judgment/Cognitive Skills: Take Action
Integrated Process: Communication and Documentation
Content Area: Foundations of Care: Communication
Health Problem: Mental Health: Therapeutic Communication

Answer: 2
Rationale: The correct option is an open-ended statement and makes no assumptions about the client's physiological or emotional state. Options 1 and 3 are incorrect because these options do not elicit all needed information when assessing pain. False reassurance is never therapeutic, which makes option 4 incorrect.
Priority Nursing Tip: Therapeutic communication between nurse and client must be conducted in a sensitive manner to achieve appropriate client care outcomes.

Test-Taking Strategy: Focus on the **data in the question** and the **strategic word,** *initial.* Use **therapeutic communication techniques** to direct you to option 2. Remember to focus on the client's feelings.

---

207. An intermittently confused client started on oral anticoagulant therapy while hospitalized to treat atrial fibrillation is now being discharged to home. The nurse determines that the client will have the **best** support system for successful anticoagulant therapy monitoring when what intervention has been implemented?

1 Having a home health aide coming to the house for 9 weeks
2 Accepting her daughter and son-in-law's offer to live with them
3 Arranging for required blood work to be drawn in the home by a local laboratory
4 Paying a good friend who lives next door to take the client to follow-up appointments

Level of Cognitive Ability: Evaluating
Client Needs: Psychosocial Integrity
Clinical Judgment/Cognitive Skills: Evaluate Outcomes
Integrated Process: Nursing Process/Evaluation
Content Area: Adult Health: Cardiovascular
Health Problem: Adult Health: Cardiovascular: Dysrhythmias

Answer: 2
Rationale: Successful anticoagulant therapy has three components: taking the medication properly, having proper follow-up medical care, and doing serial follow-up blood work. Option 1 facilitates only reminding the client to take the medication, option 3 facilitates only blood work, and option 4 facilitates only medical care. The client who is intermittently confused may need support systems in place to enhance adherence to therapy. The correct option presents the most comprehensive support system.
Priority Nursing Tip: The care of cognitively impaired individuals is best handled by prepared, loving family members whenever possible.

Test-Taking Strategy: Note the **strategic word,** *best,* and focus on the **subject,** the best support system for the client; this will direct you to the option that is most comprehensive.

---

208. A client who has undergone successful femoral-popliteal bypass grafting to the leg says to the nurse, "I hope everything goes well after this and that I don't lose my leg. I'm so afraid that I'll have gone through this for nothing." The nurse presents the **most appropriate** response to the client's concerns when making what statement?

1 "I can understand what you mean. I'd be nervous, too, if I were you."
2 "This surgery is so successful that I wouldn't be concerned if I were you."
3 "Stress isn't helpful for you. You need to just relax and try not to worry unless something actually happens."
4 "Complications are possible, but you have a good deal of control if you make the lifestyle adjustments we talked about."

Level of Cognitive Ability: Applying
Client Needs: Psychosocial Integrity
Clinical Judgment/Cognitive Skills: Take Action
Integrated Process: Communication and Documentation
Content Area: Adult Health: Cardiovascular
Health Problem: Adult Health: Cardiovascular: Vascular Disorders

Answer: 4
Rationale: Clients frequently fear that they will ultimately lose a limb or become debilitated in some other way. The correct option has the nurse reassuring the client that participation in exercise, diet, and medication therapy, along with smoking cessation, can limit further plaque development. Option 1 feeds into the client's anxiety and is nontherapeutic. Option 2 gives false reassurance, which is incorrect. Option 3 is meant to be reassuring but offers no suggestions to empower the client.
Priority Nursing Tip: Intermittent claudication, the most common symptom of peripheral arterial disease, results from gradual narrowing of a leg artery. It is a painful, aching, cramping, or tired feeling in the muscles of the leg.

Test-Taking Strategy: Note the **strategic words,** *most appropriate.* Focus on the **data in the question,** and use **therapeutic communication techniques** to address the client's concerns. The correct option acknowledges the client's concerns and empowers the client to improve health, which will ultimately reduce concern about the risk of complications.

---

209. A client is scheduled to undergo pericardiocentesis for pericardial effusion. The nurse plans to alleviate the client's apprehension by implementing what intervention?

1 Encouraging the client to watch television during the procedure as a distraction
2 Talking to the client from the foot of the bed so as to be available to get added supplies
3 Staying beside the client and giving information and encouragement during the procedure
4 Promising to be available to the client when the procedure is complete

Level of Cognitive Ability: Applying
Client Needs: Psychosocial Integrity
Clinical Judgment/Cognitive Skills: Take Action
Integrated Process: Nursing Process/Implementation
Content Area: Adult Health: Cardiovascular
Health Problem: Mental Health: Coping

Answer: 3
Rationale: Staying with the client and giving information and encouragement is most supportive to the client who is apprehensive about a procedure. Options 1 and 2 distance the nurse from a client in the psychosocial as well as the physical sense. It is nontherapeutic to make promises to a client.
Priority Nursing Tip: Providing appropriate physical contact and support is a nursing responsibility.

Test-Taking Strategy: Focus on the **subject,** providing the client with the necessary support during the procedure. Remembering that providing support to the client includes both physical and emotional interventions will direct you to the correct option. Also note that the incorrect options distance the client from the nurse.

210. An adolescent is hospitalized for the evaluation and treatment of Tourette's syndrome. Which statements from the family support the presence of the manifestations of this disorder? **Select all that apply.**

- ❒ 1 "My brother makes grunting sounds for no reason."
- ❒ 2 "My son is very conscious that his tongue often protrudes."
- ❒ 3 "Rhyming speech is often the way my grandson talks to us."
- ❒ 4 "We've been told his habit of repeating what I say is called echolalia."
- ❒ 5 "You'll notice my brother has a habit of involuntarily blinking his eye often."

Level of Cognitive Ability: Evaluating
Client Needs: Psychosocial Integrity
Clinical Judgment/Cognitive Skills: Analyze Cues
Integrated Process: Nursing Process/Data Collection
Content Area: Mental Health
Health Problem: Mental Health: Neurocognitive Impairment

Answer: 1, 2, 4, 5

Rationale: Tourette's syndrome involves motor and verbal tics that can cause marked distress and significant impairment in a client's social and occupational functioning. Individuals with this disorder may experience different symptoms. Motor tics usually involve the head but can also involve the torso and limbs. The most frequent first symptom is a single tic such as eye blinking. Other motor tics include tongue protrusion, touching, squatting, hopping, skipping, retracing steps, and twirling when walking. Vocal tics include words and sounds such as barks, grunts, yelps, clicks, snorts, sniffs, and coughs. Rhyming speech is not associated with Tourette's syndrome.

Priority Nursing Tip: Tourette's syndrome involves involuntary vocal and muscular symptoms and often includes compulsive utterances of obscenities.

Test-Taking Strategy: Focus on the **subject,** the manifestations of Tourette's syndrome. It is necessary to understand this disorder and its manifestations to answer correctly. Thinking about its psychophysiology and pathophysiology will assist in answering correctly.

---

211. The nurse is planning to reinforce education with a hospitalized client who is recovering from the signs and symptoms of autonomic dysreflexia. The nurse initiates the conversation with what statement?

1 "It's unfortunate that this happened because it is preventable."
2 "Now that this problem is taken care of, I'm sure you'll be fine."
3 "I have time and I'd like to talk with you about what happened to you."
4 "I want to be sure you understand the importance of preventing this from occurring."

Level of Cognitive Ability: Applying
Client Needs: Psychosocial Integrity
Clinical Judgment/Cognitive Skills: Take Action
Integrated Process: Communication and Documentation
Content Area: Adult Health: Neurological
Health Problem: Adult Health: Neurological: Spinal Cord Injury

Answer: 3

Rationale: Offering time to the client encourages the client to discuss feelings. Options 1, 2, and 4 are blocks to communication. Options 1 and 4 show disapproval, and option 2 gives false reassurance.

Priority Nursing Tip: Autonomic dysreflexia is a syndrome in which there is a sudden onset of excessively high blood pressure. It is more common in people with spinal cord injuries that involve the thoracic nerves of the spine or above (T6 or above).

Test-Taking Strategy: Focus on the **subject,** initiating conversation with a client to prevent autonomic dysreflexia. Select the option that uses **therapeutic communication techniques** effectively. The correct option demonstrates caring and an effective communication approach.

---

212. The nurse is assisting a client with a spinal cord injury to accomplish activities of daily living. How would the nurse respond when the client states, "I can't do this; I wish I were dead"?

1 "Why do you say that?"
2 "You wish you were dead?"
3 "I'm sure you don't really want to die."
4 "I'm sure you are frustrated, but don't give up."

Level of Cognitive Ability: Applying
Client Needs: Psychosocial Integrity
Clinical Judgment/Cognitive Skills: Take Action
Integrated Process: Communication and Documentation
Content Area: Foundations of Care: Communication
Health Problem: Adult Health: Neurological: Spinal Cord Injury

Answer: 2
Rationale: With clarifying, such as in the correct option, the nurse is using a therapeutic technique that involves restating what was said to obtain additional information. By using the word *why,* the nurse puts the client on the defensive. Other options either change the subject or provide false reassurance. Options 1, 3, and 4 are nontherapeutic and block communication.
Priority Nursing Tip: Any statement that even vaguely implies hopelessness requires further clarification.

Test-Taking Strategy: Note the **data in the question** and then use **therapeutic communication techniques** to address the client's statement. The correct option involves clarifying and restating and is the only option that will encourage the client to verbalize feelings and concerns.

---

213. A client says to the nurse, "I want to die, and I think about it often but I don't want to hurt my loving partner." Care for this client is based on what fact?

1 The suicidal risk for this individual is minimal.
2 A love for family will likely prevent any attempt.
3 All suicide attempts are well planned out in advance.
4 Continued data collection is needed because a risk for suicide exists.

Level of Cognitive Ability: Analyzing
Client Needs: Psychosocial Integrity
Clinical Judgment/Cognitive Skills: Analyze Cues
Integrated Process: Nursing Process/Data Collection
Content Area: Mental Health
Health Problem: Mental Health: Suicide

Answer: 4
Rationale: The words *I want to die* indicate a suicide risk. Any self-harm language must be viewed as serious, as suggested in the correct option. Option 1 requires additional assessment to evaluate the risk. Options 2 and 3 are inaccurate interpretations in light of the client's statements.
Priority Nursing Tip: All statements regarding a desire to die must be taken seriously and assessed further.

Test-Taking Strategy: Focus on the **data in the question,** especially the statement made by the client. Note the words *I want to die* and *I think about it often.* These words will direct you to the correct option.

---

214. Parents awaiting the news of their child's condition after a suicide attempt are tearful. The nurse meets their needs by making what statement?

1 "I can see you are worried."
2 "Everything possible is being done."
3 "Remember that you have nothing to feel guilty about."
4 "I'll let you know as soon as you can see your child."

Answer: 1
Rationale: The nursing statement in the correct option uses the therapeutic technique of clarifying. Options 2, 3, and 4 are communication blocks. Option 2 uses a cliché and false reassurance. Option 3 labels the family's behavior without their validation. Option 4 focuses on an important subject at an inappropriate time (i.e., when family members are tearful).
Priority Nursing Tip: Suicide and suicide attempts cause emotional trauma to all those involved with the depressed individual.

Level of Cognitive Ability: Applying
Client Needs: Psychosocial Integrity
Clinical Judgment/Cognitive Skills: Take Action
Integrated Process: Communication and Documentation
Content Area: Mental Health
Health Problem: Mental Health: Therapeutic Communication

Test-Taking Strategy: Focus on the **subject,** the parents' needs. Use **therapeutic communication techniques.** The correct option identifies clarifying and is the only option that will encourage the family to verbalize feelings and concerns.

---

215. Which intervention would be included in the plan of care for an 11-year-old child who has been physically abused?

1 Encouraging the child to confront the abuser
2 Providing an environment that allows for the development of trust
3 Persuading the child to identify the individual who was responsible for the abuse
4 Teaching the child to make wise choices when confronted with an abusive situation

Answer: 2
Rationale: The abused child usually requires long-term therapeutic support. The environment during the child's healing must be one in which trust and caring are provided for the child. Options 3 and 4 ask the child to behave with a maturity beyond that which would be expected for an 11-year-old child. Option 1 reinforces fear.
Priority Nursing Tip: Abuse recovery requires long-term, age-appropriate therapy.

Test-Taking Strategy: Focus on the **subject,** child abuse, and the components of a therapeutic nurse–client relationship. The correct option is the appropriate one because it provides the child with a nurturing and supportive environment in which to begin the healing process.

Level of Cognitive Ability: Applying
Client Needs: Psychosocial Integrity
Clinical Judgment/Cognitive Skills: Generate Solutions
Integrated Process: Caring
Content Area: Mental Health
Health Problem: Mental Health: Violence

---

216. The nurse collects data from an older client and monitors for signs of potential abuse. The nurse understands that which factors place the client at risk for abuse? **Select all that apply.**

❒ **1** Diagnosed with osteoporosis and hypertension 5 years ago
❒ **2** Relies on family to provide weekly allowance to pay bills
❒ **3** Exhibits signs and symptoms of fatigue, flat affect, and low energy
❒ **4** Is totally dependent on family members for both food and medicine
❒ **5** Was seen in the urgent care clinic with multiple bruising over body on three occasions

Answer: 2, 4, 5
Rationale: Elder abuse is sometimes the result of the frustration of adult children who find themselves caring for dependent parents. Dependence and evidence suggesting injury are triggers for further assessment. Option 1 is a physiological condition. Option 3, signs and symptoms of depression, do not specifically indicate abuse.
Priority Nursing Tip: Increasing demands by parents for care and financial support can cause resentment and may be burdensome, resulting in abusive behaviors.

Test-Taking Strategy: Focus on the **subject,** signs of potential elder abuse and risk for abuse. Note the words *relies, dependent,* and *multiple bruising* to direct you to the correct options.

Level of Cognitive Ability: Analyzing
Client Needs: Psychosocial Integrity
Clinical Judgment/Cognitive Skills: Analyze Cues
Integrated Process: Nursing Process/Data Collection
Content Area: Mental Health
Health Problem: Mental Health: Violence

---

217. The nurse caring for a terminally ill client with lung cancer is asked, "What would you say if I asked you to be the executor of my will?" How would the nurse respond?

1 "Why, I'd be honored to be the executor of your will."
2 "Is there any money in it? I adore money, but I am honest."
3 "I'd say, 'Great!' Don't worry. I'll carry out your will just as you want me to."
4 "Let's talk more about this. I would like to understand more about your wishes."

Level of Cognitive Ability: Applying
Client Needs: Psychosocial Integrity
Clinical Judgment/Cognitive Skills: Take Action
Integrated Process: Communication and Documentation
Content Area: Leadership/Management: Ethical/Legal
Health Problem: Adult Health: Cancer: Laryngeal and Lung

Answer: 4
Rationale: In the correct option, the nurse uses the therapeutic communication of seeking clarification. In option 1, the nurse responds with a social communication with no assessment of the consequences, which demonstrates a lack of critical thinking and of the exploration of the client's motivation or needs. In option 2, the nurse uses histrionic language and crass ideation. In option 3, the nurse provides false reassurance, which is nontherapeutic.
Priority Nursing Tip: The nurse would not accept the role of acting as an executor of a client's will.

Test-Taking Strategy: Focus on the **subject,** the ethical and legal issues related to executing wills. Use **therapeutic communication techniques.** The correct option is the only one that is therapeutic and that seeks to clarify the client's request.

---

218. A client who is experiencing urticaria and pruritus shares with the nurse, "What am I going to do? I'm getting married next week and I'll probably be covered in this rash and itching like crazy." How would the nurse respond to **best** address the client's concerns?

1 "It's probably just due to prewedding jitters."
2 "Don't worry; chances are no one will even notice."
3 "You're troubled that this won't resolve before your wedding."
4 "The antihistamine will help a great deal. Just you wait and see."

Level of Cognitive Ability: Applying
Client Needs: Psychosocial Integrity
Clinical Judgment/Cognitive Skills: Take Action
Integrated Process: Communication and Documentation
Content Area: Adult Health: Integumentary
Health Problem: Adult Health: Integumentary: Inflammations/Infections

Answer: 3
Rationale: The therapeutic communication technique that the nurse uses is reflection, and that will encourage the client to further discuss concerns about the hives and rash. In option 1, the nurse minimizes the client's anxiety and fear. In option 4, the nurse talks about antihistamines and asks the client to wait; this is nontherapeutic because the nurse is making promises that may not be kept and because the response is closed-ended and shuts off the client's expression of feelings. In option 2, the nurse tells the client not to worry, which is inappropriate; additionally, this statement is nontherapeutic.
Priority Nursing Tip: Client concerns are initially addressed by clarifying the concern and identifying the cause of the concern.

Test-Taking Strategy: Note the **strategic word,** *best.* Use **therapeutic communication techniques.** The correct option is the only one that encourages the client to express feelings.

---

219. Which comment made by a client diagnosed with a spinal cord injury (SCI) **requires follow-up** by the nurse?

1 "I'm so angry that this happened to me."
2 "I'm concerned about going home like this."
3 "I know I will have to make major adjustments in my life."
4 "I would like my family members to be here for my teaching sessions."

Level of Cognitive Ability: Evaluating
Client Needs: Psychosocial Integrity
Clinical Judgment/Cognitive Skills: Analyze Cues
Integrated Process: Nursing Process/Evaluation
Content Area: Adult Health: Neurological
Health Problem: Adult Health: Neurological: Spinal Cord Injury

Answer: 1
Rationale: It is important to allow a client with an SCI to verbalize feelings. If the client indicates a desire to discuss feelings, the nurse would respond therapeutically. The words *I'm so angry that this happened to me* indicate the client's need to discuss feelings. Options 2 and 4 indicate that the client understands that changes will be occurring and that family involvement is best. Option 3 does not require further intervention.
Priority Nursing Tip: Anger, although a normal response to a traumatic situation, needs to be addressed so that it can be managed in a way that will allow for mentally healthy adjustment.

Test-Taking Strategy: Note the **strategic words,** *requires follow-up.* These words indicate a **negative event query.** Options 2, 3, and 4 are **comparable or alike** in that the client expresses positive acceptance of the injury. Option 1 expresses need for follow-up, but it is a common reaction to the situation.

---

220. The home care nurse asks an adult client, "Were you able to walk to the store as we discussed?" The nurse documents that the client exhibited a form of confabulation based on what client response?

1 "Why do you care so much?"
2 "I just don't like walking outside."
3 "Walk, walk to the store. All you think about is walking."
4 "You said I need to walk here in the house, not walk to the store."

Level of Cognitive Ability: Evaluating
Client Needs: Psychosocial Integrity
Clinical Judgment/Cognitive Skills: Evaluate Outcomes
Integrated Process: Nursing Process/Data Collection
Content Area: Mental Health
Health Problem: Mental Health: Neurocognitive Impairment

Answer: 4
Rationale: Confabulation is a defensive maneuver and an unconscious attempt to maintain self-esteem, especially related to memory loss. None of the other options provides a response related to confabulation.
Priority Nursing Tip: Confabulation is defined as the spontaneous production of false memories: either memories for events that never occurred or memories of actual events that are displaced in space or time.

Test-Taking Strategy: Focus on the **data in the question.** Eliminate options 1 and 3 first because they are **comparable or alike.** Next, think about the definition of confabulation to assist in answering correctly.

---

221. An agoraphobic client has been hospitalized for treatment. The nurse concludes that the client's behavior is improved when the client engages in which activity?

1 The client is sleeping 8 hours a night.
2 The client eats all meals in the unit cafeteria.
3 The client seeks out staff members for constructive feedback and advice.
4 The client regularly accepts telephone calls and text messages from family and friends.

Answer: 2
Rationale: Agoraphobia is the extreme or irrational fear of crowded spaces or enclosed public places. The behaviors in the correct option demonstrate the ability to tolerate being in a public space—an improvement for a client diagnosed with agoraphobia. None of the other options are associated with the characteristics of agoraphobia.
Priority Nursing Tip: Agoraphobia is a condition that results in a panic reaction to places and situations perceived to be difficult to escape.

Level of Cognitive Ability: Evaluating
Client Needs: Psychosocial Integrity
Clinical Judgment/Cognitive Skills: Evaluate Outcomes
Integrated Process: Nursing Process/Evaluation
Content Area: Mental Health
Health Problem: Mental Health: Phobias

Test-Taking Strategy: Focus on the **subject,** improvement in a client's agoraphobia. Recalling that the definition of agoraphobia is the extreme or irrational fear of crowded spaces or enclosed public places will help direct you to the correct option.

---

222. An examination of a 14-year-old child reveals bruises and bleeding in the genital area and multiple old fractures. The child says, "I want to go home, but I'm afraid! My stepfather will be angry with me for telling on him!" What response would the nurse provide to address the teen's expressed concerns?

1 "You are right. You can't go back there with that man."
2 "Your presence in the house will only tease your stepfather more."
3 "We'll keep this just between you and me until I can find a safe place for you."
4 "I am sorry that this has happened to you. You will be safe here at the hospital for now."

Answer: 4
Rationale: A child who is found to be physically and sexually assaulted would be admitted to the hospital. This will provide time for a more comprehensive evaluation while simultaneously protecting the child from further abuse. In option 1, the nurse does not respond with a calm and reassuring communication style or maintain a professional attitude. Option 2 accuses the victim of "teasing" the stepfather and is incorrect; it is also judgmental, controlling, and demeaning. The nurse's suggestion in option 3 is inappropriate, and the statement is collusive and passive in its stance.
Priority Nursing Tip: Most states have laws that require local staff to contact authorities in certain situations, such as if there is a child or vulnerable adult who is in danger of abuse.

Test-Taking Strategy: Focus on the **data in the question** and the **subject,** sexual abuse. Recalling that the priority issue is to protect the victim from the abuser will direct you to the correct option.

Level of Cognitive Ability: Applying
Client Needs: Psychosocial Integrity
Clinical Judgment/Cognitive Skills: Take Action
Integrated Process: Communication and Documentation
Content Area: Mental Health
Health Problem: Mental Health: Violence

---

223. The nurse is caring for a 15-year-old female client admitted to the hospital suspected of being physically and sexually abused by her father. That evening, the father angrily approaches the nurse and says, "I'm taking my daughter home. She's told me what you people are up to, and we're out of here!" What is the nurse's **most appropriate** response to the situation?

1 "If you attempt to take your daughter from this unit, the police will only bring her back."
2 "She will stay until the doctor says differently. I'll notify hospital security if you do not leave."

Answer: 3
Rationale: When a child subjected to abuse is admitted to a facility for further evaluation and protection, the primary health care provider attempts to get the parents to agree to the admission, as in the correct option. If the parents refuse, the hospital can request an immediate court order to retain the child for a specific length of time. In option 1, the nurse is somewhat demanding. In option 2, the nurse is angry and verbally abusive, and it is clear that the nurse has decided that the father is guilty of child abuse. In addition, the nurse is so aggressive and challenging that it may antagonize the father to the point that the nurse will become a victim of violence as well. Option 4 is pompous and lecturing.

3 "You seem very upset. I'm sure you want to help your daughter. It will be best if you agree to let your daughter stay here for now."
4 "Your daughter is ill and needs to be here. I know you want to help her recover and that you will work to help everyone straighten out the circumstances that caused this."

Level of Cognitive Ability: Applying
Client Needs: Psychosocial Integrity
Clinical Judgment/Cognitive Skills: Take Action
Integrated Process: Communication and Documentation
Content Area: Mental Health
Health Problem: Mental Health: Violence

Priority Nursing Tip: The child's physical and emotional well-being always has priority in cases of suspected abuse.

Test-Taking Strategy: Note the **strategic words,** *most appropriate.* Use **therapeutic communication techniques.** The correct option is the only one that addresses the father's behavior as it relates to the child's needs.

---

224. The nurse collects data from a 12-year-old client seen in the health care clinic. Which data suggest to the nurse that the client is experiencing developmentally appropriate responses? **Select all that apply.**

❒ 1 The client has over 600 friends on an online network site.
❒ 2 The client works most weekends babysitting for children.
❒ 3 The client reports being involved in a sexual relationship.
❒ 4 The client devotes 2 hours a day to mastering video games.
❒ 5 The client reports earning mostly A's and B's in school classes.

Level of Cognitive Ability: Applying
Client Needs: Psychosocial Integrity
Clinical Judgment/Cognitive Skills: Evaluate Outcomes
Integrated Process: Nursing Process/Data Collection
Content Area: Developmental Stages: Preschool and School Age
Health Problem: N/A

Answer: 1, 2, 4, 5
Rationale: A sense of industry is appropriate for this age group and demonstrated by having a part-time job. The increase in self-esteem associated with skill mastery is an important part of development for the school-age child. Positive peer interaction and school success is also appropriate. The formation of an intimate relationship would not occur until early adulthood.
Priority Nursing Tip: Individuals progress through age-appropriate developmental stages. Engaging in inappropriate behaviors can lead to emotional dysfunction.

Test-Taking Strategy: Focus on the **subject,** normal growth and development for the client. Note the age of the client in the question; this will assist you with eliminating option 3.

---

225. An infant diagnosed with hyaline membrane disease is being prepared for surfactant replacement therapy (SRT) via an endotracheal tube. The parent states, "This is making me so nervous because I'm not sure about having this done to my baby." The nurse helps prepare the parent by providing what response?

1 "We do this procedure safely all the time and on many babies."
2 "It seems you have concerns about this procedure for your baby."
3 "You have definitely made the right decision for your baby's health."
4 "You may be more comfortable if you wait outside during the procedure."

Level of Cognitive Ability: Applying
Client Needs: Psychosocial Integrity
Clinical Judgment/Cognitive Skills: Take Action
Integrated Process: Communication and Documentation
Content Area: Foundations of Care: Communication
Health Problem: Mental Health: Therapeutic Communication

Answer: 2

Rationale: When planning for this infant's care and for the well-being of the parents, it is important to apply the techniques of therapeutic communication. By paraphrasing the parent's concern, the nurse restates the message in his or her own words and thus encourages discussion on the concerning topic. Option 1 involves false reassurance, which will block communication. Option 3 is a communication block that denies the parents the right to their opinion. Option 4 is incorrect because it does not address the parent's nervousness and because the parents have every right to be present during the procedure.

Priority Nursing Tip: SRT is used in the treatment of neonatal respiratory distress syndrome and severe meconium aspiration syndrome in infants.

Test-Taking Strategy: Focus on the **subject,** the parent's concerns. Use **therapeutic communication techniques** to answer the question. Select the option that enhances communication. Option 2 addresses the use of a therapeutic communication technique and addresses the needs of the parents.

---

226. The parents of a postterm newborn ask the nurse, "Why does our baby have such a worried facial expression?" How would the nurse answer the parents' question?

1 "New parents have many concerns."
2 "It's not unusual for babies to look like that."
3 "Do you have reason to believe your baby is ill?"
4 "You have concerns about the baby's facial expression?"

Level of Cognitive Ability: Applying
Client Needs: Psychosocial Integrity
Clinical Judgment/Cognitive Skills: Take Action
Integrated Process: Communication and Documentation
Content Area: Maternity: Newborn
Health Problem: Mental Health: Therapeutic Communication

Answer: 4

Rationale: Paraphrasing is restating the parents' message in the nurse's own words. The technique used in the correct option encourages the parents to clarify the concern. In option 2, the nurse is offering false reassurance, which blocks communication. Options 1 and 3 involve communication blocks as well because they do not address the subject of the client's concern, and option 3 suggests illness; the parents' question did not suggest such a concern.

Priority Nursing Tip: New parents have many questions and need to be encouraged to express them.

Test-Taking Strategy: Focus on the **subject,** the parents' concerns. Use **therapeutic communication techniques** to answer the question. Only the correct option reflects the use of a **therapeutic communication technique.**

---

227. The nurse is caring for a client who is at risk for violent behavior. Which interventions will assist in preventing violent behavior if the client becomes agitated? **Select all that apply.**

❒ 1 Speak in a calm, low voice.
❒ 2 Use short, simple sentences.
❒ 3 Maintain consistent, direct eye contact.
❒ 4 Avoid laughing and smiling inappropriately.
❒ 5 Assume a supportive stance that is at least 3 feet from the client.
❒ 6 Face the client with the arms across the chest to maintain control of the situation.

Level of Cognitive Ability: Applying
Client Needs: Psychosocial Integrity
Clinical Judgment/Cognitive Skills: Take Action
Integrated Process: Nursing Process/Implementation
Content Area: Mental Health
Health Problem: Mental Health: Violence

Answer: 1, 2, 4, 5

Rationale: Speaking to the client in a calm, low voice can help decrease the client's agitation. Agitated clients often speak loudly and use profanity. It is important that nurses not respond by raising their voices, as the client perceives this as competition and will further escalate a volatile situation. The nurse would use short, simple sentences and avoid laughing and smiling inappropriately. The nurse can help reduce agitation by acknowledging the client's feelings and reassuring the client that the staff is there to help. To avoid intimidation, the nurse would assume a nonthreatening posture. Placing the hands on the hips and crossing the arms across the chest are intimidating and communicate emotional distance and an unwillingness to help. The nurse would avoid intense direct eye contact. However, altering position so that the nurse's eyes are at the same level as those of the client allows the client to communicate from an equal rather than an inferior position. In addition, the nurse would assume a supportive stance that is at least 3 feet from the client, because a client perceives intrusion of personal space as a threat and may provoke aggression and violence.

Priority Nursing Tip: The nurse's best intervention when attempting to deescalate an agitated client is to achieve a calm, quiet, controlled but nonthreatening presence.

Test-Taking Strategy: Focus on the **subject,** preventing violent behavior in a client. Recalling that interventions in this situation should strengthen the therapeutic alliance with the client and remain nonthreatening will assist you with identifying the correct interventions.

CHAPTER

9

Physiological Integrity Practice Questions

1. The nurse is assisting in caring for a client who is receiving a blood transfusion. Which clinical manifestation would alert the nurse to fluid volume overload?
   1 Fatigue
   2 Back pain
   3 Shortness of breath
   4 Flattened neck veins

Level of Cognitive Ability: Applying
Client Needs: Physiological Integrity
Clinical Judgment/Cognitive Skills: Recognize Cues
Integrated Process: Nursing Process/Data Collection
Content Area: Complex Care: Blood Administration
Health Problem: N/A

Answer: 3
Rationale: Fluid volume overload can result from a blood transfusion, and those who have cardiac or renal compromise are at increased risk for this adverse reaction. Some signs and symptoms of this complication include shortness of breath caused by increased fluid entering the lungs; swelling in the ankles, feet, wrist, or face; high blood pressure; and heart rhythm problems. Fatigue, although it could occur, is nonspecific to fluid volume overload, and weakness is the more likely manifestation. Back pain is often associated with a hemolytic transfusion reaction. Flattened neck veins occur with hypovolemia.
Priority Nursing Tip: There are various types of blood transfusion reactions, including hemolytic, allergic or anaphylactic, and hypervolemia, each with its own set of presenting signs and symptoms. It is important to be able to differentiate among these.

Test-Taking Strategy: Focus on the **subject**, fluid volume overload as a complication of blood transfusion. Recalling the various types of transfusion reactions will direct you to the correct option.

---

2. The nurse is assisting in caring for a client who is receiving blood transfusion therapy. Which clinical manifestations would alert the nurse to a hemolytic transfusion reaction? **Select all that apply.**
   1 Headache
   2 Tachycardia
   3 Hypertension
   4 Apprehension
   5 Distended neck veins
   6 A sense of impending doom

Level of Cognitive Ability: Analyzing
Client Needs: Physiological Integrity
Clinical Judgment/Cognitive Skills: Recognize Cues
Integrated Process: Nursing Process/Data Collection
Content Area: Complex Care: Blood Administration
Health Problem: Adult Health: Immune: Hypersensitivity Reactions and Allergies

Answer: 1, 2, 4, 6
Rationale: Hemolytic transfusion reactions are caused by blood type or Rh incompatibility. When blood containing antigens different from the client's own antigens is infused, antigen–antibody complexes are formed in the client's blood. These complexes destroy the transfused cells and start inflammatory responses in the client's blood vessel walls and organs. The reaction may include fever and chills or may be life threatening with disseminated intravascular coagulation and circulatory collapse. Other manifestations include headache, tachycardia, apprehension, a sense of impending doom, chest pain, low back pain, tachypnea, hypotension, and hemoglobinuria. The onset may be immediate or may not occur until subsequent units have been transfused. Distended neck veins are characteristic of circulatory overload.
Priority Nursing Tip: The nurse would suspect a transfusion reaction if the client develops any symptom or complains of anything unusual while receiving the blood transfusion.

Test-Taking Strategy: Focus on the **subject,** a hemolytic transfusion reaction. Recall the pathophysiology of this type of reaction to select the correct options. Also think about other types of transfusion reactions that can occur, and recall that distended neck veins are characteristic of circulatory overload.

---

3. A client has an arteriovenous (AV) fistula in place in the right upper extremity for hemodialysis treatments. When planning care for this client, which measure would the nurse implement to promote client safety?
   1 Use the right arm blood pressure measurement.
   2 Use the fistula for all venipunctures and intravenous infusions.
   3 Ensure that small clamps are attached to the AV fistula dressing.
   4 Check the fistula for the presence of a bruit and thrill every 4 hours.

Level of Cognitive Ability: Applying
Client Needs: Physiological Integrity
Clinical Judgment/Cognitive Skills: Generate Solutions
Integrated Process: Nursing Process/Planning
Content Area: Adult Health: Renal and Urinary
Health Problem: Adult Health: Renal and Urinary: Chronic Kidney Disease

Answer: 4
Rationale: AV fistulas are created by anastomosis of an artery and a vein within the subcutaneous tissues to create access for hemodialysis. Fistulas need to be evaluated for presence of thrills (palpate over the area) and bruits (auscultate with a stethoscope) to determine patency. Blood pressures or venipunctures are not done on the extremity with the fistula because of the risk of clotting, infection, or damage to the fistula. The fistula is not used for venipunctures or intravenous infusions for the same reason. Clamps may be needed for an external device such as an AV shunt, but the AV fistula is internal.
Priority Nursing Tip: For the client receiving hemodialysis, the AV fistula is the client's lifeline. The client's hemodynamic status needs to be closely monitored. Clients need teaching on which medications to avoid before dialysis.

Test-Taking Strategy: Focus on the **subject,** an AV fistula and safety. Eliminate option 3 first because this refers to care of an AV shunt, in which there is an external cannula that can become disconnected. If accidental disconnection occurs, the small clamps can be used to occlude the ends of the cannula. Blood pressure measurement, insertion of intravenous access, and venipuncture would never be performed on the affected extremity because of the potential for infection and clotting of the fistula; therefore, eliminate options 1 and 2. The only option that relates to the subject of this question is option 4.

---

4. The nurse is assisting in caring for a client diagnosed with both a wound infection and osteomyelitis who is to receive hyperbaric oxygen therapy. During the therapy, which **priority** intervention would the nurse implement?
   1 Maintaining an intravenous access
   2 Ensuring that oxygen is being delivered
   3 Administering sedation to prevent claustrophobia
   4 Providing emotional support to the client's family

Level of Cognitive Ability: Applying
Client Needs: Physiological Integrity
Clinical Judgment/Cognitive Skills: Take Action
Integrated Process: Nursing Process/Implementation
Content Area: Skills: Oxygenation
Health Problem: Adult Health: Integumentary: Wounds

Answer: 2
Rationale: Hyperbaric oxygen therapy is a process by which oxygen is administered at greater than atmospheric pressure. When oxygen is inhaled under pressure, the level of tissue oxygen is greatly increased. The high levels of oxygen promote the action of phagocytes and promote healing of the wound. Because the client is placed in a closed chamber, the administration of oxygen is of primary importance. Although options 1, 3, and 4 may be appropriate interventions, option 2 is the priority.
Priority Nursing Tip: Hyperbaric oxygen therapy may be a treatment measure for chronic osteomyelitis to increase tissue perfusion and promote healing.

Test-Taking Strategy: Note the **strategic word,** *priority.* Use the **ABCs—airway, breathing, and circulation**—to direct you to option 2, which addresses oxygen. Also note the relationship of the words *hyperbaric oxygen* in the question and *oxygen* in the correct option.

---

5. A client is scheduled for hydrotherapy for a burn dressing change. Which action would the nurse take to ensure that the client is comfortable during the procedure?
   1 Ensure that the client is appropriately dressed.
   2 Administer an opioid analgesic 30 to 60 minutes before therapy.
   3 Schedule the therapy at a time when the client generally takes a nap.
   4 Assign an assistive personnel (AP) to stay with the client during the procedure.

Level of Cognitive Ability: Applying
Client Needs: Physiological Integrity
Clinical Judgment/Cognitive Skills: Take Action
Integrated Process: Nursing Process/ Implementation
Content Area: Skills: Vital Signs
Health Problem: Adult Health: Integumentary: Burns

Answer: 2
Rationale: The client needs to receive pain medication approximately 30 to 60 minutes before a burn dressing change. This will help the client tolerate an otherwise painful procedure. None of the remaining options addresses the issue of pain effectively.
Priority Nursing Tip: A burn injury is extremely painful, and the client is adequately medicated before a burn dressing change to reduce pain and prevent fear of future dressing changes. Strict aseptic technique is used for dressing changes because of the risk of infection.

Test-Taking Strategy: Use **Maslow's Hierarchy of Needs theory** (physiological needs are the priority). This will direct you to option 2, which addresses pain management.

---

6. The nurse is assisting in caring for a client diagnosed with heart failure who has a magnesium level of 0.75 mEq/L. Which action would the nurse take?
   1 Monitor the client for irregular heart rhythms.
   2 Encourage the intake of antacids with phosphate.
   3 Teach the client to avoid foods high in magnesium.
   4 Provide a diet of ground beef, eggs, and chicken breast.

Level of Cognitive Ability: Applying
Client Needs: Physiological Integrity
Clinical Judgment/Cognitive Skills: Take Action
Integrated Process: Nursing Process/ Implementation
Content Area: Foundations of Care: Laboratory Tests
Health Problem: Adult Health: Cardiovascular: Heart Failure

Answer: 1
Rationale: The normal magnesium level ranges from 1.8 to 2.6 mEq/L; therefore, this client is experiencing hypomagnesemia. The client needs to be monitored for dysrhythmias because magnesium plays an important role in myocardial nerve cell impulse conduction; thus, hypomagnesemia increases the client's risk of ventricular dysrhythmias. The nurse avoids administering phosphate in the presence of hypomagnesemia because it aggravates the condition. The nurse instructs the client to consume foods high in magnesium; ground beef, eggs, and chicken breast are low in magnesium.
Priority Nursing Tip: The client with hypomagnesemia is at risk for seizures. Therefore, the nurse needs to initiate seizure precautions if the magnesium level is low.

Test-Taking Strategy: Focus on the **subject**, a client with heart failure who has a magnesium level of 0.75 mEq/L. Recalling the normal magnesium level and noting that the client is experiencing hypomagnesemia will direct you to option 1. Also, the use of the **ABCs—airway, breathing, and circulation**—will direct you to the correct option.

---

7. The nurse is collecting data on a pregnant client with a diagnosis of abruptio placentae. Which manifestations of this condition would the nurse expect to note? **Select all that apply.**

1 Uterine irritability
2 Uterine tenderness
3 Painless vaginal bleeding
4 Abdominal and low back pain
5 Strong and frequent contractions
6 Nonreassuring fetal heart rate patterns

Level of Cognitive Ability: Analyzing
Client Needs: Physiological Integrity
Clinical Judgment/Cognitive Skills: Recognize Cues
Integrated Process: Nursing Process/Data Collection
Content Area: Maternity: Intrapartum
Health Problem: Maternity: Abruptio Placentae

Answer: 1, 2, 4, 6

Rationale: Placental abruption, also referred to as *abruptio placentae,* is the separation of a normally implanted placenta before the fetus is born. It occurs when there is bleeding and formation of a hematoma on the maternal side of the placenta. Manifestations include uterine irritability with frequent low-intensity contractions, uterine tenderness that may be localized to the site of the abruption, aching and dull abdominal and low back pain, painful vaginal bleeding, and a high uterine resting tone identified by the use of an intrauterine pressure catheter. Additional signs include nonreassuring fetal heart rate patterns, signs of hypovolemic shock, and fetal death. Painless vaginal bleeding is a sign of placenta previa.

Priority Nursing Tip: It is important to know the differences between the manifestations of abruptio placentae and placenta previa. In abruptio placentae, dark red vaginal bleeding, uterine pain and/or tenderness, and uterine rigidity are characteristic. In placenta previa, there is painless, bright red vaginal bleeding, and the uterus is soft, relaxed, and nontender.

Test-Taking Strategy: Focus on the **subject,** manifestations of abruptio placentae. Think about the word *abrupt.* Recalling the pathophysiology associated with this hemorrhagic condition will assist in selecting the correct options. Remember that placental abruption occurs when there is separation of the placenta and bleeding and formation of a hematoma on the maternal side of the placenta.

---

8. The nurse is caring for a client diagnosed with a herniated lumbar intervertebral disk who is experiencing low back pain. Which position would the nurse place the client in to minimize the pain?

1 Supine with the knees slightly raised
2 High Fowler's position with the foot of the bed flat
3 Semi-Fowler's position with the foot of the bed flat
4 Semi-Fowler's position with the knees slightly raised

Level of Cognitive Ability: Applying
Client Needs: Physiological Integrity
Clinical Judgment/Cognitive Skills: Take Action
Integrated Process: Nursing Process/Implementation
Content Area: Adult Health: Musculoskeletal
Health Problem: Adult Health: Neurological: Intervertebral Disk

Answer: 4

Rationale: Clients with low back pain are often more comfortable in the semi-Fowler's position with the knees raised sufficiently to flex the knees (William's position). This relaxes the muscles of the lower back and relieves pressure on the spinal nerve root. Keeping the bed flat or lying in a supine position with the knees raised would excessively stretch the lower back. Keeping the foot of the bed flat will enhance extension of the spine.

Priority Nursing Tip: A physical therapist will work with a client with a herniated lumbar intervertebral disk to develop an individualized exercise program, and the type of exercises prescribed depends on the location and nature of the injury and the type of pain. The client does not begin exercise until acute pain is reduced.

Test-Taking Strategy: Focus on the **subject,** a client with a herniated lumbar intervertebral disk who is experiencing low back pain. Visualize each of the positions, noting that option 4 places the least amount of pressure on the spine.

---

9. A client with myasthenia gravis admitted to the hospital has been prescribed pyridostigmine. When checking the client for side effects of the medication, the nurse would ask the client about the presence of which occurrence?

1 Mouth ulcers
2 Muscle cramps
3 Feelings of depression
4 Unexplained weight gain

Level of Cognitive Ability: Applying
Client Needs: Physiological Integrity
Clinical Judgment/Cognitive Skills: Recognize Cues
Integrated Process: Nursing Process/Data Collection
Content Area: Pharmacology: Neurological: Antimyasthenics
Health Problem: Adult Health: Neurological: Myasthenia gravis

Answer: 2

Rationale: Pyridostigmine is an acetylcholinesterase inhibitor used to treat myasthenia gravis, a neuromuscular disorder. Muscle cramps and small muscle contractions are side effects and occur as a result of overstimulation of neuromuscular receptors. Mouth ulcers, depression, and weight gain are not associated with this medication.

Priority Nursing Tip: Indicators of a therapeutic response to pyridostigmine include increased muscle strength, decreased fatigue, and improved chewing and swallowing functions.

Test-Taking Strategy: Focus on the **subject,** the side effects of pyridostigmine. Note that this medication is used to treat myasthenia gravis, a neuromuscular disorder. Select the option that is most closely associated with this disorder. This will direct you to the correct option.

---

10. A client who experienced a fractured right ankle has a short leg cast applied in the emergency department. During discharge teaching, which information would the nurse reinforce to the client to prevent complications?

1 Trim the rough edges of the cast after it is dry.
2 Weight bearing on the right leg is allowed once the cast feels dry.
3 Expect burning and tingling sensations under the cast for 3 to 4 days.
4 Keep the right ankle elevated above the heart level with pillows for 24 hours.

Level of Cognitive Ability: Applying
Client Needs: Physiological Integrity
Clinical Judgment/Cognitive Skills: Take Action
Integrated Process: Teaching and Learning
Content Area: Adult Health: Musculoskeletal
Health Problem: Adult Health: Musculoskeletal: Skeletal Injury

Answer: 4

Rationale: Leg elevation is important to increase venous return and decrease edema. Edema can cause compartment syndrome, a major complication of fractures and casting. The client and/or family may be taught how to "petal" the cast to prevent skin irritation and breakdown, but rough edges, if trimmed, can fall into the cast and cause a break in skin integrity. Weight bearing on a fractured extremity is prescribed by the orthopedic specialist during follow-up examination, after radiographs are obtained. Additionally, a walking heel or cast shoe may be added to the cast if the client is allowed to bear weight and walk on the affected leg. Although the client may feel heat after the cast is applied, burning and/or tingling sensations indicate nerve damage or ischemia and are not expected. These complaints need to be reported immediately.

Priority Nursing Tip: Circulation impairment and peripheral nerve damage can result from tightness of the cast applied to an extremity. The client needs to be taught to check for adequate circulation, including the ability to move the area distal to the casted extremity.

Test-Taking Strategy: Focus on the **subject,** measures to prevent complications with a short leg cast. Use the **ABCs—airway, breathing, and circulation.** Option 4 is associated with maintenance of circulation.

---

11. An adult client who experienced a fractured left tibia has a long leg cast and is using crutches to ambulate. In caring for the client, the nurse checks for which sign/symptom that indicates a complication associated with crutch walking?
   1 Left leg discomfort
   2 Weak biceps brachii
   3 Triceps muscle spasms
   4 Forearm muscle weakness

Level of Cognitive Ability: Analyzing
Client Needs: Physiological Integrity
Clinical Judgment/Cognitive Skills: Recognize Cues
Integrated Process: Nursing Process/Data Collection
Content Area: Skills: Activity/Mobility
Health Problem: Adult Health: Musculoskeletal: Skeletal Injury

Answer: 4
Rationale: Forearm muscle weakness is a sign of radial nerve injury caused by crutch pressure on the axillae. When a client lacks upper body strength, especially in the flexor and extensor muscles of the arms, he or she frequently allows weight to rest on the axillae and on the crutch pads instead of using the arms for support while ambulating with crutches. Leg discomfort is expected as a result of the injury. Weak biceps brachii is not a complication of crutch walking. Triceps muscle spasms may occur as a result of increased muscle use but are not a complication of crutch walking.
Priority Nursing Tip: To prevent pressure on the axillary nerve from the use of crutches, the client needs to keep two to three fingerbreadths between the axilla and the top of the crutch when the crutch tip is at least 6 inches diagonally in front of the foot. The crutch is adjusted so that the elbow is flexed no more than 30 degrees when the palm is on the handle.

Test-Taking Strategy: Focus on the **subject,** a complication of crutch walking. When asked about a complication of the use of crutches, think about nerve injury caused by crutch pressure on the axillae. This will direct you to option 4.

---

12. A client with myasthenia gravis is experiencing prolonged periods of weakness, and the neurologist prescribes an edrophonium test, also known as a *Tensilon test.* A test dose is administered by the neurologist, and the client becomes weaker. How would the nurse interpret these results?
   1 Myasthenic crisis is present.
   2 Cholinergic crisis is present.
   3 This result is a normal finding.
   4 This result is a positive finding.

Level of Cognitive Ability: Analyzing
Client Needs: Physiological Integrity
Clinical Judgment/Cognitive Skills: Analyze Cues
Integrated Process: Nursing Process/Data Collection
Content Area: Foundations of Care: Diagnostic Tests
Health Problem: Adult Health: Neurological: Myasthenia Gravis

Answer: 2
Rationale: An edrophonium test may be performed to determine whether increasing weakness in a client with previously diagnosed myasthenia gravis is a result of cholinergic crisis (overmedication) with anticholinesterase medications or myasthenic crisis (undermedication). Worsening of the symptoms after the test dose of medication is administered indicates a cholinergic crisis.
Priority Nursing Tip: Although rare, the edrophonium test can cause ventricular fibrillation and cardiac arrest. Atropine sulfate is the antidote for edrophonium and needs to be available when the test is performed in case these complications occur.

Test-Taking Strategy: Focus on the **subject,** a client who becomes weaker after edrophonium is administered. Recalling that edrophonium is a short-acting anticholinesterase and that the treatment for myasthenia gravis includes administration of an anticholinesterase will assist in answering the question. If the client's symptoms worsen after administration of edrophonium, then the client is likely experiencing overmedication.

---

13. When tranylcypromine is prescribed for a client, which food items would the nurse instruct the client to avoid? **Select all that apply.**

1 Figs
2 Apples
3 Bananas
4 Broccoli
5 Sauerkraut
6 Baked chicken

Level of Cognitive Ability: Applying
Client Needs: Physiological Integrity
Clinical Judgment/Cognitive Skills: Take Action
Integrated Process: Teaching and Learning
Content Area: Pharmacology: Psychiatric Medications: Monoamine Oxidase Inhibitors (MAOIs)
Health Problem: Mental Health: Mood Disorders

Answer: 1, 3, 5
Rationale: Tranylcypromine is a monoamine oxidase inhibitor (MAOI) used to treat depression. Foods that contain tyramine need to be avoided because of the risk of hypertensive crisis associated with use of this medication. Foods to avoid include figs; bananas; sauerkraut; avocados; soybeans; meats or fish that are fermented, smoked, or otherwise aged; some cheeses; yeast extract; and some beers and wine.
Priority Nursing Tip: Hypertensive crisis is characterized by an extreme increase in blood pressure resulting in an increased risk for stroke, headache, anxiety, and shortness of breath.

Test-Taking Strategy: Focus on the **subject,** foods to avoid with an MAOI. Focus on the name of the medication, and recall that tranylcypromine is an MAOI. Next, recall the foods that contain tyramine to answer the question. Remember that figs, bananas, and sauerkraut are high in tyramine.

---

14. The nurse notes an isolated premature ventricular contraction (PVC) on the cardiac monitor of a hospitalized client recovering from anesthesia. Which action would the nurse take?

1 Prepare for defibrillation.
2 Continue to monitor the rhythm.
3 Prepare to administer lidocaine hydrochloride.
4 Notify the primary health care provider immediately.

Level of Cognitive Ability: Analyzing
Client Needs: Physiological Integrity
Clinical Judgment/Cognitive Skills: Take Action
Integrated Process: Nursing Process/Implementation
Content Area: Adult Health: Cardiovascular
Health Problem: Adult Health: Cardiovascular: Dysrhythmias

Answer: 2
Rationale: As an isolated occurrence, the PVC is not life threatening. In this situation, the nurse needs to let the registered nurse (RN) know about the finding and then continue to monitor the client. It is unnecessary to notify the primary health care provider (PHCP) immediately. In addition, the RN would be the person to contact the PHCP if that is necessary. Frequent PVCs, however, may be precursors of more life-threatening rhythms, such as ventricular tachycardia and ventricular fibrillation. If this occurs, the primary health care provider needs to be notified. Defibrillation is done to treat ventricular fibrillation. Lidocaine hydrochloride is not needed to treat isolated PVCs; it may be used to treat frequent PVCs in a client who is symptomatic and is experiencing decreased cardiac output.
Priority Nursing Tip: Ventricular tachycardia can progress to ventricular fibrillation, a life-threatening condition.

Test-Taking Strategy: Focus on the **subject,** the action to take for an isolated PVC. Noting the word *isolated* would direct you to the option that addresses continued monitoring. Also, use of the **ABCs—airway, breathing, and circulation**—will direct you to the correct option.

---

15. The clinic nurse prepares to collect data from a client who is in the second trimester of pregnancy. When measuring the fundal height, what would the nurse expect to note with this measurement regarding gestational age?

1 It is less than gestational age.
2 It correlates with gestational age.
3 It is greater than gestational age.
4 It has no correlation with gestational age.

Level of Cognitive Ability: Applying
Client Needs: Physiological Integrity
Clinical Judgment/Cognitive Skills: Recognize Cues
Integrated Process: Nursing Process/Data Collection
Content Area: Maternity: Antepartum
Health Problem: N/A

Answer: 2
Rationale: Until the third trimester, the measurement of fundal height will, on average, correlate with the gestational age. Therefore, options 1, 3, and 4 are incorrect.
Priority Nursing Tip: Usually a paper tape is used to measure fundal height. Consistency in performing the measurement technique is important to ensure reliability in the findings. If possible, the same person needs to examine the pregnant client at each prenatal visit.

Test-Taking Strategy: Focus on the **subject,** fundal height in the second trimester. Recall the correlation of fundal height and gestational age to direct you to the correct option.

---

16. A pregnant client tells the nurse that they felt wetness on their peripad and found some clear fluid. The nurse inspects the perineum and notes the presence of the umbilical cord. What is the **immediate** nursing action?

1 Monitor the fetal heart rate.
2 Notify the registered nurse.
3 Transfer the client to the delivery room.
4 Place the client in Trendelenburg's position.

Level of Cognitive Ability: Applying
Client Needs: Physiological Integrity
Clinical Judgment/Cognitive Skills: Take Action
Integrated Process: Nursing Process/Implementation
Content Area: Complex Care: Emergency Situations/Management
Health Problem: Maternity: Prolapsed Umbilical Cord

Answer: 4
Rationale: On inspection of the perineum, if the umbilical cord is noted, the nurse immediately places the client in Trendelenburg's position while gently holding the presenting part upward to relieve the cord compression. This position is maintained and the registered nurse is notified, who will intervene and contact the obstetrician. The fetal heart rate also needs to be monitored to check for fetal distress. The client is transferred to the delivery room when prescribed by the obstetrician.
Priority Nursing Tip: Relieving cord compression is the priority goal if the umbilical cord is protruding from the vagina. The nurse never attempts to push the cord back into the vagina.

Test-Taking Strategy: Note the **strategic word,** *immediate,* which indicates the immediate action on the nurse's part to prevent or relieve cord compression. The only action that will achieve this is option 4.

---

17. On data collection of a newborn being admitted to the nursery, the nurse palpates the anterior fontanel and notes that it feels soft. The nurse determines that this finding indicates which condition?

1 Dehydration
2 A normal finding
3 Increased intracranial pressure
4 Decreased intracranial pressure

Answer: 2
Rationale: The anterior fontanel is normally 2 to 3 cm in width, 3 to 4 cm in length, and diamond-like in shape. It can be described as soft, which is normal, or full and bulging, which could indicate increased intracranial pressure. Conversely, a depressed fontanel could mean that the infant is dehydrated.
Priority Nursing Tip: The anterior fontanel is a diamond-shaped area where the frontal and parietal bones meet. It closes between 12 and 18 months of age. Vigorous crying may cause the fontanel to bulge, which is a normal finding.

Level of Cognitive Ability: Applying
Client Needs: Physiological Integrity
Clinical Judgment/Cognitive Skills: Analyze Cues
Integrated Process: Nursing Process/Data Collection
Content Area: Maternity: Newborn
Health Problem: N/A

Test-Taking Strategy: Focus on the **subject**, an anterior fontanel that is soft. Recalling the normal physiological finding in the newborn will direct you to the correct option.

---

18. The parent explains that after meals the infant has been vomiting, and now it is becoming more frequent and forceful. During data collection, the nurse notes visible peristaltic waves moving from left to right across the infant's abdomen. On the basis of these findings, which condition would the nurse suspect?

1 Colic
2 Intussusception
3 Congenital megacolon
4 Hypertrophic pyloric stenosis

Level of Cognitive Ability: Analyzing
Client Needs: Physiological Integrity
Clinical Judgment/Cognitive Skills: Analyze Cues
Integrated Process: Nursing Process/Data Collection
Content Area: Pediatrics: Gastrointestinal
Health Problem: Pediatric-Specific: Developmental GI Defects

Answer: 4
Rationale: In pyloric stenosis, the vomitus contains sour, undigested food but no bile; the child is constipated; and visible peristaltic waves move from left to right across the abdomen. A movable, palpable, firm, olive-shaped mass in the right upper quadrant may be noted. Crying during the evening hours and appearing to be in pain but eating well and gaining weight are clinical manifestations of colic. An infant who suddenly becomes pale, cries out, and draws the legs up to the chest is demonstrating physical signs of intussusception. Ribbon-like stool, bile-stained emesis, the absence of peristalsis, and abdominal distention are symptoms of congenital megacolon (Hirschsprung's disease).
Priority Nursing Tip: In pyloric stenosis, the nurse needs to monitor for signs of dehydration and electrolyte imbalances.

Test-Taking Strategy: Focus on the **subject**, an infant who is vomiting after meals with increasing force and frequency. Note all of the child's assessment data and the possible diagnoses. Consider each condition presented in the options, and think about the clinical manifestations of each. Recalling the manifestations associated with pyloric stenosis will direct you to the correct option. Also, recalling that stenosis means "narrowing" will direct you to the correct option.

---

19. During the postoperative period, the client who underwent a pelvic exenteration reports pain in the calf area. What action would the nurse take?

1 Ask the client to walk and observe the gait.
2 Lightly massage the calf area to relieve the pain.
3 Check the calf area for temperature, color, and size.
4 Administer PRN (as needed) morphine sulfate as prescribed for postoperative pain.

Level of Cognitive Ability: Applying
Client Needs: Physiological Integrity
Clinical Judgment/Cognitive Skills: Take Action
Integrated Process: Nursing Process/Implementation
Content Area: Foundations of Care: Perioperative Care
Health Problem: Adult Health: Cardiovascular: Vascular Disorders

Answer: 3
Rationale: The nurse monitors the postoperative client for complications such as deep vein thrombosis, pulmonary emboli, and wound infection. Pain in the calf area could indicate a deep vein thrombosis. Change in color, temperature, or size of the client's calf could also indicate this complication. Options 1 and 2 could result in an embolus if in fact the client had a deep vein thrombosis. Administering pain medication for this client is not the appropriate nursing action because further data collection needs to take place.
Priority Nursing Tip: The primary signs of deep vein thrombosis are calf or groin tenderness and pain and sudden onset of unilateral swelling of the leg.

Test-Taking Strategy: Focus on the **information in the question** and use the **steps of the nursing process.** Data collection is the first step. Option 3 is the only option that addresses data collection.

---

20. A primary health care provider prescribes acetaminophen liquid 450 mg orally every 4 hours PRN (as needed) for pain. The medication label reads 160 mg/5 mL. The nurse prepares how many milliliters (mL) to administer 1 dose? **Fill in the blank and record your answer to the nearest whole number.**
Answer: ______ mL

Level of Cognitive Ability: Applying
Client Needs: Physiological Integrity
Clinical Judgment/Cognitive Skills: Generate Solutions
Integrated Process: Nursing Process/Implementation
Content Area: Skills: Dosage Calculations
Health Problem: N/A

Answer: 14
Rationale: Use the formula for calculating medication dosages.
Formula:

$$\frac{\text{Desired} \times \text{Volume}}{\text{Available}} = \text{mL per dose}$$

$$\frac{450 \text{ mg} \times 5 \text{ mL}}{160 \text{ mg}} = 14 \text{ mL}$$

Priority Nursing Tip: After performing a medication calculation, ensure that the amount calculated is a reasonable amount.

Test-Taking Strategy: Focus on the **subject,** a medication calculation. Identify the components of the question and what the question is asking. In this case, the question asks for milliliters per dose. Set up the formula, knowing that the desired dose is 450 mg and that what is available is 160 mg per 5 mL. Verify the answer using a calculator, and be sure that the answer makes sense.

---

21. The client is prescribed sotalol 80 mg orally twice daily. Which finding indicates that the client is experiencing an adverse effect of the medication?
1 Dry mouth
2 Palpitations
3 Diaphoresis
4 Difficulty swallowing

Level of Cognitive Ability: Analyzing
Client Needs: Physiological Integrity
Clinical Judgment/Cognitive Skills: Recognize Cues
Integrated Process: Nursing Process/Data Collection
Content Area: Pharmacology: Cardiovascular: Beta Blockers
Health Problem: N/A

Answer: 2
Rationale: Sotalol is a beta-adrenergic blocking agent that may be prescribed to treat chronic angina pectoris. Adverse effects include palpitations, bradycardia, an irregular heartbeat, difficulty breathing, signs of heart failure, and cold hands and feet. Gastrointestinal disturbances, anxiety and nervousness, and unusual tiredness and weakness can also occur. Options 1, 3, and 4 are not adverse effects of this medication.
Priority Nursing Tip: For the client taking a beta-adrenergic blocking agent, monitor the blood pressure for hypotension and the apical pulse rate for bradycardia. If the client's blood pressure is lower than the client's baseline or the heart rate is below 60 beats per minute, notify the primary health care provider before administration.

Test-Taking Strategy: Focus on the **subject,** adverse effects of sotalol. Remember that medication names ending with the letters *-lol* (sotalol) are beta blockers, which are commonly used for cardiac disorders. Note that option 2 is the only option that is directly cardiac related.

---

22. What would the nurse do when assisting the registered nurse to perform a venipuncture to initiate continuous intravenous (IV) therapy?
1 Apply a cool compress to the affected area.
2 Inspect the IV solution and expiration date.
3 Secure a padded arm board above the IV site.
4 Apply a tourniquet below the venipuncture site.

Answer: 2
Rationale: IV solutions need to be free of particles or precipitates to prevent trauma to veins or a thromboembolic event; in addition, the nurse avoids administering IV solutions whose expiration date has passed to prevent infection. Cool compresses cause vasoconstriction, making the vein less visible, smaller, and more difficult to puncture. Arm boards are applied after the IV is started and are used only if necessary. A tourniquet is applied above the chosen vein site to halt venous return and engorge the vein; this makes the vein easier to puncture.

Level of Cognitive Ability: Applying
Client Needs: Physiological Integrity
Clinical Judgment/Cognitive Skills: Recognize Cues
Integrated Process: Nursing Process/ Implementation
Content Area: Foundations of Care: Safety
Health Problem: N/A

Priority Nursing Tip: Administration of an IV solution provides immediate access to the vascular system. Check the primary health care provider's prescription, and ensure that the correct solution and flow rate are administered as prescribed.

Test-Taking Strategy: Use the **steps of the nursing process.** Option 2 is the only option that reflects data collection, the first step of the nursing process.

---

23. The nurse is caring for a client who is receiving tacrolimus daily. Which finding indicates to the nurse that the client is experiencing an adverse effect of the medication?

1 Hypotension
2 Photophobia
3 Profuse sweating
4 Decrease in urine output

Answer: 4

Rationale: Tacrolimus is an immunosuppressant medication used in the prophylaxis of organ rejection in clients receiving allogenic liver transplants. Adverse reactions and toxic effects include nephrotoxicity and pleural effusion. Nephrotoxicity is characterized by an increasing serum creatinine level and a decrease in urine output. Frequent side effects include headache, tremor, insomnia, paresthesia, diarrhea, nausea, constipation, vomiting, abdominal pain, and hypertension. None of the other options are associated with an adverse reaction to this medication.

Priority Nursing Tip: Check the renal status of the client before administering tacrolimus because the medication is nephrotoxic.

Level of Cognitive Ability: Analyzing
Client Needs: Physiological Integrity
Clinical Judgment/Cognitive Skills: Recognize Cues
Integrated Process: Nursing Process/Data Collection
Content Area: Pharmacology: Immune: Immunosuppressants
Health Problem: N/A

Test-Taking Strategy: Focus on the **subject,** an adverse effect of tacrolimus. First, determine the medication classification. This will assist in identifying the medication classification as immunosuppressant. Next, recalling that nephrotoxicity is an adverse effect of the medication will direct you to the correct option.

---

24. A client was admitted to the hospital 24 hours ago after sustaining blunt chest trauma. Which is the **earliest** clinical manifestation of acute respiratory distress syndrome (ARDS) the nurse needs to monitor for?

1 Cyanosis with accompanying pallor
2 Diffuse crackles and rhonchi on chest auscultation
3 Increase in respiratory rate from 18 to 30 breaths per minute
4 Haziness or "white-out" appearance of lungs on chest radiograph

Answer: 3

Rationale: ARDS usually develops within 24 to 48 hours after an initiating event, such as chest trauma. In most cases, tachypnea and dyspnea are the earliest clinical manifestations as the body compensates for mild hypoxemia through hyperventilation. Cyanosis and pallor are late findings and are the result of severe hypoxemia. Breath sounds in the early stages of ARDS are usually clear but then progress to diffuse crackles and rhonchi as pulmonary edema occurs. Chest radiographic findings may be normal during the early stages but will show diffuse haziness or "white-out" appearance in the later stages.

Priority Nursing Tip: If the client sustains a chest injury, check the respiratory status of the client, and provide respiratory treatments as needed. This is followed by the treatment of life-threatening conditions.

Level of Cognitive Ability: Analyzing
Client Needs: Physiological Integrity
Clinical Judgment/Cognitive Skills: Recognize Cues
Integrated Process: Nursing Process/Data Collection
Content Area: Adult Health: Respiratory
Health Problem: Adult Health: Respiratory: Acute Respiratory Distress Syndrome

Test-Taking Strategy: Note the **strategic word,** *earliest.* Remember that with ARDS initial presenting symptoms are tachypnea, dyspnea, and restlessness as hypoxia develops. Knowing the definition of tachypnea and possible etiologies will direct you to the correct option.

---

25. The nurse caring for a client with Buck's traction is monitoring the client for associated complications. Which finding indicates a complication of this form of traction?

1 Weak pedal pulses
2 Drainage at the pin sites
3 Complaints of leg discomfort
4 Toes demonstrating a brisk capillary refill

Level of Cognitive Ability: Analyzing
Client Needs: Physiological Integrity
Clinical Judgment/Cognitive Skills: Recognize Cues
Integrated Process: Nursing Process/Data Collection
Content Area: Adult Health: Musculoskeletal
Health Problem: Adult Health: Musculoskeletal: Skeletal Injury

Answer: 1

Rationale: Buck's traction is skin traction. Weak pedal pulses are a sign of vascular compromise, which can be caused by pressure on the tissues of the leg by the elastic bandage or prefabricated boot used to secure this type of traction. Skeletal (not skin) traction uses pins. Discomfort is expected. Warm toes with brisk capillary refill are a normal finding.

Priority Nursing Tip: If the client in traction exhibits signs of neurovascular compromise such as changes in temperature, sensation, or the ability to move digits of the affected extremity, the primary health care provider needs to be notified immediately.

Test-Taking Strategy: Use the **ABCs—airway, breathing, and circulation**—to direct you to option 1, indicative of vascular compromise. Also eliminate option 2 because Buck's traction does not use pins. Options 3 and 4 can be eliminated because they are **comparable or alike** and are both normal findings.

---

26. A prenatal client has been diagnosed with a vaginal infection from the organism *Candida albicans*. What would the nurse expect to note on data collection of the client?

1 Costovertebral-angle pain
2 Absence of any observable signs
3 Pain, itching, and vaginal discharge
4 Proteinuria, hematuria, and hypertension

Level of Cognitive Ability: Analyzing
Client Needs: Physiological Integrity
Clinical Judgment/Cognitive Skills: Recognize Cues
Integrated Process: Nursing Process/Data Collection
Content Area: Maternity: Antepartum
Health Problem: Maternity: Infections/Inflammations

Answer: 3

Rationale: Clinical manifestations of a *Candida* infection include pain; itching; and a thick, white vaginal discharge. Proteinuria and hypertension are signs of preeclampsia. Costovertebral-angle pain, proteinuria, and hematuria are clinical manifestations associated with upper urinary tract infections.

Priority Nursing Tip: *Candida albicans* is a fungal infection of the skin and mucous membranes. Common areas of occurrence include the mucous membranes of the mouth, perineum, vagina, axilla, and under the breasts.

Test-Taking Strategy: Focus on the **subject**, vaginal infection. Note the relationship between the subject and the correct option.

---

27. A prenatal client has a suspected diagnosis of iron-deficiency anemia. On data collection, which finding would the nurse expect to note as a result of this condition?
   1 Dehydration
   2 Overhydration
   3 A high hematocrit level
   4 A low hemoglobin level

Level of Cognitive Ability: Analyzing
Client Needs: Physiological Integrity
Clinical Judgment/Cognitive Skills: Recognize Cues
Integrated Process: Nursing Process/Data Collection
Content Area: Maternity: Antepartum
Health Problem: Adult Health: Hematological: Anemias

Answer: 4
Rationale: Pathological anemia of pregnancy is primarily caused by iron deficiency. When the hemoglobin level is below 11 mg/dL, iron deficiency is suspected. An indirect index of the oxygen-carrying capacity is determined via a packed red blood cell volume or hematocrit level. Dehydration and overhydration are not specifically associated with iron-deficiency anemia.
Priority Nursing Tip: The ferritin level is a laboratory test that is used to diagnose iron-deficiency anemia. For a female, a ferritin level of less than 10 ng/mL confirms the diagnosis.

Test-Taking Strategy: Focus on the **subject,** manifestations of iron-deficiency anemia. Note the relationship between the words *deficiency* in the diagnosis and *low* in the correct option.

---

28. The nurse caring for a postpartum client would suspect that the client is experiencing endometritis if which is noted?
   1 Breast engorgement
   2 Elevated white blood cell count
   3 Lochia rubra on the second day postpartum
   4 Fever over 38°C (100.4°F), beginning 2 days postpartum

Level of Cognitive Ability: Analyzing
Client Needs: Physiological Integrity
Clinical Judgment/Cognitive Skills: Recognize Cues
Integrated Process: Nursing Process/Data Collection
Content Area: Maternity: Postpartum
Health Problem: Maternity: Infections/Inflammations

Answer: 4
Rationale: Endometritis is a common cause of postpartum infection. The presence of fever of 38°C (100.4°F) or more on 2 successive days of the first 10 postpartum days (not counting the first 24 hours after birth) is indicative of a postpartum infection. Breast engorgement is a normal response in the postpartum period and is not associated with endometritis. The white blood cell count of a postpartum woman is normally elevated; thus, this method of detecting infection is not of great value in the puerperium. Lochia rubra on the second day postpartum is a normal finding.
Priority Nursing Tip: A postpartum infection may also be termed a *puerperal infection* and is described as an infection of the genital canal that occurs within 28 days after a miscarriage, induced abortion, or childbirth.

Test-Taking Strategy: Focus on the **subject,** endometritis. Recalling the normal findings in the postpartum period will assist in eliminating options 1, 2, and 3.

---

29. The nurse is collecting data on a postterm infant. Which physical characteristic would the nurse expect to observe in this infant?
 1 Peeling of the skin
 2 Smooth soles without creases
 3 Lanugo covering the entire body
 4 Vernix that covers the body in a thick layer

Level of Cognitive Ability: Analyzing
Client Needs: Physiological Integrity
Clinical Judgment/Cognitive Skills: Recognize Cues
Integrated Process: Nursing Process/Data Collection
Content Area: Maternity: Newborn
Health Problem: Newborn: Preterm and Postterm Newborn

Answer: 1
Rationale: The postterm infant (born after the 42nd week of gestation) exhibits dry, peeling, cracked, almost leather-like skin over the body, which is called *desquamation*. The preterm infant (born between 24 and 37 weeks of gestation) exhibits smooth soles without creases, lanugo covering the entire body, and thick vernix covering the body.
Priority Nursing Tip: The postterm infant may exhibit meconium staining on the fingernails, long nails and hair, and the absence of vernix.

Test-Taking Strategy: Focus on the **subject,** the postterm infant. Think about the physiology associated with the postterm infant. Recalling that the postterm infant is born after the 42nd week of gestation will assist in directing you to the correct option.

---

30. A postterm infant, delivered vaginally, is exhibiting tachypnea, grunting, retractions, and nasal flaring. The nurse interprets that these findings are indicative of which condition?
 1 Hypoglycemia
 2 Respiratory distress syndrome
 3 Meconium aspiration syndrome
 4 Transient tachypnea of the newborn

Level of Cognitive Ability: Analyzing
Client Needs: Physiological Integrity
Clinical Judgment/Cognitive Skills: Analyze Cues
Integrated Process: Nursing Process/Data Collection
Content Area: Maternity: Newborn
Health Problem: Newborn: Respiratory Problems

Answer: 3
Rationale: Tachypnea, grunting, retractions, and nasal flaring are symptoms of respiratory distress related to meconium aspiration syndrome (MAS). MAS occurs often in postterm infants and develops when meconium in the amniotic fluid enters the lungs during fetal life or at birth. The symptoms noted in the question are unrelated to hypoglycemia. Respiratory distress syndrome is a complication of preterm infants. Transient tachypnea of the newborn is primarily found in infants delivered via cesarean section.
Priority Nursing Tip: The obstetrician is notified if meconium is noted in the amniotic fluid during labor. Although meconium is sterile, aspiration can lead to lung damage, which promotes the growth of bacteria; thus, the newborn needs to be closely monitored for infection.

Test-Taking Strategy: Focus on the **subject,** a postterm infant, and note the symptoms identified in the question. Option 1 is eliminated first because hypoglycemia is not a respiratory condition. From the remaining options, recalling the complications that can occur in a postterm infant will direct you to the correct option.

---

31. The nurse is caring for a client who had an orthopedic injury of the leg that required surgery and the application of a cast. Postoperatively, which nursing intervention is of **highest priority** to ensure client safety?
 1 Monitoring for heel breakdown
 2 Monitoring for bladder distention
 3 Monitoring for extremity shortening
 4 Monitoring for blanching ability of toe nail beds

Answer: 4
Rationale: With cast application, concern for compartment syndrome development is of the highest priority. If postsurgical edema compromises circulation, the client will demonstrate numbness, tingling, loss of blanching of toe nail beds, and pain that will not be relieved by opioids. Although heel breakdown, bladder distention, or extremity lengthening or shortening can occur, these complications are not potentially life threatening.
Priority Nursing Tip: Monitor the client with a cast for early signs of compartment syndrome. Check the client for the "six P's," which include pain, pressure, paralysis, paresthesia, pallor, and pulselessness.

Level of Cognitive Ability: Analyzing
Client Needs: Physiological Integrity
Clinical Judgment/Cognitive Skills: Prioritize Hypotheses
Integrated Process: Nursing Process/Data Collection
Content Area: Adult Health: Musculoskeletal
Health Problem: Adult Health: Musculoskeletal: Skeletal Injury

Test-Taking Strategy: Note the **strategic words,** *highest priority.* Use the **ABCs—airway, breathing, and circulation**—to answer the question. Checking for circulation to the foot, including observations for numbness, tingling, and the ability of the nail beds to blanch, will direct you to the correct option.

---

32. The nurse is sending an arterial blood gas (ABG) specimen to the laboratory for analysis. What information would the nurse include on the laboratory requisition? **Select all that apply.**

1 Ventilator settings
2 A list of client allergies
3 The client's temperature
4 The date and time the specimen was drawn
5 Any supplemental oxygen the client is receiving
6 Extremity from which the specimen was obtained

Level of Cognitive Ability: Applying
Client Needs: Physiological Integrity
Clinical Judgment/Cognitive Skills: Take Action
Integrated Process: Communication and Documentation
Content Area: Foundations of Care: Laboratory Tests
Health Problem: N/A

Answer: 1, 3, 4, 5
Rationale: An ABG requisition usually contains information about the date and time the specimen was drawn, the client's temperature, whether the specimen was drawn on room air or using supplemental oxygen, and the ventilator settings if the client is on a mechanical ventilator. The client's allergies and the extremity from which the specimen was drawn do not have a direct bearing on the laboratory results.
Priority Nursing Tip: An ABG specimen must be transported to the laboratory for processing within 15 minutes from the time that it was obtained.

Test-Taking Strategy: Focus on the **subject,** procedures for preparing an ABG draw. Review the pieces of information from the viewpoint of the relevance of the item to the client's airway status or oxygen use. The only pieces of information that do not relate to airway status or oxygen use are the client's allergies and the extremity from which the specimen was drawn.

---

33. The nurse is reviewing the laboratory results for a client who is receiving torsemide 5 mg orally daily. What value would indicate to the nurse that the client might be experiencing an adverse effect of the medication?

1 A chloride level of 98 mEq/L
2 A sodium level of 135 mEq/L
3 A potassium level of 3.1 mEq/L
4 A blood urea nitrogen (BUN) level of 15 mg/dL

Level of Cognitive Ability: Analyzing
Client Needs: Physiological Integrity
Clinical Judgment/Cognitive Skills: Analyze Cues
Integrated Process: Nursing Process/Data Collection
Content Area: Pharmacology: Cardiovascular: Diuretics
Health Problem: N/A

Answer: 3
Rationale: Torsemide is a loop diuretic. The medication can produce acute, profound water loss; volume and electrolyte depletion; dehydration; decreased blood volume; and circulatory collapse. Option 3 is the only option that indicates electrolyte depletion because the normal potassium level is 3.5 to 5.0 mEq/L. The normal chloride level is 98 to 106 mEq/L. The normal sodium level is 135 to 145 mEq/L. The normal BUN level ranges from 10 to 20 mg/dL.
Priority Nursing Tip: Nursing interventions for a client taking a loop diuretic include monitoring the blood pressure, weight, intake and output, and serum electrolytes (especially potassium) and checking the client for any hearing abnormality.

Test-Taking Strategy: Focus on the **subject,** adverse effects of torsemide. Recall knowledge of normal laboratory values to assist in selecting option 3, which is the only abnormal laboratory value presented.

---

34. During history taking of a client admitted with newly diagnosed Hodgkin's disease, which symptom would the nurse expect the client to report?

1 Weight gain
2 Night sweats
3 Severe lymph node pain
4 Headache with minor visual changes

Level of Cognitive Ability: Analyzing
Client Needs: Physiological Integrity
Clinical Judgment/Cognitive Skills: Recognize Cues
Integrated Process: Nursing Process/Data Collection
Content Area: Adult Health: Oncology
Health Problem: Adult Health: Cancer/ Lymphoma: Hodgkin's and Non-Hodgkin's

Answer: 2

Rationale: Data collection of a client with Hodgkin's disease most often reveals night sweats; enlarged, painless lymph nodes; fever; and malaise. Weight loss may be present if metastatic disease occurs. Headache and visual changes may occur if brain metastasis is present.

Priority Nursing Tip: The most common finding in Hodgkin's disease is the presence of a large and painless lymph node(s), often located in the neck. Biopsy of the node reveals the presence of Reed–Sternberg cells.

Test-Taking Strategy: Focus on the **subject,** symptoms associated with Hodgkin's disease. Eliminate options 3 and 4 first because they are **comparable or alike** in that they relate to discomfort. Weight gain is rarely the symptom of a cancer diagnosis, so it would be eliminated.

---

35. The nurse is collecting data on a 3-day-old preterm neonate with a diagnosis of respiratory distress syndrome (RDS). Which finding indicates that the neonate's respiratory condition is improving?

1 Edema of the hands and feet
2 Urine output of 3 mL/kg/hr
3 Presence of a systolic murmur
4 Respiratory rate between 60 and 70 breaths per minute

Level of Cognitive Ability: Evaluating
Client Needs: Physiological Integrity
Clinical Judgment/Cognitive Skills: Evaluate Outcomes
Integrated Process: Nursing Process/Evaluation
Content Area: Maternity: Newborn
Health Problem: Newborn: Respiratory Problems

Answer: 2

Rationale: RDS is a serious lung disorder caused by immaturity and the inability to produce surfactant, resulting in hypoxia and acidosis. Lung fluid, which occurs in RDS, moves from the lungs into the bloodstream as the condition improves and the alveoli open. This extra fluid circulates to the kidneys, which results in increased voiding. Therefore, normal urination is an early sign that the neonate's respiratory condition is improving (normal urinary output is 2 to 5 mL/kg/hr). Edema of the hands and feet occurs within the first 24 hours after the development of RDS as a result of low protein concentrations, a decrease in colloidal osmotic pressure, and transudation of fluid from the vascular system to the tissues. Systolic murmurs usually indicate the presence of a patent ductus arteriosus, which is a common complication of RDS. Respiratory rates above 60 are indicative of tachypnea, which is a sign of respiratory distress.

Priority Nursing Tip: Surfactant replacement therapy is used to treat RDS. The surfactant is instilled into the endotracheal tube.

Test-Taking Strategy: Note the **subject,** sign of improvement of a preterm neonate with a diagnosis of RDS. Option 2 is the only normal finding and indicates a normal urine output, which would indicate resolution of excess lung fluid.

---

36. The nurse is assisting in caring for a term newborn. Which finding would predispose the newborn to the occurrence of jaundice?
 1 Presence of a cephalohematoma
 2 Infant blood type of O negative
 3 Birth weight of 8 pounds, 6 ounces
 4 A negative direct Coombs' test result

Level of Cognitive Ability: Analyzing
Client Needs: Physiological Integrity
Clinical Judgment/Cognitive Skills: Recognize Cues
Integrated Process: Nursing Process/Data Collection
Content Area: Complex Care: Emergency Situations/Management
Health Problem: Newborn: Cephalohematoma

Answer: 1
Rationale: A cephalohematoma is swelling caused by bleeding into an area between the bone and its periosteum (does not cross over the suture line). Enclosed hemorrhage, such as with cephalohematoma, predisposes the newborn to jaundice by producing an increased bilirubin load as the cephalohematoma resolves (usually within 6 weeks) and is absorbed into the circulatory system. The classic Rh incompatibility situation involves an Rh-negative parent with an Rh-positive fetus/newborn. The birth weight in option 3 is within the acceptable range for a term newborn and therefore does not contribute to an increased bilirubin level. A negative direct Coombs' test result indicates that there are no maternal antibodies on fetal erythrocytes.
Priority Nursing Tip: Normal or physiological jaundice appears after the first 24 hours in a full-term newborn. Jaundice occurring before this time is known as *pathological jaundice* and warrants pediatrician notification.

Test-Taking Strategy: Focus on the **subject,** a term newborn's predisposition to jaundice. Recalling the risk factors associated with jaundice and the association between hemorrhage and jaundice will direct you to the correct option.

---

37. To ensure client safety, which is **most important** for the nurse to assess before advancing a client from liquid to solid food?
 1 Bowel sounds
 2 Chewing ability
 3 Current appetite
 4 Food preferences

Level of Cognitive Ability: Analyzing
Client Needs: Physiological Integrity
Clinical Judgment/Cognitive Skills: Recognize Cues
Integrated Process: Nursing Process/Data Collection
Content Area: Foundations of Care: Safety
Health Problem: N/A

Answer: 2
Rationale: The nurse needs to check the client's chewing ability before advancing a client from liquid to solid food. It may be necessary to modify a client's diet to a soft or mechanical chopped diet if the client has difficulty chewing, because of the risk of aspiration. Bowel sounds need to be present before introducing any diet, including liquids. Appetite will affect the amount of food eaten but not the type of diet prescribed. Food preferences need to be ascertained on admission assessment.
Priority Nursing Tip: The consistency of food would be altered based on the client's ability to chew or swallow. Liquid can be added to food to alter its consistency, but the liquid used needs to complement the food and its original flavor.

Test-Taking Strategy: Note the **strategic words,** *most important.* Also, focusing on the **subject,** advancing a diet from liquid to solid, will direct you to the correct option because the primary difference between a liquid and a solid diet is that the food needs mechanical processing (chewing) before it can be safely swallowed.

---

38. The licensed practical nurse (LPN) assisting in caring for a client in the active stage of labor is monitoring the fetal status and notes that the monitor strip shows a late deceleration. Based on this observation, which action would the LPN plan to take **immediately**?

1 Document the findings.
2 Prepare for immediate birth.
3 Increase the rate of an oxytocin infusion.
4 Administer oxygen to the client via face mask.

Level of Cognitive Ability: Analyzing
Client Needs: Physiological Integrity
Clinical Judgment/Cognitive Skills: Take Action
Integrated Process: Nursing Process/Implementation
Content Area: Complex Care: Emergency Situations/Management
Health Problem: Maternity: Fetal Distress/Demise

Answer: 4
Rationale: Late decelerations are caused by uteroplacental insufficiency as the result of decreased blood flow and oxygen transfer to the fetus through the intervillous space during the uterine contractions. This causes hypoxemia; therefore, oxygen is necessary. Although the finding needs to be documented, documentation is not the priority action in this situation. Late decelerations are considered an ominous sign but do not necessarily require immediate birth of the baby. The oxytocin infusion needs to be discontinued when a late deceleration is noted. The oxytocin would cause further hypoxemia because the medication stimulates contractions and leads to increased uteroplacental insufficiency.
Priority Nursing Tip: Late decelerations are nonreassuring patterns that reflect impaired placental exchange or uteroplacental insufficiency. The patterns look similar to early decelerations, but they begin well after the contraction begins and return to baseline after the contraction ends.

Test-Taking Strategy: Note the **strategic word,** *immediately.* Use the **ABCs—airway, breathing, and circulation**—to direct you to the correct option.

---

39. The nurse is caring for an obese client on a weight-loss program. Which method would the nurse use to **most** accurately determine the program's **effectiveness**?

1 Monitor the client's weight.
2 Monitor the client's intake and output.
3 Calculate the client's daily caloric intake.
4 Frequently check the client's serum protein levels.

Level of Cognitive Ability: Evaluating
Client Needs: Physiological Integrity
Clinical Judgment/Cognitive Skills: Evaluate Outcomes
Integrated Process: Nursing Process/Evaluation
Content Area: Foundations of Care: Therapeutic Diets
Health Problem: Adult Health: Gastrointestinal: Nutrition Problems

Answer: 1
Rationale: The most accurate measurement of weight loss is weighing of the client. This needs to be done at the same time of the day, in the same clothes, and using the same scale. Options 2, 3, and 4 measure nutrition and hydration status but are not associated with effectiveness of the weight-loss program.
Priority Nursing Tip: Clothing and shoes affect the obtained weight measurement. It is important to make a notation about any clothing, shoes, accessories (heavy jewelry), or other items such as casts or braces worn by the client while obtaining the weight.

Test-Taking Strategy: Focus on the **subject,** weight loss, and note the **strategic words,** *most* and *effectiveness.* Checking weight will most accurately identify weight changes. Also note that options 2, 3, and 4 are **comparable or alike** and measure nutrition and hydration status.

---

40. A client has fallen and sustained a leg injury. Which question would the nurse ask to help determine whether the client sustained a fracture?

1 "Is the pain a dull ache?"
2 "Is the pain sharp and continuous?"
3 "Does the discomfort feel like a cramp?"
4 "Does the pain feel as if the muscle was stretched?"

Level of Cognitive Ability: Applying
Client Needs: Physiological Integrity
Clinical Judgment/Cognitive Skills: Take Action
Integrated Process: Nursing Process/Data Collection
Content Area: Skills: Vital Signs
Health Problem: Adult Health: Musculoskeletal: Skeletal Injury

Answer: 2
Rationale: Fracture pain is generally described as sharp, continuous, and increasing in frequency. Bone pain is often described as a dull, deep ache. Muscle injury is often described as an aching or cramping pain, or soreness. Strains result from trauma to a muscle body or the attachment of a tendon from overstretching or overextension.
Priority Nursing Tip: Some fractures can be identified on inspection and exhibit manifestations such as an obvious deformity, edema, and bruising; others are detected only on x-ray examination.

Test-Taking Strategy: Focus on the **subject**, manifestations of a fracture. Recalling that pain from a new injury such as a fracture is more likely to be described as sharp will direct you to the correct option.

---

41. Which arterial blood gas (ABG) values would the nurse anticipate in the client with a nasogastric tube attached to continuous suction?

1 pH 7.25, $Paco_2$ 55, HCO_3 24
2 pH 7.30, $Paco_2$ 38, HCO_3 20
3 pH 7.48, $Paco_2$ 30, HCO_3 23
4 pH 7.49, $Paco_2$ 38, HCO_3 30

Level of Cognitive Ability: Analyzing
Client Needs: Physiological Integrity
Clinical Judgment/Cognitive Skills: Analyze Cues
Integrated Process: Nursing Process/Data Collection
Content Area: Foundations of Care: Acid-Base
Health Problem: Adult Health: Gastrointestinal: Upper GI Disorders

Answer: 4
Rationale: The anticipated ABG finding in the client with a nasogastric tube to continuous suction is metabolic alkalosis resulting from loss of acid. In uncompensated metabolic alkalosis, the pH will be elevated (greater than 7.45), bicarbonate will be elevated (greater than 28 mEq/mL), and the $Paco_2$ will most likely be within normal limits (35 to 45 mm Hg). Therefore, options 1, 2, and 3 are incorrect.
Priority Nursing Tip: The normal pH is 7.35 to 7.45. A pH level below 7.35 indicates an acidotic condition. A pH greater than 7.45 indicates an alkalotic condition.

Test-Taking Strategy: Focus on the **subject,** the acid–base imbalance that occurs in a client with continuous nasogastric suctioning. Note that the question addresses a gastrointestinal situation. Eliminate options 1 and 3 because they both identify a respiratory imbalance (opposite effects between the pH and the $Paco_2$). From the remaining options, remember that acid will be removed with nasogastric suctioning, so an alkalotic condition will result. This will direct you to the correct option.

---

42. The nurse is monitoring a client who was recently prescribed total parenteral nutrition (TPN). Which action would the nurse take when obtaining a finger-stick glucose reading of 425 mg/dL?

1 Stop the TPN.
2 Administer insulin.
3 Notify the registered nurse.
4 Decrease the flow rate of the TPN.

Answer: 3
Rationale: Hyperglycemia is a complication of TPN, and the nurse needs to report abnormalities to the registered nurse, who will then contact the primary health care provider. Options 1, 2, and 4 are not done without a primary health care provider's prescription.
Priority Nursing Tip: When a client is receiving TPN, the risk of hyperglycemia exists because of the high concentration of dextrose (glucose) in the solution.

Level of Cognitive Ability: Applying
Client Needs: Physiological Integrity
Clinical Judgment/Cognitive Skills: Take Action
Integrated Process: Nursing Process/Implementation
Content Area: Complex Care: Emergency Situations/Management
Health Problem: Adult Health: Gastrointestinal: Nutrition Problems

Test-Taking Strategy: Focus on the **subject,** a finger-stick glucose reading of 425 mg/dL. Note that options 1, 2, and 4 are **comparable or alike** and are not within the scope of nursing practice and require a primary health care provider's prescription. A blood glucose of 425 mg/dL requires notification of the primary health care provider.

---

43. The nurse provides information to a preoperative client who will be receiving relaxation therapy. What effects would the nurse teach the client to expect regarding this type of therapy? **Select all that apply.**

1 Increased heart rate
2 Improved well-being
3 Lowered blood pressure
4 Increased respiratory rate
5 Decreased muscle tension
6 Increased neural impulses to the brain

Level of Cognitive Ability: Applying
Client Needs: Physiological Integrity
Clinical Judgment/Cognitive Skills: Take Action
Integrated Process: Teaching and Learning
Content Area: Foundations of Care: Perioperative Care
Health Problem: N/A

Answer: 2, 3, 5
Rationale: Relaxation is the state of generalized decreased cognitive, physiological, and/or behavioral arousal. Relaxation elongates the muscle fibers, reduces the neural impulses to the brain, and thus decreases the activity of the brain and other systems. The effects of relaxation therapy include improved well-being; lowered blood pressure, heart rate, and respiratory rate; decreased muscle tension; and reduced symptoms of distress in persons who need to undergo treatments, those experiencing complications from medical treatment or disease, or those grieving the loss of a significant other. This therapy does not cause an increased heart rate, increased respiratory rate, or increased neural impulses to the brain.
Priority Nursing Tip: A simple relaxation exercise would be incorporated into the daily routine of an individual's life to decrease stress levels; stress can be a significant factor in the development of disease.

Test-Taking Strategy: Focus on the **subject,** the effects of relaxation therapy. Thinking about the definition of relaxation and recalling that it is the state of generalized decreased cognitive, physiological, and/or behavioral arousal will assist in directing you to the correct options.

---

44. A client has developed atrial fibrillation resulting in a ventricular rate of 150 beats per minute. The nurse would check the client for which effects of this cardiac occurrence? **Select all that apply.**

1 Dyspnea
2 Flat neck veins
3 Nausea and vomiting
4 Chest pain or discomfort
5 Hypotension and dizziness
6 Hypertension and headache

Level of Cognitive Ability: Analyzing
Client Needs: Physiological Integrity
Clinical Judgment/Cognitive Skills: Recognize Cues
Integrated Process: Nursing Process/Data Collection
Content Area: Adult Health: Cardiovascular
Health Problem: Adult Health: Cardiovascular: Dysrhythmias

Answer: 1, 4, 5
Rationale: The client with uncontrolled atrial fibrillation with a ventricular rate over 100 beats per minute is at risk for low cardiac output caused by loss of atrial kick. The nurse needs to check the client for palpitations, chest pain or discomfort, hypotension, pulse deficit, fatigue, weakness, dizziness, syncope, shortness of breath, and distended neck veins. Neither headache nor nausea and vomiting are associated with the effects of uncontrolled atrial fibrillation.
Priority Nursing Tip: Clients with atrial fibrillation are at risk for thromboembolism. Monitor the client closely for signs of this life-threatening situation.

Test-Taking Strategy: Focus on the **subject,** the effects of uncontrolled atrial fibrillation. Recalling that flat neck veins are normal or indicate hypovolemia will assist you in eliminating option 2. Remembering that nausea and vomiting are associated with vagus nerve activity, not a tachycardic state, will assist you in eliminating option 3. From the remaining options, thinking of the effects of a falling cardiac output will direct you to the correct options.

45. A preschooler with a history of cleft palate repair comes to the clinic for a routine well-child checkup. To determine whether this child is experiencing a long-term effect of cleft palate, which question would the nurse ask the parent?

1 "Does the child play with an imaginary friend?"
2 "Was the child recently treated for pneumonia?"
3 "Does the child respond when called by name?"
4 "Has the child had any difficulty in swallowing food?"

Level of Cognitive Ability: Analyzing
Client Needs: Physiological Integrity
Clinical Judgment/Cognitive Skills: Recognize Cues
Integrated Process: Nursing Process/Data Collection
Content Area: Pediatrics: Gastrointestinal
Health Problem: Pediatric-Specific: Disorders of Prenatal Development

Answer: 3
Rationale: A child with cleft palate is at risk for developing frequent otitis media, which can result in hearing loss. Unresponsiveness may be an indication that the child is experiencing hearing loss. Option 1 is normal behavior for a preschool child. Many preschoolers with vivid imaginations have imaginary friends. Options 2 and 4 are unrelated to cleft palate after repair.
Priority Nursing Tip: After a cleft palate repair, avoid the use of oral suction or the placement of objects in the child's mouth, such as a tongue depressor, thermometer, straws, spoons, forks, or pacifiers.

Test-Taking Strategy: Focus on the **subject,** a long-term effect of cleft palate. Think about the anatomy of this disorder and the pathophysiology associated with it. Recalling that hearing loss can occur in a child with cleft palate will direct you to the correct option.

---

46. The nurse is collecting data on the respiratory system of a client being treated for an asthma attack. The nurse determines that the client's respiratory status is worsening based on which finding?

1 Loud wheezing
2 Wheezing on expiration
3 Noticeably diminished breath sounds
4 Increased displays of emotional apprehension

Level of Cognitive Ability: Evaluating
Client Needs: Physiological Integrity
Clinical Judgment/Cognitive Skills: Evaluate Outcomes
Integrated Process: Nursing Process/Evaluation
Content Area: Adult Health: Respiratory
Health Problem: Adult Health: Respiratory: Asthma

Answer: 3
Rationale: Noticeably diminished breath sounds are an indication of severe obstruction and impending respiratory failure. Wheezing is not a reliable manifestation to determine the severity of an asthma attack. Clients with minor attacks may experience loud wheezes, whereas others with severe attacks may not wheeze. The client with a severe asthma attack may have no audible wheezing because of the decrease of airflow. For wheezing to occur, the client must be able to move sufficient air to produce breath sounds. Emotional apprehension is likely whatever the degree of respiratory distress being experienced.
Priority Nursing Tip: During an acute asthma attack, position the client in a high-Fowler's or sitting position to aid in breathing.

Test-Taking Strategy: Note the **subject,** evidence of worsening respiratory status in a client being treated for an asthma attack. Use **Maslow's Hierarchy of Needs theory** to eliminate option 4. Next, use the **ABCs—airway, breathing, and circulation.** Remember that diminished breath sounds indicate obstruction and impending respiratory failure; this will direct you to the correct option. Also note that options 1 and 2 are **comparable or alike** and address wheezing.

---

47. The nurse is checking the casted extremity of a client for signs of infection. Which finding is indicative of the presence of an infection?

1 Dependent edema
2 Diminished distal pulse
3 Coolness and pallor of the skin
4 Presence of warm areas on the cast

Level of Cognitive Ability: Analyzing
Client Needs: Physiological Integrity
Clinical Judgment/Cognitive Skills: Analyze Cues
Integrated Process: Nursing Process/Data Collection
Content Area: Adult Health: Musculoskeletal
Health Problem: Adult Health: Musculoskeletal: Skeletal Injury

Answer: 4
Rationale: Manifestations of infection under a casted area include a musty odor or purulent drainage from the cast or the presence of areas on the cast that are warmer than others. The primary health care provider needs to be notified if any of these occur. Dependent edema, diminished arterial pulse, and coolness and pallor of the skin all signify impaired circulation in the distal extremity.
Priority Nursing Tip: Teach the client and family to monitor for signs of infection under a casted area. Teach them to monitor for warm areas on the cast and to smell the area for a musty or unpleasant odor, which would indicate the presence of infected material.

Test-Taking Strategy: Focus on the **subject,** manifestations of infection under the cast. Eliminate options 1, 2, and 3 because edema, diminished distal pulse, and coolness and pallor of the skin are **comparable or alike,** and all signify impaired circulation in the distal extremity. Also thinking about the signs of infection (i.e., redness, swelling, heat, and drainage) will direct you to the correct option.

---

48. The home-care nurse checks a client diagnosed with chronic obstructive pulmonary disease (COPD) who is reporting increased dyspnea. The client is on home oxygen via a concentrator at 2 L/min and has a respiratory rate of 22 breaths per minute. Which action would the nurse take?

1 Determine the need to increase the oxygen.
2 Reassure the client that there is no need to worry.
3 Collect further data about the respiratory status.
4 Call emergency services to take the client to the emergency department.

Level of Cognitive Ability: Applying
Client Needs: Physiological Integrity
Clinical Judgment/Cognitive Skills: Take Action
Integrated Process: Nursing Process/Implementation
Content Area: Adult Health: Respiratory
Health Problem: Adult Health: Respiratory: Obstructive Pulmonary Disease

Answer: 3
Rationale: With the client's respiratory rate at 22 breaths per minute, the nurse needs to obtain further data. Oxygen is not increased without the approval of the primary health care provider, especially because the client with COPD can retain carbon dioxide. Reassuring the client that there is "no need to worry" is inappropriate. Calling emergency services is a premature action.
Priority Nursing Tip: For some clients with COPD, a low concentration of oxygen may be prescribed (1 to 2 L/min) by the primary health care provider because the stimulus to breathe is a low arterial Pa_{O_2} instead of an increased Pa_{CO_2}.

Test-Taking Strategy: Focus on the **subject,** the action to take for a client with COPD experiencing increased dyspnea. Eliminate option 2 first because it is an inappropriate communication technique and dismisses the client's complaint of dyspnea. Option 4 can be eliminated because calling emergency services is a premature action and there are no data to support the notion that an emergency exists. Remember that oxygen is not increased without primary health care provider approval, and there is no evidence to support that the client is exhibiting tissue hypoxia. Also, use the **steps of the nursing process** to direct you to the correct option.

49. The nurse reviews the client's vital signs in the client's chart. Based on these data findings, what is the client's pulse pressure? **Refer to chart. Fill in the blank.**

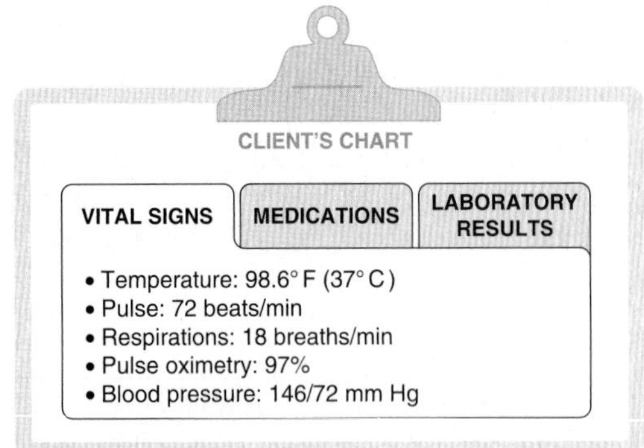

CLIENT'S CHART
VITAL SIGNS
MEDICATIONS
LABORATORY RESULTS
• Temperature: 98.6° F (37° C)
• Pulse: 72 beats/min
• Respirations: 18 breaths/min
• Pulse oximetry: 97%
• Blood pressure: 146/72 mm Hg

Answer: ______

Level of Cognitive Ability: Applying
Client Needs: Physiological Integrity
Clinical Judgment/Cognitive Skills: Analyze Cues
Integrated Process: Nursing Process/Data Collection
Content Area: Skills: Vital Signs
Health Problem: N/A

Answer: 74
Rationale: The difference between the systolic and diastolic blood pressure is the pulse pressure. Therefore, if the client has a blood pressure of 146/72 mm Hg, then the pulse pressure is 74.
Priority Nursing Tip: The pulse pressure value is an indirect measure of cardiac output. A narrow pulse pressure is seen in clients with heart failure, hypovolemia, or shock. An increased pulse pressure is noted in clients with hypertension, increased intracranial pressure, slow heart rate, aortic regurgitation, atherosclerosis, and aging.

Test-Taking Strategy: Focus on the **subject,** determining the pulse pressure. Recall that the pulse pressure is the difference between the systolic and diastolic blood pressure, and then use simple mathematics to subtract 72 from 146 to yield 74.

---

50. The home-care nurse is making a follow-up visit to a client who received a renal transplant. Which data support the possible existence of acute graft rejection? **Select all that apply.**

1 Pale skin color
2 Urine output of 45 mL/hr
3 Blood pressure of 164/98 mm Hg
4 Temperature of 102.4°F (39.1°C)
5 Client reporting "feeling so very tired"
6 Client reporting that graft site is tender when touched

Level of Cognitive Ability: Analyzing
Client Needs: Physiological Integrity
Clinical Judgment/Cognitive Skills: Analyze Cues
Integrated Process: Nursing Process/Data Collection
Content Area: Adult Health: Immune
Health Problem: Adult Health: Immune: Transplantation

Answer: 3, 4, 5, 6
Rationale: Acute rejection usually occurs within the first 3 months after transplant, although it can occur for up to 2 years after transplant. The client exhibits fever, hypertension, malaise, and graft tenderness. Treatment is immediately begun with corticosteroids and possibly also with monoclonal antibodies and antilymphocytic agents. None of the other options present symptomatology associated with acute graft rejection.
Priority Nursing Tip: The priority focus of care for the renal transplant recipient is the prevention and early recognition of graft rejection. Goals of care include preventing infection and rejection, maintaining hydration, promoting diuresis, and avoiding fluid overload.

Test-Taking Strategy: Focus on the **subject,** the manifestations of acute graft rejection. Think about the pathophysiology that occurs with acute graft rejection. Eliminate option 1 because pale skin color is related to low hemoglobin and hematocrit status or vascular status rather than acute rejection. Option 2 can be eliminated because an output of 45 mL/hr is adequate (output needs to be at least 30 mL/hr).

---

51. The licensed practical nurse (LPN) is assisting the registered nurse (RN) in caring for a client who is receiving tobramycin sulfate intravenously every 8 hours. Which result would indicate to the LPN that the client is experiencing an adverse effect of the medication?

1 A total bilirubin of 0.5 mg/dL
2 A blood urea nitrogen (BUN) of 30 mg/dL
3 An erythrocyte sedimentation rate of 15 mm/hr
4 A white blood cell count (WBC) of 6000 mm^3

Level of Cognitive Ability: Analyzing
Client Needs: Physiological Integrity
Clinical Judgment/Cognitive Skills: Analyze Cues
Integrated Process: Nursing Process/Data Collection
Content Area: Pharmacology: Immune: Aminoglycosides
Health Problem: N/A

Answer: 2
Rationale: Tobramycin sulfate is an aminoglycoside antibiotic. Adverse effects or toxic effects of tobramycin sulfate include nephrotoxicity, as evidenced by an increased BUN and serum creatinine; irreversible ototoxicity, as evidenced by tinnitus, dizziness, ringing or roaring in the ears, and reduced hearing; and neurotoxicity, as evidenced by headaches, dizziness, lethargy, tremors, and visual disturbances. The normal BUN ranges from 10 to 20 mg/dL, depending on the laboratory. The normal total bilirubin level ranges from 0.3 to 1.0 mg/dL. The normal sedimentation rate for a male is ≤ 15 mm/hr and for a female is ≤ 20 mm/hr. A normal WBC count is 5000 to 10,000 mm^3.
Priority Nursing Tip: Aminoglycoside antibiotics are potentially nephrotoxic substances.

Test-Taking Strategy: Focus on the **subject**, an adverse effect of tobramycin sulfate. Think about these adverse effects and recall knowledge of normal laboratory values to assist in directing you to the correct option, which is the only abnormal laboratory value presented in the options.

---

52. A client's telemetry monitor displays ventricular tachycardia. Upon reaching the client's bedside, which action would the nurse take **first**?

1 Call a code.
2 Prepare for cardioversion.
3 Prepare to defibrillate the client.
4 Check the client's level of consciousness.

Level of Cognitive Ability: Analyzing
Client Needs: Physiological Integrity
Clinical Judgment/Cognitive Skills: Prioritize Hypotheses
Integrated Process: Nursing Process/Implementation
Content Area: Complex Care: Emergency Situations/Management
Health Problem: Adult Health: Cardiovascular: Dysrhythmias

Answer: 4
Rationale: Determining unresponsiveness is the first action to take. When a client is in ventricular tachycardia, there is a significant decrease in cardiac output. However, checking for unresponsiveness helps determine whether the client is affected by the decreased cardiac output. If the client is unconscious, then cardiopulmonary resuscitation is initiated.
Priority Nursing Tip: For the client with stable ventricular tachycardia (with a pulse and no signs or symptoms of decreased cardiac output), oxygen and antidysrhythmics may be prescribed.

Test-Taking Strategy: Note the **strategic word,** ***first.*** Use the **steps of the nursing process,** remembering that data collection is the first action.

---

53. Which data collection question would be asked to help determine the client's risk for developing malignant hyperthermia in the perioperative period?

1 "Have you ever had heat exhaustion or heat stroke?"
2 "What is the normal range for your body temperature?"
3 "Do you or any of your family members have frequent infections?"
4 "Do you or any of your family members have problems with general anesthesia?"

Level of Cognitive Ability: Analyzing
Client Needs: Physiological Integrity
Clinical Judgment/Cognitive Skills: Recognize Cues
Integrated Process: Nursing Process/Data Collection
Content Area: Foundations of Care: Perioperative Care
Health Problem: Adult Health: Neurological: Thermoregulation

Answer: 4
Rationale: Malignant hyperthermia is a genetic disorder in which a combination of anesthetic agents (the muscle relaxant succinylcholine and inhalation agents such as halothanes) triggers uncontrolled skeletal muscle contractions that can quickly lead to a potentially fatal hyperthermia. Questioning the client about the family history of general anesthesia problems may reveal this as a risk for the client. Options 1, 2, and 3 are unrelated to this surgical complication.
Priority Nursing Tip: Early indicators of malignant hyperthermia include masseter muscle contractions and tachycardia. An elevated temperature is a late sign.

Test-Taking Strategy: Focus on the **subject,** malignant hyperthermia. Think about the pathophysiology associated with this disorder. Recalling that this disorder is genetic will direct you to the correct option.

---

54. A client has developed oral mucositis as a result of radiation to the head and neck. Which measure would the nurse teach the client to incorporate in a daily home-care routine to help manage this condition?

1 A glass of wine per day will introduce useful bacteria to the oral cavity.
2 High-protein foods such as peanut butter should be incorporated in the diet.
3 Clean teeth and rinse mouth with a weak saline and water solution before and after each meal.
4 Oral hygiene, including brushing and flossing, should be performed in the morning and evening.

Level of Cognitive Ability: Applying
Client Needs: Physiological Integrity
Clinical Judgment/Cognitive Skills: Take Action
Integrated Process: Teaching and Learning
Content Area: Adult Health: Oncology
Health Problem: Adult Health: Integumentary: Inflammations/Infections

Answer: 3
Rationale: Oral mucositis (irritation, inflammation, and/or ulceration of the mucosa), also known as *stomatitis,* commonly occurs in clients receiving radiation to the head and neck. Measures need to be taken to soothe the mucosa and provide effective cleansing of the oral cavity. A combination of a weak saline and water solution is an effective cleansing agent. Oral hygiene needs to be performed more frequently than in the morning and evening. Alcohol would dry and irritate the mucosa and not affect the oral bacteria. Peanut butter has a thick consistency and will stick to the irritated mucosa.
Priority Nursing Tip: Special "swish and spit" mixtures are available to treat mucositis (stomatitis), and many contain a local anesthetic combined with antiinflammatory agents. The client would be taught not to swallow these mixtures.

Test-Taking Strategy: Focus on the **subject,** oral mucositis. Knowing the definition of mucositis will help you eliminate the incorrect options. First, eliminate option 1, knowing that alcohol will have a further drying and irritating effect on the mucosa. Next, eliminate option 2, knowing that although high-protein foods are necessary, peanut butter would not be a good choice because of its consistency. From the remaining options, choose option 3 over option 4 because of the frequency noted in option 4.

---

55. The licensed practical nurse (LPN) is assisting the registered nurse (RN) in caring for a client who is being treated for heart failure. The client has the following vital signs: blood pressure (BP), 85/50 mm Hg; pulse, 96 beats per minute; respirations, 26 breaths per minute. The cardiologist prescribes digoxin. To evaluate a therapeutic response to this medication, which changes in the client's vital signs would the LPN expect?

1 BP 85/50 mm Hg, pulse 60 beats per minute, respirations 26 breaths per minute
2 BP 98/60 mm Hg, pulse 80 beats per minute, respirations 24 breaths per minute
3 BP 130/70 mm Hg, pulse 104 beats per minute, respirations 20 breaths per minute
4 BP 110/40 mm Hg, pulse 110 beats per minute, respirations 20 breaths per minute

Level of Cognitive Ability: Evaluating
Client Needs: Physiological Integrity
Clinical Judgment/Cognitive Skills: Evaluate Outcomes
Integrated Process: Nursing Process/Evaluation
Content Area: Adult Health: Cardiovascular
Health Problem: Adult Health: Cardiovascular: Heart Failure

Answer: 2
Rationale: The main function of digoxin is inotropic. It produces increased myocardial contractility that is associated with an increased cardiac output. This causes a rise in the BP in a client with heart failure. Digoxin also has a negative chronotropic effect (decreases heart rate) and will therefore cause a slowing of the heart rate. As cardiac output improves, there would be an improvement in respirations as well. The remaining choices do not reflect the physiological changes attributed to this medication.
Priority Nursing Tip: The nurse needs to monitor the client taking digoxin for digoxin toxicity. A normal serum digoxin level is 0.8 to 2.0 ng/mL.

Test-Taking Strategy: Focus on the **subject,** the physiological changes that occur with digoxin administration. Recalling that digoxin slows the heart rate will assist in eliminating options 3 and 4, which show an increase in the heart rate. Next, recalling that digoxin improves cardiac output will assist in eliminating option 1, which does not show improvement in blood pressure.

---

56. A client has been taking a prescribed calcium channel blocker therapy for approximately 2 months. The nurse monitoring the effects of therapy would determine that medication tolerance has developed if which is noted in the client?

1 Decrease in weight
2 Increased joint pain
3 Output greater than intake
4 Gradual rise in blood pressure

Level of Cognitive Ability: Analyzing
Client Needs: Physiological Integrity
Clinical Judgment/Cognitive Skills: Recognize Cues
Integrated Process: Nursing Process/Data Collection
Content Area: Pharmacology: Cardiovascular: Calcium Channel Blockers
Health Problem: N/A

Answer: 4
Rationale: Medication tolerance can develop in a client taking an antihypertensive such as a calcium channel blocker, which is evident by rising blood pressure levels. The registered nurse is notified, who then will contact the primary health care provider, who may then increase the medication dosage, change medication, or add a diuretic to the medication regimen. The client is also at risk of developing fluid retention, which would be manifested as dependent edema, intake greater than output, and an increase in weight. This would also warrant adding a diuretic to the course of therapy. Joint pain is not associated with this form of tolerance.
Priority Nursing Tip: Hypertension is a major risk factor for coronary, cerebral, renal, and peripheral vascular disease.

Test-Taking Strategy: Focus on the **subject,** medication tolerance with antihypertensives such as calcium channel blockers. Recall the definition of medication tolerance; that is, as one adjusts to a medication, the therapeutic effect diminishes. These concepts will direct you to the correct option.

---

57. A client with a known history of panic disorder comes to the emergency department and states to the nurse, "Please help me. I think I'm having a heart attack." What is the **priority** nursing action?

1 Check the client's vital signs.
2 Encourage the client to use relaxation techniques.
3 Identify the manifestations related to the panic disorder.
4 Determine what the client's activity involved when the pain started.

Level of Cognitive Ability: Analyzing
Client Needs: Physiological Integrity
Clinical Judgment/Cognitive Skills: Prioritize Hypotheses
Integrated Process: Nursing Process/Implementation
Content Area: Mental Health
Health Problem: Mental Health: Anxiety Disorder

Answer: 1
Rationale: Clients with a panic disorder can experience acute physical symptoms, such as chest pain and palpitations. The priority is to assess the client's physical condition to rule out a physiological disorder for these signs and symptoms. Although options 2, 3, and 4 may be appropriate at some point in the care of the client, they are not the priority.
Priority Nursing Tip: A client complaint of chest pain is always a priority. Immediate assessment and treatment are needed.

Test-Taking Strategy: Note the **strategic word,** *priority.* Focus on **Maslow's Hierarchy of Needs theory,** recalling that physiological needs are the priority. Also, use the **ABCs—airway, breathing, and circulation**—as well as the **steps of the nursing process** to direct you to the correct option.

---

58. A client experiencing trigeminal neuralgia (tic douloureux) asks the nurse for a snack and something to drink. Which is the **best** selection the nurse would provide for the client?

1 Hot cocoa with honey and toast
2 Vanilla pudding and lukewarm milk
3 Hot herbal tea with graham crackers
4 Iced coffee and peanut butter and crackers

Level of Cognitive Ability: Analyzing
Client Needs: Physiological Integrity
Clinical Judgment/Cognitive Skills: Take Action
Integrated Process: Nursing Process/Implementation
Content Area: Adult Health: Neurological
Health Problem: Adult Health: Neurological: Trigeminal Neuralgia

Answer: 2
Rationale: Because mild tactile stimulation of the face of clients with trigeminal neuralgia can trigger pain, the client needs to eat or drink lukewarm, nutritious foods that are soft and easy to chew. Extremes of temperature will cause trigeminal pain.
Priority Nursing Tip: Monitor the nutritional status of the client with trigeminal neuralgia closely. Because of the facial pain associated with the disorder, the client may not eat enough to meet her or his daily nutritional needs.

Test-Taking Strategy: Focus on the **strategic word,** *best.* Note that options 1, 3, and 4 are **comparable or alike** because these options contain hot or iced items and foods that are mechanically difficult to chew and swallow.

---

59. An adolescent is admitted to the orthopedic nursing unit after spinal rod insertion for the treatment of scoliosis. Which assessments are **most important** in the immediate postoperative period when considering the client's neurovascular status? **Select all that apply.**

1 Pain level
2 Urinary output
3 Ability to move all extremities
4 Capillary refill in all extremities
5 Ability to flex and extend the feet
6 Ability to detect sensations in all extremities

Level of Cognitive Ability: Analyzing
Client Needs: Physiological Integrity
Clinical Judgment/Cognitive Skills: Recognize Cues
Integrated Process: Nursing Process/Data Collection
Content Area: Pediatrics: Neurological
Health Problem: Pediatric-Specific: Scoliosis

Answer: 3, 4, 5, 6

Rationale: When the spinal column is manipulated during surgery, altered neurovascular status is a possible complication; therefore, neurovascular checks, including circulation, sensation, and motion, would be done at least every 2 hours. Level of pain and urinary output are important postoperative assessments, but are not specifically related to neurovascular status.

Priority Nursing Tip: The surgeon is notified immediately if signs of neurovascular impairment are noted in a postoperative client or a client with a cast, traction, or brace.

Test-Taking Strategy: Note the **strategic words,** *most important.* Focus on the **subject,** neurovascular status. Use the **ABCs—airway, breathing, and circulation**—to lead you to the correct options because they address circulatory status.

---

60. The licensed practical nurse (LPN) has just finished assisting the primary health care provider in placing a central intravenous (IV) line. Which is a **priority** intervention to ensure the client's safety?

1 Checking the client's pain level
2 Checking the client's temperature
3 Preparing the client for a chest x-ray
4 Monitoring the client's blood pressure (BP)

Level of Cognitive Ability: Analyzing
Client Needs: Physiological Integrity
Clinical Judgment/Cognitive Skills: Take Action
Integrated Process: Nursing Process/Implementation
Content Area: Complex Care: Intravenous Therapy
Health Problem: N/A

Answer: 3

Rationale: A major risk associated with central line placement is the possibility of a pneumothorax developing from an accidental puncture of the lung. Checking the results of a chest radiograph is one of the best methods to determine whether this complication has occurred and to verify catheter tip placement before initiating IV therapy. A temperature elevation related to central line insertion would not likely occur immediately after placement. Pain management is important but is not the priority at this point. Although BP assessment is always important in checking a client's status after an invasive procedure, fluid volume overload is not a concern until IV fluids are started.

Priority Nursing Tip: A chest x-ray is needed to ensure that the tip of a newly inserted central IV catheter resides in the superior vena cava. IV solutions would not be infused into the catheter until this is verified.

Test-Taking Strategy: Note the **strategic word,** *priority.* Recall that checking accurate placement is essential before initiating IV therapy.

---

61. A child sustains a greenstick fracture of the humerus from a fall out of a tree house. The nurse describes this type of fracture to the parents and would provide them with which picture? **Refer to the figures.**

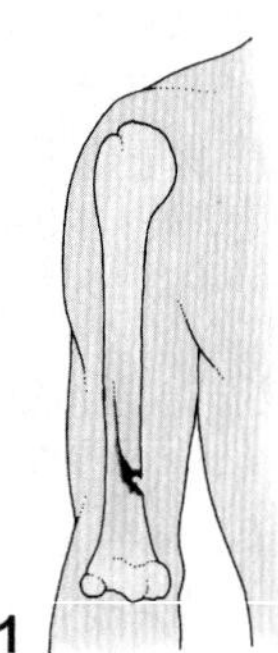
1

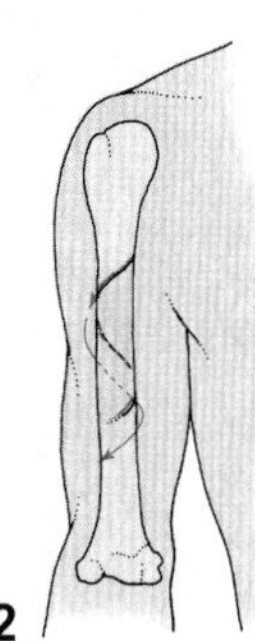
2

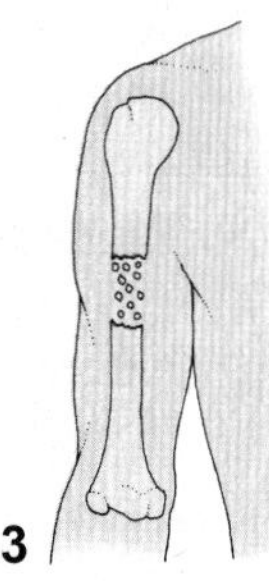
3

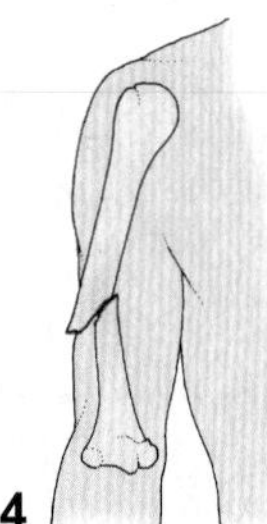
4

(From Ignatavicius D, Workman M: *Medical-surgical nursing: patient-centered collaborative care,* ed 8, St. Louis, 2015, Saunders.)

Level of Cognitive Ability: Analyzing
Client Needs: Physiological Integrity
Clinical Judgment/Cognitive Skills: Take Action
Integrated Process: Nursing Process/Implementation
Content Area: Pediatrics: Musculoskeletal
Health Problem: Pediatric-Specific: Fractures

Answer: 1
Rationale: A greenstick fracture is a break that occurs through the periosteum on one side of the bone with only bowing or buckling on the other side. A spiral fracture (option 2) is characterized by a twisted or circular break that affects the length rather than the width. In a comminuted fracture (option 3), the bone is splintered into pieces. In an open (compound) fracture (option 4), the skin surface over the fracture is disrupted, causing an external wound.
Priority Nursing Tip: The nurse would closely monitor the client's affected extremity. Of particular importance are color, sensation, and motion of the affected limb. Compartment syndrome, which occurs when pressure builds within the muscle, causing decreased blood flow and oxygen delivery, is a common complication associated with breaks and fractures.

Test-Taking Strategy: Focus on the **subject,** greenstick fracture. Recalling that the definition of a greenstick fracture is a break that occurs through the periosteum on one side of the bone with only bowing or buckling on the other side will assist in directing you to the correct option.

62. A 2-year-old toddler has just returned from surgery where a hip spica cast was applied. Which nursing action will **best** maintain the child's skin integrity?

1 Changing the toddler's diapers every 2 hours
2 Keeping the toddler's genital area open to the air
3 Implementing a 3-hour turning schedule for the toddler
4 Checking the toddler's perineal area for redness regularly

Level of Cognitive Ability: Applying
Client Needs: Physiological Integrity
Clinical Judgment/Cognitive Skills: Take Action
Integrated Process: Nursing Process/Implementation
Content Area: Pediatrics: Integumentary
Health Problem: Pediatric-Specific: Developmental Dysplasia of Hip

Answer: 1

Rationale: The spica cast is often needed to treat developmental hip dysplasia or after hip/pelvis surgery. The cast encases the child's trunk and one or both legs while leaving access to the genital area. Considering the age of the child, diapers will be in use and will need to be changed at least every 2 hours during the day and every 3 to 4 hours during the night to help minimize the effect of urine and feces on the child's diaper area. Exposing the genital and perineal area to the air is an intervention that is implemented to assist in healing damaged skin tissue. Turning the child regularly is appropriate care but has no impact on the major issue of incontinence. Checking the skin is necessary but may not identify skin breakdown until after it has begun.

Priority Nursing Tip: If a hip spica cast is placed, the cast edges around the perineum and buttocks may need to be taped with waterproof tape to prevent the cast from becoming wet or soiled during elimination.

Test-Taking Strategy: Focus on the **subject,** skin care for the client in a hip spica cast. Note the **strategic word,** *best.* Eliminate options that reflect interventions that are directed toward addressing skin breakdown once it occurs.

---

63. The licensed practical nurse (LPN) assists the registered nurse to perform a Glasgow Coma Scale assessment on a client with a brainstem injury. Which additional interventions would the LPN be prepared to assist with? **Select all that apply.**

1 Assisting with arterial blood gases
2 Assisting with a lumbar puncture
3 Assessing cranial nerve functioning
4 Assessing respiratory rate and rhythm
5 Assessing pulmonary wedge pressure
6 Assessing cognitive abilities, including memory

Level of Cognitive Ability: Applying
Client Needs: Physiological Integrity
Clinical Judgment/Cognitive Skills: Take Action
Integrated Process: Nursing Process/Implementation
Content Area: Adult Health: Neurological
Health Problem: Adult Health: Neurological: Head Injury/Trauma

Answer: 3, 4

Rationale: Assessment would be specific to the area of the brain involved. Assessing the respiratory status and cranial nerve function is a critical component of the assessment process in a client with a brainstem injury because the respiratory center is located in the brainstem. Options 1, 2, 5, and 6 are not necessary based on the data in the question.

Priority Nursing Tip: For a client with a head injury, priority is given to maintaining a patent airway, breathing, and circulation.

Test-Taking Strategy: Focus on the **data in the question** to assist in selecting option 3. Next, use the **ABCs—airway, breathing, and circulation.** Recall the anatomical location of the respiratory center to direct you to option 4. Remember that the respiratory center is located in the brainstem.

---

64. A client has had a nasointestinal (NI) tube in place for 24 hours. Which finding indicates that the tube is properly located in the intestine?

1 Bowel sounds are absent.
2 The client denies being nauseous.
3 Aspirate from the tube has a pH of 7.
4 The abdominal x-ray indicates that the end of the tube is above the pylorus.

Level of Cognitive Ability: Analyzing
Client Needs: Physiological Integrity
Clinical Judgment/Cognitive Skills: Analyze Cues
Integrated Process: Nursing Process/Data Collection
Content Area: Skills: Tube Care
Health Problem: Adult Health: Gastrointestinal: Lower GI Disorders

Answer: 3

Rationale: The nasogastric or NI tube is used to decompress the intestine and correct a bowel obstruction. Nausea would subside as decompression is accomplished. The pH of the gastric fluid is acidic, and the pH of the intestinal fluid is alkaline (7 or higher). Although bowel sounds will be abnormal in the presence of obstruction, the presence or absence of bowel sounds is not associated with the location of the tube. The end of the tube would be located in the intestine (below the pylorus). Location of the tube can also be determined by radiographs.

Priority Nursing Tip: The client who has had an intestinal tube inserted needs to be positioned on her or his right side to facilitate passage of the weighted bag in the tube through the pylorus of the stomach and into the small intestine.

Test-Taking Strategy: Focus on the **subject**, an NI tube and determining its intestinal location. Recalling that intestinal fluid is alkaline will direct you to the correct option.

---

65. A client diagnosed with myxedema reports having experienced a lack of energy, cold intolerance, and puffiness around the eyes and face. The nurse plans care, knowing that these clinical manifestations are caused by a lack of production of which hormones? **Select all that apply.**

1 Thyroxine (T_4)
2 Prolactin (PRL)
3 Triiodothyronine (T_3)
4 Growth hormone (GH)
5 Luteinizing hormone (LH)
6 Adrenocorticotropic hormone (ACTH)

Level of Cognitive Ability: Applying
Client Needs: Physiological Integrity
Clinical Judgment/Cognitive Skills: Generate Solutions
Integrated Process: Nursing Process/Planning
Content Area: Adult Health: Endocrine
Health Problem: Adult Health: Endocrine: Thyroid Disorders

Answer: 1, 3

Rationale: Although all of these hormones originate from the anterior pituitary, only T_3 and T_4 are associated with the client's symptoms. Myxedema results from inadequate thyroid hormone levels (T_3 and T_4). Low levels of thyroid hormone result in an overall decrease in the basal metabolic rate, affecting virtually every body system and leading to weakness, fatigue, and a decrease in heat production. PRL stimulates breast milk production by the mammary glands, and GH affects bone and soft tissue by promoting growth through protein anabolism and lipolysis. A decrease in LH results in the loss of secondary sex characteristics. A decrease in ACTH is seen in Addison's disease.

Priority Nursing Tip: Myxedema is a rare but serious disorder that results from severe or prolonged thyroid deficiency.

Test-Taking Strategy: Focus on the **subject**, myxedema. Recalling that myxedema is associated with the thyroid gland (hypothyroidism) will assist in connecting the subject of the question, the client's symptoms, to the correct options.

---

66. A client is admitted to the hospital with a suspected diagnosis of Graves' disease. On data collection, which manifestation related to the client's menstrual cycle would the nurse expect the client to report?

1 Amenorrhea
2 Menorrhagia
3 Metrorrhagia
4 Dysmenorrhea

Answer: 1

Rationale: Amenorrhea, or a decreased menstrual flow, is common in the client with Graves' disease. Menorrhagia, metrorrhagia, and dysmenorrhea are also disorders related to the female reproductive system; however, they do not manifest in the presence of Graves' disease.

Priority Nursing Tip: Graves' disease is also known as *toxic diffuse goiter* and results in a hyperthyroid state from the hypersecretion of thyroid hormones.

Test-Taking Strategy: Focus on the **subject,** Graves' disease. Thinking about the pathophysiology associated with Graves' disease will direct you to the correct option.

Level of Cognitive Ability: Applying
Client Needs: Physiological Integrity
Clinical Judgment/Cognitive Skills: Recognize Cues
Integrated Process: Nursing Process/Data Collection
Content Area: Adult Health: Endocrine
Health Problem: Adult Health: Endocrine: Thyroid Disorders

---

67. A client diagnosed with gestational hypertension has just been admitted and is in early active labor. Which finding would the nurse **most likely** expect to note?

1 Increased urine output
2 Increased blood pressure
3 Decreased fetal heart rate
4 Decreased brachial reflexes

Answer: 2

Rationale: The major manifestation of gestational hypertension is increased blood pressure. As the disease progresses, it is possible that increased brachial reflexes, decreased fetal heart rate and variability, and decreased urine output will occur, particularly during labor.

Priority Nursing Tip: Gestational hypertension can lead to preeclampsia. Manifestations of preeclampsia are hypertension and proteinuria. However, note that proteinuria is not always a reliable indicator of preeclampsia.

Test-Taking Strategy: Note the **strategic words,** *most likely,* and focus on the **subject,** gestational hypertension. Noting the name of the disorder will easily direct you to the correct option.

Level of Cognitive Ability: Analyzing
Client Needs: Physiological Integrity
Clinical Judgment/Cognitive Skills: Recognize Cues
Integrated Process: Nursing Process/Data Collection
Content Area: Maternity: Intrapartum
Health Problem: Maternity: Gestational hypertension/preeclampsia and eclampsia

---

68. The nurse has just administered a purified protein derivative (PPD) tuberculin skin test (Mantoux test) to a client who is at low risk for developing tuberculosis. The nurse determines that the test is positive if which occurs?

1 An induration of 15 mm
2 The presence of a wheal
3 A large area of erythema
4 Itching at the injection site

Answer: 1

Rationale: An induration of 10 mm or more is considered positive for clients in low-risk groups. The presence of a wheal would indicate that the skin test was administered appropriately. Erythema or itching at the site is not indicative of a positive reaction.

Priority Nursing Tip: A positive Mantoux test does not mean that active tuberculosis is present, but rather indicates previous exposure to tuberculosis or the presence of inactive (dormant) disease.

Level of Cognitive Ability: Applying
Client Needs: Physiological Integrity
Clinical Judgment/Cognitive Skills: Analyze Cues
Integrated Process: Nursing Process/Data Collection
Content Area: Foundations of Care: Diagnostic Tests
Health Problem: Adult Health: Respiratory: Tuberculosis

Test-Taking Strategy: Focus on the **subject,** a positive Mantoux test, and note that the client is at low risk for developing tuberculosis. This will direct you to the correct option.

---

69. The nurse is reviewing the results of an otoscopic examination done on a client with a suspected diagnosis of mastoiditis. Which finding would the nurse expect to note documented if this disorder was present?

1 A dull red tympanic membrane
2 A mobile tympanic membrane
3 A transparent tympanic membrane
4 A pearly colored tympanic membrane

Answer: 1

Rationale: Otoscopic examination of a client with mastoiditis reveals a red, dull, thick, and immobile tympanic membrane, with or without perforation. Options 2, 3, and 4 indicate normal findings in an otoscopic examination.
Priority Nursing Tip: Mastoiditis may be acute or chronic and results from untreated or inadequately treated chronic or acute otitis media. Interventions focus on stopping the infection before it spreads to other structures.

Test-Taking Strategy: Focus on the **subject,** manifestations of mastoiditis. Recall knowledge of normal findings on an ear examination to direct you to the correct option, the only abnormal finding.

Level of Cognitive Ability: Applying
Client Needs: Physiological Integrity
Clinical Judgment/Cognitive Skills: Recognize Cues
Integrated Process: Nursing Process/Data Collection
Content Area: Adult Health: Ear
Health Problem: Adult Health: Ear: Inflammatory/Infections/Structural Problems

---

70. The nurse is reviewing the record of a client with a disorder involving the inner ear. Which finding would the nurse **most likely** note in this client?

1 Tinnitus
2 Burning in the ear
3 Itching in the affected ear
4 Severe pain in the affected ear

Answer: 1

Rationale: Tinnitus is the most common complaint of clients with ear disorders, especially disorders involving the inner ear. Manifestations of tinnitus can range from mild ringing in the ear that can go unnoticed during the day to a loud roaring in the ear that can interfere with the client's thinking process and attention span. The findings noted in options 2, 3, and 4 are not specifically noted in the client with an inner ear disorder.
Priority Nursing Tip: The inner ear contains the semicircular canals, cochlea, and the distal end of the eight cranial nerves and maintains a sense of balance or equilibrium.

Test-Taking Strategy: Note the **strategic words,** *most likely.* Focus on the **subject,** inner ear disorder. Recalling the function of the inner ear will direct you to the correct option.

Level of Cognitive Ability: Applying
Client Needs: Physiological Integrity
Clinical Judgment/Cognitive Skills: Recognize Cues
Integrated Process: Nursing Process/Data Collection
Content Area: Adult Health: Ear
Health Problem: Adult Health: Ear: Inflammatory/Infections/Structural Problems

---

71. The nurse has a prescription to administer hydroxyzine to a client by the intramuscular route. Before administering the medication, what information would the nurse share with the client?

1 Excessive salivation is a side effect.
2 There will be some pain at the injection site.
3 There would be relief from nausea within 5 minutes.
4 The client may experience increased agitation for about 2 hours.

Level of Cognitive Ability: Applying
Client Needs: Physiological Integrity
Clinical Judgment/Cognitive Skills: Take Action
Integrated Process: Nursing Process/Implementation
Content Area: Pharmacology: Gastrointestinal: Antiemetics
Health Problem: N/A

Answer: 2
Rationale: Hydroxyzine is an antiemetic and sedative/hypnotic that may be used in conjunction with opioid analgesics for added effect. The injection can be painful. Hydroxyzine causes dry mouth and drowsiness as side effects. Agitation is not a usual side effect. Medications administered by the intramuscular route generally take 20 to 30 minutes to become effective.
Priority Nursing Tip: In an adult, a maximum of 3 mL of solution would be administered by the intramuscular route. Larger volumes are difficult for the injection site to absorb and, if prescribed, need to be verified.

Test-Taking Strategy: Focus on the **subject**, intramuscular injection of hydroxyzine. Read each option carefully. Recalling that the medication is an antiemetic and sedative/hypnotic, eliminate options 1 and 4 first because they are the least likely effects. From the remaining options, noting that the medication is administered by the intramuscular route will direct you to the correct option.

---

72. A client with a diagnosis of diabetes mellitus has a blood glucose level of 644 mg/dL. The nurse interprets that this client is at risk of developing which type of acid–base imbalance?

1 Metabolic acidosis
2 Metabolic alkalosis
3 Respiratory acidosis
4 Respiratory alkalosis

Level of Cognitive Ability: Analyzing
Client Needs: Physiological Integrity
Clinical Judgment/Cognitive Skills: Analyze Cues
Integrated Process: Nursing Process/Data Collection
Content Area: Adult Health: Endocrine
Health Problem: Adult Health: Endocrine: Diabetes Mellitus

Answer: 1
Rationale: Diabetes mellitus can lead to metabolic acidosis. When the body does not have sufficient circulating insulin, the blood glucose level rises. At the same time, the cells of the body use all available glucose. The body then breaks down glycogen and fat for fuel. The by-products of fat metabolism are acidotic and can lead to the condition known as *diabetic ketoacidosis.* Options 2, 3, and 4 are incorrect.
Priority Nursing Tip: In metabolic acidosis, to compensate for the acidosis, hyperpnea with Kussmaul's respiration occurs as the lungs attempt to exhale excess carbon dioxide (CO_2), an acidotic by-product of respiration.

Test-Taking Strategy: Focus on the **subject**, diabetes mellitus. Noting the client's diagnosis will assist in eliminating options 3 and 4. From the remaining options, remember that the client with diabetes mellitus is at risk for developing acidosis.

---

73. The nurse reviews the client's most recent blood gas results, which include a pH of 7.43, Pco_2 of 31 mm Hg, and HCO_3 of 21 mEq/L. In analyzing these results, the nurse determines that which acid–base imbalance is present?

1 Compensated metabolic acidosis
2 Compensated respiratory alkalosis
3 Uncompensated respiratory acidosis
4 Uncompensated metabolic alkalosis

Level of Cognitive Ability: Analyzing
Client Needs: Physiological Integrity
Clinical Judgment/Cognitive Skills: Analyze Cues
Integrated Process: Nursing Process/Data Collection
Content Area: Foundations of Care: Acid-Base
Health Problem: N/A

Answer: 2

Rationale: The normal pH is 7.35 to 7.45, the normal Pco_2 is 35 to 45 mm Hg, and the normal HCO_3 is 22 to 27 mEq/L. The pH is elevated in alkalosis and low in acidosis. In a respiratory condition, the pH and the Pco_2 move in opposite directions; that is, the pH rises and the Pco_2 drops (alkalosis) or vice versa (acidosis). In a metabolic condition, the pH and the bicarbonate move in the same direction; if the pH is low, the bicarbonate level will be low also. In this client, the pH is at the high end of normal, indicating compensation and alkalosis. The Pco_2 is low, indicating a respiratory condition (opposite direction of the pH).

Priority Nursing Tip: If the client has a condition that causes overstimulation of the respiratory system, monitor the client for respiratory alkalosis.

Test-Taking Strategy: Focus on the **subject**, an acid–base imbalance. Remember that in a respiratory imbalance you will find that the pH and Pco_2 move in opposite directions. Therefore, options 1 and 4 are eliminated first. Next, remember that the pH is elevated with alkalosis, but compensation has occurred if the pH is within normal range. Option 2 reflects a respiratory alkalotic condition and compensation because the Pco_2 is below normal, but the pH is at the high end of normal.

---

74. The nurse is caring for a client with a nasogastric tube that is attached to low suction. If the client's HCO_3^- is 30, which additional value is **most likely** to be noted in this client's test result?

1 pH 7.52
2 pH 7.36
3 pH 7.25
4 pH 7.20

Level of Cognitive Ability: Analyzing
Client Needs: Physiological Integrity
Clinical Judgment/Cognitive Skills: Analyze Cues
Integrated Process: Nursing Process/Data Collection
Content Area: Foundations of Care: Acid-Base
Health Problem: N/A

Answer: 1

Rationale: Loss of gastric fluid via nasogastric suction or vomiting causes metabolic alkalosis because of the loss of hydrochloric acid (HCl), an acid secreted in the stomach. This occurs as HCO_3 rises above normal. Thus, the loss of hydrogen ions in the HCl results in alkalosis. A pH above 7.45 would be noted.

Priority Nursing Tip: Monitor the client experiencing excessive vomiting or the client with gastrointestinal suctioning for manifestations of metabolic alkalosis.

Test-Taking Strategy: Note the **strategic words,** *most likely,* and focus on the **subject,** complications of gastrointestinal suctioning and acid–base disorders. Eliminate options 3 and 4 first because the loss of HCl would cause an alkalotic condition. Next, note that the pH in option 2 is within normal range.

---

75. The nurse reviews the results of a blood chemistry profile for a client who is experiencing late-stage salicylate poisoning and metabolic acidosis. Which serum study would the nurse review for data about the client's acid–base balance?

1 Sodium
2 Potassium
3 Magnesium
4 Phosphorus

Level of Cognitive Ability: Applying
Client Needs: Physiological Integrity
Clinical Judgment/Cognitive Skills: Recognize Cues
Integrated Process: Nursing Process/Data Collection
Content Area: Complex Care: Poisoning
Health Problem: N/A

Answer: 2
Rationale: A client with late-stage salicylate poisoning is at risk for metabolic acidosis because acetylsalicylic acid increases the client's hydrogen ion (H^+) concentration, decreases the pH, and creates a bicarbonate deficit. Hyperkalemia develops as the body attempts to compensate for the influx of H^+ by moving H^+ into the cell and potassium out of the cell; thus, potassium accumulates in the extracellular space. Clinical manifestations of metabolic acidosis include the clinical indicators of hyperkalemia, including hyperpnea, central nervous system depression, twitching, and seizures. Options 1, 3, and 4 are not primary concerns.
Priority Nursing Tip: In acidosis, the potassium moves out of the cell to make room for the hydrogen ions; thus, the potassium level increases. In alkalosis, the potassium moves into the cell and the potassium level decreases.

Test-Taking Strategy: Focus on the **subject,** an acid–base imbalance and salicylate poisoning. Specific knowledge about the effect of an influx of H^+ in an acid–base disorder and the potassium shifts that occur will direct you to the correct option.

---

76. The licensed practical nurse (LPN) is assisting the emergency room registered nurse in care for a child diagnosed with acetaminophen overdose. The LPN reviews the primary health care provider's prescriptions and prepares to assist to administer which medication?

1 Succimer
2 Vitamin K
3 Acetylcysteine
4 Protamine sulfate

Level of Cognitive Ability: Analyzing
Client Needs: Physiological Integrity
Clinical Judgment/Cognitive Skills: Generate Solutions
Integrated Process: Nursing Process/Planning
Content Area: Complex Care: Poisoning
Health Problem: Pediatric-Specific: Poisoning

Answer: 3
Rationale: Acetylcysteine is the antidote for acetaminophen overdose. It is administered orally or via nasogastric tube in a diluted form with water, juice, or soda. It can also be administered intravenously (undiluted). Protamine sulfate is the antidote for heparin. Succimer is used in the treatment of lead poisoning. Vitamin K is the antidote for warfarin.
Priority Nursing Tip: When used as an antidote via oral administration, dilute acetylcysteine in juice or soda because of its offensive odor.

Test-Taking Strategy: Focus on the **subject,** acetaminophen overdose management. Specific knowledge regarding the antidote for acetaminophen overdose is required to answer this question. Remember that acetylcysteine is the antidote for acetaminophen overdose.

---

77. What would the nurse consider when determining whether a client diagnosed with a respiratory disease could tolerate and benefit from active progressive relaxation? **Select all that apply.**

1 Social status
2 Financial status
3 Functional status
4 Medical diagnosis
5 Ability to expend energy
6 Motivation of the individual

Answer: 3, 4, 5, 6
Rationale: Active progressive relaxation training teaches the client how to effectively rest and reduce tension in the body. Some important considerations when choosing the type of relaxation technique are the client's physiological and psychological status. Because active progressive relaxation training requires a moderate expenditure of energy, the nurse needs to consider the client's functional status, medical diagnosis, and ability to expend energy. For example, a client with advanced respiratory disease may not have sufficient energy reserves to participate in active progressive relaxation techniques. The client needs to be motivated to participate

Level of Cognitive Ability: Applying
Client Needs: Physiological Integrity
Clinical Judgment/Cognitive Skills: Generate Solutions
Integrated Process: Nursing Process/Planning
Content Area: Adult Health: Respiratory
Health Problem: N/A

in this form of alternative therapy to obtain beneficial results. The client's social or financial status has no connection to an ability to tolerate and benefit from active progressive relaxation.
Priority Nursing Tip: Relaxation techniques are important to learn and integrate into daily activities to aid in the prevention of potential stress-related disease processes.

Test-Taking Strategy: Focus on the **subject**, determining whether a client could tolerate and benefit from active progressive relaxation. Use teaching and learning principles to determine whether client motivation is a key factor in the learning process. From the remaining options, noting the word *active* will assist in determining that options 3, 4, and 5 would be considered.

---

78. An adult client has undergone a lumbar puncture to obtain cerebrospinal fluid (CSF) for analysis. After reviewing the results of the analysis, the nurse recognizes that the CSF is normal when which element is negative?

1 Protein
2 Glucose
3 Red blood cells
4 White blood cells

Level of Cognitive Ability: Applying
Client Needs: Physiological Integrity
Clinical Judgment/Cognitive Skills: Recognize Cues
Integrated Process: Nursing Process/Data Collection
Content Area: Foundations of Care: Laboratory Tests
Health Problem: N/A

Answer: 3
Rationale: The adult with a normal CSF has no red blood cells in the CSF. Protein (15–45 mg/dL) and glucose (50–75 mg/dL) are normally present in CSF. The client may have small levels of white blood cells (0–5 cells/mcL).
Priority Nursing Tip: Cerebrospinal fluid is normally clear. A pink or red specimen may be caused by the presence of red blood cells.

Test-Taking Strategy: Focus on the **subject,** normal CSF analysis. Recalling that the presence of red blood cells is abnormal and would indicate blood vessel rupture or meningeal irritation will direct you to the correct option.

---

79. A client who has sustained a burn injury receives a prescription for a regular diet. Which is the **best** meal for the nurse to provide to the client to promote wound healing?

1 Peanut butter and jelly sandwich, apple, tea
2 Chicken breast, broccoli, strawberries, milk
3 Veal chop, boiled potatoes, Jell-O, orange juice
4 Pasta with tomato sauce, garlic bread, ginger ale

Level of Cognitive Ability: Analyzing
Client Needs: Physiological Integrity
Clinical Judgment/Cognitive Skills: Take Action
Integrated Process: Nursing Process/Implementation
Content Area: Foundations of Care: Therapeutic Diets
Health Problem: Adult Health: Integumentary: Burns

Answer: 2
Rationale: The meal with the best potential to promote wound healing includes nutrient-rich food choices, including protein, such as chicken and milk, and vitamin C, such as broccoli and strawberries. The remaining options include one or more items with a low nutritional value, especially the tea, jelly, Jell-O, and ginger ale.
Priority Nursing Tip: Depending on the extent of the injury, the basal metabolic rate is 40 to 100 times higher than normal in a client with a burn.

Test-Taking Strategy: Note the **strategic word,** *best.* Focus on the **subject,** nutrition for a client with a burn injury. Knowledge that protein and vitamin C are necessary for wound healing assists in selecting the option that contains those nutrients, and the option with the most nutrients is the best choice. Eliminate options 1 and 3 first because jelly, tea, and Jell-O have no nutritional value related to healing. From the remaining options, select option 2 over option 4 because option 2 contains foods with greater nutritional value.

---

80. The nurse is assisting in developing a care plan for a client experiencing urge urinary incontinence. Which interventions would be helpful for this type of incontinence? **Select all that apply.**

1 Surgery
2 Bladder retraining
3 Scheduled toileting
4 Dietary modifications
5 Pelvic muscle exercises
6 Intermittent catheterization

Level of Cognitive Ability: Applying
Client Needs: Physiological Integrity
Clinical Judgment/Cognitive Skills: Generate Solutions
Integrated Process: Nursing Process/Planning
Content Area: Skills: Elimination
Health Problem: N/A

Answer: 2, 3, 4, 5
Rationale: Urge incontinence is the involuntary passage of urine after a strong sense of the urgency to void. It is characterized by urinary urgency, often with frequency (more often than every 2 hours); bladder spasm or contraction; and voiding in either small amounts (less than 100 mL) or large amounts (greater than 500 mL). It can be caused by decreased bladder capacity, irritation of the bladder stretch receptors, infection, or alcohol or caffeine ingestion. Interventions to assist the client with urge incontinence include bladder retraining, scheduled toileting, dietary modifications such as eliminating alcohol and caffeine intake, and pelvic muscle exercises to strengthen the muscles. Surgery and urinary catheterization are invasive measures and will not assist in the treatment of urge incontinence.
Priority Nursing Tip: During bladder retraining, to aid in ensuring complete bladder emptying, teach the client to urinate as much as possible, relax for a few moments, then attempt to urinate again. This is known as *double-voiding*.

Test-Taking Strategy: Focus on the **subject,** urge urinary incontinence, and recall the definition of this type of incontinence. Also note that options 1 and 6 are invasive measures, and these types of measures are avoided.

---

81. The nurse caring for a client diagnosed with a stroke is planning care to maintain nutritional status. The nurse is concerned about the client's swallowing ability. Which food item would the nurse eliminate from this client's diet?

1 Spinach
2 Custard
3 Scrambled eggs
4 Mashed potatoes

Level of Cognitive Ability: Applying
Client Needs: Physiological Integrity
Clinical Judgment/Cognitive Skills: Generate Solutions
Integrated Process: Nursing Process/Planning
Content Area: Foundations of Care: Therapeutic Diets
Health Problem: Adult Health: Neurological: Stroke

Answer: 1
Rationale: Raw vegetables; chunky vegetables such as diced beets; and stringy vegetables such as spinach, corn, and peas are foods commonly excluded from the diet of a client with a poor swallowing reflex. In general, flavorful, warm, or well-chilled foods with texture stimulate the swallowing reflex. Soft and semisoft foods such as custards or puddings, egg dishes, and potatoes are usually effective.
Priority Nursing Tip: Pureed foods may be necessary as a means of providing nutritional intake to a client with an altered swallowing ability. Molding the pureed food into the shape of the original food can enhance the appeal of the food item and thus enhance the client's appetite.

Test-Taking Strategy: Focus on the **subject,** altered swallowing ability. Select option 1 as the food that is stringy and with the least amount of substance or consistency.

---

82. An adult client arrives in the emergency department with burns to both entire legs and the perineal area. Using the rule of nines, the nurse would determine that approximately what percentage of the client's body surface has been burned? **Fill in the blank.**

Answer: ____%

Level of Cognitive Ability: Applying
Client Needs: Physiological Integrity
Clinical Judgment/Cognitive Skills: Recognize Cues
Integrated Process: Nursing Process/Data Collection
Content Area: Adult Health: Integumentary
Health Problem: Adult Health: Integumentary: Burns

Answer: 37

Rationale: The most rapid method used to calculate the size of a burn injury in adult clients whose weights are in normal proportion to their heights is the rule of nines. This method divides the body into areas that are multiples of 9%, except for the perineum. Each entire leg is 18%, each arm is 9%, and the head is 9%. The trunk is 36%, and the perineal area is 1%. Both legs and perineal area equal 37%.

Priority Nursing Tip: The rule of nines gives an inaccurate estimate of the extent of the burn injury in a child because of the difference in body proportion between children and adults. Instead, the extent of the burn is expressed as a percentage of the total body surface area using age-related charts.

Test-Taking Strategy: Focus on the **subject,** rule of nines. Knowledge regarding the percentages associated with this method of calculating burn injuries is required to answer this question. Remember that each leg is 18%, each arm is 9%, the head is 9%, the trunk is 36%, and the perineal area is 1%.

---

83. A client is resuming a diet after a Billroth II procedure. To minimize complications associated with eating, which actions would the nurse teach the client? **Select all that apply.**

1 Lying down after eating
2 Eating a diet high in protein
3 Drinking liquids with meals
4 Eating six small meals per day
5 Eating concentrated sweets only between meals

Level of Cognitive Ability: Applying
Client Needs: Physiological Integrity
Clinical Judgment/Cognitive Skills: Take Action
Integrated Process: Nursing Process/Implementation
Content Area: Foundations of Care: Therapeutic Diets
Health Problem: Adult Health: Gastrointestinal: Nutrition Problems

Answer: 1, 2, 4

Rationale: The client who has had a Billroth II procedure is at risk for dumping syndrome. The client would lie down after eating and avoid drinking liquids with meals to prevent this syndrome. The client would be placed on a dry diet that is high in protein, moderate in fat, and low in carbohydrates. Frequent small meals are encouraged, and the client would avoid concentrated sweets.

Priority Nursing Tip: Dumping syndrome is a complication of gastric resection and results from the rapid emptying of the gastric contents into the small intestine after eating.

Test-Taking Strategy: Focusing on the **subject,** Billroth II procedure, and recalling that dumping syndrome is a complication of this surgical procedure will direct you to the correct options. Eliminate option 5 because of the **closed-ended word** "only." Also thinking about the pathophysiology associated with dumping syndrome will assist in answering correctly.

---

84. The nurse is ambulating a client for the first time after having abdominal surgery. What clinical manifestations would indicate to the nurse that the client may be experiencing orthostatic hypotension? **Select all that apply.**

1 Nausea
2 Dizziness
3 Bradycardia
4 Light-headedness
5 Flushing of the face
6 Reports of seeing spots

Level of Cognitive Ability: Analyzing
Client Needs: Physiological Integrity
Clinical Judgment/Cognitive Skills: Analyze Cues
Integrated Process: Nursing Process/Data Collection
Content Area: Foundations of Care: Perioperative Care
Health Problem: N/A

Answer: 1, 2, 4, 6

Rationale: Orthostatic hypotension occurs when a normotensive person develops symptoms of low blood pressure when rising to an upright position. Whenever the nurse gets a client up and out of a bed or chair, there is a risk for orthostatic hypotension. Symptoms of nausea, dizziness, light-headedness, tachycardia, pallor, and reports of seeing spots are characteristic of orthostatic hypotension. A drop of approximately 15 mm Hg in the systolic blood pressure and 10 mm Hg in the diastolic blood pressure also occurs. Fainting can result without intervention, which includes immediately assisting the client to a lying position.

Priority Nursing Tip: Baroreceptors (located in the walls of the aortic arch and carotid sinuses) are specialized nerve endings affected by changes in blood pressure. Increases in the arterial pressure stimulate baroreceptors to decrease the pressure. Conversely, decreases in arterial pressure reduce stimulation, and the blood pressure increases.

Test-Taking Strategy: Focus on the **subject,** the manifestations of orthostatic hypotension. As you read each option, think about the physiological changes that occur when the blood pressure drops. This will assist in answering the question.

---

85. After closely monitoring a child with a head injury who has been exhibiting decorticate (flexor) posturing, the nurse notes that the child suddenly exhibits decerebrate (extensor) posturing. The nurse interprets that this change in the child's posturing indicates what?

1 An insignificant finding
2 An improvement in condition
3 Decreasing intracranial pressure
4 Deteriorating neurological function

Level of Cognitive Ability: Analyzing
Client Needs: Physiological Integrity
Clinical Judgment/Cognitive Skills: Analyze Cues
Integrated Process: Nursing Process/Data Collection
Content Area: Pediatrics: Neurological
Health Problem: Pediatric-Specific: Head Injury

Answer: 4

Rationale: The progression from decorticate to decerebrate posturing usually indicates deteriorating neurological function and warrants the need to notify the registered nurse, who will then contact the neurologist. Options 1, 2, and 3 are inaccurate interpretations.

Priority Nursing Tip: Posturing indicates deterioration in the client's neurological status.

Test-Taking Strategy: Focus on the **subject,** decorticate and decerebrate posturing. Eliminate options 2 and 3 first because they are **comparable or alike.** From the remaining options, recalling the significance of decerebrate posturing will assist in eliminating option 1.

---

86. While caring for a hospitalized infant being monitored for increased intracranial pressure (ICP), the nurse notes that the anterior fontanel bulges when the infant cries. Based on this finding, which conclusion would the nurse draw?

1 No action is required.
2 The head of the bed needs to be lowered.
3 The infant needs to be placed on NPO status.
4 The registered nurse would be notified immediately.

Level of Cognitive Ability: Applying
Client Needs: Physiological Integrity
Clinical Judgment/Cognitive Skills: Take Action
Integrated Process: Nursing Process/Implementation
Content Area: Health Assessment/Physical Exam: Neurological
Health Problem: N/A

Answer: 1

Rationale: The anterior fontanel is diamond shaped and located on the top of the head. It would be soft and flat in a normal infant, and it normally closes by 12 to 18 months of age. The posterior fontanel closes by 2 to 3 months of age. A bulging or tense fontanel may result from crying or increased ICP. Noting a bulging fontanel when the infant cries is a normal finding that requires no action. It is unnecessary to notify the registered nurse immediately. Options 2 and 3 are inappropriate actions.

Priority Nursing Tip: A full or bulging anterior fontanel in a quiet infant may indicate increased ICP.

Test-Taking Strategy: Focus on the **subject,** bulging anterior fontanel. Note that the question states that the anterior fontanel bulges when the infant cries. Remember that a bulging or tense fontanel may result from crying; therefore, it is a normal finding.

---

87. The nurse checking the vital signs of a 3-year-old child hospitalized with a diagnosis of croup notes that the respiratory rate is 28 breaths per minute. Based on this finding, which nursing action is appropriate?

1 Notify the registered nurse immediately.
2 Begin to administer supplemental oxygen.
3 Document the findings according to facility policies.
4 Reassess the respiratory rate, rhythm, and depth in 15 minutes.

Level of Cognitive Ability: Applying
Client Needs: Physiological Integrity
Clinical Judgment/Cognitive Skills: Take Action
Integrated Process: Nursing Process/Implementation
Content Area: Pediatrics: Throat/Respiratory
Health Problem: Pediatric-Specific: Croup

Answer: 3

Rationale: The normal respiratory rate for a 3-year-old child is approximately 20 to 30 breaths per minute. Because the respiratory rate is normal, options 1, 2, and 4 are unnecessary actions. The nurse would document the findings.

Priority Nursing Tip: Nasal flaring, sternal retractions, and inspiratory stridor are signs of a compromised airway and respiratory distress.

Test-Taking Strategy: Focus on the **subject,** pediatric vital signs. Recalling that the normal respiratory rate for a 3-year-old child is approximately 20 to 30 breaths per minute will direct you to the correct option.

---

88. The nurse is collecting data from a client who is suspected of having mittelschmerz. Which subjective finding supports the possibility of this condition?

1 Experiences pain during intercourse
2 Has pain at the onset of menstruation
3 Experiences profuse vaginal bleeding
4 Has sharp pelvic pain during ovulation

Level of Cognitive Ability: Applying
Client Needs: Physiological Integrity
Clinical Judgment/Cognitive Skills: Recognize Cues
Integrated Process: Nursing Process/Data Collection
Content Area: Adult Health: Reproductive
Health Problem: Adult Health: Reproductive: Menstruation Problems/Fertility/Infertility

Answer: 4

Rationale: Mittelschmerz (middle pain) refers to pelvic pain that occurs midway between menstrual periods or at the time of ovulation. The pain is caused by a growth follicle within the ovary, or rupture of the follicle and subsequent spillage of follicular fluid and blood into the peritoneal space. The pain is fairly sharp and is felt on the right or left side of the pelvis. It generally lasts 1 to 3 days, and slight vaginal bleeding may accompany the discomfort.
Priority Nursing Tip: The discomfort that occurs with mittelschmerz is usually relieved with a mild analgesic.

Test-Taking Strategy: Focus on the **subject,** mittelschmerz. Recalling that mittelschmerz is "middle pain" will direct you to the correct option.

---

89. During data collection, the client tells the nurse that she was diagnosed with endometriosis. Which explanation presented by the client demonstrates an understanding of the description of the condition?

1 "Endometriosis is known as primary dysmenorrhea."
2 "Endometriosis is what causes the pain when I ovulate."
3 "Endometriosis is the condition that has caused me to stop menstruating."
4 "Endometriosis means that I have uterine tissue growing outside my uterus."

Level of Cognitive Ability: Evaluating
Client Needs: Physiological Integrity
Clinical Judgment/Cognitive Skills: Evaluate Outcomes
Integrated Process: Nursing Process/Implementation
Content Area: Adult Health: Reproductive
Health Problem: Adult Health: Reproductive: Inflammatory/Infectious Problems

Answer: 4

Rationale: *Endometriosis* is defined as the presence of tissue outside the uterus that resembles the endometrium in structure, function, and response to estrogen and progesterone during the menstrual cycle. *Mittelschmerz* refers to pelvic pain that occurs midway between menstrual periods coinciding with ovulation. *Primary dysmenorrhea* refers to menstrual pain without identified pathology. *Amenorrhea,* the cessation of menstruation for a period of at least three cycles or 6 months in a woman who has established a pattern of menstruation, can result from a variety of causes.
Priority Nursing Tip: Nonpharmacological measures such as rest and the application of heat to the lower abdomen will assist in relieving the discomfort associated with menstrual discomfort.

Test-Taking Strategy: Focus on the **subject,** endometriosis. Specific knowledge about this disorder is needed to answer correctly. It is necessary to know that this condition refers to tissue outside the uterus that resembles the endometrium.

---

90. The primary health care provider prescribes 250 mg of amikacin sulfate every 12 hours. How many milliliters (mL) would the nurse prepare to administer 1 dose? **Refer to the figure. Fill in the blank.**

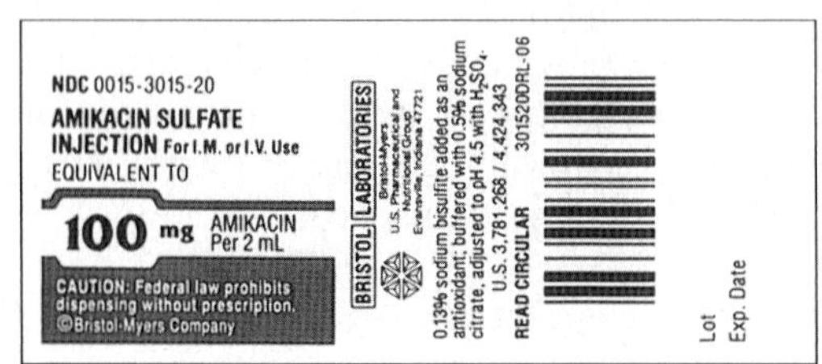

(From Kee J, Marshall S: *Clinical calculations*, ed 7, St. Louis, 2012, Saunders.)

Answer: _______ mL

Level of Cognitive Ability: Applying
Client Needs: Physiological Integrity
Clinical Judgment/Cognitive Skills: Generate Solutions
Integrated Process: Nursing Process/Implementation
Content Area: Skills: Dosage Calculations
Health Problem: N/A

Answer: 5
Rationale: Use the medication calculation formula.
Formula:

$$\frac{\text{Desired} \times \text{mL}}{\text{Available}} = \text{mL per dose}$$

$$\frac{250\text{ mg} \times 2\text{ mL}}{100\text{ mg}} = 5\text{ mL per dose}$$

Priority Nursing Tip: Amikacin sulfate is an aminoglycoside that can cause ototoxicity and renal toxicity as adverse effects.

Test-Taking Strategy: Focus on the **subject,** amikacin sulfate, and note the data on the medication label. Follow the formula for calculating the correct dose. Once you have performed the calculation, recheck your work with a calculator and ensure that the answer makes sense.

---

91. A hepatitis B screen is performed on a postpartum client, and the results indicate the presence of antigens in the maternal blood. Which intervention would the nurse anticipate to be prescribed for the neonate? **Select all that apply.**

1 Obtaining serum liver enzymes
2 Administering hepatitis vaccine
3 Supporting breast-feeding every 5 hours
4 Repeating hepatitis B screen in 1 week
5 Administering hepatitis B immune globulin
6 Administering antibiotics while hospitalized

Level of Cognitive Ability: Applying
Client Needs: Physiological Integrity
Clinical Judgment/Cognitive Skills: Generate Solutions
Integrated Process: Nursing Process/Planning
Content Area: Maternity: Newborn
Health Problem: Newborn: Infections

Answer: 2, 5
Rationale: A hepatitis B screen is performed to detect the presence of antigens in maternal blood. If antigens are present, the neonate would receive the hepatitis vaccine and hepatitis B immune globulin within 12 hours after birth. Obtaining serum liver enzymes, retesting the maternal blood in a week, breast-feeding every 5 hours, and administering antibiotics are inappropriate actions that would not decrease the chance of the neonate contracting the hepatitis B virus.
Priority Nursing Tip: The risks of prematurity, low birth weight, and neonatal death increase if the parent has hepatitis B infection.

Test-Taking Strategy: Focus on the **subject,** hepatitis B in pregnancy, and the **data in the question.** Eliminate the remaining options because they are actions that would not decrease the chance of the neonate contracting the hepatitis B virus. Recall that the concern is the effect on the fetus and neonate, which will lead you to the correct option.

92. The nurse is reinforcing information to the family of a terminally ill client about palliative care. The nurse identifies which goals as being those of palliative care? **Select all that apply.**

1 The delay of the impending death
2 Offering a caring support system
3 Providing measures focused on pain management
4 Introduction of interventions that enhance the quality of life
5 Expanding the focus of care to both the client and the family
6 Addressing the expressed spiritual needs of the client and the family

Level of Cognitive Ability: Applying
Client Needs: Physiological Integrity
Clinical Judgment/Cognitive Skills: Take Action
Integrated Process: Caring
Content Area: Developmental Stages: End-of-Life Care
Health Problem: N/A

Answer: 2, 3, 4, 5, 6
Rationale: Palliative care is a philosophy of total care. Palliative care goals include the following: offering a support system to help the client live as actively as possible until death; providing relief from pain and other distressing symptoms; enhancing the quality of life; offering a support system to help families cope during the client's illness and their own bereavement; affirming life and regarding dying as a normal process, neither hastening nor postponing death; and integrating psychological and spiritual aspects of client care.
Priority Nursing Tip: Palliative care is designed to assist the client and family in achieving the best quality of life during the entire course of an illness.

Test-Taking Strategy: Focus on the **subject,** goals of palliative care. Recall that palliative care interventions are designed to relieve or reduce the intensity of uncomfortable symptoms, but not to produce a cure, and that palliative care is a philosophy of total care. With this in mind, read each option and determine if it meets this description.

---

93. A pregnant client reports that their last menstrual period was February 9, 2022. Using Naegele's rule, what will the nurse determine as the estimated date of birth?

1 October 7, 2022
2 October 16, 2022
3 November 7, 2022
4 November 16, 2022

Level of Cognitive Ability: Applying
Client Needs: Physiological Integrity
Clinical Judgment/Cognitive Skills: Analyze Cues
Integrated Process: Nursing Process/Data Collection
Content Area: Maternity: Antepartum
Health Problem: N/A

Answer: 4
Rationale: Accurate use of Naegele's rule requires that the woman has a regular 28-day menstrual cycle. To calculate the estimated date of birth, the nurse would subtract 3 months from the first day of the last menstrual period, add 7 days, and then adjust the year as appropriate. First day of last menstrual period: February 9, 2022; subtract 3 months: November 9, 2021; add 7 days: November 16, 2021; and add 1 year, November 16, 2022.
Priority Nursing Tip: Several formulas can be used by the obstetrician to determine the estimated date of birth. Naegele's rule is reasonably accurate and is the method that is usually used.

Test-Taking Strategy: Focus on the **subject,** Naegele's rule, to answer this question. Be careful when following the steps to determine the estimated date of birth using this rule. Read all of the options carefully, noting the dates and years before selecting an option.

---

94. The nurse is assisting in developing a plan of care for a client who suffered a pelvic fracture after a motor vehicle crash (MVC). Which interventions would be included in the nursing care plan to prevent skin breakdown? **Select all that apply.**

1. Minimize the force and friction applied to the skin.
2. Massage vigorously over bony prominences twice daily.
3. Perform a systematic skin inspection at least once a day.
4. Cleanse the skin at the time of soiling and at routine intervals.
5. Use pillows to keep the knees and other bony prominences from direct contact with one another.
6. Use hot water and a mild cleansing agent that minimizes irritation and dryness of the skin when bathing the client.

Answer: 1, 3, 4, 5

Rationale: The client in this question is at high risk for pressure injury. Interventions for prevention of pressure injuries include minimizing the force and friction applied to the skin; performing a systematic skin inspection at least once a day, giving particular attention to the bony prominences; cleansing the skin at the time of soiling and at routine intervals; avoiding the use of hot water; and using a mild cleansing agent that minimizes irritation and dryness of the skin. Pillows would be used to keep the knees and other bony prominences from direct contact with one another, because skin contact can promote breakdown. Massaging over bony prominences (especially vigorous massage) can be harmful to at-risk skin surfaces.

Priority Nursing Tip: The skin is the first line of defense against infection; therefore, a major role of the nurse is to prevent skin breakdown.

Test-Taking Strategy: Focus on the **subject,** preventing skin breakdown. Visualize each of the options in terms of how it will prevent or promote skin breakdown. Eliminate option 2 because of the word *vigorously,* and eliminate option 6 because of the word *hot.*

Level of Cognitive Ability: Applying
Client Needs: Physiological Integrity
Clinical Judgment/Cognitive Skills: Generate Solutions
Integrated Process: Nursing Process: Planning
Content Area: Adult Health: Integumentary
Health Problem: Adult Health: Musculoskeletal: Skeletal Injury

---

95. The nurse is preparing to assist to measure the fundal height of a client whose fetus is 28 weeks' gestation. In what position would the nurse place the client to perform the procedure?

1. In a standing position
2. In Trendelenburg's position
3. Supine with the head of the bed elevated to 45 degrees
4. Supine with their head on a pillow and knees slightly flexed

Answer: 4

Rationale: When measuring fundal height, the client lies in a supine (back) position with their head on a pillow and knees slightly flexed. The standing position, Trendelenburg's (head lowered), or supine with the head of the bed elevated to 45 degrees would prevent the nurse from getting an accurate measurement.

Priority Nursing Tip: During the second and third trimesters of pregnancy (weeks 18 to 30), fundal height in centimeters (cm) approximately equals fetal age in weeks plus 2 cm.

Test-Taking Strategy: Focus on the **subject,** measuring fundal height. Visualize this data collection technique to direct you to the correct option. Options 1, 2, or 3 would not give an accurate measurement.

Level of Cognitive Ability: Applying
Client Needs: Physiological Integrity
Clinical Judgment/Cognitive Skills: Take Action
Integrated Process: Nursing Process/Data Collection
Content Area: Maternity: Antepartum
Health Problem: N/A

96. The nurse is assisting to measure the fundal height on a client who is 36 weeks' gestation when the client reports feeling light-headed. What would the nurse expect is occurring when collecting data from the client?

1 Fear
2 Anemia
3 A full bladder
4 Compression of the vena cava

Level of Cognitive Ability: Analyzing
Client Needs: Physiological Integrity
Clinical Judgment/Cognitive Skills: Analyze Cues
Integrated Process: Nursing Process/Data Collection
Content Area: Maternity: Antepartum
Health Problem: Maternity: Supine Hypotension

Answer: 4

Rationale: Compression of the inferior vena cava and aorta by the uterus may cause supine hypotension syndrome (vena cava syndrome) late in pregnancy. Having the client turn onto their left side or elevating the left buttock during fundal height measurement will prevent the problem. Options 1, 2, and 3 are unrelated to this syndrome.

Priority Nursing Tip: Signs of supine hypotension (vena cava syndrome) in a pregnant client include pallor, light-headedness, breathlessness, tachycardia, hypotension, sweating, cool and damp skin, and fetal distress.

Test-Taking Strategy: Focus on the **subject,** vena cava syndrome. Recalling that compression of the inferior vena cava and aorta by the uterus may cause supine hypotension syndrome will direct you to the correct option.

---

97. The nurse in the prenatal clinic is assisting in monitoring a client who is pregnant with twins. The nurse monitors the client closely for which **priority** complication that is associated with a twin pregnancy?

1 Hemorrhoids
2 Postterm labor
3 Maternal anemia
4 Costovertebral-angle tenderness

Level of Cognitive Ability: Applying
Client Needs: Physiological Integrity
Clinical Judgment/Cognitive Skills: Recognize Cues
Integrated Process: Nursing Process/Data Collection
Content Area: Maternity: Antepartum
Health Problem: N/A

Answer: 3

Rationale: Maternal anemia often occurs in twin pregnancies because of a greater demand for iron by the fetuses. Options 1 and 4 occur in a twin pregnancy but would not be as high a priority as anemia. Option 2 is incorrect because twin pregnancies often end in prematurity.

Priority Nursing Tip: The woman with a multifetal pregnancy needs to be monitored closely for signs of anemia. Adequate nutrition is critical, and supplemental vitamins are prescribed to meet the needs of each fetus without depleting maternal stores.

Test-Taking Strategy: Focus on the **subject,** twin pregnancy, and note the **strategic word,** *priority.* Thinking about the physiological occurrences of a twin pregnancy will direct you to the correct option.

---

98. A nurse is collecting data from a prenatal client who has been diagnosed with heart disease. The nurse carefully checks the client's vital signs, weight, and fluid and nutritional status to detect for complications caused by which pregnancy-related concern?

1 Rh incompatibility
2 Fetal cardiomegaly
3 Increase in circulating blood volume
4 Hypertrophy and increased contractility of the heart

Level of Cognitive Ability: Analyzing
Client Needs: Physiological Integrity
Clinical Judgment/Cognitive Skills: Recognize Cues
Integrated Process: Nursing Process/Data Collection
Content Area: Maternity: Antepartum
Health Problem: Maternity: Cardiac Disease

Answer: 3

Rationale: Pregnancy taxes the circulating system of every woman because the blood volume increases, which causes the cardiac output to increase. Stroke volume × heart rate = cardiac output (SV × HR = CO). Options 1, 2, and 4 are not directly associated with pregnancy in a client with a cardiac condition.

Priority Nursing Tip: A pregnant client with cardiac disease may be unable to physiologically cope with the added blood volume that occurs during pregnancy.

Test-Taking Strategy: Focus on the **subject,** a prenatal client with heart disease. Eliminate options 1 and 2 first because they address the fetus, not the prenatal client. From the remaining options, recalling the changes that take place in the woman during pregnancy will direct you to the correct option. Also, remember that hypertrophy of the heart may occur in cardiac disease, but the outcome would be a decrease in contractility, not an increase.

---

99. The nurse is providing care for a client who has just experienced a liver biopsy performed at the bedside. Which position would the nurse place the client in after the biopsy?

1 Supine with the head elevated on one pillow
2 Semi-Fowler's with two pillows under the legs
3 Left side-lying with a small pillow under the puncture site
4 Right side-lying with a folded towel under the puncture site

Level of Cognitive Ability: Applying
Client Needs: Physiological Integrity
Clinical Judgment/Cognitive Skills: Take Action
Integrated Process: Nursing Process/Implementation
Content Area: Foundations of Care: Diagnostic Tests
Health Problem: N/A

Answer: 4

Rationale: The liver is located on the right side of the body. After a liver biopsy, the nurse positions the client on the right side with a small pillow or folded towel under the puncture site for 2 hours. This position compresses the liver against the abdominal wall at the biopsy site to tamponade bleeding from the puncture site.

Priority Nursing Tip: Because of the concern for bleeding after a liver biopsy, coagulation blood studies (prothrombin time, partial thromboplastin time, platelet count) are performed before the procedure is done.

Test-Taking Strategy: Focus on the **subject,** liver biopsy. Use knowledge regarding the anatomy of the body and principles of hemostasis to answer this question. Remember that the liver is on the right side of the body, and by applying pressure at the puncture site, the nurse helps prevent the escape of blood or bile.

100. A client has a prescription to receive an enema before bowel surgery. The nurse assists the client into which **best** position to administer the enema? **Refer to the figures.**

1 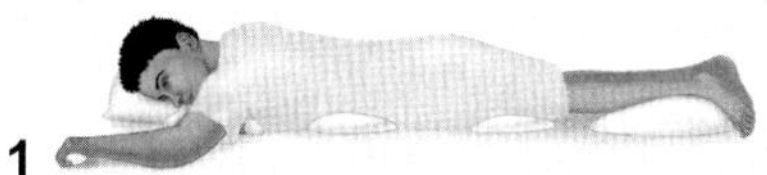

2 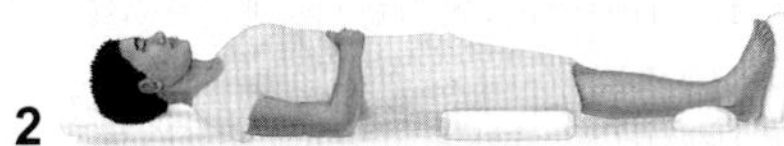

3 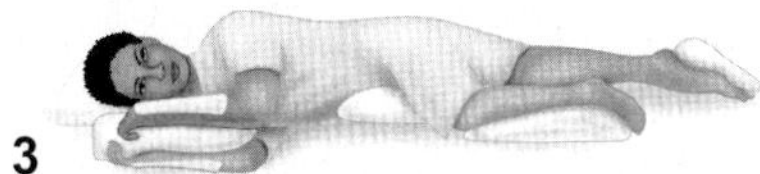

4 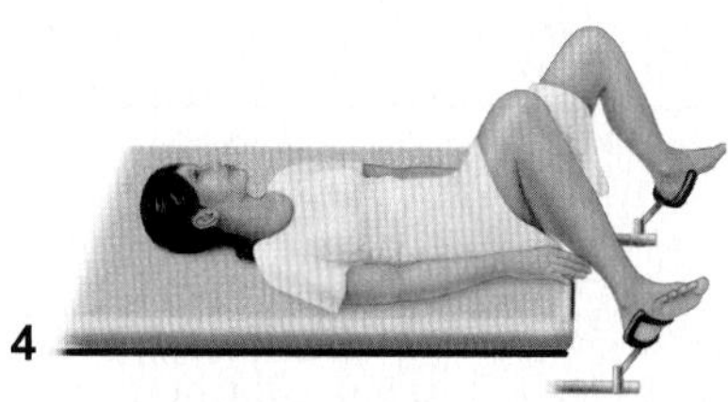

Level of Cognitive Ability: Applying
Client Needs: Physiological Integrity
Clinical Judgment/Cognitive Skills: Take Action
Integrated Process: Nursing Process/Implementation
Content Area: Skills: Elimination
Health Problem: N/A

Answer: 3

Rationale: When administering an enema, the nurse places the client in a modified lateral recumbent position (option 3), exposing the rectal area and allowing the enema solution to flow by gravity in the natural direction of the colon. In the prone position (option 1), the client is lying on the stomach. In the supine position (option 2), the client is lying on the back. The lithotomy position (option 4) is used for performing a pelvic examination.

Priority Nursing Tip: Administering an enema with the client sitting on the toilet can cause injury to the rectal mucosa because the rectal tubing is curved and could scratch the tissue.

Test-Taking Strategy: Note the **strategic word,** *best.* Focus on the **subject,** enema administration. Use knowledge regarding the anatomy of the bowel to answer the question. This will assist in eliminating options 2 and 4. From the remaining options, visualize the procedure for administering an enema and eliminate option 1 because, in the prone position, the client is lying on the stomach.

101. The nurse is assisting in monitoring a client who is receiving cyclosporine after a kidney transplant. Which condition indicates to the nurse that the client is experiencing an adverse effect of the medication?

1 Acne
2 Sweating
3 Joint pain
4 Hyperkalemia

Answer: 4

Rationale: Cyclosporine is an immunosuppressant medication used in the prophylaxis of organ rejection. Adverse effects include nephrotoxicity, infection, hepatotoxicity, hypomagnesemia, coma, hypertension, tremor, and hirsutism. Additionally, neurotoxicity, gastrointestinal effects, hyperkalemia, and hyperglycemia can occur. Options 1, 2, and 3 are not associated with this medication.

Priority Nursing Tip: Monitor the urine output and the potassium level if a client is receiving a medication that is nephrotoxic.

Test-Taking Strategy: Focus on the **subject**, cyclosporine. Recall that this medication is an immunosuppressant used to prevent organ rejection. Next, remember that this medication is nephrotoxic and causes hyperkalemia. This will direct you to the correct option.

Level of Cognitive Ability: Analyzing
Client Needs: Physiological Integrity
Clinical Judgment/Cognitive Skills: Recognize Cues
Integrated Process: Nursing Process/Data Collection
Content Area: Pharmacology: Immune: Immunosuppressants
Health Problem: Adult Health: Immune: Transplantation

---

102. The nurse tells the parents of a newborn that it is standard routine to instill the ophthalmic ointment form of which medication into the eyes of a newborn infant as a preventive measure against ophthalmia neonatorum?

1 Penicillin
2 Neomycin
3 Vitamin K
4 Erythromycin

Answer: 4

Rationale: Ophthalmic erythromycin 0.5% ointment is a broad-spectrum antibiotic and is used prophylactically to prevent ophthalmia neonatorum, an eye infection acquired from the newborn infant's passage through the birth canal. Infection from these organisms can cause blindness or serious eye damage. Erythromycin is effective against *Neisseria gonorrhoeae* and *Chlamydia trachomatis.* Vitamin K is administered in an injectable form to the newborn infant to prevent abnormal bleeding, and it promotes the liver's formation of the clotting factors II, VII, IX, and X. Options 1 and 2 are incorrect and are not medications routinely used in the newborn.

Priority Nursing Tip: Administer prophylactic eye medication to a newborn within 1 hour after birth.

Test-Taking Strategy: Focus on the **subject,** eye medication used for the prophylaxis of ophthalmia neonatorum. This will assist in eliminating option 3, an injection. From the remaining options, recalling that erythromycin is a broad-spectrum antibiotic will direct you to the correct option.

Level of Cognitive Ability: Applying
Client Needs: Physiological Integrity
Clinical Judgment/Cognitive Skills: Take Action
Integrated Process: Teaching and Learning
Content Area: Maternity: Newborn
Health Problem: Newborn: Infections

---

103. The nurse is reviewing the records of recently admitted clients to the postpartum unit. The nurse determines that which clients would have an increased risk for developing a puerperal infection? **Select all that apply.**

1 A client with a history of previous infections
2 A client who has given birth to a set of twins
3 A client who had numerous vaginal examinations
4 A client who has experienced three previous miscarriages
5 A client who underwent a vaginal delivery of the newborn
6 A client who experienced prolonged rupture of the membranes

Level of Cognitive Ability: Analyzing
Client Needs: Physiological Integrity
Clinical Judgment/Cognitive Skills: Analyze Cues
Integrated Process: Nursing Process/Data Collection
Content Area: Maternity: Antepartum
Health Problem: Maternity: Infections/Inflammations

Answer: 1, 3, 6

Rationale: Risk factors associated with puerperal infection include a history of previous infections, excessive number of vaginal examinations, cesarean births, prolonged rupture of the membranes, prolonged labor, trauma, and retained placental fragments. A vaginal delivery, a history of miscarriages, and the delivery of twins are not considered risk factors for developing a puerperal infection.

Priority Nursing Tip: The temperature may be elevated during the first 24 hours postpartum because of the dehydrating effects of labor. However, a temperature higher than 100.4°F needs to be reported to the obstetrician because it is an indication of infection.

Test-Taking Strategy: Focus on the **subject,** risks for developing a puerperal infection. Think about the causes of infection, and select the options that present a pathway for bacteria to enter into the woman's body.

---

104. After assisting with a vaginal delivery, what would the nurse do to prevent heat loss via conduction in the newborn?

1 Wrap the newborn in a blanket.
2 Close the doors to the delivery room.
3 Dry the newborn with a warm blanket.
4 Place the newborn on a warm crib pad.

Level of Cognitive Ability: Applying
Client Needs: Physiological Integrity
Clinical Judgment/Cognitive Skills: Take Action
Integrated Process: Nursing Process/Implementation
Content Area: Maternity: Newborn
Health Problem: Newborn: Thermoregulation

Answer: 4

Rationale: Hypothermia caused by conduction occurs when the newborn is on a cold surface, such as a cold pad or mattress. Warming the crib pad will assist in preventing hypothermia by conduction. Radiation occurs when heat from the newborn radiates to a colder surface. Convection occurs as air moves across the newborn's skin from an open door and heat is transferred to the air. Evaporation of moisture from a wet body dissipates heat along with the moisture. Keeping the newborn dry by drying the wet newborn at birth will prevent hypothermia via evaporation.

Priority Nursing Tip: Newborns do not shiver to produce heat. Instead, they have brown fat deposits, which produce heat.

Test-Taking Strategy: Focus on the **subject,** preventing heat loss in the newborn. Note the word *conduction* in the question to assist in selecting the correct option. Recalling that conduction occurs when a baby is on a cold surface will assist in directing you to the correct option.

---

105. After data collection and diagnostic evaluation, it has been determined that the client has a diagnosis of Lyme disease, stage II. The nurse checks the client for which manifestation that is **most** indicative of this stage?

1 Lethargy
2 Headache
3 Erythematous rash
4 Cardiac dysrhythmias

Level of Cognitive Ability: Analyzing
Client Needs: Physiological Integrity
Clinical Judgment/Cognitive Skills: Recognize Cues
Integrated Process: Nursing Process/Data Collection
Content Area: Adult Health: Immune
Health Problem: Adult Health: Immune: Lyme Disease

Answer: 4

Rationale: Stage II of Lyme disease develops within 1 to 3 months in most untreated individuals. The most serious problems in this stage include cardiac dysrhythmias, dyspnea, dizziness, and neurological disorders such as Bell's palsy and paralysis. These problems are not usually permanent. Flulike symptoms (headache and lethargy), muscle pain and stiffness, and a rash appear in stage I.

Priority Nursing Tip: The typical ring-shaped rash of Lyme disease does not occur in all clients. Additionally, if a rash does occur, it can occur anywhere on the body, not only at the site of the tick bite.

Test-Taking Strategy: Note the **strategic word,** *most.* Focus on the **subject,** Lyme disease. Recalling that a rash and flulike symptoms occur in stage I will assist you in eliminating options 1, 2, and 3 and direct you to the correct option.

---

106. The nurse is caring for a client with a diagnosis of pemphigus vulgaris. On data collection of the client, the nurse would look for which sign characteristic of this condition?

1 Turner's sign
2 Chvostek's sign
3 Nikolsky's sign
4 Trousseau's sign

Level of Cognitive Ability: Analyzing
Client Needs: Physiological Integrity
Clinical Judgment/Cognitive Skills: Recognize Cues
Integrated Process: Nursing Process/Data Collection
Content Area: Adult Health: Immune
Health Problem: Adult Health: Immune: Autoimmune Disease

Answer: 3

Rationale: A hallmark sign of pemphigus vulgaris is Nikolsky's sign, which occurs when the epidermis can be rubbed off by slight friction or injury. Other characteristics include flaccid bullae that rupture easily and emit a foul-smelling drainage, leaving crusted, denuded skin. The lesions are common on the face, back, chest, and umbilicus. Even slight pressure on an intact blister may cause spread to adjacent skin. *Turner's sign* refers to a grayish discoloration of the flanks and is seen in clients with acute pancreatitis. *Chvostek's sign,* seen in tetany, is a spasm of the facial muscles elicited by tapping the facial nerve in the region of the parotid gland. *Trousseau's sign* is a sign for tetany, in which carpal spasm can be elicited by compressing the upper arm with a blood pressure cuff inflated above the systolic pressure and causing ischemia to the nerves distally.

Priority Nursing Tip: Pemphigus vulgaris is a rare autoimmune disease that causes blister (bullae) formation. The nurse needs to provide gentle care to prevent disruption of the skin lesions.

Test-Taking Strategy: Focus on the **subject,** pemphigus vulgaris. Eliminate options 2 and 4 first because they are **comparable or alike** and both relate to tetany. From the remaining options, recalling that Turner's sign is related to pancreatitis will direct you to the correct option.

---

107. The nurse is caring for a child recovering from a tonsillectomy. Which fluid or food item would be offered to the child?

1 Green Jell-O
2 Cold soda pop
3 Butterscotch pudding
4 Cool cherry-flavored Kool-Aid

Level of Cognitive Ability: Applying
Client Needs: Physiological Integrity
Clinical Judgment/Cognitive Skills: Take Action
Integrated Process: Nursing Process/Implementation
Content Area: Pediatrics: Throat/Respiratory
Health Problem: Pediatric-Specific: Tonsillitis and Adenoiditis

Answer: 1
Rationale: After tonsillectomy, clear, cool liquids would be administered. Citrus, carbonated, and extremely hot or cold liquids need to be avoided because they may irritate the throat. Milk and milk products (pudding) are avoided because they coat the throat and cause the child to clear the throat, thus increasing the risk of bleeding. Red liquids need to be avoided because they give the appearance of blood if the child vomits.
Priority Nursing Tip: After tonsillectomy, position the client prone or side-lying to facilitate mouth drainage.

Test-Taking Strategy: Focus on the **subject**, care after tonsillectomy. Avoiding foods and fluids that may irritate or cause bleeding is the concern. This will assist in eliminating options 2 and 3. The words *cherry-flavored* in option 4 would be the clue that this is not an appropriate food item.

---

108. The nurse is reinforcing information to a new parent on newborn care. When teaching cord care, the nurse would instruct the parent to take which action?

1 If antibiotic ointment has been applied to the cord, it is not necessary to do anything else to it.
2 All that is necessary is to wash the cord with antibacterial soap and allow it to air-dry once a day.
3 Apply alcohol thoroughly to the cord, being careful not to move the cord because it will cause pain to the newborn infant.
4 Apply the prescribed cleansing agent to the cord, ensuring that all areas around the cord are cleaned 2 to 3 times a day.

Level of Cognitive Ability: Applying
Client Needs: Physiological Integrity
Clinical Judgment/Cognitive Skills: Take Action
Integrated Process: Teaching and Learning
Content Area: Maternity: Newborn
Health Problem: N/A

Answer: 4
Rationale: The cord and base would be cleansed with alcohol (or another substance as prescribed) thoroughly, 2 to 3 times per day. The steps are: (1) lift the cord; (2) wipe around the cord, starting at the top; (3) clean the base of the cord; and (4) fold the diaper below the umbilical cord to allow the cord to air-dry and prevent contamination from urine. Antibiotic ointment is not normally prescribed. Continuation of cord care is necessary until the cord falls off within 7 to 14 days. Water and soap are not necessary; in fact, the cord needs to be kept from getting wet. The infant does not feel pain in this area.
Priority Nursing Tip: The nurse needs to teach the parents of a newborn about the importance of providing cord care because the umbilical cord stump provides a medium for bacterial growth and can easily become infected.

Test-Taking Strategy: Focus on the **subject**, umbilical cord care. Simply recalling that the cord needs to be cleansed 2 to 3 times a day will direct you to the correct option. Also, note the words *prescribed cleansing agent* in the correct option.

---

109. The nurse assisting in monitoring a preterm newborn infant for manifestations of respiratory distress syndrome (RDS) would check the infant for which manifestations? **Select all that apply.**

1 Cyanosis
2 Tachypnea
3 Retractions
4 Nasal flaring
5 Acrocyanosis
6 Grunting respirations

Answer: 1, 2, 3, 4, 6
Rationale: The newborn infant with RDS may present with clinical manifestation of cyanosis, tachypnea or apnea, chest wall retractions, audible grunts, or nasal flaring. Acrocyanosis, the bluish discoloration of the hands and feet, is associated with immature peripheral circulation and is not uncommon in the first few hours of life.
Priority Nursing Tip: The presence of retractions indicates respiratory distress and possible hypoxemia.

Level of Cognitive Ability: Analyzing
Client Needs: Physiological Integrity
Clinical Judgment/Cognitive Skills: Recognize Cues
Integrated Process: Nursing Process/Data Collection
Content Area: Maternity: Newborn
Health Problem: Newborn: Respiratory Problems

Test-Taking Strategy: Focus on the **subject**, respiratory distress syndrome. Recalling that acrocyanosis may be a normal sign in a newborn infant will assist in eliminating it as an option.

---

110. The nurse checking the apical heart rates of several different newborn infants notes that which heart rate is normal for this newborn population?

1 90 beats per minute
2 140 beats per minute
3 180 beats per minute
4 190 beats per minute

Answer: 2
Rationale: The normal heart rate in a newborn infant is approximately 100 to 160 beats per minute. Options 1, 3, and 4 are incorrect. Option 1 indicates bradycardia, and options 3 and 4 indicate tachycardia (more than 160 beats per minute).
Priority Nursing Tip: To measure the apical heart rate of a newborn infant, the nurse would place the stethoscope at the fourth intercostal space and auscultate for 1 full minute.

Level of Cognitive Ability: Applying
Client Needs: Physiological Integrity
Clinical Judgment/Cognitive Skills: Recognize Cues
Integrated Process: Nursing Process/Data Collection
Content Area: Maternity: Newborn
Health Problem: N/A

Test-Taking Strategy: Focus on the **subject**, a newborn infant heart rate. Recalling the normal heart rate for a newborn infant will direct you to the correct option.

---

111. A child is admitted to the pediatric unit with a diagnosis of acute gastroenteritis. The licensed practical nurse (LPN) assists the registered nurse to monitor the child for signs of hypovolemic shock as a result of fluid and electrolyte losses that have occurred in the child. Which finding would indicate the presence of compensated shock?

1 Bradycardia
2 Hypotension
3 Profuse diarrhea
4 Capillary refill time longer than 2 seconds

Answer: 4
Rationale: Shock may be classified as compensated or decompensated. In compensated shock, the child becomes tachycardic in an effort to increase the cardiac output. The blood pressure remains normal. The capillary refill time may be prolonged and more than 2 seconds, and the child may become irritable as a result of increasing hypoxia. The most prevalent cause of hypovolemic shock is fluid and electrolyte losses associated with gastroenteritis. Diarrhea is not a sign of shock; rather, it is a cause of the fluid and electrolyte imbalance.
Priority Nursing Tip: Rotavirus is a cause of serious gastroenteritis and is a nosocomial (hospital-acquired) pathogen that is most severe in children 3 to 24 months old. Children younger than 3 months have some protection because of maternally acquired antibodies.

Level of Cognitive Ability: Synthesizing
Client Needs: Physiological Integrity
Clinical Judgment/Cognitive Skills: Analyze Cues
Integrated Process: Nursing Process/Data Collection
Content Area: Critical Care: Shock
Health Problem: Pediatric-Specific: GI and Rectal Problems

Test-Taking Strategy: Focus on the **subject**, compensated shock. Recalling that hypotension is a late sign of shock in children will assist you with eliminating option 2. Recalling that tachycardia rather than bradycardia occurs in shock will assist you with eliminating option 1. From the remaining choices, focusing on the subject, signs of shock, will direct you to the correct option.

---

112. The nurse assisting in managing a client's postsupratentorial craniotomy care would ensure that the client is maintained in which position?

1 Prone
2 Supine
3 Semi-Fowler's
4 Dorsal recumbent

Level of Cognitive Ability: Applying
Client Needs: Physiological Integrity
Clinical Judgment/Cognitive Skills: Take Action
Integrated Process: Nursing Process/Implementation
Content Area: Adult Health: Neurological
Health Problem: Adult Health: Neurological: Head Injury/Trauma

Answer: 3
Rationale: After supratentorial surgery (surgery above the brain's tentorium), the client's head is usually elevated 30 degrees to promote venous outflow through the jugular veins and modulate intracranial pressure (ICP). Options 1, 2, and 4 are incorrect positions after this surgery because they are likely to increase ICP.
Priority Nursing Tip: To prevent increased ICP, position the client to avoid extreme hip or neck flexion and maintain the head in a midline, neutral position.

Test-Taking Strategy: Focus on the **subject,** supratentorial craniotomy. A helpful strategy is to remember the following: supra, above the brain's tentorium, head up. Also note that options 1 and 2 are **comparable or alike** in that they are flat positions; option 4 is eliminated because the increased intra-abdominal pressure from this position is more likely to inhibit venous return from the brain.

---

113. An infant has been found to be human immunodeficiency virus (HIV) positive. When teaching condition-specific care, which action would the nurse reinforce to the parent to take to minimize the child's risk for condition-related injury?

1 Check the anterior fontanel for bulging and the sutures for widening each day.
2 Feed the infant in an upright position with the head and chest tilted slightly back to avoid aspiration.
3 Provide meticulous skin care to the infant and change the infant's diaper after each voiding or stool.
4 Feed the infant with a special nipple and burp the infant frequently to decrease the tendency to swallow air.

Level of Cognitive Ability: Applying
Client Needs: Physiological Integrity
Clinical Judgment/Cognitive Skills: Take Action
Integrated Process: Teaching and Learning
Content Area: Pediatrics: Immune
Health Problem: Pediatric-Specific: Immunodeficiency Disease

Answer: 3
Rationale: Meticulous skin care helps protect the HIV-infected infant from secondary infections. Bulging fontanels, feeding the infant in an upright position, and using a special nipple are unrelated to the pathology associated with HIV.
Priority Nursing Tip: Newborns born to HIV-positive clients may test positive because the parent's antibodies may persist in the newborn for 18 months after birth.

Test-Taking Strategy: Focus on the **subject,** a newborn with HIV. Read the question carefully. The question specifically asks for instructions to be given to the parent regarding HIV. Although options 1, 2, and 4 may be correct or partially correct, the content does not specifically relate to care of the infant infected with HIV.

114. The nurse is checking postoperative prescriptions and planning care for a 110-pound child after surgery to treat scoliosis. Morphine sulfate, 8 mg subcutaneously every 4 hours PRN for pain, is prescribed. The pediatric medication reference states that the safe dose is 0.1 to 0.2 mg/kg/dose every 3 to 4 hours. From this information, the nurse determines what about the prescription?
1 The dose is too low.
2 The dose is too high.
3 The dose is within the safe dosage range.
4 There is not enough information to determine the safe dose.

Level of Cognitive Ability: Analyzing
Client Needs: Physiological Integrity
Clinical Judgment/Cognitive Skills: Generate Solutions
Integrated Process: Nursing Process/Planning
Content Area: Skills: Dosage Calculations
Health Problem: Pediatric-Specific: Scoliosis

Answer: 3
Rationale: Use the formula to determine the dosage parameters. Convert pounds to kilograms by dividing weight by 2.2. Therefore, 110 lb ÷ 2.2 = 50 kg.
Dosage parameters:

$$0.1 \text{mg/kg/dose} \times 50 \text{ kg} = 5 \text{ mg}$$

$$0.2 \text{mg/kg/dose} \times 50 \text{ kg} = 10 \text{ mg}$$

The dosage is within the safe range.
Priority Nursing Tip: Conversion is the first step in the calculation of medication doses.

Test-Taking Strategy: Focus on the **subject,** a medication calculation. Identify the important components of the question and what the question is asking. In this case, the question asks for the safe dosage range for a medication. Change pounds to kilograms. Calculate the dosage parameters using the safe dosage range identified in the question and the child's weight in kilograms. Use a calculator to verify the answer.

---

115. What action would the nurse take to check the pharyngeal reflex on a child?
1 Ask the client to swallow.
2 Pull down on the lower eyelid.
3 Shine a light toward the bridge of the nose.
4 Stimulate the back of the throat with a tongue depressor.

Level of Cognitive Ability: Applying
Client Needs: Physiological Integrity
Clinical Judgment/Cognitive Skills: Recognize Cues
Integrated Process: Nursing Process/Data Collection
Content Area: Health Assessment/Physical Exam: Neurological
Health Problem: N/A

Answer: 4
Rationale: The pharyngeal (gag) reflex is tested by touching the back of the throat with an object, such as a tongue depressor. A positive response to this reflex is considered normal. Asking the client to swallow checks the swallowing reflex. To check the palpebral conjunctiva, the nurse would pull down and evert the lower eyelid. The corneal light reflex is tested by shining a penlight toward the bridge of the nose at a distance of 12 to 15 inches (light reflection would be symmetrical in both corneas).
Priority Nursing Tip: If a client receives a local throat anesthetic for a diagnostic or other procedure, the client must remain NPO until the gag reflex returns.

Test-Taking Strategy: Focus on the **subject,** pharyngeal reflex. Recalling that *pharyngeal* refers to the pharynx, or back of the throat, will assist in determining how this reflex is tested and direct you to the correct option.

---

116. Which clinical manifestation signifies the **most** common complication of mumps?
1 Pain
2 Nuchal rigidity
3 Impaired hearing
4 A red swollen testicle

Level of Cognitive Ability: Analyzing
Client Needs: Physiological Integrity
Clinical Judgment/Cognitive Skills: Recognize Cues
Integrated Process: Nursing Process/Data Collection
Content Area: Pediatrics: Infectious and Communicable Diseases
Health Problem: Pediatric-Specific: Communicable Diseases

Answer: 2
Rationale: The most common complication of mumps is aseptic meningitis, with the virus being identified in the cerebrospinal fluid. Common signs of aseptic meningitis include nuchal rigidity, lethargy, and vomiting. Muscular pain, parotid pain, or testicular pain may occur, but pain does not indicate a sign of aseptic meningitis. Although mumps is one of the leading causes of unilateral nerve deafness, it does not occur frequently. A red swollen testicle may be indicative of orchitis. Although orchitis appears to cause most concern among parents, it is not the most common complication. Swollen and tender salivary glands under the ears on one or both sides of the head (parotitis) are the most common sign of mumps.
Priority Nursing Tip: Transmission of mumps is via direct contact or droplet spread from an infected person.

Test-Taking Strategy: Focus on the **subject,** mumps, and the **strategic word,** *most.* Recalling that aseptic meningitis is the most common complication of mumps will direct you to the correct option.

---

117. An adolescent is hospitalized with a diagnosis of Rocky Mountain spotted fever (RMSF). The nurse assisting in caring for the adolescent anticipates that which medication will be prescribed?
1 Ganciclovir
2 Amantadine
3 Doxycycline
4 Amphotericin B

Level of Cognitive Ability: Analyzing
Client Needs: Physiological Integrity
Clinical Judgment/Cognitive Skills: Generate Solutions
Integrated Process: Nursing Process/Planning
Content Area: Pediatrics: Infectious and Communicable Diseases
Health Problem: Pediatric-Specific: Communicable Diseases

Answer: 3
Rationale: The nursing care of an adolescent with RMSF includes the administration of doxycycline. An alternative medication is chloramphenicol. Ganciclovir is used to treat cytomegalovirus. Amantadine is used to treat Parkinson's disease. Amphotericin B is used for fungal infections.
Priority Nursing Tip: The agent that causes RMSF is *Rickettsia rickettsii;* transmission is via the bite of an infected tick.

Test-Taking Strategy: Focus on the **subject,** RMSF. Knowledge regarding the treatment plan associated with RMSF is required to answer this question. Remember that this condition is treated with doxycycline.

---

118. A nursing student is assigned to present a clinical conference to other nursing students about brain tumors in children younger than 3 years. The nursing student would include which information in the presentation?

1 Radiation is the treatment of choice.
2 The most significant symptoms are headache and vomiting.
3 Head shaving is not required before removal of the brain tumor.
4 Surgery is not normally performed because of the increased risk of functional deficits.

Level of Cognitive Ability: Applying
Client Needs: Physiological Integrity
Clinical Judgment/Cognitive Skills: Take Action
Integrated Process: Teaching and Learning
Content Area: Pediatrics: Oncological
Health Problem: Pediatric-Specific: Cancers

Answer: 2

Rationale: The classic symptoms of children with brain tumors are headaches and vomiting. The treatment of choice is total surgical removal of the tumor. Before surgery, the child's head will be shaved, although every effort is made to shave only as much hair as is necessary. Radiation therapy is avoided in children younger than 3 years because of the toxic side effects on the developing brain, particularly in very young children.

Priority Nursing Tip: The headache associated with a brain tumor in a child is worse on awakening and improves during the day.

Test-Taking Strategy: Focus on the **subject,** brain tumors in children. Eliminate options 3 and 4 first because of the **closed-ended word** "not." From the remaining options, recalling that radiation therapy is avoided in children younger than 3 years because of the toxic side effects on the developing brain will lead you to the correct option.

---

119. The nurse assisting in caring for a child admitted to the hospital with a diagnosis of viral pneumonia describes the treatment plan to the parents. The nurse determines the **need for further teaching** when the parents make which statement regarding the treatment?

1 "We need to be very careful because oxygen is extremely flammable."
2 "It's important that the child isn't allergic to the antibiotic that is prescribed."
3 "It's difficult to watch the needle be inserted when intravenous fluids are needed."
4 "Chest physiotherapy will loosen the congestion, so coughing will clear the lungs."

Level of Cognitive Ability: Evaluating
Client Needs: Physiological Integrity
Clinical Judgment/Cognitive Skills: Evaluate Outcomes
Integrated Process: Teaching and Learning
Content Area: Pediatrics: Throat/Respiratory
Health Problem: Pediatric-Specific: Pneumonia

Answer: 2

Rationale: The therapeutic management for viral pneumonia is supportive. Antibiotics are not given unless the pneumonia is bacterial. More severely ill children may be hospitalized and given oxygen, chest physiotherapy, and intravenous fluids.

Priority Nursing Tip: If a specimen culture is prescribed, the culture is obtained before prescribed antibiotics are initiated.

Test-Taking Strategy: Note the **strategic words,** *need for further teaching.* These words indicate a **negative event query** and ask you to select an option that is an incorrect statement. Also note the word *viral* in the question. Recalling that viral infections are not treated with antibiotics will direct you to option 2. Oxygen, intravenous fluids, and chest physiotherapy are all appropriate interventions for this child.

---

120. Tretinoin gel has been prescribed for a client with acne. What is the nurse's response when the client calls the prescriber's office and reports that the treated skin has become very red and is beginning to peel?

1 "Discontinue the medication immediately."
2 "Come to the clinic immediately for an assessment."
3 "I'll notify your primary health care provider of these results."
4 "This is a normal occurrence with the use of this medication."

Level of Cognitive Ability: Applying
Client Needs: Physiological Integrity
Clinical Judgment/Cognitive Skills: Take Action
Integrated Process: Nursing Process/Implementation
Content Area: Pharmacology: Integumentary: Acne Products
Health Problem: Adult Health: Integumentary: Inflammations/Infections

Answer: 4

Rationale: Tretinoin decreases cohesiveness of the epithelial cells, increasing cell mitosis and turnover. It is potentially irritating, particularly when used correctly. Within 48 hours of use, the skin generally becomes red and begins to peel. Options 1, 2, and 3 are incorrect statements to the client.

Priority Nursing Tip: Tretinoin is a derivative of vitamin A; therefore, vitamin A supplements need to be discontinued during therapy with tretinoin.

> ***Test-Taking Strategy:*** Focus on the **subject**, tretinoin. Options 2 and 3 can be eliminated first because they are **comparable or alike.** Eliminate option 1 next because it is not within the scope of nursing practice to advise a client to discontinue a medication.

---

121. A child hospitalized with a diagnosis of lead poisoning is prescribed chelation therapy. The nurse assisting in caring for the child anticipates that which medication will be prescribed?

1 Ipecac syrup
2 Activated charcoal
3 Sodium bicarbonate
4 Calcium disodium edetate (EDTA)

Level of Cognitive Ability: Applying
Client Needs: Physiological Integrity
Clinical Judgment/Cognitive Skills: Generate Solutions
Integrated Process: Nursing Process/Planning
Content Area: Complex Care: Poisoning
Health Problem: Pediatric-Specific: Poisoning

Answer: 4

Rationale: EDTA is a chelating agent that is used to treat lead poisoning. Ipecac syrup may be prescribed by the primary health care provider for use in the hospital setting but would not be used to treat lead poisoning. Activated charcoal is used to decrease absorption in certain poisoning situations. Sodium bicarbonate may be used in salicylate poisoning.

Priority Nursing Tip: During chelation therapy, provide adequate hydration and monitor kidney function for nephrotoxicity because the medication is excreted via the kidneys.

> ***Test-Taking Strategy:*** Focus on the **subject,** treatment related to lead poisoning. Think about the classifications of the medications in the options. Recalling that EDTA is a chelating agent will direct you to the correct option.

---

122. The nurse is performing pin-site care on a client in skeletal traction. Which normal finding would the nurse expect to note when checking the pin sites?

1 Loose but intact pin sites
2 Clear drainage from the pin sites
3 Purulent drainage from the pin sites
4 Redness and swelling around the pin sites

Level of Cognitive Ability: Analyzing
Client Needs: Physiological Integrity
Clinical Judgment/Cognitive Skills: Recognize Cues
Integrated Process: Nursing Process/Data Collection
Content Area: Adult Health: Musculoskeletal
Health Problem: Adult Health: Musculoskeletal: Skeletal Injury

Answer: 2
Rationale: A small amount of clear drainage ("weeping") may be expected after cleaning and removing crusting around the pin sites of skeletal traction. Pins should not be loose; if this is noted, the primary health care provider needs to be notified. Purulent drainage, redness, and swelling around the pin sites may be indicative of an infection.
Priority Nursing Tip: Skeletal traction is applied mechanically to the bone with pins, wires, or tongs. Because skin integrity is disrupted, the client is at risk for infection.

Test-Taking Strategy: Focus on the **subject,** pin-site care. Option 1 is not an expected finding and can be eliminated first because loose pins would not provide a secure hold with the traction. Eliminate options 3 and 4 next because they are **comparable or alike** and indicate signs of infection.

---

123. The nurse is assisting in caring for a client who has been placed in Buck's extension traction while awaiting surgical repair of a fractured femur. As part of the care the nurse would help in performing a complete neurovascular assessment of the affected extremity, including which interventions? **Select all that apply.**

1 Vital signs
2 Bilateral lung sounds
3 Pulse in the affected extremity
4 Level of pain in the affected leg
5 Skin color of the affected extremity
6 Capillary refill of the affected toes

Level of Cognitive Ability: Applying
Client Needs: Physiological Integrity
Clinical Judgment/Cognitive Skills: Recognize Cues
Integrated Process: Nursing Process/Data Collection
Content Area: Adult Health: Musculoskeletal
Health Problem: Adult Health: Musculoskeletal: Skeletal Injury

Answer: 3, 4, 5, 6
Rationale: A complete neurovascular assessment of an extremity includes color, sensation, movement, capillary refill, and pulse of the affected extremity. Options 1 and 2 are unrelated to neurovascular assessment.
Priority Nursing Tip: Buck's extension traction is a type of skin traction used to alleviate muscle spasms and immobilize a lower limb. It is applied by using elastic bandages or adhesive, a foam boot, or a sling and counterweights; the foot of the bed is elevated to provide the traction.

Test-Taking Strategy: Focus on the **subject,** a complete neurovascular assessment. Eliminate options that are not considered components of a neurovascular assessment. Also, use the **ABCs—airway, breathing, and circulation**—to direct you to the correct option.

124. The nurse prepares to transfer the client with a newly applied arm cast into the bed using which method?

1 Placing ice on top of the cast
2 Supporting the cast with the fingertips only
3 Asking the client to support the cast during transfer
4 Using the palms of the hands and soft pillows to support the cast

Level of Cognitive Ability: Applying
Client Needs: Physiological Integrity
Clinical Judgment/Cognitive Skills: Generate Solutions
Integrated Process: Nursing Process/Planning
Content Area: Adult Health: Musculoskeletal
Health Problem: Adult Health: Musculoskeletal: Skeletal Injury

Answer: 4
Rationale: The palms or the flat surface of the extended fingers would be used when moving a wet cast to prevent indentations. Pillows are used to support the curves of the cast to prevent cracking or flattening of the cast from the weight of the body. Half-full bags of ice may be placed next to the cast to prevent swelling, but this would be done after the client is placed in bed. Asking the client to support the cast during transfer is inappropriate.
Priority Nursing Tip: Instruct the client with a cast not to stick objects inside the cast because the object can disrupt skin integrity and result in infection. If the skin under the cast is itchy, instruct the client to direct cool air from a hair dryer inside the cast.

Test-Taking Strategy: Focus on the **subject,** cast care. Eliminate option 1 because ice can be used for swelling after the client is placed in bed. Eliminate option 2 because of the **closed-ended word** "only" in this option. Eliminate option 3 because it is inappropriate to ask the client to support the cast.

---

125. A magnetic resonance imaging (MRI) scan is prescribed for a client with a suspected brain tumor. Which prescription would the nurse anticipate may be prescribed for the client before the procedure?

1 An opioid
2 A sedative
3 A corticosteroid
4 An antihistamine

Level of Cognitive Ability: Analyzing
Client Needs: Physiological Integrity
Clinical Judgment/Cognitive Skills: Generate Solutions
Integrated Process: Nursing Process/Planning
Content Area: Foundations of Care: Diagnostic Tests
Health Problem: Adult Health: Cancer: Brain Tumors

Answer: 2
Rationale: An MRI scan is a noninvasive diagnostic test that visualizes the body's tissues, structure, and blood flow. For an MRI, the client is positioned on a padded table and moved into a cylinder-shaped scanner. Relaxation techniques, an eye mask, and sedation may be used before the procedure to reduce claustrophobic effects; however, because the client must remain very still during the scan, the nurse avoids oversedating the client to ensure client cooperation. There is no useful purpose for administering an opioid, corticosteroid, or antihistamine. Open MRI systems are available in some diagnostic facilities, and this method of testing can be used for clients with claustrophobia.
Priority Nursing Tip: In a magnetic resonance scan, magnetic fields are used to produce an image. Therefore, all metallic objects such as a watch, other jewelry, clothing with metal fasteners, and metal hair fasteners must be removed.

Test-Taking Strategy: Focus on the **subject,** MRI scan. Recalling that claustrophobia is a concern will direct you to the correct option.

---

126. A low dose of ondansetron is prescribed for a client receiving chemotherapy. The nurse assisting in the care of the client anticipates that the primary health care provider will prescribe the medication by which route?

1 Oral
2 Intranasal
3 Intravenous
4 Subcutaneous

Answer: 3
Rationale: Ondansetron is an antiemetic used to control nausea, vomiting, and motion sickness. It is available for administration by the oral, intramuscular (IM), or intravenous (IV) routes. The IV route is used when relief of nausea is needed in the client receiving chemotherapy. The IM route may be used when the medication is used as an adjunct to anesthesia. Option 1 would not be used in clients who are nauseated. Options 2 and 4 are not routes of administration for this medication.
Priority Nursing Tip: Antiemetics can cause drowsiness and hypotension; therefore, a priority intervention is to protect the client from injury.

Level of Cognitive Ability: Applying
Client Needs: Physiological Integrity
Clinical Judgment/Cognitive Skills: Generate Solutions
Integrated Process: Nursing Process/Planning
Content Area: Pharmacology: Gastrointestinal: Antiemetics
Health Problem: N/A

Test-Taking Strategy: Focus on the **subject,** ondansetron administration to a client receiving chemotherapy. Noting that the client is receiving chemotherapy will direct you to the correct option.

---

127. The nurse is assisting in teaching the parents of a child diagnosed with celiac disease about dietary measures. The nurse would instruct the parents to take which measure?

1 Restrict corn and rice in the diet.
2 Restrict fresh vegetables in the diet.
3 Substitute grain cereals with pasta products.
4 Avoid foods that are hidden sources of gluten.

Answer: 4
Rationale: Gluten is found primarily in the grains of wheat, rye, barley, and oats. Gluten is added to many foods as hydrolyzed vegetable protein that is derived from cereal grains; therefore, labels need to be read. Corn and rice, as well as vegetables, are acceptable in a gluten-free diet, and corn and rice become substitute foods. Many pasta products contain gluten. Grains are frequently added to processed foods for thickness or fillers.
Priority Nursing Tip: Celiac crisis is precipitated by fasting, infection, or the ingestion of gluten. It causes profuse watery diarrhea and vomiting, leading to rapid dehydration, electrolyte imbalance, and severe acidosis.

Level of Cognitive Ability: Applying
Client Needs: Physiological Integrity
Clinical Judgment/Cognitive Skills: Take Action
Integrated Process: Teaching and Learning
Content Area: Foundations of Care: Therapeutic Diets
Health Problem: Pediatric-Specific: Nutrition Problems

Test-Taking Strategy: Focus on the **subject,** celiac diet. Recall that a gluten-free diet is required in celiac disease. Select option 4 because it is the **umbrella option.**

---

128. A client admitted to the hospital for evaluation of recurrent runs of ventricular tachycardia is scheduled for electrophysiology studies (EPS). Which statement would the nurse include when reinforcing information about this test to the client?

1 "You will continue to take your medications until the morning of the test."
2 "You will be sedated during the procedure and will not remember what has happened."
3 "This test is a noninvasive method of determining the effectiveness of your medication regimen."
4 "The test uses a special wire to increase the heart rate and produce the irregular beats that cause your signs and symptoms."

Answer: 4
Rationale: The purpose of EPS is to study the heart's electrical system. During this invasive procedure, a special wire is introduced into the heart to produce dysrhythmias. To prepare for this procedure, the client needs to be NPO for 6 to 8 hours before the test, and all antidysrhythmics are held for at least 24 hours before the test to study the dysrhythmias without the influence of medications. Because the client's verbal responses to the rhythm changes are extremely important, sedation is avoided if possible.
Priority Nursing Tip: Inducing a dysrhythmia during EPS assists the cardiologist in making a diagnosis and determining the appropriate treatment.

Level of Cognitive Ability: Applying
Client Needs: Physiological Integrity
Clinical Judgment/Cognitive Skills: Take Action
Integrated Process: Nursing Process/Implementation
Content Area: Foundations of Care: Diagnostic Tests
Health Problem: Adult Health: Cardiovascular: Dysrhythmias

Test-Taking Strategy: Focus on the **subject,** EPS. Note the relationship between the words *recurrent runs of ventricular tachycardia* in the question and *produce the irregular beats* in option 4.

---

129. The nurse reinforcing diet teaching to a client experiencing heart failure instructs the client to avoid which food item?

1 Sherbet
2 Steak sauce
3 Apple juice
4 Leafy green vegetables

Answer: 2
Rationale: Steak sauce is high in sodium. Leafy green vegetables, any juice (except tomato or V8 brand vegetable), and sherbet are all low in sodium. Clients with heart failure need to monitor sodium intake.
Priority Nursing Tip: Clients with heart failure need to monitor sodium intake because sodium causes the retention of fluid.

Level of Cognitive Ability: Applying
Client Needs: Physiological Integrity
Clinical Judgment/Cognitive Skills: Take Action
Integrated Process: Teaching and Learning
Content Area: Foundations of Care: Therapeutic Diets
Health Problem: Adult Health: Cardiovascular: Heart Failure

Test-Taking Strategy: Focus on the **subject,** a client with heart failure. Note the word *avoid.* This word asks you to select an inappropriate food choice. Note that options 1, 3, and 4 are **comparable or alike** in that they are low-sodium foods. Recalling that the client with heart failure needs to limit sodium intake will direct you to the correct option.

---

130. The nurse is assisting in developing a plan of care for an older client diagnosed with type 1 diabetes mellitus who is also experiencing acute gastroenteritis. To maintain food and fluid intake to prevent dehydration, which action would the nurse plan to include?

1 Offering only water until the client is able to tolerate solid foods
2 Withholding all fluids until vomiting has ceased entirely for at least 4 hours
3 Encouraging the client to take 8 to 12 ounces of fluid every hour while awake
4 Maintaining a clear liquid diet for at least 5 days before advancing to solid foods

Answer: 3
Rationale: Dehydration needs to be prevented in the client with type 1 diabetes mellitus because of the risk of diabetic ketoacidosis (DKA). Small amounts of fluid may be tolerated, even when vomiting is present. The client would be offered liquids containing both glucose and electrolytes. The diet would be advanced as tolerated and include a minimum of 100 to 150 g of carbohydrates daily. Offering water only and maintaining liquids for 5 days will not prevent dehydration but may promote it in this client.
Priority Nursing Tip: DKA is a life-threatening complication of type 1 diabetes mellitus that develops when a severe insulin deficiency occurs.

Level of Cognitive Ability: Applying
Client Needs: Physiological Integrity
Clinical Judgment/Cognitive Skills: Generate Solutions
Integrated Process: Nursing Process/Planning
Content Area: Foundations of Care: Fluids & Electrolytes
Health Problem: Adult Health: Endocrine: Diabetes Mellitus

Test-Taking Strategy: Focus on the **subject,** type 1 diabetes mellitus. Eliminate options 1 and 2 because of the **closed-ended words** "only" and "all" in these options, respectively. From the remaining options, note the words *for at least 5 days* in option 4. Thinking about the **subject,** a client with diabetes mellitus and preventing dehydration, will assist in eliminating this option.

---

131. The nurse in the postpartum unit is checking for signs of breast-feeding problems demonstrated by either the newborn or the parent. Which findings indicate a problem? **Select all that apply.**

1 The infant exhibits dimpling of the cheeks.
2 The infant makes smacking or clicking sounds.
3 The parent's breast gets softer during a feeding.
4 Milk drips from the parent's breast occasionally.
5 The infant falls asleep after feeding less than 5 minutes.
6 The infant can be heard swallowing frequently during a feeding.

Level of Cognitive Ability: Analyzing
Client Needs: Physiological Integrity
Clinical Judgment/Cognitive Skills: Analyze Cues
Integrated Process: Nursing Process/Data Collection
Content Area: Maternity: Postpartum
Health Problem: Newborn: Newborn Feeding

Answer: 1, 2, 5

Rationale: It is important for the nurse to identify breast-feeding problems while the parent is hospitalized so that the nurse can teach the parent how to prevent and treat any problems. Infant signs of breast-feeding problems include dimpling of the cheeks; making smacking or clicking sounds; falling asleep after feeding less than 5 minutes; refusing to breast-feed; tongue thrusting; failing to open the mouth at latch-on; turning the lower lip in; making short, choppy motions of the jaw; and not swallowing audibly. Softening of the breast during feeding, noting milk in the infant's mouth or dripping from the parent's breast occasionally, and hearing the infant swallow are signs that the infant is receiving adequate nutrition.

Priority Nursing Tip: If the parent is breast-feeding, calorie needs increase by 200 to 500 calories per day; increased fluids and the continuance of prenatal vitamins and minerals are important.

Test-Taking Strategy: Focus on the **subject,** signs of breast-feeding problems. Think about the process of feeding and visualize the effect of each observation identified in the options. This will direct you to the correct options.

---

132. The nurse has completed tracheostomy care for a client whose tracheostomy tube has a nondisposable inner cannula. Which intervention will the nurse implement **immediately** before reinserting the inner cannula?

1 Rinsing it in sterile water
2 Suctioning the client's airway
3 Tapping it gently against a sterile basin
4 Drying it with the provided pipe cleaners

Level of Cognitive Ability: Analyzing
Client Needs: Physiological Integrity
Clinical Judgment/Cognitive Skills: Take Action
Integrated Process: Nursing Process/Implementation
Content Area: Skills: Tube Care
Health Problem: Adult Health: Respiratory: Upper Airway

Answer: 4

Rationale: After washing and rinsing the inner cannula, the nurse taps it dry to remove large water droplets and then uses pipe cleaners specifically for use with a tracheostomy to dry it; then the nurse inserts the cannula into the tracheostomy and turns it clockwise to lock it into place. The nurse would avoid shaking or tapping the inner cannula to prevent contamination. A wet cannula would not be inserted into a tracheostomy because water is a lung irritant. Suctioning is not performed without an inner cannula in place.

Priority Nursing Tip: Keep a tracheostomy obturator and a tracheostomy tube of the same size for emergency replacement if the tracheostomy is dislodged.

Test-Taking Strategy: Note the **strategic word,** *immediately.* Also note the word *nondisposable* and visualize the procedure. Eliminate option 1 because a wet cannula would not be inserted and option 2 because you would not suction a client without the inner cannula in place. Eliminate option 3 because tapping could deposit debris.

---

133. The nurse suspects that an air embolism has occurred when the client's central venous catheter disconnects from the intravenous (IV) tubing. The nurse **immediately** places the client on her or his left side in which position?

1 High Fowler's
2 Trendelenburg's
3 Lateral recumbent
4 Reverse Trendelenburg's

Level of Cognitive Ability: Applying
Client Needs: Physiological Integrity
Clinical Judgment/Cognitive Skills: Take Action
Integrated Process: Nursing Process/Implementation
Content Area: Complex Care: Emergency Situations/Management
Health Problem: N/A

Answer: 2

Rationale: If the client develops an air embolism, the immediate action is to place the client in Trendelenburg's position on the left side. This position raises the client's feet higher than the head and traps any air in the right atrium. If necessary, the air can then be directly removed by intracardiac aspiration. Options 1 and 4 are incorrect positions because both positions elevate the head, put the air in a dependent position, and increase the risk of a cerebral embolism; lying flat in the lateral position does not help trap the air in the right atrium.

Priority Nursing Tip: If an air embolism is suspected, the IV tubing is clamped off immediately.

Test-Taking Strategy: Focus on the **subject,** air embolism. Note the **strategic word,** *immediately.* Visualize each position in the options and recall cardiac anatomy. Recalling that the goal of action is to trap air in the right atrium will direct you to the correct option.

---

134. An anxious client enters the emergency department seeking treatment for a laceration of the finger. The client's vital signs are pulse 106 beats per minute, blood pressure (BP) 158/88 mm Hg, and respirations 28 breaths per minute. After cleansing the injury and reassuring the client, the nurse rechecks the vital signs and notes a pulse of 82 beats per minute, BP 130/80 mm Hg, and respirations 20 breaths per minute. Which factor likely accounts for the change in vital signs?

1 Cooling effects of the cleansing agent
2 Client's adaptation to the air conditioning
3 Early clinical indicators of cardiogenic shock
4 Decline in sympathetic nervous system discharge

Level of Cognitive Ability: Synthesizing
Client Needs: Physiological Integrity
Clinical Judgment/Cognitive Skills: Analyze Cues
Integrated Process: Nursing Process/Data Collection
Content Area: Adult Health: Integumentary
Health Problem: Adult Health: Integumentary: Wounds

Answer: 4

Rationale: Physical or emotional stress triggers sympathetic nervous system stimulation. Increased epinephrine and norepinephrine cause tachycardia, high blood pressure, and tachypnea. Stress reduction then returns these parameters to baseline as the sympathetic discharge falls. Options 1 and 2 are unrelated to the changes in vital signs. Because the client's vital signs remain within normal limits, the client exhibits no indication of cardiogenic shock.

Priority Nursing Tip: Anxiety can cause an increase in the pulse rate, respiratory rate, and blood pressure.

Test-Taking Strategy: Focus on the **subject,** stress effects on vital signs. Eliminate options 1 and 2 first because they are **comparable or alike** in that they are unrelated to factors that could notably change the vital signs. Next, note that the client is anxious and has an injury. These two pieces of information guide you to think about the body's response to stress. Recalling the relationship of stress to the sympathetic nervous system will direct you to the correct option.

---

135. An echocardiogram, chest x-ray (CXR), and computed axial tomography (CAT) scan are prescribed for a client with heart failure who has activity intolerance. In which order would the nurse expect these tests to be scheduled to meet the needs of this client safely and **effectively**?

1. CAT scan and CXR in the morning and echocardiogram on the following morning
2. CXR and echocardiogram together in the morning and CAT scan in the afternoon of the same day
3. Echocardiogram in the morning and CXR and CAT scans together in the afternoon of the same day
4. CXR in the morning, echocardiogram in the afternoon, and CAT scan in the morning of the following day

Level of Cognitive Ability: Analyzing
Client Needs: Physiological Integrity
Clinical Judgment/Cognitive Skills: Generate Solutions
Integrated Process: Nursing Process/Planning
Content Area: Foundations of Care: Diagnostic Tests
Health Problem: Adult Health: Cardiovascular: Heart Failure

Answer: 4

Rationale: CAT scans are always performed in radiology, and CXR and echocardiograms can be done at the bedside; however, the best results usually occur when the test is performed in the related department. As long as the client is stable and transportation is provided, the nurse can schedule each procedure in its department with two procedures on the first day separated by a rest period and the remaining procedure the next day. The nurse would plan the CXR and echocardiogram on the same day because if the client's condition deteriorates after the first procedure, the nurse can obtain a portable CXR or echocardiogram.

Priority Nursing Tip: The nurse would instruct the client with heart failure to balance periods of rest and activity and avoid performing isometric activities because they increase pressure in the heart.

Test-Taking Strategy: Focus on the **subject**, scheduling multiple diagnostic procedures for the client with heart failure who has activity intolerance. Note the **strategic word,** *effectively.* Recalling that the client will do best if activities are spaced will direct you to the correct option.

---

136. The licensed practical nurse (LPN) is assisting the registered nurse (RN) with preparing to initiate an intravenous nitroglycerin drip on a client who has experienced an acute myocardial infarction. In the absence of an invasive (arterial) monitoring line, the LPN anticipates the need to have which piece of equipment for use by the RN at the bedside to help ensure the client's safety?

1. Defibrillator
2. Pulse oximeter
3. Central venous pressure (CVP) tray
4. Noninvasive blood pressure monitor

Level of Cognitive Ability: Analyzing
Client Needs: Physiological Integrity
Clinical Judgment/Cognitive Skills: Generate Solutions
Integrated Process: Nursing Process/Planning
Content Area: Complex Care: Emergency Situations/Management
Health Problem: Adult Health: Cardiovascular: Myocardial Infarction

Answer: 4

Rationale: Nitroglycerin dilates arteries and veins (vasodilator), causing peripheral blood pooling, thus reducing preload, afterload, and myocardial workload. This action accounts for the primary side effect of nitroglycerin, which is hypotension. In the absence of an arterial monitoring line, the nurse needs to have a noninvasive blood pressure monitor for use at the bedside. None of the other options would monitor blood pressure. Additionally, the client would be on a cardiac monitor.

Priority Nursing Tip: An intravenous infusion device such as a pump or controller must be used when administering nitroglycerin via the intravenous route.

Test-Taking Strategy: Focus on the **subject,** initiating an intravenous nitroglycerin drip on a client with acute myocardial infarction. Note the words *absence of an invasive (arterial) monitoring line.* Recalling the purpose of this type of monitoring device and the action of nitroglycerin will direct you to the correct option.

137. A client in labor has a diagnosis of sickle cell anemia. Which action will the nurse plan to take to assist in preventing the client from experiencing a sickling crisis during labor?

1 Being reassuring
2 Administering oxygen
3 Preventing bearing down
4 Maintaining strict asepsis

Level of Cognitive Ability: Applying
Client Needs: Physiological Integrity
Clinical Judgment/Cognitive Skills: Generate Solutions
Integrated Process: Nursing Process/Implementation
Content Area: Maternity: Intrapartum
Health Problem: Adult Health: Hematological: Anemias

Answer: 2
Rationale: During the labor process, the client with sickle cell anemia is at high risk for being unable to meet the oxygen demands of labor. Administering oxygen will prevent sickle cell crisis during labor. Intravenous fluid therapy will also reduce the risk of a sickle cell crisis. Options 1 and 4 are appropriate actions but are unrelated to sickle cell crisis. Option 3 is inappropriate.
Priority Nursing Tip: During labor, the client with sickle cell anemia needs to receive oxygen and fluids to prevent hypoxemia and dehydration because these conditions stimulate the sickling process.

Test-Taking Strategy: Focus on the client's diagnosis and use the **ABCs—airway, breathing, and circulation**—to direct you to the correct option.

---

138. A client is scheduled for computed tomography (CT) with contrast of the kidneys to rule out renal disease. Which would the nurse check the client for before the procedure to **best** ensure the client's safety?

1 Allergies
2 Familial renal disease
3 Frequent antibiotic use
4 Long-term diuretic therapy

Level of Cognitive Ability: Analyzing
Client Needs: Physiological Integrity
Clinical Judgment/Cognitive Skills: Recognize Cues
Integrated Process: Nursing Process/Data Collection
Content Area: Foundations of Care: Diagnostic Tests
Health Problem: N/A

Answer: 1
Rationale: The client undergoing any type of diagnostic testing involving possible dye administration needs to be questioned about allergies, specifically an allergy to shellfish or iodine. This is essential to identify the risk for potential allergic reaction to contrast dye, which may be used. The other items are also useful as part of data collection but are not as critical as the allergy determination in the preprocedure period in the attempt to maximize client safety.
Priority Nursing Tip: The nurse would ask the client if he or she ever had an allergic reaction to contrast media used for diagnostic testing. If so, the client is at high risk for experiencing another reaction if contrast media is administered.

Test-Taking Strategy: Note the **strategic word,** *best,* and focus on the **subject,** preprocedural CT scan. Because the question indicates that CT of the kidneys is planned, the items in the options are evaluated against their potential connection to this aspect of care. Recalling that contrast dye may be used during CT to enhance visualization of the kidneys will direct you to the correct option.

---

139. The nurse assists a client diagnosed with a renal disorder in collecting a 24-hour urine specimen. Which intervention does the nurse implement to ensure proper collection of the 24-hour urine specimen?

1 Have the client void at the start time and discard the specimen.
2 Strain the specimen before pouring the urine into the container.
3 Save all urine, beginning with the urine voided at the start time.
4 Once completed, refrigerate the urine collection until picked up by the laboratory.

Level of Cognitive Ability: Applying
Client Needs: Physiological Integrity
Clinical Judgment/Cognitive Skills: Take Action
Integrated Process: Nursing Process/ Implementation
Content Area: Skills: Specimen Collection
Health Problem: N/A

Answer: 1
Rationale: The nurse asks the client to void at the beginning of the collection period and discards this urine sample because this urine has been stored in the bladder for an undetermined length of time. All urine thereafter is saved in an iced or refrigerated container. The client is asked to void at the finish time, and this sample is the last specimen added to the collection. Straining the urine is contraindicated for timed urine collections. The container is labeled, placed on fresh ice, and sent to the laboratory immediately after the 24-hour urine collection has ended.
Priority Nursing Tip: If the client is collecting a 24-hour urine specimen, check with the laboratory about the need to restrict certain foods or avoid taking certain medications before and during the collection. Some foods and medications affect test results.

Test-Taking Strategy: Focusing on the **subject**, a 24-hour urine collection, will assist in eliminating options 2 and 4. Straining the urine is contraindicated, and the urine must be sent to the laboratory immediately after the collection time has ended. For the remaining options, think about the procedure. Remember that it is best to discard the first specimen.

---

140. The nurse is assisting in caring for a client in active labor. Which intervention would the nurse implement to prevent fetal heart rate decelerations?

1 Discourage the client from walking.
2 Increase the rate of the oxytocin infusion.
3 Monitor the fetal heart rate every 30 minutes.
4 Encourage upright or side-lying maternal positions.

Level of Cognitive Ability: Analyzing
Client Needs: Physiological Integrity
Clinical Judgment/Cognitive Skills: Take Action
Integrated Process: Nursing Process/ Implementation
Content Area: Maternity: Intrapartum
Health Problem: Maternity: Fetal Distress/ Demise

Answer: 4
Rationale: If fetal heart rate decelerations occur, the nurse immediately notifies the registered nurse. There are nursing actions to prevent fetal heart rate decelerations without necessitating surgical intervention. Side-lying and upright positions such as walking, standing, and squatting can improve venous return and encourage effective uterine activity. Monitoring the fetal heart rate every 30 minutes will not prevent fetal heart rate decelerations. An oxytocin infusion would be discontinued in the presence of fetal heart rate decelerations, thereby reducing uterine activity and increasing uteroplacental perfusion.
Priority Nursing Tip: Early fetal heart rate decelerations are not associated with fetal compromise and require no intervention. Late decelerations indicate impaired placental exchange or uteroplacental insufficiency.

Test-Taking Strategy: Focus on the **subject**, preventing fetal heart rate decelerations. Options 1, 2, and 3 will not prevent fetal heart rate decelerations. Side-lying and upright positions will improve venous return and encourage effective uterine activity.

---

141. A client diagnosed with diabetes mellitus is at 36 weeks' gestation. The client has had weekly reactive nonstress tests for the last 3 weeks. This week, the nonstress test was nonreactive after 40 minutes. Based on these results, the nurse would prepare the client for which intervention?

1 A contraction stress test
2 Immediate induction of labor
3 Hospitalization with continuous fetal monitoring
4 A return appointment in 2 days to repeat the nonstress test

Level of Cognitive Ability: Analyzing
Client Needs: Physiological Integrity
Clinical Judgment/Cognitive Skills: Generate Solutions
Integrated Process: Nursing Process/Planning
Content Area: Maternity: Antepartum
Health Problem: Maternity: Diabetes

Answer: 1
Rationale: A nonreactive nonstress test needs further assessment. A contraction stress test is the next test needed to further assess the fetal status. There are not enough data in the question to indicate that the procedures in options 2 and 3 are necessary at this time. To send the client home for 2 days may place the fetus in jeopardy.
Priority Nursing Tip: A nonstress test is performed to assess placental function and oxygenation and evaluate the fetal heart rate response to fetal movement.

Test-Taking Strategy: Focus on the **subject**, a change in nonstress test results from reactive to nonreactive. Options 2 and 3 can be eliminated first because they are unnecessary at this time. Option 4 can be eliminated next because repeating the test at a later time is not a safe intervention, especially considering the fact that previous test results were reactive.

---

142. The nurse is assisting in the care of a client experiencing severe preeclampsia who is receiving magnesium sulfate. What intervention would the nurse implement during the administration of magnesium sulfate for this client?

1 Schedule a daily ultrasound to assess fetal movement.
2 Schedule a nonstress test every 4 hours to assess fetal well-being.
3 Check the client's temperature every 2 hours because the client is at high risk for infection.
4 Check for signs and symptoms of labor because the client's level of consciousness may be altered.

Level of Cognitive Ability: Applying
Client Needs: Physiological Integrity
Clinical Judgment/Cognitive Skills: Take Action
Integrated Process: Nursing Process/Implementation
Content Area: Pharmacology: Maternity/Newborn: Magnesium Sulfate
Health Problem: Maternity: Gestational Hypertension/Preeclampsia and Eclampsia

Answer: 4
Rationale: Magnesium sulfate is a central nervous system depressant and anticonvulsant. Because of the sedative effect of the magnesium sulfate, the client may not perceive labor. Daily ultrasounds are not necessary for this client. A nonstress test may be done, but not every 4 hours. This client is not at high risk for infection.
Priority Nursing Tip: Calcium gluconate is the antidote to magnesium sulfate.

Test-Taking Strategy: Focus on the **subject**, magnesium sulfate administration. Use the **steps of the nursing process** to answer the question. Data collection is the first step; therefore, eliminate options 1 and 2. From the remaining options, knowledge that the client is not at high risk for infection will assist in directing you to the correct option.

---

143. When a client's nasogastric (NG) tube stops draining, which intervention would the nurse implement to maintain client safety?

1 Instill 10 to 20 mL of fluid to dislodge any clots.
2 Verify the tube placement according to agency procedure.
3 Clamp the tube for 2 hours to allow the drainage to accumulate.
4 Retract the tube by 2 inches to be above any possible obstruction.

Level of Cognitive Ability: Applying
Client Needs: Physiological Integrity
Clinical Judgment/Cognitive Skills: Take Action
Integrated Process: Nursing Process/Implementation
Content Area: Skills: Tube Care
Health Problem: N/A

Answer: 2

Rationale: If a client's NG tube stops draining, the nurse verifies placement first to ensure that the tube remains in the stomach. After checking placement and verifying a prescription for tube irrigation, the nurse irrigates the tube with 30 to 60 mL of the fluid per agency procedure. Clamping the tube increases the risk of aspiration and is contraindicated; besides, this intervention cannot unclog a tube. Retracting the tube may displace the tube and place the client at risk for aspiration. Replacement of the tube is the last step if other actions are unsuccessful.

Priority Nursing Tip: Accurate placement of a gastrointestinal tube is always checked before instilling feeding solutions, medications, or any other solution.

Test-Taking Strategy: Focus on the **subject,** an NG tube that has stopped draining. Eliminate options 1, 3, and 4 because these interventions increase client risk of aspiration. Also use the **steps of the nursing process;** option 2 is the only data collection action.

---

144. The nurse is planning to give a tepid tub bath to a child experiencing hyperthermia. Which action would the nurse plan to perform?

1 Obtain isopropyl alcohol to add to the bathwater.
2 Allow 5 minutes for the child to soak in the bathwater.
3 Have cool water available to add to the warm bathwater.
4 Warm the water to the same body temperature as the child's.

Level of Cognitive Ability: Applying
Client Needs: Physiological Integrity
Clinical Judgment/Cognitive Skills: Generate Solutions
Integrated Process: Nursing Process/Planning
Content Area: Pediatrics: Metabolic/Endocrine
Health Problem: Pediatric-Specific: Fever

Answer: 3

Rationale: Adding cool water to an already warm bath allows the water temperature to slowly drop. The child is able to gradually adjust to the changing water temperature and will not experience chilling. Alcohol is toxic, can cause peripheral vasoconstriction, and is contraindicated for tepid sponge or tub baths. The child needs to be in a tepid tub bath for 20 to 30 minutes to achieve maximum results. To achieve the best cooling results, the water temperature needs to be at least 2 degrees lower than the child's body temperature.

Priority Nursing Tip: The nurse would assist in performing a complete assessment on a child with a fever. Assessment findings associated with the fever provide important indications of the seriousness of the fever.

Test-Taking Strategy: Focus on the **subject,** tepid water bath. Eliminate option 1, recalling that alcohol is toxic, as well as irritating to the skin. Eliminate option 4 because water that is the same as body temperature will not reduce hyperthermia. Eliminate option 2 because of the 5-minute time frame.

---

145. The nurse is assigned to assist in the care of an infant on the first postoperative day after a surgical repair of a cleft lip. Which nursing intervention would the nurse plan to take when caring for this child's surgical incision?

1 Rinsing the incision with sterile water after feeding
2 Cleaning the incision only when serous exudate forms
3 Rubbing the incision gently with a sterile cotton-tipped swab
4 Replacing the Logan bar carefully after cleaning the incision

Level of Cognitive Ability: Applying
Client Needs: Physiological Integrity
Clinical Judgment/Cognitive Skills: Generate Solutions
Integrated Process: Nursing Process/ Implementation
Content Area: Pediatrics: Gastrointestinal
Health Problem: Pediatric-Specific: Disorders of Prenatal Development

Answer: 1
Rationale: The incision would be rinsed with sterile water after every feeding. Rubbing alters the integrity of the suture line. Rather, the incision needs to be patted or dabbed. The purpose of the Logan bar is to maintain the integrity of the suture line. Removing the Logan bar on the first postoperative day would increase tension on the surgical incision.
Priority Nursing Tip: After cleft lip repair, avoid positioning the infant on the side of the repair or in the prone position because these positions can cause rubbing of the surgical site on the mattress.

Test-Taking Strategy: Focus on the **subject**, cleft lip repair. Eliminate options 2 and 3 first because of the words *only* in option 2 and *rubbing* in option 3. Focus on the words *first postoperative day*. This would assist in eliminating option 4.

---

146. A 3-week-old infant is brought to the well-baby clinic for a phenylketonuria (PKU) screening test. The nurse reviews the results of the serum phenylalanine levels and notes that the level is 1.0 mg/dL. What is the nurse's **priority** action?

1 Report the test as inconclusive.
2 Tell the parent that the test is normal.
3 Prepare to perform another test on the client.
4 Notify the pediatrician that the test is moderately elevated.

Level of Cognitive Ability: Analyzing
Client Needs: Physiological Integrity
Clinical Judgment/Cognitive Skills: Take Action
Integrated Process: Nursing Process/ Implementation
Content Area: Maternity: Newborn
Health Problem: N/A

Answer: 2
Rationale: The normal PKU level is 0.8 to 1.8 mg/dL. With early postpartum discharge, screening is often performed when the infant is less than 2 days old because of the concern that the infant will be lost to follow-up. Infants need to be rescreened by the time they are 14 days old if the initial screening was done when the infant was 24 to 48 hours old.
Priority Nursing Tip: All 50 states require routine screening of all newborns for phenylketonuria.

Test-Taking Strategy: Focus on the **strategic word,** *priority,* and the **subject,** the normal phenylalanine level. Recalling that the normal level is 0.8 to 1.8 mg/dL will direct you to option 2. Also note that the remaining options are **comparable or alike** and indicate an other-than-normal finding.

---

147. The nurse is assisting in the care of a client receiving total parenteral nutrition (TPN) via a central venous catheter (CVC) who is scheduled to receive an intravenous (IV) antibiotic. Which intervention would the nurse anticipate being done before the antibiotic is administered?

1 Turning off the TPN for 30 minutes
2 Ensuring a separate IV access route
3 Flushing the CVC with normal saline
4 Checking for compatibility with TPN

Level of Cognitive Ability: Applying
Client Needs: Physiological Integrity
Clinical Judgment/Cognitive Skills: Take Action
Integrated Process: Nursing Process/Implementation
Content Area: Skills: Medication Administration
Health Problem: N/A

Answer: 2

Rationale: The TPN line is used only for the administration of the TPN solution to prevent crystallization in the CVC tubing and disruption of the TPN infusion. Any other IV medication must be administered through a separate IV access site, including a separate infusion port of the CVC catheter. Therefore, options 1, 3, and 4 are incorrect actions.

Priority Nursing Tip: Parenteral nutrition solutions that are cloudy or darkened would not be used for administration and would be returned to the pharmacy.

Test-Taking Strategy: Focus on the **subject,** total parenteral nutrition. Eliminate options 1, 3, and 4 because they are **comparable or alike** in that they involve using the TPN line for the administration of the antibiotic.

---

148. The nurse monitoring a postoperative client would recognize which behaviors as indicators that the client is in pain? **Select all that apply.**

1 Gasping
2 Lip biting
3 Muscle tension
4 Pacing activities
5 Staring out the window
6 Asking for the television to be turned off

Level of Cognitive Ability: Analyzing
Client Needs: Physiological Integrity
Clinical Judgment/Cognitive Skills: Recognize Cues
Integrated Process: Nursing Process/Data Collection
Content Area: Skills: Vital Signs
Health Problem: N/A

Answer: 1, 2, 3, 4

Rationale: The nurse needs to check verbalization, vocal response, facial and body movements, and social interaction as indicators of pain. Behavioral indicators of pain include gasping, lip biting (facial expressions), muscle tension, pacing activities, moaning, crying, grunting (vocalizations), grimacing, clenching teeth, wrinkling the forehead, tightly closing or widely opening the eyes or mouth, restlessness, immobilization, increased hand and finger movements, rhythmic or rubbing motions, protective movements of body parts (body movement), avoidance of conversation, focusing only on activities for pain relief, avoiding social contacts and interactions, and reduced attention span. Options 5 and 6 are not to be assumed as pain-related behaviors because there can be a variety of reasons for such actions.

Priority Nursing Tip: It is important for the nurse to monitor for behavioral indicators of pain, particularly if the client is unable to verbalize the presence of pain.

Test-Taking Strategy: Focus on the **subject,** behavioral indicators of pain. Think about the physiological and psychosocial responses that occur during the pain experience as you read each option. This will assist in answering correctly.

---

149. Which conditions place the client receiving enteral nutrition at increased risk for aspiration? **Select all that apply.**

1 Sedation
2 Coughing
3 An artificial airway
4 Head-elevated position
5 Nasotracheal suctioning
6 Decreased level of consciousness

Level of Cognitive Ability: Analyzing
Client Needs: Physiological Integrity
Clinical Judgment/Cognitive Skills: Generate Solutions
Integrated Process: Nursing Process/Planning
Content Area: Foundations of Care: Safety
Health Problem: N/A

Answer: 1, 2, 3, 5, 6

Rationale: A serious complication associated with enteral feedings is aspiration of formula into the tracheobronchial tree. Some common conditions that increase the risk of aspiration include sedation, coughing, an artificial airway, nasotracheal suctioning, decreased level of consciousness, and lying flat. A head-elevated position does not increase the risk of aspiration.

Priority Nursing Tip: The nurse must check the client for conditions that place him or her at risk of aspiration. Aspiration can result in airway obstruction.

Test-Taking Strategy: Focus on the **subject,** the risks associated with aspiration. Recall that aspiration is the inhalation of foreign material into the tracheobronchial tree. Next, read each option and think about the effect it produces with regard to aspiration. This will direct you to the correct options.

---

150. A client experiencing a sudden onset of chest pain and dyspnea is diagnosed with a pulmonary embolus. The nurse assisting in caring for the client prepares to **immediately** implement which expected prescriptions for this client? **Select all that apply.**

1 Supplemental oxygen
2 High Fowler's position
3 Semi-Fowler's position
4 Morphine sulfate intravenously
5 Two tablets of acetaminophen with codeine
6 Meperidine hydrochloride intravenously

Level of Cognitive Ability: Applying
Client Needs: Physiological Integrity
Clinical Judgment/Cognitive Skills: Take Action
Integrated Process: Nursing Process/Implementation
Content Area: Complex Care: Emergency Situations/Management
Health Problem: Adult Health: Respiratory: Pulmonary Embolism

Answer: 1, 3, 4

Rationale: Standard therapeutic intervention for the client with pulmonary embolus includes proper positioning, oxygen, and intravenous analgesics. The head of the bed is placed in semi-Fowler's position. Fowler's is avoided because extreme hip flexure slows venous return from the legs and increases the risk of new thrombi. The usual analgesic of choice is morphine sulfate administered intravenously. This medication reduces pain, alleviates anxiety, and can diminish congestion of blood in the pulmonary vessels because it causes peripheral venous dilation.

Priority Nursing Tip: Clients prone to pulmonary embolism are those at risk for deep vein thrombosis.

Test-Taking Strategy: Note the **strategic word,** *immediately.* Eliminate option 2 first because a high-Fowler's position could place the client at risk for development of new thrombi. From the remaining options, recall that morphine is used for its vasodilating effects as well as its opioid effects for a client experiencing chest pain.

---

151. A client is scheduled to have a percutaneous transluminal coronary angioplasty (PTCA). What information about the balloon-tipped catheter would the nurse plan to include when reinforcing client education concerning the procedure?

1 A meshlike device within the catheter will be inflated, causing it to spring open.
2 The catheter will be used to compress the plaque against the coronary blood vessel wall.
3 The catheter will cut away the plaque from the coronary vessel wall using an embedded blade.
4 The catheter will be positioned in a coronary artery to take pressure measurements in the vessel.

Level of Cognitive Ability: Applying
Client Needs: Physiological Integrity
Clinical Judgment/Cognitive Skills: Take Action
Integrated Process: Teaching and Learning
Content Area: Adult Health: Cardiovascular
Health Problem: Adult Health: Cardiovascular: Coronary Artery Disease

Answer: 2
Rationale: In PTCA, a balloon-tipped catheter is used to compress the plaque against the coronary blood vessel wall. Option 1 describes placement of a coronary stent, option 3 describes coronary atherectomy, and option 4 describes part of the process used in cardiac catheterization.
Priority Nursing Tip: Complications of PTCA include arterial dissection or rupture, embolization of plaque fragments, spasm, and acute myocardial infarction.

Test-Taking Strategy: Focus on the **subject,** PTCA. Look at the name of the procedure. *Angioplasty* refers to repair of a blood vessel; this will assist in eliminating options 1 and 4. From the remaining options, recalling that a procedure that cuts something away would have the suffix *-ectomy* will assist in eliminating option 3.

---

152. The nurse is caring for a client who has been placed in skin traction. Which action by the nurse provides for countertraction to reduce shear and friction?

1 Using a footboard
2 Providing an overhead trapeze
3 Slightly elevating the foot of the bed
4 Slightly elevating the head of the bed

Level of Cognitive Ability: Applying
Client Needs: Physiological Integrity
Clinical Judgment/Cognitive Skills: Take Action
Integrated Process: Nursing Process/Implementation
Content Area: Adult Health: Musculoskeletal
Health Problem: Adult Health: Musculoskeletal: Skeletal Injury

Answer: 3
Rationale: The part of the bed under an area in traction is usually elevated to aid in countertraction. For the client in skin traction (which is applied to a leg), the foot of the bed is elevated. Option 3 provides a force that opposes the traction force effectively without harming the client. A footboard, an overhead trapeze, and elevation of the head of the bed are not measures used to provide countertraction.
Priority Nursing Tip: The surgeon's prescription is always followed regarding the amount of weight applied to the traction device. For Buck's extension, traction of usually not more than 8 to 10 pounds is prescribed.

Test-Taking Strategy: Focus on the **subject,** countertraction for skin traction. Eliminate option 4, recalling that skin extension traction is applied to the leg. From the remaining options, focus on the subject to eliminate options 1 and 2.

---

153. The nurse is preparing to initiate a bolus enteral feeding via nasogastric (NG) tube to a client. Which action represents safe practice by the nurse?

1 Checking the volume of the residual after administering the bolus feeding
2 Aspirating gastric contents before initiating the feeding to ensure that pH is greater than 9
3 Elevating the head of the bed to 25 degrees and maintaining that position for 30 minutes after feeding
4 Verifying correct NG tube position with aspiration and administration of air bolus with auscultation

Level of Cognitive Ability: Applying
Client Needs: Physiological Integrity
Clinical Judgment/Cognitive Skills: Take Action
Integrated Process: Nursing Process/ Implementation
Content Area: Skills: Tube Care
Health Problem: N/A

Answer: 4
Rationale: After initial radiographic confirmation of NG tube placement, methods used to verify NG tube placement include measuring the length of the tube from the point it protrudes from the nose to the end, injecting 10 to 30 mL of air into the tube and auscultating over the left upper quadrant of the abdomen, and aspirating the secretions and checking to see whether the pH is less than 3.5 (safest method). Residual needs to be checked before administration of the next feeding. Fowler's position is recommended for bolus feedings, if permitted, and would be maintained for 1 hour after instillation.
Priority Nursing Tip: Residual volumes are checked every 4 hours, before each feeding or the instillation of any solution, and before giving medications.

Test-Taking Strategy: Focus on the **subject,** bolus enteral feedings via NG tube. Note the words *safe practice*. Knowing that the pH of gastric contents needs to be between 1 and 5 will assist you in eliminating option 2. Option 3 can be eliminated because the head of the bed elevation would be at a minimum of 30 degrees for all types of enteral feedings to prevent aspiration. From the remaining two options, use knowledge of when to check residuals to assist you in eliminating option 1.

---

154. The nurse is reviewing the laboratory analysis of cerebrospinal fluid (CSF) obtained during a lumbar puncture from a child who is suspected of having bacterial meningitis. Which result would **most likely** confirm this diagnosis?

1 Clear CSF with low protein and low glucose
2 Cloudy CSF with low protein and low glucose
3 Cloudy CSF with high protein and low glucose
4 Decreased pressure and cloudy CSF with high protein

Level of Cognitive Ability: Analyzing
Client Needs: Physiological Integrity
Clinical Judgment/Cognitive Skills: Analyze Cues
Integrated Process: Nursing Process/Data Collection
Content Area: Pediatrics: Neurological
Health Problem: Pediatric Specific: Meningitis

Answer: 3
Rationale: A diagnosis of meningitis is made by testing CSF obtained by lumbar puncture. In the case of bacterial meningitis, findings usually include increased pressure and cloudy CSF with high protein and low glucose. Therefore, options 1, 2, and 4 are incorrect.
Priority Nursing Tip: Pneumococcal conjugate vaccine is recommended for all children beginning at age 2 months to protect against meningitis.

Test-Taking Strategy: Focus on the **subject,** laboratory analysis results of CSF associated with bacterial meningitis. Note the **strategic words,** *most likely*. Eliminate options 1 and 4 because clear CSF and decreased pressure are unlikely to be found with an infectious process such as meningitis. From the remaining choices, recalling that high protein indicates a possible diagnosis of meningitis will direct you to the correct option.

---

155. The nurse is caring for a client with a terminal condition who is dying. Which respiratory findings would indicate to the nurse that death is imminent? **Select all that apply.**

1 Dyspnea
2 Cyanosis
3 Tachypnea
4 Kussmaul's respiration
5 Irregular respiratory pattern
6 Adventitious bubbling lung sounds

Level of Cognitive Ability: Analyzing
Client Needs: Physiological Integrity
Clinical Judgment/Cognitive Skills: Recognize Cues
Integrated Process: Nursing Process/Data Collection
Content Area: Developmental Stages: End-of-Life Care
Health Problem: N/A

Answer: 1, 2, 5, 6

Rationale: Respiratory findings that indicate death is imminent include poor gas exchange as evidenced by hypoxia, dyspnea, or cyanosis; altered patterns of respiration, such as slow, labored, irregular, or Cheyne–Stokes pattern (alternating periods of apnea and deep, rapid breathing); increased respiratory secretions and adventitious bubbling lung sounds (death rattle); and irritation of the tracheobronchial airway as evidenced by hiccups, chest pain, fatigue, or exhaustion. Kussmaul's respirations are abnormally deep, very rapid sighing respirations characteristic of diabetic ketoacidosis. Tachypnea is defined as rapid breathing. In an adult, it would indicate a respiratory rate of over 20 breaths per minute.

Priority Nursing Tip: As death approaches, metabolism is reduced, and the body gradually slows down until all function ends.

Test-Taking Strategy: Focus on the **subject,** respiratory findings that occur near death. Think about the physiological processes that occur in the dying person as you read each option. This will assist in answering the question correctly.

---

156. An infant diagnosed with spina bifida cystica (meningomyelocele type) has had the sac surgically removed. The nurse plans for which intervention in the postoperative period to maintain the infant's safety?

1 Covering the back dressing with a binder
2 Placing the infant in a head-down position
3 Strapping the infant in a baby seat, sitting up
4 Elevating the head with the infant in the prone position

Level of Cognitive Ability: Applying
Client Needs: Physiological Integrity
Clinical Judgment/Cognitive Skills: Generate Solutions
Integrated Process: Nursing Process/Planning
Content Area: Pediatrics: Neurological
Health Problem: Pediatric-Specific: Neural Tube Defects

Answer: 4

Rationale: Spina bifida is a central nervous system defect that results from failure of the neural tube to close during embryonic development. Care of the operative site is carried out under the direction of the surgeon and includes close observation for signs of leakage of cerebrospinal fluid. The prone position is maintained after surgical closure to decrease the pressure on the surgical site on the back; however, many surgeons allow side-lying or partial side-lying position unless it aggravates a coexisting hip dysplasia or permits undesirable hip flexion. This offers an opportunity for position changes, which reduces the risk of pressure sores and facilitates feeding. Elevating the head will decrease the chance of cerebrospinal fluid collecting in the cranial cavity. If permitted, the infant can be held upright against the body with care taken to avoid pressure on the operative site. Binders and a baby seat would not be used because of the pressure they would exert on the surgical site.

Priority Nursing Tip: In the preoperative period, the myelomeningocele sac is protected by covering it with a sterile, moist (normal saline), nonadherent dressing to maintain the moisture of the sac and contents.

Test-Taking Strategy: Focus on the **subject,** postoperative care for an infant with spina bifida who had the sac removed. Recall that preventing pressure on the surgical site and preventing intracranial cerebrospinal fluid collection are goals for the postoperative period. Options 1 and 3 would increase pressure on the surgical site, and option 2 would not promote drainage of cerebrospinal fluid from the cranial cavity.

157. The nurse is checking a client who is being treated with a beta-adrenergic blocker. Which findings would indicate that the client may be experiencing dose-related side effects of the medication? **Select all that apply.**

1 Dizziness
2 Bradycardia
3 Chest pain
4 Reflex tachycardia
5 Sexual dysfunction
6 Cardiac dysrhythmias

Level of Cognitive Ability: Analyzing
Client Needs: Physiological Integrity
Clinical Judgment/Cognitive Skills: Analyze Cues
Integrated Process: Nursing Process/Data Collection
Content Area: Pharmacology: Cardiovascular: Beta Blockers
Health Problem: N/A

Answer: 1, 2, 5

Rationale: Beta-adrenergic blockers, commonly called *beta blockers,* are useful in treating cardiac dysrhythmias, mild hypertension, mild tachycardia, and angina pectoris. Side effects commonly associated with beta blockers are usually dose related and include dizziness (hypotensive effect), bradycardia, hypotension, and sexual dysfunction (impotence). Options 3, 4, and 6 are reasons for prescribing a beta blocker; however, these are general side effects of alpha-adrenergic blockers.

Priority Nursing Tip: Advise the client with diabetes mellitus who is taking beta-adrenergic blockers that the medication can mask the early signs of hypoglycemia such as nervousness and tachycardia.

Test-Taking Strategy: Focus on the **subject,** beta blockers. Specific knowledge regarding the side effects of beta blockers is needed to select the correct options. However, if you can remember that beta blockers are useful in treating cardiac dysrhythmias, mild hypertension, mild tachycardia, and angina pectoris, you will be able to eliminate the incorrect options.

---

158. A client at risk for respiratory failure is receiving oxygen via nasal cannula at 6 L/min. Arterial blood gas (ABG) results indicate pH 7.29, PCO_2 49 mm Hg, PO_2 58 mm Hg, and HCO_3 18 mEq/L. The nurse assists with care, anticipating that the primary health care provider will prescribe which intervention for respiratory support for this client?

1 Intubating for mechanical ventilation
2 Keeping the oxygen at 6 L/min via nasal cannula
3 Lowering the oxygen to 4 L/min via nasal cannula
4 Adding a partial rebreather mask to the current prescription

Level of Cognitive Ability: Synthesizing
Client Needs: Physiological Integrity
Clinical Judgment/Cognitive Skills: Generate Solutions
Integrated Process: Nursing Process/Planning
Content Area: Complex Care: Emergency Situations/Management
Health Problem: Adult Health: Respiratory: Acute Respiratory Distress Syndrome/Failure

Answer: 1

Rationale: If respiratory failure occurs and supplemental oxygen cannot maintain acceptable PO_2 and PCO_2 levels, endotracheal intubation and mechanical ventilation are necessary. The client is exhibiting respiratory acidosis, metabolic acidosis, and hypoxemia. Lowering or keeping the oxygen at the same liter flow will not improve the client's condition. A partial rebreather mask will raise CO_2 levels even further.

Priority Nursing Tip: The manifestations of respiratory failure are related to the extent and rapidity of change in the PO_2 and PCO_2.

Test-Taking Strategy: Focus on the **subject,** ABG analysis in a client at risk for respiratory failure. Note the ABG values. Noting that the oxygen level is low will eliminate options 2 and 3. Knowing that the PCO_2 is high will eliminate option 4 because a partial rebreather mask will raise CO_2 levels even further.

159. The nurse is preparing to check the respirations of several newborns in the nursery. The nurse performs the procedure and determines that the respiratory rate is normal if which finding is noted?

1 A respiratory rate of 30 breaths per minute in a crying newborn
2 A respiratory rate of 46 breaths per minute in an awake newborn
3 A respiratory rate of 60 breaths per minute in a sleeping newborn
4 A respiratory rate of 76 breaths per minute in a newly delivered newborn

Level of Cognitive Ability: Analyzing
Client Needs: Physiological Integrity
Clinical Judgment/Cognitive Skills: Recognize Cues
Integrated Process: Nursing Process/Data Collection
Content Area: Maternity: Newborn
Health Problem: N/A

Answer: 2
Rationale: Normal respiratory rate varies from 30 to 50 breaths per minute when the infant is not crying. Respirations need to be counted for 1 full minute to ensure an accurate measurement because the newborn infant may be a periodic breather. Observing and palpating respirations while the infant is quiet promotes accurate assessment. Palpation aids observation in determining the respiratory rate. Option 1 indicates bradypnea, and options 3 and 4 indicate tachypnea.
Priority Nursing Tip: The newborn infant's respiratory rate and apical heart rate are counted for 1 full minute to detect irregularities in rate or rhythm.

Test-Taking Strategy: Focus on the **subject,** newborn respiratory rate. Recall knowledge regarding the normal respiratory rate for a newborn infant to answer this question. Remember that the normal respiratory rate varies from 30 to 50 breaths per minute.

---

160. During a routine prenatal visit, a client in the third trimester of pregnancy reports having frequent calf pain when walking. The nurse suspects superficial thrombophlebitis and checks for which sign associated with this condition?

1 Severe chills
2 Kernig's sign
3 Brudzinski's sign
4 Palpable hard thrombus

Level of Cognitive Ability: Analyzing
Client Needs: Physiological Integrity
Clinical Judgment/Cognitive Skills: Recognize Cues
Integrated Process: Nursing Process/Data Collection
Content Area: Maternity: Antepartum
Health Problem: Adult Health: Cardiovascular: Vascular Disorders

Answer: 4
Rationale: Pain in the calf during walking could indicate venous thrombosis or peripheral arterial disease. The manifestations of superficial thrombophlebitis include a palpable thrombus that feels bumpy and hard, tenderness and pain in the affected lower extremity, and a warm and pinkish red color over the thrombus area. Severe chills can occur in a variety of inflammatory or infectious conditions and are also a manifestation of pelvic thrombophlebitis. Brudzinski's sign and Kernig's sign test for meningeal irritability.
Priority Nursing Tip: If a thrombus is suspected, never massage the site because of the risk of dislodging it and causing it to travel to the pulmonary system.

Test-Taking Strategy: Focus on the **subject,** thrombophlebitis. Eliminate options 2 and 3 first because they are **comparable or alike** and both test for meningeal irritation. From the remaining options, focus on the words *frequent calf pain when she walks* and *thrombophlebitis* to assist in directing you to the correct option.

---

161. The nurse evaluates the patency of a peripheral intravenous (IV) site and suspects an infiltration. Which action would the nurse take to determine whether the IV has infiltrated?

1 Strip the tubing and check for a blood return.
2 Check the regional tissue for redness and warmth.
3 Increase the infusion rate and observe for swelling.
4 Gently palpate regional tissue for edema and coolness.

Level of Cognitive Ability: Applying
Client Needs: Physiological Integrity
Clinical Judgment/Cognitive Skills: Take Action
Integrated Process: Nursing Process/ Implementation
Content Area: Skills: Complex Care: Intravenous Therapy
Health Problem: N/A

Answer: 4
Rationale: When checking an IV for clinical indicators of infiltration, it is important to check the site for edema and coolness, signifying leakage of the IV fluid into the surrounding tissues. Stripping the tubing will not cause a blood return but will force IV fluid into the surrounding tissues, which can increase the risk of tissue damage. Redness and warmth are more likely to indicate infection or phlebitis. The nurse would notify the registered nurse of the occurrence. Increasing the IV flow rate can further damage the tissues if the IV has infiltrated. Additionally, a prescription is needed to increase an IV flow rate.
Priority Nursing Tip: If an IV infiltration occurs, the IV device is removed from the client's vein; if IV therapy is still needed, a new IV device is inserted into a vein in a different extremity.

Test-Taking Strategy: Focus on the **subject,** IV infiltration. Recalling that the site will feel cool will direct you to the correct option. Also note the word *gently* in the correct option.

---

162. A client who has sustained a neck injury is unresponsive and pulseless. What would the emergency department nurse do to open the client's airway?

1 Insert an oropharyngeal airway.
2 Tilt the head and lift the chin.
3 Place in the recovery position.
4 Stabilize the skull and push up the jaw.

Level of Cognitive Ability: Applying
Client Needs: Physiological Integrity
Clinical Judgment/Cognitive Skills: Take Action
Integrated Process: Nursing Process/ Implementation
Content Area: Complex Care: Emergency Situations/Management
Health Problem: Adult Health: Neurological: Head Injury/Trauma

Answer: 4
Rationale: The health care team uses the jaw-thrust maneuver to open the airway until a radiograph confirms that the client's cervical spine is stable to avoid potential aggravation of a cervical spine injury. Options 1 and 2 require manipulation of the spine to open the airway, and option 3 can be ineffective for opening the airway.
Priority Nursing Tip: If a neck injury is suspected in a victim who sustained an injury, the jaw-thrust maneuver (rather than the head-tilt chin-lift) is used to open the airway to prevent further spine damage.

Test-Taking Strategy: Focus on the **ABCs—airway, breathing, and circulation.** Recalling the principles related to airway management will assist in eliminating options 1 and 2. From the remaining options, visualize each and eliminate option 3 because this action can be ineffective if the client is unable to maintain the airway.

---

163. The nurse is caring for a child diagnosed with Reye's syndrome. The nurse monitors for manifestations of which condition associated with this syndrome?

1 Protein in the urine
2 Symptoms of hyperglycemia
3 Increased intracranial pressure
4 A history of a *Staphylococcus* infection

Level of Cognitive Ability: Analyzing
Client Needs: Physiological Integrity
Clinical Judgment/Cognitive Skills: Recognize Cues
Integrated Process: Nursing Process/Data Collection
Content Area: Pediatrics: Neurological
Health Problem: Pediatric-Specific: Reye's Syndrome

Answer: 3

Rationale: Reye's syndrome is an acute encephalopathy that follows a viral illness and is characterized pathologically by cerebral edema and fatty changes in the liver. Intracranial pressure and encephalopathy are major problems associated with Reye's syndrome. Protein is not present in the urine. Reye's syndrome is related to a history of viral infections, and hypoglycemia is a symptom of this disease.

Priority Nursing Tip: The administration of aspirin and non–aspirin- containing salicylates is not recommended for a child with a febrile illness or a child with varicella or influenza because of its association with Reye's syndrome.

Test-Taking Strategy: Focus on the **subject,** Reye's syndrome. Recalling that Reye's syndrome is an acute encephalopathy will assist in directing you to the correct option.

---

164. The nurse analyzed an electrocardiogram (ECG) strip for a client demonstrating left-sided heart failure and interprets the ECG strip as which rhythm? **Refer to the figure.**

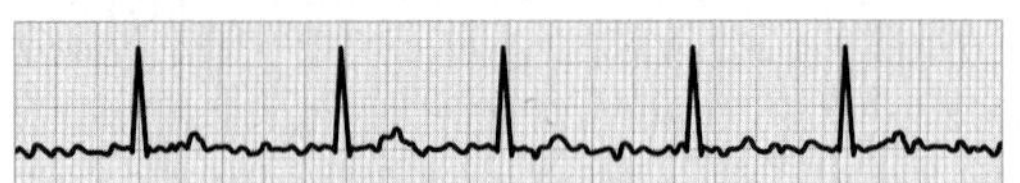

1 Atrial fibrillation
2 Sinus dysrhythmia
3 Ventricular fibrillation
4 Third-degree heart block

Level of Cognitive Ability: Synthesizing
Client Needs: Physiological Integrity
Clinical Judgment/Cognitive Skills: Analyze Cues
Integrated Process: Nursing Process/Data Collection
Content Area: Adult Health: Cardiovascular
Health Problem: Adult Health: Cardiovascular: Dysrhythmias

Answer: 1

Rationale: Atrial fibrillation is characterized by rapid, chaotic atrial depolarization. Ventricular rates may be less than 100 beats per minute (controlled) or more than 100 beats per minute (uncontrolled). The ECG reveals chaotic or no identifiable P waves and an irregular ventricular rhythm. A sinus dysrhythmia has a normal P wave and PR interval and QRS complex. In ventricular fibrillation, there are no identifiable P waves, QRS complexes, or T waves. In third-degree heart block, the atria and ventricles beat independently, and the PR interval varies in length.

Priority Nursing Tip: The client with atrial fibrillation is at risk for pulmonary embolism because thrombi can form in the right atrium as a result of atrial quivering and travel from the right atrium to the lungs.

Test-Taking Strategy: Focus on the **subject,** ECG interpretation. Look at the rhythm and compare it to what a normal rhythm would look like. Recall that in atrial fibrillation the P wave is usually absent or chaotic and the ventricular rhythm is irregular. This will direct you to the correct option.

---

165. The nurse is assisting with the admission of a client with a suspected diagnosis of bulimia nervosa. While collecting admission data, the nurse expects to elicit which data about the client's beliefs?

1 Is accepting of body size
2 Views purging as an accepted behavior
3 Overeats for the enjoyment of eating food
4 Overeats in response to losing control of diet

Level of Cognitive Ability: Applying
Client Needs: Physiological Integrity
Clinical Judgment/Cognitive Skills: Recognize Cues
Integrated Process: Nursing Process/Data Collection
Content Area: Mental Health
Health Problem: Mental Health: Eating Disorders

Answer: 2
Rationale: Individuals with bulimia nervosa develop cycles of binge eating, followed by purging. They seldom attempt to diet and have no sense of loss of control. Options 1, 3, and 4 are true of the obese person who may binge eat (not purge).
Priority Nursing Tip: The client with an eating disorder experiences an altered body image.

Test-Taking Strategy: Focus on the **subject,** bulimia nervosa. Eliminate options 3 and 4 because they are **comparable or alike** because both involve overeating. From the remaining options, recalling the definition of bulimia will direct you to the correct option.

---

166. The nurse is caring for a client who develops compartment syndrome as a result of a severely fractured arm. When the client asks why this happens, how would the nurse respond?

1 A bone fragment has injured the nerve supply in the area.
2 An injured artery causes impaired arterial perfusion through the compartment.
3 Bleeding and swelling cause increased pressure in an area that cannot expand.
4 The fascia expands with injury, causing pressure on underlying nerves and muscles.

Level of Cognitive Ability: Applying
Client Needs: Physiological Integrity
Clinical Judgment/Cognitive Skills: Take Action
Integrated Process: Nursing Process/Implementation
Content Area: Adult Health: Musculoskeletal
Health Problem: Adult Health: Musculoskeletal: Skeletal Injury

Answer: 3
Rationale: Compartment syndrome is caused by bleeding and swelling within a compartment, which is lined by fascia that does not expand. The bleeding and swelling place pressure on the nerves, muscles, and blood vessels in the compartment, triggering the symptoms. Therefore, options 1, 2, and 4 are incorrect statements.
Priority Nursing Tip: Within 4 to 6 hours after the onset of compartment syndrome, neurovascular damage is irreversible if untreated.

Test-Taking Strategy: Focus on the **subject,** compartment syndrome. Option 2 is eliminated first because this syndrome is not caused by an arterial injury. Knowing that the fascia cannot expand eliminates option 4. From the remaining options, it is necessary to know that bleeding and swelling (not a nerve injury) cause the symptoms.

---

167. A client with an extremity burn injury has undergone a fasciotomy. The nurse assisting in the care of the client anticipates that which type of wound care will be prescribed for the fasciotomy site?

1 Dry sterile dressings
2 Hydrocolloid dressings
3 Wet sterile saline dressings
4 One-half-strength povidone–iodine dressings

Level of Cognitive Ability: Applying
Client Needs: Physiological Integrity
Clinical Judgment/Cognitive Skills: Generate Solutions
Integrated Process: Nursing Process/Planning
Content Area: Skills: Wound Care
Health Problem: Adult Health: Integumentary: Burns

Answer: 3

Rationale: A fasciotomy is an incision made extending through the subcutaneous tissue and fascia. The fasciotomy site is not sutured but is left open to relieve pressure and edema. The site is covered with wet sterile saline dressings. After 3 to 5 days, when perfusion is adequate and edema subsides, the wound is debrided and closed. A hydrocolloid dressing is not indicated for use with clean, open incisions. The incision is clean, not dirty, so there would be no reason to require povidone–iodine. Additionally, povidone–iodine can be irritating to normal tissues.

Priority Nursing Tip: After fasciotomy, check pulses, color, movement, and sensation of the affected extremity, and control any bleeding with pressure.

Test-Taking Strategy: Focus on the **subject,** fasciotomy. Recall knowledge of what a fasciotomy involves and the basics of wound care. Recall that the skin is not sutured closed but left open for pressure relief. Remembering that moist tissue needs to remain moist will direct you to the correct option.

---

168. The nurse is caring for a client who was recently admitted with a diagnosis of anorexia nervosa. When the nurse enters the room, the client is engaged in rigorous push-ups. Which nursing action would the nurse implement?

1 Allow the client to complete the exercise program.
2 Interrupt the client and weigh the client immediately.
3 Interrupt the client and offer to take the client for a walk.
4 Tell the client that he or she is not allowed to exercise rigorously.

Level of Cognitive Ability: Applying
Client Needs: Physiological Integrity
Clinical Judgment/Cognitive Skills: Take Action
Integrated Process: Nursing Process/Implementation
Content Area: Mental Health
Health Problem: Mental Health: Eating Disorders

Answer: 3

Rationale: Clients with anorexia nervosa are frequently preoccupied with rigorous exercise and push themselves beyond normal limits to work off caloric intake. The nurse must provide for appropriate exercise, as well as place limits on rigorous activities. Allowing the client to complete the exercise program could be harmful. Weighing the client reinforces the altered self-concept that the client experiences and the client's need to control weight. Telling the client that he or she is not allowed to exercise rigorously will increase his or her anxiety.

Priority Nursing Tip: The client with an eating disorder experiences an altered body image.

Test-Taking Strategy: Focus on the **subject,** a client with anorexia nervosa. Focus on the need for the nurse to set limits with clients who have this disorder. Also, recalling that the nurse needs to provide and guide the client to perform appropriate exercise will direct you to the correct option.

---

169. The nurse checks a peripheral intravenous (IV) dressing and notes that it is damp and the tape is loose. What action would the nurse take **initially**?

1 Stop the infusion immediately.
2 Apply a sterile, occlusive dressing.
3 Ensure all IV tubing connections are tight.
4 Gather the supplies needed to insert a new IV.

Level of Cognitive Ability: Analyzing
Client Needs: Physiological Integrity
Clinical Judgment/Cognitive Skills: Prioritize Hypotheses
Integrated Process: Nursing Process/Implementation
Content Area: Foundations of Care: Safety
Health Problem: N/A

Answer: 3

Rationale: To determine subsequent nursing interventions, the nurse checks all connections to ensure tight seals while the IV infuses to help locate the source of the leak. If the leak is at the insertion site, the nurse stops the infusion, removes the IV, and inserts a new IV catheter. The nurse applies a new sterile occlusive dressing after resolving the source of the leak.

Priority Nursing Tip: Administration of an IV solution provides immediate access to the vascular system. Always ensure that the correct solution is administered as prescribed.

Test-Taking Strategy: Note the **strategic word,** *initially,* and recall that the nurse needs to determine the cause of the leaking. Use the **steps of the nursing process** and remember that data collection is the first step. Read each option carefully to determine which option indicates data collection to direct you to the correct option.

---

170. The nurse assists the primary health care provider with the removal of a chest tube. During the procedure, the nurse would instruct the client to perform which action?

1 Inhale quickly twice.
2 Breathe normally.
3 Breathe out forcefully.
4 Take a deep breath and hold it.

Level of Cognitive Ability: Applying
Client Needs: Physiological Integrity
Clinical Judgment/Cognitive Skills: Take Action
Integrated Process: Nursing Process/Implementation
Content Area: Skills: Tube Care
Health Problem: N/A

Answer: 4

Rationale: The client is instructed to take a deep breath and hold it for chest tube removal. This maneuver will increase intrathoracic pressure, thereby lessening the potential for air to enter the pleural space. Therefore, options 1, 2, and 3 are incorrect.

Priority Nursing Tip: Never clamp a chest tube without a written prescription from the primary health care provider. Additionally, agency policy regarding clamping a chest tube needs to be followed.

Test-Taking Strategy: Focus on the **subject,** chest tube removal. Eliminate options 1 and 2 because they are **comparable or alike** in that breathing will cause air to enter the pleural space. From the remaining options, eliminate option 3 because of the word *forcefully*.

---

171. The nurse checks the water seal chamber of a closed chest drainage system and notes fluctuations in the chamber. What intervention would the nurse implement?

1 Unkink the tubing.
2 Check for an air leak.
3 Document that the lung has reexpanded.
4 Document that the lung has not yet reexpanded.

Level of Cognitive Ability: Analyzing
Client Needs: Physiological Integrity
Clinical Judgment/Cognitive Skills: Take Action
Integrated Process: Nursing Process/Implementation
Content Area: Skills: Tube Care
Health Problem: N/A

Answer: 4

Rationale: Fluctuations (tidaling) in the water seal chamber are normal during inhalation and exhalation until the lung reexpands and the client no longer requires chest drainage. If fluctuations are absent, it could indicate occlusion of the tubing or that the lung has reexpanded. Excessive bubbling in the water seal chamber indicates that an air leak is present.

Priority Nursing Tip: In the water seal chamber, the tip of the tube is underwater, allowing fluid and air to drain from the pleural space and preventing air from entering the pleural space.

Test-Taking Strategy: Focus on the **subject,** chest tube system. Recalling the normal expectations related to the functioning of chest tube drainage systems will direct you to the correct option.

---

172. The nurse is assisting in developing a care plan for an older client being admitted to a long-term care facility. Which information would the nurse use to plan interventions for this client? **Select all that apply.**

1 Older clients tend to be incontinent.
2 Older clients are at risk for dehydration.
3 Depression is a normal part of the aging process.
4 Age-related skin changes require special monitoring.
5 Older clients are at risk for complications of immobility.
6 Confusion and cognitive changes are common findings in the older population.

Answer: 2, 4, 5
Rationale: Older clients are at risk for dehydration and complications related to immobility. Another normal physiological change that occurs during the aging process is loss of skin integrity. Incontinence, depression, confusion, and cognitive changes are not normal parts of the aging process.
Priority Nursing Tip: During the aging process, normal physiological body changes occur.

Test-Taking Strategy: Focus on the **subject,** an older client being admitted to a long-term care facility. Read each option carefully and recall normal manifestations of the aging process to lead you to the correct options.

Level of Cognitive Ability: Applying
Client Needs: Physiological Integrity
Clinical Judgment/Cognitive Skills: Generate Solutions
Integrated Process: Nursing Process/Planning
Content Area: Developmental Stages: Early Adulthood to Later Adulthood
Health Problem: N/A

---

173. The nurse assists in planning care for a client requiring intravenous (IV) fluids and electrolytes, understanding that which findings correlate with the need for this type of therapy? **Select all that apply.**

1 Hyponatremia
2 Bounding pulse rate
3 Chronic kidney disease
4 Isolated syncope episodes
5 Rapid, weak, and thready pulse
6 Abnormal serum and urine osmolality levels

Answer: 1, 5, 6
Rationale: Abnormal findings of major body systems offer clues to fluid and electrolyte imbalances. Rapid, weak, and thready pulse is an abnormality found with fluid and electrolyte imbalances, such as hyponatremia. Abnormal serum and urine osmolality are laboratory tests that are helpful in identifying the presence of or risk of fluid imbalances. Isolated episodes of syncope are not indicators for IV therapy unless fluid and electrolyte imbalances are identified. A bounding pulse rate is a manifestation of fluid volume excess; therefore, IV fluids are not indicated. Clients with chronic kidney disease experience the inability of the kidneys to regulate the body's water balance; fluid restrictions may be used.
Priority Nursing Tip: Clinical data noted from the data collection process are necessary to consider before IV therapy is initiated.

Test-Taking Strategy: Focus on the **subject,** clinical indicators of IV fluid and electrolyte therapy. Think about the purpose of IV therapy and circumstances in which it is prescribed to lead you to the correct options.

Level of Cognitive Ability: Analyzing
Client Needs: Physiological Integrity
Clinical Judgment/Cognitive Skills: Generate Solutions
Integrated Process: Nursing Process/Planning
Content Area: Foundations of Care: Fluids & Electrolytes
Health Problem: N/A

---

174. A child is admitted to the hospital with a diagnosis of rheumatic fever. The nurse assisting in the care of the child reviews the blood laboratory findings, knowing that which finding will confirm the likelihood of this disorder?

1 Increased leukocyte count
2 Decreased hemoglobin count
3 Increased antistreptolysin-O (ASO titer)
4 Decreased erythrocyte sedimentation rate

Level of Cognitive Ability: Analyzing
Client Needs: Physiological Integrity
Clinical Judgment/Cognitive Skills: Recognize Cues
Integrated Process: Nursing Process/Data Collection
Content Area: Pediatrics: Cardiovascular
Health Problem: Pediatric-Specific: Rheumatic Fever

Answer: 3

Rationale: Children suspected of having rheumatic fever are tested for streptococcal antibodies. The most reliable and best standardized test to confirm the diagnosis is the ASO titer. An elevated level indicates the presence of rheumatic fever. The remaining options are unrelated to diagnosing rheumatic fever. Additionally, an increased leukocyte count indicates the presence of infection but is not specific in confirming a particular diagnosis.

Priority Nursing Tip: Rheumatic fever manifests 2 to 6 weeks after a group A beta-hemolytic streptococcal infection of the upper respiratory tract.

Test-Taking Strategy: Note the word *confirm*. Focusing on the **subject**, rheumatic fever, will assist in eliminating options 2 and 4. From the remaining options, recall that an increased leukocyte count indicates the presence of infection but is not specific in confirming a particular diagnosis.

---

175. The nurse assisting in the care of a 5-year-old with a history of tetralogy of Fallot notes that the child has clubbed fingers. This finding is indicative of which associated condition?

1 Tissue hypoxia
2 Chronic hypertension
3 Delayed physical growth
4 Destruction of bone marrow

Level of Cognitive Ability: Analyzing
Client Needs: Physiological Integrity
Clinical Judgment/Cognitive Skills: Recognize Cues
Integrated Process: Nursing Process/Data Collection
Content Area: Pediatrics: Cardiovascular
Health Problem: Pediatric-Specific: Congenital Cardiac Defects

Answer: 1

Rationale: Clubbing, a thickening and flattening of the tips of the fingers and toes, is thought to occur because of chronic tissue hypoxia and polycythemia. Options 2, 3, and 4 do not cause clubbing.

Priority Nursing Tip: Hypercyanotic spells (acute episodes of cyanosis and hypoxia) are also called *blue spells* or *tet spells* and occur when the child's oxygen requirements exceed the blood supply, such as during feeding, crying, or defecating.

Test-Taking Strategy: Focus on the **subject**, the child's diagnosis. Use the **ABCs—airway, breathing, and circulation.** Hypoxia relates to oxygenation, which is a concern with this disorder.

---

176. The nurse assists in planning care for a client diagnosed with end-stage renal disease (ESRD). Which findings does the nurse expect to note documented in the client's medical record? **Select all that apply.**

1 Edema
2 Anemia
3 Polyuria
4 Bradycardia
5 Hypotension
6 Osteoporosis

Answer: 1, 2

Rationale: The manifestations of ESRD are the result of impaired kidney function. Two functions of the kidney are maintenance of water balance in the body and the secretion of erythropoietin, which stimulates red blood cell formation in bone marrow. Impairment of these functions results in edema and anemia. Kidney failure results in decreased urine production and increased blood pressure. Tachycardia is a result of increased fluid load on the heart. Osteoporosis is not a common finding with ESRD.

Priority Nursing Tip: The manifestations of kidney failure are primarily caused by the retention of nitrogenous wastes, the

Level of Cognitive Ability: Analyzing
Client Needs: Physiological Integrity
Clinical Judgment/Cognitive Skills: Recognize Cues
Integrated Process: Nursing Process/Data Collection
Content Area: Adult Health: Renal and Urinary
Health Problem: Adult Health: Renal and Urinary: Chronic Kidney Disease

retention of fluids, and the inability of the kidneys to regulate electrolytes.

Test-Taking Strategy: Focus on the **subject,** ESRD. Recalling the anatomy and physiology of the renal system and focusing on how the kidney functions and pathophysiology of ESRD will lead you to the correct options.

---

177. The nurse is performing range-of-motion (ROM) exercises on a client when the client unexpectedly develops spastic muscle contractions. Which interventions would the nurse implement? **Select all that apply.**

1 Stop movement of the affected part.
2 Massage the affected part vigorously.
3 Force movement of the joint supporting the muscle.
4 Notify the primary health care provider immediately.
5 Ask the client to stand and walk rapidly around the room.
6 Place continuous gentle pressure on the muscle group until it relaxes.

Level of Cognitive Ability: Applying
Client Needs: Physiological Integrity
Clinical Judgment/Cognitive Skills: Take Action
Integrated Process: Nursing Process/Implementation
Content Area: Skills: Activity/Mobility
Health Problem: N/A

Answer: **1, 6**
Rationale: ROM exercises would put each joint through as full a range of motion as possible without causing discomfort. An unexpected outcome is the development of spastic muscle contraction during ROM exercises. If this occurs, the nurse would stop movement of the affected part and place continuous gentle pressure on the muscle group until it relaxes. Once the contraction subsides, the exercises are resumed using slow, steady movement. Massaging the affected part vigorously may worsen the contraction. There is no need to notify the primary health care provider unless intervention is ineffective. The nurse would never force movement of a joint. Asking the client to stand and walk rapidly around the room is an inappropriate measure. Additionally, if the client is able to walk, ROM exercises are probably unnecessary.
Priority Nursing Tip: ROM exercises provide adequate muscle use and maintain strength and flexibility of the muscles and joints.

Test-Taking Strategy: Focus on the **subject,** interventions to relieve spastic muscle contractions. Eliminate option 2 because of the word *vigorously,* option 3 because of the word *force,* and option 4 because of the word *immediately.* Next eliminate option 5 because if the client is able to walk, ROM exercises are probably unnecessary.

---

178. A client has been admitted to the hospital with a diagnosis of acute glomerulonephritis. During history taking, the nurse would ask the client about a recent history of which event?

1 Bleeding ulcer
2 Myocardial infarction
3 Deep vein thrombosis
4 Streptococcal infection

Level of Cognitive Ability: Applying
Client Needs: Physiological Integrity
Clinical Judgment/Cognitive Skills: Take Action
Integrated Process: Nursing Process/Data Collection
Content Area: Adult Health: Renal and Urinary
Health Problem: Adult Health: Renal and Urinary: Inflammations/Infections

Answer: **4**
Rationale: The predominant cause of acute glomerulonephritis is infection with beta-hemolytic *Streptococcus* 3 weeks before the onset of symptoms. In addition to bacteria, other infectious agents that could trigger the disorder include viruses, fungi, and parasites. Bleeding ulcer, myocardial infarction, and deep vein thrombosis are not precipitating causes.
Priority Nursing Tip: Edema, hematuria, and proteinuria are manifestations of glomerulonephritis.

Test-Taking Strategy: Focus on the **subject,** glomerulonephritis. Recalling that infection is a common trigger for glomerulonephritis assists in eliminating options 1, 2, and 3. It is also necessary to know that streptococcal infections are a common cause of this problem.

---

179. A client has just been admitted to the emergency department with chest pain. Serum cardiac enzyme levels are drawn, and the results indicate an elevated serum creatine kinase (CK)-MB isoenzyme, troponin T, and troponin I. The nurse assisting in the care of the client concludes that these results are compatible with what diagnosis?

1 Stable angina
2 Unstable angina
3 Prinzmetal's angina
4 New-onset myocardial infarction (MI)

Level of Cognitive Ability: Analyzing
Client Needs: Physiological Integrity
Clinical Judgment/Cognitive Skills: Analyze Cues
Integrated Process: Nursing Process/Data Collection
Content Area: Foundations of Care: Laboratory Tests
Health Problem: Adult Health: Cardiovascular: Myocardial Infarction

Answer: 4
Rationale: CK-MB isoenzyme is a sensitive indicator of myocardial damage. Levels begin to rise 3 to 6 hours after the onset of chest pain, peak at approximately 24 hours, and return to normal in about 3 days. Troponin is a regulatory protein found in striated muscle (skeletal and myocardial). Increased amounts of troponins are released into the bloodstream when an infarction causes damage to the myocardium. Troponin I is particularly sensitive to myocardial muscle injury; therefore, the client's results are compatible with new-onset MI. Options 1, 2, and 3 all refer to angina. These levels would not be elevated in angina.
Priority Nursing Tip: Troponin I has a high affinity for myocardial injury. The level rises within 3 hours after injury and persists up to 7 to 10 days.

Test-Taking Strategy: Focus on the **subject,** cardiac enzymes. Eliminate options 1, 2, and 3 because they are **comparable or alike** and all refer to angina.

---

180. As part of cardiac assessment, to palpate the apical pulse, the nurse would place the fingertips at which location?

1 At the left midclavicular line at the fifth intercostal space
2 At the left midclavicular line at the third intercostal space
3 To the right of the left midclavicular line at the fifth intercostal space
4 To the right of the left midclavicular line at the third intercostal space

Level of Cognitive Ability: Applying
Client Needs: Physiological Integrity
Clinical Judgment/Cognitive Skills: Take Action
Integrated Process: Nursing Process/Data Collection
Content Area: Health Assessment/Physical Exam: Heart and Peripheral Vascular
Health Problem: N/A

Answer: 1
Rationale: The point of maximal impulse (PMI), where the apical pulse is palpated, is normally located in the fourth or fifth intercostal space, at the left midclavicular line. Options 2, 3, and 4 are not descriptions of the location for palpation of the apical pulse.
Priority Nursing Tip: The apical impulse may not be palpable in obese clients or clients with thick chest walls.

Test-Taking Strategy: Focus on the **subject,** PMI. Recalling that the PMI corresponds to the left ventricular apex and visualizing each position in the options will direct you to the correct option.

---

181. The nurse is caring for a client receiving bolus feedings via a nasogastric (NG) tube. The nurse would place the client in which position to administer the feeding?

1 Supine
2 Semi-Fowler's
3 Trendelenburg's
4 Lateral recumbent

Level of Cognitive Ability: Applying
Client Needs: Physiological Integrity
Clinical Judgment/Cognitive Skills: Take Action
Integrated Process: Nursing Process/Implementation
Content Area: Skills: Nutrition
Health Problem: N/A

Answer: 2
Rationale: Clients are at high risk for aspiration during an NG tube feeding because the tube bypasses a protective mechanism, the gag reflex. The head of the bed is elevated 35 to 40 degrees (semi-Fowler's) to prevent this complication by facilitating gastric emptying. The remaining options increase the risk of aspiration by blunting the effect of gravity on gastric emptying.
Priority Nursing Tip: Check the expiration date on the formula before administering the NG tube feeding.

Test-Taking Strategy: Focus on the **subject,** NG tube feeding. Eliminate options 1, 3, and 4 because they are **comparable or alike** and increase the risk of aspiration.

---

182. The nurse monitors a client with acute pancreatitis. Which finding indicates that paralytic ileus has developed?

1 Inability to pass flatus
2 Loss of anal sphincter control
3 Severe, constant pain with rapid onset
4 Firm, nontender mass palpable at the lower right costal margin

Level of Cognitive Ability: Applying
Client Needs: Physiological Integrity
Clinical Judgment/Cognitive Skills: Recognize Cues
Integrated Process: Nursing Process/Data Collection
Content Area: Adult Health: Gastrointestinal
Health Problem: Adult Health: Gastrointestinal: GI Accessory Organs

Answer: 1
Rationale: An inflammatory reaction such as acute pancreatitis can cause paralytic ileus, the common form of nonmechanical obstruction. Inability to pass flatus is a clinical manifestation of paralytic ileus. Loss of sphincter control is not a sign of paralytic ileus. Pain is associated with paralytic ileus, but the pain usually presents as a more constant generalized discomfort. Pain that is severe, constant, and rapid in onset is more likely caused by strangulation of the bowel. Option 4 is the description of the physical finding of liver enlargement. The liver is usually enlarged in the client with cirrhosis or hepatitis. An enlarged liver is not a sign of paralytic ileus.
Priority Nursing Tip: Cullen's sign (discoloration of the abdomen and periumbilical area) and Turner's sign (bluish discoloration of the flanks) are indicative of pancreatitis.

Test-Taking Strategy: Focus on the **subject,** a sign of paralytic ileus. Recalling the definition of this complication and noting the word *paralytic* will direct you to the correct option.

---

183. After collecting data on a client with a diagnosis of cholelithiasis, the nurse documents that the bowel sounds are normal. When asked, how would the nurse describe this finding to the client?

1 Waves of loud gurgles auscultated in all four quadrants
2 Soft gurgling or clicking sounds auscultated in all four quadrants
3 Low-pitched swishing sounds auscultated in one or two quadrants
4 Very high-pitched loud rushes auscultated, especially in one or two quadrants

Answer: 2
Rationale: Although frequency and intensity of bowel sounds will vary depending on the phase of digestion, normal bowel sounds are relatively soft gurgling or clicking sounds that occur irregularly 5 to 35 times per minute. Loud gurgles (borborygmi) indicate hyperperistalsis. A swishing or buzzing sound represents turbulent blood flow associated with a bruit. No aortic bruits would be heard. Bowel sounds will be higher pitched and loud (hyperresonance) when the intestines are under tension, as in intestinal obstruction.
Priority Nursing Tip: Murphy's sign (the client cannot take a deep breath when the examiner's fingers are passed below the hepatic margin because of pain) is a characteristic of cholecystitis.

Level of Cognitive Ability: Applying
Client Needs: Physiological Integrity
Clinical Judgment/Cognitive Skills: Take Action
Integrated Process: Nursing Process/Data Collection
Content Area: Health Assessment: Physical Exam: Abdomen
Health Problem: Adult Health: Gastrointestinal: GI Accessory Organs

Test-Taking Strategy: Focus on the **subject,** normal bowel sounds. Normally, bowel sounds would be audible in all four quadrants; therefore, options 3 and 4 can be eliminated. From the remaining options, select option 2 because of the word *soft* in this option.

---

184. Which important parameter would the nurse check on a daily basis for a client diagnosed with nephrotic syndrome?

1 Weight
2 Albumin levels
3 Activity tolerance
4 Blood urea nitrogen (BUN) level

Answer: 1
Rationale: The client with nephrotic syndrome typically presents with edema, hypoalbuminemia, and proteinuria. The nurse carefully checks the fluid balance of the client, which includes daily monitoring of weight, intake and output, edema, and girth measurements. Albumin levels are monitored as they are prescribed, as are the BUN and creatinine levels. The client's activity level is adjusted according to the amount of edema and water retention. As edema increases, the client's activity level needs to be restricted.
Priority Nursing Tip: In nephrotic syndrome, the blood pressure may be normal or slightly decreased from normal.

Level of Cognitive Ability: Applying
Client Needs: Physiological Integrity
Clinical Judgment/Cognitive Skills: Recognize Cues
Integrated Process: Nursing Process/Data Collection
Content Area: Adult Health: Renal and Urinary
Health Problem: Adult Health: Renal and Urinary: Inflammation and Infections

Test-Taking Strategy: Focus on the **subject,** a client with nephrotic syndrome. Note the words *daily basis.* Recalling that the typical signs of nephrotic syndrome are edema, hypoalbuminemia, and proteinuria will direct you to the correct option.

---

185. A client is being admitted to the hospital with a diagnosis of urolithiasis and ureteral colic. The nurse assisting in the care of the client expects to note which finding on pain assessment?

1 Dull and aching pain in the costovertebral area
2 Aching and cramplike pain throughout the abdomen
3 Pain that is sharp and radiating posteriorly to the spinal column
4 Pain that is excruciating, wavelike, and radiating toward the genitalia

Answer: 4
Rationale: The pain of ureteral colic is caused by movement of a stone through the ureter and is sharp, excruciating, and wavelike, radiating to the genitalia and thigh. The stone causes reduced flow of urine, and the urine also contains blood because of the stone's abrasive action on urinary tract mucosa. Stones in the renal pelvis cause pain that is a dull ache in the costovertebral area. Renal colic is characterized by pain that is acute, with tenderness over the costovertebral area. Options 1, 2, and 3 are not characteristics of urolithiasis and ureteral colic.
Priority Nursing Tip: For the client with renal calculi, strain all urine for the presence of stones and send the stones to the laboratory for analysis.

Level of Cognitive Ability: Analyzing
Client Needs: Physiological Integrity
Clinical Judgment/Cognitive Skills: Recognize Cues
Integrated Process: Nursing Process/Data Collection
Content Area: Skills: Vital Signs
Health Problem: Adult Health: Renal and Urinary: Obstructive Problems

Test-Taking Strategy: Focus on the **subject,** urolithiasis and ureteral colic. Recall the anatomical location of the kidneys and the ureters. Because the kidneys are located in the posterior abdomen near the rib cage, pain in the costovertebral area is more likely to be associated with stones in the renal pelvis. On the other hand, sharp wavelike pain that radiates toward the genitalia is more consistent with the location of the ureters in the abdomen.

186. The client with heart failure states the need to use three pillows under the head and upper torso at night to be able to breathe comfortably while sleeping. The nurse documents that the client is experiencing which clinical finding?

1 Orthopnea
2 Dyspnea at rest
3 Dyspnea on exertion
4 Paroxysmal nocturnal dyspnea

Level of Cognitive Ability: Applying
Client Needs: Physiological Integrity
Clinical Judgment/Cognitive Skills: Analyze Cues
Integrated Process: Communication and Documentation
Content Area: Foundations of Care: Sleep & Rest
Health Problem: Adult Health: Cardiovascular: Heart Failure

Answer: 1

Rationale: Dyspnea is a subjective complaint that can range from an awareness of breathing to physical distress and does not necessarily correlate with the degree of heart failure. Dyspnea can be exertional or at rest. Orthopnea is a more severe form of dyspnea, requiring the client to assume a "three-point" position while upright and use pillows to support the head and upper torso at night. Paroxysmal nocturnal dyspnea is a severe form of dyspnea occurring suddenly at night because of rapid fluid reentry into the vasculature from the interstitium during sleep.

Priority Nursing Tip: Signs of left-sided heart failure are evident in the pulmonary system. Signs of right-sided heart failure are evident in the systemic circulation.

Test-Taking Strategy: Focus on the **subject**, a client with left-sided heart failure who has trouble breathing while sleeping. Recall knowledge of the different degrees of dyspnea. Eliminate options 3 and 4 because the question mentions nothing about exertion or a sudden (paroxysmal) event. From the remaining options, select option 1 because the client is breathing "comfortably" with the use of pillows.

---

187. The nurse assists in the care of a client admitted to the hospital who is in sickle cell crisis. The nurse would prepare for which intervention as a **priority** in the management of the client?

1 Pain management with an opioid
2 Intravenous fluid therapy
3 Oxygen administration
4 Blood transfusion

Level of Cognitive Ability: Applying
Client Needs: Physiological Integrity
Clinical Judgment/Cognitive Skills: Generate Solutions
Integrated Process: Nursing Process/Planning
Content Area: Adult Health: Hematological
Health Problem: Adult Health: Hematological: Anemias

Answer: 3

Rationale: The priority nursing intervention for a client in sickle cell crisis is to administer supplemental oxygen because the client is hypoxemic, and as a result, the red blood cells change to the sickle shape. In addition, oxygen is the priority because airway and breathing are more important than circulatory needs. The nurse also plans for fluid therapy to promote hydration and reverse the agglutination of sickled cells, opioid analgesics for relief from severe pain, and blood transfusions (rather than iron administration) to increase the blood's oxygen-carrying capacity.

Priority Nursing Tip: In sickle cell anemia, situations that precipitate sickling include fever, dehydration, and emotional and physical stress.

Test-Taking Strategy: Focus on the **subject,** sickle cell crisis, and focus on the **strategic word,** *priority.* Recalling the **ABCs—airway, breathing, and circulation**—will assist in answering correctly. Recalling that clumping of sickled cells occurs when the sickle cell client is hypoxemic will direct you to the correct option.

---

188. The nurse suspecting that a client is developing cardiogenic shock would check for which peripheral vascular manifestation of this complication? **Select all that apply.**

1 Warm, moist skin
2 Flushed, dry skin
3 Cool, clammy skin
4 Irregular pedal pulses
5 Bounding pedal pulses
6 Weak or thready pedal pulses

Level of Cognitive Ability: Analyzing
Client Needs: Physiological Integrity
Clinical Judgment/Cognitive Skills: Recognize Cues
Integrated Process: Nursing Process/Data Collection
Content Area: Complex Care: Shock
Health Problem: Adult Health: Cardiovascular: Myocardial Infarction

Answer: 3, 6
Rationale: Some of the manifestations of cardiogenic shock include increased pulse (weak and thready); decreased blood pressure; decreasing urinary output; signs of cerebral ischemia (confusion, agitation); and cool, clammy skin. None of the remaining options are associated with the peripheral vascular aspects of cardiogenic shock.
Priority Nursing Tip: The goals of treatment for cardiogenic shock are to maintain tissue oxygenation and perfusion and improve the pumping ability of the heart.

Test-Taking Strategy: Focus on the **subject,** cardiogenic shock. Recall the signs and symptoms of shock. The words *clammy* and *weak or thready* would direct you to the correct option.

---

189. The nurse teaching an older client with diabetes mellitus about general hygienic measures for foot and nail care would include which instructions? **Select all that apply.**

1 Wear knee-high hose to prevent edema.
2 Soak and wash the feet daily using cool water.
3 Use commercial removers for corns or calluses.
4 Use over-the-counter preparations to treat ingrown nails.
5 Apply lanolin or baby oil if dryness is noted along the feet.
6 Pat the feet dry thoroughly after washing and dry well between toes.

Level of Cognitive Ability: Applying
Client Needs: Physiological Integrity
Clinical Judgment/Cognitive Skills: Take Action
Integrated Process: Teaching and Learning
Content Area: Skills: Hygiene
Health Problem: Adult Health: Endocrine: Diabetes Mellitus

Answer: 5, 6
Rationale: The nurse would offer the following guidelines in a general hygienic foot and nail care program: Inspect the feet daily, including the tops and soles of the feet, the heels, and the areas between the toes; wash the feet daily using lukewarm water, and avoid soaks to the feet, thoroughly patting the feet dry and drying well between toes; and avoid cutting corns or calluses or using commercial removers. Additional general hygienic measures include gently rubbing lanolin, baby oil, or corn oil into the skin if dryness is noted along the feet or between the toes; filing the toenails straight across and square (do not use scissors or clippers); avoiding the use of over-the-counter preparations to treat ingrown toenails and consulting a primary health care provider for these problems; and avoiding the use of elastic stockings (unless prescribed by a health care professional), knee-high hose, or constricting garters.
Priority Nursing Tip: A complication of diabetes mellitus is peripheral neuropathy, which results in decreased sensation, particularly in the feet. A client with diabetes mellitus needs to be cautious about temperature exposure and injuries to the feet, as they may not be felt because of the decreased sensation.

Test-Taking Strategy: Focus on the **subject,** general hygienic measures for foot and nail care. Eliminate option 1, recalling that constricting items need to be avoided. Eliminate option 2 because of the words *soak* and *cool.* Eliminate options 3 and 4 because of the words *commercial removers* and *over-the-counter,* respectively.

---

190. A client diagnosed with renal cancer is being treated preoperatively with radiation therapy. The nurse determines that the client has an understanding of proper care of the skin over the treatment field when the client makes which statement?

1 "I'll be able to wash the ink marks off my skin after the initial treatment."
2 "Direct sunlight is something I'll have to really avoid exposing my skin to."
3 "I'll have my family bring me some unscented lotion to keep my skin soft."
4 "Wearing snug-fitting clothing over the skin site will help provide good support."

Level of Cognitive Ability: Evaluating
Client Needs: Physiological Integrity
Clinical Judgment/Cognitive Skills: Evaluate Outcomes
Integrated Process: Nursing Process/Evaluation
Content Area: Adult Health: Oncology
Health Problem: Adult Health: Cancer: Bladder and Kidney

Answer: 2

Rationale: The client undergoing radiation therapy must keep the affected skin protected from temperature extremes, direct sunlight, and chlorinated water (as from swimming pools). The client needs to wash the site using mild soap and warm or cool water and pat the area dry. Lines or ink marks that are placed on the skin to guide the radiation therapy need to be left in place. No lotions, creams, alcohol, perfumes, or deodorants would be placed on the skin over the treatment site. The client would wear cotton clothing over the skin site and guard against irritation from tight or rough clothing such as belts or bras.

Priority Nursing Tip: Radiation therapy is effective on tissues directly within the path of the radiation beam.

Test-Taking Strategy: Focus on the **subject,** care of the skin over the treatment field after radiation therapy. Note the words *understanding of proper care.* Recalling that the goal of care is to prevent skin irritation will direct you to the correct option.

---

191. A client diagnosed with chronic kidney disease is prescribed epoetin alfa. When discussing measures needed to support this medication therapy, the nurse would reinforce information regarding which supplement?

1 Iron
2 Zinc
3 Calcium
4 Magnesium

Level of Cognitive Ability: Applying
Client Needs: Physiological Integrity
Clinical Judgment/Cognitive Skills: Take Action
Integrated Process: Nursing Process/Data Collection
Content Area: Pharmacology: Hematological: Hematopoietic Agents
Health Problem: Adult Health: Renal and Urinary: Chronic Kidney Disease

Answer: 1

Rationale: Iron is needed for red blood cell (RBC) production; otherwise, the body cannot produce sufficient erythrocytes. In either case the client is not receiving the full benefit of epoetin alfa therapy if iron is not taken. Options 2, 3, or 4 are not prescribed for RBC production.

Priority Nursing Tip: A side effect of epoetin alfa is hypertension.

Test-Taking Strategy: Focus on the **subject,** RBC production. Note the relationship of RBC production in the question and the word *iron* in the correct option.

192. The licensed practical nurse is assisting the home health nurse in performing an initial assessment on a client who has been discharged after an insertion of a permanent pacemaker. Which client statement indicates that an understanding of self-care is evident?

1 "I will never be able to operate a microwave oven again."
2 "I need to expect occasional feelings of dizziness and fatigue."
3 "I will take my pulse in the wrist or neck daily and record it in a log."
4 "Moving my arms and shoulders vigorously helps check pacemaker functioning."

Level of Cognitive Ability: Evaluating
Client Needs: Physiological Integrity
Clinical Judgment/Cognitive Skills: Evaluate Outcomes
Integrated Process: Nursing Process/Evaluation
Content Area: Adult Health: Cardiovascular
Health Problem: Adult Health: Cardiovascular: Dysrhythmias

Answer: 3
Rationale: Clients with permanent pacemakers must be able to take their pulse in the wrist and/or neck accurately so as to note any variation in the pulse rate or rhythm that may need to be reported to the cardiologist. Clients can safely operate most appliances and tools, such as microwave ovens, video recorders, AM-FM radios, electric blankets, lawn mowers, and leaf blowers, as long as the devices are grounded and in good repair. If the client experiences any feelings of dizziness, fatigue, or an irregular heartbeat, the cardiologist is notified. The arms and shoulders would not be moved vigorously for 6 weeks after insertion.
Priority Nursing Tip: A responsibility of the nurse is to teach a client with a pacemaker how to measure the pulse rate.

Test-Taking Strategy: Focus on the **subject,** client understanding about care of a pacemaker. Recalling that a pacemaker assists in controlling cardiac rate and rhythm will direct you to the correct option.

---

193. A client experiencing a severe major depressive episode is unable to address activities of daily living (ADLs). Which nursing intervention **best** meets the client's current needs therapeutically?

1 Have the client's peers approach the client about how noncompliance in addressing ADLs affects the milieu.
2 Structure the client's day so that adequate time can be devoted to the client's assuming responsibility for ADLs.
3 Offer the client choices, and describe the consequences for failure to comply with the expectation of maintaining her or his own ADLs.
4 Feed, bathe, and dress the client as needed until the client's condition improves so that she or he can perform these activities independently.

Level of Cognitive Ability: Applying
Client Needs: Physiological Integrity
Clinical Judgment/Cognitive Skills: Take Action
Integrated Process: Nursing Process/Implementation
Content Area: Mental Health
Health Problem: Mental Health: Mood Disorders

Answer: 4
Rationale: The symptoms of major depression include depressed mood, loss of interest or pleasure, changes in appetite and sleep patterns, psychomotor agitation or retardation, fatigue, feelings of worthlessness or guilt, diminished ability to think or concentrate, and recurrent thoughts of death. Often, the client does not have the energy or interest to complete activities of daily living. Option 1 will increase the client's feelings of poor self-esteem and of unworthiness. Option 2 is incorrect because the client still lacks the energy and motivation to do these independently. Option 3 may lead to increased feelings of worthlessness as the client fails to meet expectations.
Priority Nursing Tip: For the client with depression, the nurse needs to avoid pushing the client to make decisions that the client is not ready to make. The nurse could spend time with the client to convey the client's worth and value.

Test-Taking Strategy: Focus on the **subject,** major depression. Note the **strategic word,** *best.* Use **Maslow's Hierarchy of Needs theory,** and remember that physiological needs are the priority. This will direct you to the correct option.

194. A pregnant client at 32 weeks' gestation is admitted to the obstetrical unit for observation after a motor vehicle crash. When the client begins experiencing slight vaginal bleeding and mild cramps, the licensed practical nurse (LPN) notifies the registered nurse (RN) immediately. The LPN anticipates that the RN will take which action to determine the viability of the fetus?

1. Insert an intravenous line and begin an infusion at 125 mL/hr.
2. Administer oxygen to the client via a face mask at 7 to 10 L/min.
3. Position and connect the ultrasound transducer to the external fetal monitor.
4. Position and connect a spiral electrode to the fetal monitor for internal fetal monitoring.

Answer: 3

Rationale: External fetal monitoring will allow the nurse to determine any change in the fetal heart rate and rhythm that would indicate that the fetus is in jeopardy. The amount of bleeding described is insufficient to require intravenous fluid replacement. Because fetal distress has not been determined at this time, oxygen administration is premature. Internal monitoring is contraindicated when there is vaginal bleeding, especially in preterm labor.

Priority Nursing Tip: Internal fetal monitoring is invasive and requires rupturing of the membranes and attaching an electrode to the presenting part of the fetus.

Test-Taking Strategy: Focus on the **subject,** determining viability of the fetus. Next use the **steps of the nursing process,** and note that option 3 is a data collection action and a noninvasive measure.

Level of Cognitive Ability: Applying
Client Needs: Physiological Integrity
Clinical Judgment/Cognitive Skills: Take Action
Integrated Process: Nursing Process/Implementation
Content Area: Maternity: Antepartum
Health Problem: Maternity: Fetal Distress/Demise

---

195. The nurse is reviewing the results of a sweat test performed on a child diagnosed with cystic fibrosis (CF). Which finding would the nurse identify as supporting this diagnosis?

1. An evening sweat potassium concentration greater than 60 mEq/L
2. A sweat chloride concentration that is consistently greater 60 mEq/L
3. An early morning sweat chloride concentration of less than 40 mEq/L
4. A sweat potassium concentration that is consistently less than 40 mEq/L

Answer: 2

Rationale: Cystic fibrosis is a chronic multisystem disorder characterized by exocrine gland dysfunction. A consistent finding of abnormally high chloride concentrations in the sweat is a unique characteristic of CF. Normally the sweat chloride concentration is less than 40 mEq/L. A sweat chloride concentration greater than 60 mEq/L is diagnostic of CF. Potassium concentration is unrelated to the sweat test.

Priority Nursing Tip: Usually more than 75 mg of sweat is needed to perform the sweat test. This amount is difficult to obtain from an infant; therefore, an immunoreactive trypsinogen analysis and direct deoxyribonucleic acid (DNA) analysis for mutant genes may be done to test for CF.

Test-Taking Strategy: Focus on the **subject,** sweat test. Eliminate options 1 and 4 first because they are **comparable or alike** and the potassium level is unrelated to the sweat test. From the remaining options, note that option 2 indicates a greater value.

Level of Cognitive Ability: Applying
Client Needs: Physiological Integrity
Clinical Judgment/Cognitive Skills: Analyze Cues
Integrated Process: Nursing Process/Data Collection
Content Area: Foundations of Care: Diagnostic Tests
Health Problem: Pediatric-Specific: Cystic Fibrosis

---

196. The licensed practical nurse (LPN) is assisting an emergency department nurse in assessing a client who abruptly discontinued benzodiazepine therapy and is experiencing withdrawal. Which manifestations of withdrawal would the nurse expect to note? **Select all that apply.**

1 Tremors
2 Sweating
3 Lethargy
4 Agitation
5 Nervousness
6 Muscle weakness

Level of Cognitive Ability: Analyzing
Client Needs: Physiological Integrity
Clinical Judgment/Cognitive Skills: Recognize Cues
Integrated Process: Nursing Process/Data Collection
Content Area: Pharmacology: Psychotherapeutics: Benzodiazepines
Health Problem: N/A

Answer: 1, 2, 4, 5
Rationale: Benzodiazepines would not be abruptly discontinued because withdrawal symptoms are likely to occur. Withdrawal symptoms include tremors, sweating, agitation, nervousness, insomnia, anorexia, and muscular cramps. Withdrawal symptoms from long-term, high-dose benzodiazepine therapy include paranoia, delirium, panic, hypertension, and status epilepticus. Lethargy is not associated with benzodiazepine withdrawal.
Priority Nursing Tip: Abrupt withdrawal of benzodiazepines can be potentially life threatening, and withdrawal would occur only under medical supervision.

Test-Taking Strategy: Focus on the **subject,** benzodiazepines. Specific knowledge regarding the withdrawal symptoms of benzodiazepines is needed to select the correct options. However, if you can remember that the therapeutic effect of benzodiazepines is anxiolytic, you will be able to eliminate the incorrect options because abrupt withdrawal will produce the opposite effect of an anxiolytic.

---

197. The nurse collects neurovascular data on a client with a newly applied cast. The nurse would determine that there is a need for close observation and a **need for follow-up** if which is noted?

1 Palpable pulses distal to the cast
2 Capillary refill greater than 6 seconds
3 Blanching of the nail bed when it is depressed
4 Sensation when the area distal to the cast is pinched

Level of Cognitive Ability: Analyzing
Client Needs: Physiological Integrity
Clinical Judgment/Cognitive Skills: Recognize Cues
Integrated Process: Nursing Process/Data Collection
Content Area: Adult Health: Musculoskeletal
Health Problem: Adult Health: Musculoskeletal: Musculoskeletal Injury

Answer: 2
Rationale: To check for adequate circulation, the nail bed of each finger or toe is depressed until it blanches, and then the pressure is released. This is known as *capillary refill time.* Optimally, the color will change from white to pink rapidly (less than 3 seconds). If this does not occur, the toes or fingers will require close observation and follow-up. Palpable pulses and sensations distal to the cast are expected. However, if pulses cannot be palpated or if the client complains of numbness or tingling, the primary health care provider needs to be notified.
Priority Nursing Tip: For the client with a cast applied to an extremity, if pulses cannot be palpated or the client complains of numbness or tingling, a potential complication is compartment syndrome or circulatory impairment.

Test-Taking Strategy: Focus on the **subject,** data collection after cast application. Note the **strategic words,** *need for follow-up.* This creates a **negative event query** and requires you to select a finding that is abnormal. Eliminate options 1, 3, and 4 because these options identify normal expected findings. Option 2 identifies an abnormal or unexpected finding.

---

198. The nurse is monitoring an unconscious client who sustained a head injury. Which observed positioning supports the suspicion that the client sustained an upper brainstem injury?

1 Abnormal involuntary flexion of the extremities
2 Abnormal involuntary extension of the extremities
3 Upper extremity extension with lower extremity flexion
4 Upper extremity flexion with lower extremity extension

Level of Cognitive Ability: Analyzing
Client Needs: Physiological Integrity
Clinical Judgment/Cognitive Skills: Recognize Cues
Integrated Process: Nursing Process/Data Collection
Content Area: Adult Health: Neurological
Health Problem: Adult Health: Neurological: Head Injury/Trauma

Answer: 2
Rationale: Decerebrate posturing, which can occur with upper brainstem injury, is characterized by abnormal involuntary extension of the extremities. Options 1, 3, and 4 are incorrect descriptions of this type of posturing.
Priority Nursing Tip: Decerebrate or decorticate posturing is an indication of neurological deterioration warranting immediate notification of the neurologist.

Test-Taking Strategy: Focus on the **data in the question** and note the **subject,** decerebrate posturing. Remember that decerebrate may also be known as *extension.* Recalling this concept will direct you to the correct option.

---

199. The nurse assisting in caring for a client after right radical mastectomy plans to include which intervention in the nursing plan of care for this client?

1 Takes blood pressures in the right arm only
2 Draws serum laboratory samples from the right arm only
3 Positions the client supine and flat with the right arm elevated on a pillow
4 Checks the right posterior axilla area when assessing the surgical dressing

Level of Cognitive Ability: Applying
Client Needs: Physiological Integrity
Clinical Judgment/Cognitive Skills: Generate Solutions
Integrated Process: Nursing Process/Planning
Content Area: Adult Health: Oncology
Health Problem: Adult Health: Cancer: Breast

Answer: 4
Rationale: If there is drainage or bleeding from the surgical site after mastectomy, gravity will cause the drainage to seep down and soak the posterior axillary portion of the dressing first. The nurse checks this area to detect early bleeding. Blood pressure measurement, venipuncture, and intravenous sites would not involve use of the operative arm. The client would be positioned with the head in semi-Fowler's position and the arm on the operative side elevated on pillows to decrease edema. Edema is likely to occur because lymph drainage channels have been resected during the surgical procedure.
Priority Nursing Tip: Breast self-examination (BSE) needs to be done monthly, 7 to 10 days after menses. Postmenopausal clients need to select a specific day of the month and perform BSE monthly on that day.

Test-Taking Strategy: Focus on the **subject,** postmastectomy care. Eliminate options 1 and 2 first because of the words *right arm only.* From the remaining options, use knowledge of the effects of gravity to direct you to the correct option.

---

200. The nurse is assisting a client diagnosed with hepatic encephalopathy to fill out the dietary menu. The nurse advises the client to avoid which entree item?

1 Tomato soup
2 Fresh fruit plate
3 Vegetable lasagna
4 Ground beef patty

Answer: 4
Rationale: Clients with hepatic encephalopathy have impaired ability to convert ammonia to urea and must limit intake of protein and ammonia-containing foods in the diet. The client needs to avoid foods such as chicken, beef, ham, cheese, milk, peanut butter, and gelatin. The food items in options 1, 2, and 3 are acceptable to eat.

Level of Cognitive Ability: Applying
Client Needs: Physiological Integrity
Clinical Judgment/Cognitive Skills: Take Action
Integrated Process: Nursing Process/Implementation
Content Area: Foundations of Care: Therapeutic Diets
Health Problem: Adult Health: Gastrointestinal: GI Accessory Organs

Priority Nursing Tip: Some food sources of protein include bread and cereal products, dairy products, beans, eggs, meats, fish, and poultry.

Test-Taking Strategy: Focus on the **subject,** hepatic encephalopathy, and note the word *avoid.* Note that options 1, 2, and 3 are **comparable or alike** in that they address food items of a fruit and vegetable nature.

---

201. A client with a colostomy reports gas buildup in the colostomy bag. The nurse instructs the client that consuming which food items would help prevent this problem? **Select all that apply.**

1 Yogurt
2 Broccoli
3 Cabbage
4 Crackers
5 Cauliflower
6 Toasted bread

Level of Cognitive Ability: Applying
Client Needs: Physiological Integrity
Clinical Judgment/Cognitive Skills: Take Action
Integrated Process: Teaching and Learning
Content Area: Foundations of Care: Therapeutic Diets
Health Problem: Adult Health: Gastrointestinal: Lower GI Disorders

Answer: 1, 4, 6
Rationale: Consumption of yogurt, crackers, and toasted bread can help prevent gas. Gas-forming foods include broccoli, mushrooms, cauliflower, onions, peas, and cabbage. These foods need to be avoided by the client with a colostomy until tolerance to them is determined.
Priority Nursing Tip: The best way for a client with a colostomy to control flatus is through diet. Every client is different, and the client must learn which foods will be problematic.

Test-Taking Strategy: Focus on the **subject,** prevention of gas buildup in the colostomy bag. Note the similarity between options 2, 3, and 5 in terms of their food substance to assist you in eliminating these options.

---

202. A client receiving total parenteral nutrition (TPN) reports nausea, polydipsia, and polyuria. To determine the cause of the client's report, the nurse assisting in the care of the client would check which client data?

1 Rectal temperature
2 Last serum potassium
3 Capillary blood glucose
4 Serum blood urea nitrogen and creatinine

Level of Cognitive Ability: Applying
Client Needs: Physiological Integrity
Clinical Judgment/Cognitive Skills: Recognize Cues
Integrated Process: Nursing Process/Data Collection
Content Area: Skills: Nutrition
Health Problem: N/A

Answer: 3
Rationale: Clients receiving TPN are at risk for hyperglycemia related to the increased glucose load of the solution. The symptoms exhibited by the client are consistent with hyperglycemia. The nurse would need to check the client's blood glucose level to verify these data. The other food options would not provide any information that would correlate with the client's symptoms.
Priority Nursing Tip: Hyperglycemia occurs in the client receiving TPN because of the high concentration of dextrose (glucose) in the solution.

Test-Taking Strategy: Focus on the **subject,** TPN therapy. Review the client's symptoms and think about the complications of TPN. Recalling that hyperglycemia is a complication will direct you to the correct option.

---

203. A client admitted to the hospital with a diagnosis of cirrhosis demonstrates massive ascites causing dyspnea. The nurse performs which intervention as a **priority** measure to assist the client with this complication?

1. Repositions side to side every 2 hours
2. Elevates the head of the bed 60 degrees
3. Auscultates the lung fields every 4 hours
4. Encourages deep breathing exercises every 2 hours

Level of Cognitive Ability: Applying
Client Needs: Physiological Integrity
Clinical Judgment/Cognitive Skills: Take Action
Integrated Process: Nursing Process/Implementation
Content Area: Adult Health: Gastrointestinal
Health Problem: Adult Health: Gastrointestinal: GI Accessory Organs

Answer: 2
Rationale: The client is having difficulty breathing because of upward pressure on the diaphragm from the ascitic fluid in the abdomen. Elevating the head of the bed enlists the aid of gravity in relieving pressure on the diaphragm. Although data collection is the first step of the nursing process, the question identifies the findings of ascites and difficulty breathing, so the best answer is to intervene based on the data, by elevating the head of the bed to make the client's breathing easier. The other options are general measures in the care of a client with ascites, but the priority measure is the one that relieves diaphragmatic pressure, thus assisting effective respirations.
Priority Nursing Tip: A paracentesis may be performed to remove abdominal fluid in a client with cirrhosis and ascites.

Test-Taking Strategy: Note the **strategic word,** *priority,* and the **subject,** to assist with breathing in a client with massive ascites. Recalling that elevating the head will provide immediate relief of symptoms associated with difficulty breathing will direct you to the correct option.

---

204. The nurse who practices culturally sensitive nursing care incorporates which concepts into client care? **Select all that apply.**

1. The expression of pain is affected by learned behaviors.
2. Physiologically, all individuals experience pain in a similar manner.
3. Ethnic culture has an effect on the physiological response to pain medications.
4. Clients would be checked for pain, regardless of a lack of overt symptomatology.
5. The use of a standardized pain assessment tool ensures unbiased pain assessment.

Level of Cognitive Ability: Analyzing
Client Needs: Physiological Integrity
Clinical Judgment/Cognitive Skills: Take Action
Integrated Process: Culture/Spirituality
Content Area: Foundations of Care: Spirituality, Culture, and Ethnicity
Health Problem: Adult Health: Neurological: Pain

Answer: 1, 3, 4
Rationale: Pain and its expression are often affected by an individual's ethnic culture in ways that include learned means of pain expression, the physiological response to pain medications, and attitudes regarding acceptable ways of dealing with pain. Physiologically not all individuals, even those of the same ethnic culture, will respond to pain in a similar manner, and so a standardized pain assessment tool is not effective in measuring pain in all clients.
Priority Nursing Tip: Pain and the expression of pain are individual-specific responses that are greatly influenced by an individual's ethnic culture.

Test-Taking Strategy: Focus on the **subject,** pain and cultural awareness. Considering the effects of culture on pain will direct you to the correct options. Also note the **closed-ended word** "all" in option 2 and the words *ensures unbiased* in option 5.

---

205. While gathering data, the nurse notes that the client has been prescribed tolterodine tartrate. The nurse would determine that the client is taking the medication to treat which disorder?

1 Glaucoma
2 Pyloric stenosis
3 Renal insufficiency
4 Urinary frequency and urgency

Level of Cognitive Ability: Analyzing
Client Needs: Physiological Integrity
Clinical Judgment/Cognitive Skills: Recognize Cues
Integrated Process: Nursing Process/Planning
Content Area: Pharmacology: Renal and Urinary: Anticholinergics/Antispasmodics
Health Problem: N/A

Answer: 4
Rationale: Tolterodine tartrate is an antispasmodic used to treat overactive bladder and symptoms of urinary frequency, urgency, or urge incontinence. It is contraindicated in urinary retention and uncontrolled narrow-angle glaucoma. It is used with caution in renal function impairment, bladder outflow obstruction, and gastrointestinal obstructive disease such as pyloric stenosis.
Priority Nursing Tip: Extended-release capsules of tolterodine tartrate would not be split, chewed, or crushed.

Test-Taking Strategy: Focus on the **subject,** the action and use of tolterodine tartrate. Recalling that tolterodine tartrate is an antispasmodic will direct you to the correct option.

---

206. The nurse reinforces discharge instructions to a client beginning oral hypoglycemic therapy. Which statements if made by the client indicate a **need for further teaching? Select all that apply.**

1 "If I am ill, I need to skip my daily dose."
2 "If I overeat, I will double my dosage of medication."
3 "Oral agents are effective in managing type 2 diabetes."
4 "If I become pregnant, I will discontinue my medication."
5 "Oral hypoglycemic medications will cause my urine to turn orange."
6 "My medications are used to manage my diabetes along with diet and exercise."

Level of Cognitive Ability: Evaluating
Client Needs: Physiological Integrity
Clinical Judgment/Cognitive Skills: Evaluate Outcomes
Integrated Process: Teaching and Learning
Content Area: Pharmacology: Endocrine: Oral Hypoglycemic
Health Problem: Adult Health: Endocrine: Diabetes Mellitus

Answer: 1, 2, 4, 5
Rationale: Clients are instructed that oral agents are used in addition to diet and exercise as therapy for diabetes mellitus. During illness or periods of intense stress, the client needs to be instructed to monitor her or his blood glucose level frequently and would contact the primary health care provider if the blood glucose is elevated, because insulin may be needed to prevent symptoms of acute hyperglycemia. The medication would not be skipped or the dosage would not be doubled. Taking extra medication would be avoided unless specifically prescribed by the primary health care provider. Medication would never be discontinued unless instructed to do so by the primary health care provider. However, the diabetic who becomes pregnant will need to contact their obstetrician, because the oral diabetic medication may have to be changed to insulin therapy, because some oral hypoglycemics can be harmful to the fetus. These medications do not change the color of the urine.
Priority Nursing Tip: Any changes to prescribed medication usage or amounts would not be made by clients without prior primary health care provider approval.

Test-Taking Strategy: Focus on the **subject,** oral hypoglycemic therapy. Note the **strategic words,** *need for further teaching.* These words indicate a **negative event query** and the need to select the incorrect options. Think about the pathophysiology of diabetes mellitus and its treatment, and use general medication guidelines to select the correct options.

207. The nurse evaluates a client after treatment for carbon monoxide poisoning after a burn injury. The nurse would document that the treatment was **effective** if which findings were present? **Select all that apply.**

1 The client is sleeping soundly.
2 The client is awake and talking.
3 Respiratory rate is 26 breaths/minute.
4 The client's heart rate is 84 beats/minute.
5 Carboxyhemoglobin levels are less than 5%.
6 The heart monitor shows normal sinus rhythm.

Level of Cognitive Ability: Evaluating
Client Needs: Physiological Integrity
Clinical Judgment/Cognitive Skills: Evaluate Outcomes
Integrated Process: Nursing Process/Evaluation
Content Area: Complex Care: Poisoning
Health Problem: Adult Health: Integumentary: Burns

Answer: 4, 5, 6

Rationale: Normal carboxyhemoglobin levels are less than 5% for a nonsmoking adult. Clients can be awake and talking with abnormally high levels. The symptoms of carbon monoxide poisoning are tachycardia, tachypnea, and central nervous system depression.

Priority Nursing Tip: A carbon monoxide level of 61% or above is fatal poisoning.

Test-Taking Strategy: Focus on the **subject,** carbon monoxide poisoning. Note the **strategic word,** *effective.* Note the relationship between the words *carbon monoxide poisoning* in the question and options 4, 5, and 6. These are the only options that specifically address this subject.

---

208. The nurse instructs a preoperative client about the proper use of an incentive spirometer. What result would the nurse use to determine that the client is using the incentive spirometer **effectively**?

1 Cloudy sputum
2 Shallow breathing
3 Unilateral wheezing
4 Productive coughing

Level of Cognitive Ability: Evaluating
Client Needs: Physiological Integrity
Clinical Judgment/Cognitive Skills: Evaluate Outcomes
Integrated Process: Nursing Process/Evaluation
Content Area: Skills: Oxygenation
Health Problem: N/A

Answer: 4

Rationale: Incentive spirometry helps reduce atelectasis, open airways, stimulate coughing, and mobilize secretions for expectoration via vital client participation in recovery. Cloudy sputum, shallow breathing, and wheezing indicate that the incentive spirometry has been ineffective because they point to infection, counterproductive depth of breathing, and bronchoconstriction, respectively.

Priority Nursing Tip: The client needs to assume a sitting or upright position when using an incentive spirometer.

Test-Taking Strategy: Focus on the **subject,** use of an incentive spirometer. Note the **strategic word,** *effectively.* Think about the purpose of an incentive spirometer. Eliminate options 1, 2, and 3, which indicate abnormal findings.

---

209. A client prescribed prazosin hydrochloride asks the nurse why the first dose must be taken at bedtime. Which response by the nurse is based on the understanding of the first dose of prazosin hydrochloride?

1 Treatment with prazosin hydrochloride results in drowsiness.
2 Treatment with prazosin hydrochloride can cause dependent edema.
3 Prazosin hydrochloride needs to be taken when the stomach is empty.
4 Treatment with prazosin hydrochloride can cause dizziness or possible syncope.

Level of Cognitive Ability: Applying
Client Needs: Physiological Integrity
Clinical Judgment/Cognitive Skills: Take Action
Integrated Process: Teaching and Learning
Content Area: Pharmacology: Cardiovascular: Antihypertensives
Health Problem: Adult Health: Cardiovascular: Hypertension

Answer: 4

Rationale: Prazosin is an alpha-adrenergic blocking agent. "First-dose hypotensive reaction" may occur during early therapy, which is characterized by dizziness, light-headedness, and possible loss of consciousness. The occurrence of these effects is better tolerated if the client is in bed. This also can occur when the dosage is increased. This effect usually disappears with continued use or if the dosage is decreased. Options 1, 2, and 3 are not characteristics of the medication.

Priority Nursing Tip: When prescribed, the first dose of prazosin hydrochloride would be given at bedtime. If the first dose needs to be given during the daytime, the client must remain supine for 3 to 4 hours.

Test-Taking Strategy: Focus on the **subject**, prazosin hydrochloride. Note the name of the medication. This will assist in determining that the medication is an antihypertensive agent. Recalling that orthostatic hypotension occurs with the use of antihypertensives will direct you to the correct option.

---

210. The nurse has applied the prescribed dressing to the leg of a client with an ischemic arterial leg ulcer. Which method would the nurse use to cover the dressing?

1 Apply a Kerlix roll and tape it to the skin.
2 Apply a large, soft pad and tape it to the skin.
3 Apply small Montgomery straps and tie the edges together.
4 Apply a Kling roll and tape the edge of the roll onto the bandage.

Level of Cognitive Ability: Applying
Client Needs: Physiological Integrity
Clinical Judgment/Cognitive Skills: Take Action
Integrated Process: Nursing Process/Implementation
Content Area: Skills: Wound Care
Health Problem: Adult Health: Cardiovascular: Vascular Disorders

Answer: 4

Rationale: Standard dressing technique includes the use of Kling rolls on circumferential dressings. With an arterial leg ulcer, the nurse applies tape only to the bandage. Tape is never used directly on the skin because it could cause further tissue damage. For the same reason, Montgomery straps would not be applied to the skin (although these are generally intended for use on abdominal wounds, anyway).

Priority Nursing Tip: Because swelling in the extremities prevents arterial blood flow, the client with peripheral arterial disease is instructed to elevate the feet at rest but to avoid elevating them above the level of the heart, because extreme elevation slows arterial blood flow to the feet.

Test-Taking Strategy: Focus on the **subject**, care of ischemic arterial leg ulcers. Note that options 1, 2, and 3 are **comparable or alike.** In options 1 and 2, tape is applied to the skin. For the same reason, eliminate option 3, because the Montgomery straps would need to be adhered to the skin as well.

---

211. A child is admitted to the pediatric unit with a diagnosis of celiac disease. Based on this diagnosis, the nurse expects that the child's stools will have which characteristic?

1 Malodorous
2 Dark in color
3 Unusually hard
4 Abnormally small in amount

Level of Cognitive Ability: Analyzing
Client Needs: Physiological Integrity
Clinical Judgment/Cognitive Skills: Recognize Cues
Integrated Process: Nursing Process/Data Collection
Content Area: Pediatrics: Gastrointestinal
Health Problem: Pediatric-Specific: Nutrition Problems

Answer: 1

Rationale: Celiac disease is a disorder in which the child has intolerance to gluten, the protein component of wheat, barley, rye, and oats. The stools of a child with celiac disease are characteristically malodorous, pale, large (bulky), and soft (loose). Excessive flatus is common, and bouts of diarrhea may occur.

Priority Nursing Tip: Teach the parents of a child with celiac disease to read all food labels for the presence of gluten; if the food contains gluten, it needs to be avoided.

Test-Taking Strategy: Focus on the **subject**, celiac disease. Thinking about the pathophysiology that occurs in celiac disease and the manifestations will direct you to the correct option.

---

212. A nurse is assisting in caring for a client with a suspected diagnosis of gestational hypertension. The nurse checks the client, expecting to note which set of findings if gestational hypertension is present?

1 Edema, ketonuria, and obesity
2 Edema, tachycardia, and ketonuria
3 Glycosuria, hypertension, and obesity
4 Elevated blood pressure and proteinuria

Level of Cognitive Ability: Analyzing
Client Needs: Physiological Integrity
Clinical Judgment/Cognitive Skills: Recognize Cues
Integrated Process: Nursing Process/Data Collection
Content Area: Maternity: Antepartum
Health Problem: Maternity: Gestational Hypertension/Preeclampsia and Eclampsia

Answer: 4

Rationale: Gestational hypertension is the most common hypertensive disorder in pregnancy. It is characterized by the development of hypertension and normally proteinuria. Glycosuria and ketonuria occur in diabetes mellitus. Tachycardia and obesity are not specifically related to diagnosing gestational hypertension. Edema is not specific to gestational hypertension and can occur in many disorders.

Priority Nursing Tip: Gestational hypertension can be mild or severe and can lead to preeclampsia and then eclampsia (seizures).

Test-Taking Strategy: Focus on the **subject**, gestational hypertension. Eliminate options 1 and 2 because they do not address hypertension. From the remaining options, recalling that glycosuria is an indication of diabetes mellitus will assist in directing you to the correct option.

---

213. A client who undergoes a gastric resection is at risk for developing dumping syndrome. Which manifestation would the nurse monitor the client for? **Select all that apply.**

1 Pallor
2 Dizziness
3 Diaphoresis
4 Bradycardia
5 Constipation
6 Extreme thirst

Level of Cognitive Ability: Applying
Client Needs: Physiological Integrity
Clinical Judgment/Cognitive Skills: Recognize Cues
Integrated Process: Nursing Process/Data Collection
Content Area: Adult Health: Gastrointestinal
Health Problem: Adult Health: Gastrointestinal: Upper GI Disorders

Answer: 1, 2, 3

Rationale: Dumping syndrome is the rapid emptying of the gastric contents into the small intestine that occurs after gastric resection. Early manifestations of dumping syndrome occur 5 to 30 minutes after eating. Manifestations also include vasomotor disturbances such as dizziness, tachycardia, syncope, sweating, pallor, palpitations, and the desire to lie down.

Priority Nursing Tip: The client with dumping syndrome needs to eat small meals and avoid consuming fluids with meals.

Test-Taking Strategy: Focus on the **subject,** dumping syndrome. Recalling that the symptoms of this disorder are vasomotor in nature will direct you to the correct option.

---

214. The nurse is assisting in monitoring a client in the telemetry unit who has recently been admitted with the diagnosis of chest pain and notes this heart rate pattern on the monitoring strip. What is the **initial** action to be taken by the nurse? **Refer to the figure.**

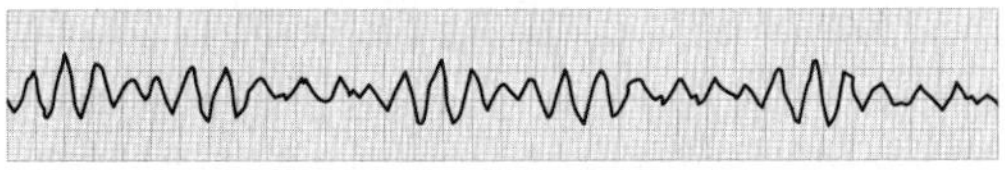

1 Notify the registered nurse.
2 Initiate cardiopulmonary resuscitation (CPR).
3 Continue to monitor the client and the heart rate patterns.
4 Administer oxygen with a face mask at 8 to 10 L/min.

Level of Cognitive Ability: Applying
Client Needs: Physiological Integrity
Clinical Judgment/Cognitive Skills: Prioritize Hypotheses
Integrated Process: Nursing Process/Implementation
Content Area: Complex Care: Emergency Situations/Management
Health Problem: Adult Health: Cardiovascular: Dysrhythmias

Answer: 2

Rationale: The monitor is showing ventricular fibrillation, a life-threatening dysrhythmia that requires CPR and defibrillation to maintain life. Although the registered nurse and primary health care provider must be notified, CPR is the initial action. Oxygen is necessary, but again the initiation of CPR is the priority because it will provide more than just oxygen to the client. Monitoring the client is necessary, but not as an initial action; emergency resuscitative treatment must be provided to the client immediately.

Priority Nursing Tip: There is no cardiac output with ventricular fibrillation, and it must be treated immediately to save the client's life.

Test-Taking Strategy: Knowledge regarding emergency care is essential. Note the **strategic word,** *initial.* Recalling that ventricular fibrillation is a life-threatening dysrhythmia that requires CPR and defibrillation to maintain life will direct you to the correct option.

---

215. Which finding indicates the presence of an inguinal hernia on a child?

1 Reports of difficulty defecating
2 Reports of a dribbling urinary stream
3 Absence of the testes within the scrotum
4 Painless groin swelling noticed when the child cries

Level of Cognitive Ability: Analyzing
Client Needs: Physiological Integrity
Clinical Judgment/Cognitive Skills: Recognize Cues
Integrated Process: Nursing Process/Data Collection
Content Area: Pediatrics: Renal and Urinary
Health Problem: Pediatric-Specific: Developmental GI Defects

Answer: 4
Rationale: Inguinal hernia is a common defect that may appear as a painless inguinal (groin) swelling when the child cries or strains. Option 1 is a symptom indicating a partial obstruction of the herniated loop of intestine. Option 2 describes a sign of phimosis, a narrowing or stenosis of the preputial opening of the foreskin. Option 3 describes cryptorchidism.
Priority Nursing Tip: An inguinal hernia is characterized by painless inguinal swelling that is reducible. Swelling may disappear during periods of rest and is most noticeable when the infant cries or coughs.

Test-Taking Strategy: Focus on the **subject,** assessment of an inguinal hernia. Note the relationship between the child's diagnosis, inguinal hernia, and the words *groin swelling* in option 4.

---

216. A client experiencing difficulty breathing and increased pulmonary congestion was prescribed furosemide 40 mg to be given intravenously. After an hour, which value indicates that the therapy has been **effective**?

1 The lungs are now clear upon auscultation.
2 The urine output has increased by 400 mL.
3 The serum potassium has decreased from 4.7 mEq to 4.1 mEq.
4 The blood pressure has decreased from 118/64 mm Hg to 106/62 mm Hg.

Level of Cognitive Ability: Evaluating
Client Needs: Physiological Integrity
Clinical Judgment/Cognitive Skills: Evaluate Outcomes
Integrated Process: Nursing Process/Evaluation
Content Area: Pharmacology: Cardiovascular: Diuretics
Health Problem: N/A

Answer: 1
Rationale: Furosemide is a diuretic. In this situation, it was given to decrease preload and reduce the pulmonary congestion and associated difficulty in breathing. Although all options may occur, option 1 is the reason that the furosemide was administered.
Priority Nursing Tip: When administering a medication, knowing its purpose will assist in evaluating its effectiveness.

Test-Taking Strategy: Focus on the **subject,** furosemide administration in a client with heart failure who was experiencing difficulty breathing and increased pulmonary congestion. Note the **strategic word,** *effective.* Specific knowledge of the use of furosemide in heart failure and its side effects is essential. Note the relationship between the words *pulmonary congestion* in the question and the correct option.

---

217. Skin closure with heterograft will be performed on a client with a burn injury. When the client asks the nurse where the heterograft comes from, the nurse would explain it is from which source?

1 A cadaver
2 Another animal species
3 The burned client, a graft from self
4 A synthetic source

Level of Cognitive Ability: Applying
Client Needs: Physiological Integrity
Clinical Judgment/Cognitive Skills: Take Action
Integrated Process: Nursing Process/Implementation
Content Area: Adult Health: Integumentary
Health Problem: Adult Health: Integumentary: Burns

Answer: 2
Rationale: Biological dressings are usually heterograft or homograft material. Heterograft is skin from another species. The most commonly used type of heterograft is pig skin because of its availability and its relative compatibility with human skin. Homograft is skin from another human, which is usually obtained from a cadaver and is provided through a skin bank. Autograft is skin from the client. Synthetic dressings are also available for covering burn wounds.
Priority Nursing Tip: Autografting provides permanent wound coverage.

Test-Taking Strategy: Focus on the **subject,** a heterograft. Also, note that options 1 and 3 are **comparable or alike** and relate to grafts from human skin. Next it is necessary to know that heterograft is skin from another species.

---

218. The nurse would place a client who sustained a head injury in which position to prevent increased intracranial pressure (ICP)?

1 In left lateral position
2 In reverse Trendelenburg's
3 With the head elevated on a small, flat pillow
4 With the head of the bed elevated at least 30 degrees

Level of Cognitive Ability: Applying
Client Needs: Physiological Integrity
Clinical Judgment/Cognitive Skills: Take Action
Integrated Process: Nursing Process/Implementation
Content Area: Adult Health: Neurological
Health Problem: Adult Health: Neurological: Head Injury/Trauma

Answer: 4
Rationale: The client with a head injury is positioned to avoid extreme flexion or extension of the neck and to maintain the head in the midline, neutral position. The head of the bed is elevated to at least 30 degrees or as recommended by the neurologist. The client is logrolled when turned to avoid extreme hip flexion. Therefore, options 1, 2, and 3 are incorrect.
Priority Nursing Tip: Altered level of consciousness is the most sensitive and earliest indication of increased ICP.

Test-Taking Strategy: Focus on the **subject,** preventing an increase in ICP. Recall that the client with a head injury is at risk for increased ICP. Bearing this in mind and considering the principles of gravity will direct you to the correct option.

---

219. A newborn infant is diagnosed with esophageal atresia. Which finding supports this diagnosis?

1 Slowed reflexes
2 Continuous drooling
3 Diaphragmatic breathing
4 Passage of large amounts of frothy stool

Level of Cognitive Ability: Analyzing
Client Needs: Physiological Integrity
Clinical Judgment/Cognitive Skills: Recognize Cues
Integrated Process: Nursing Process/Data Collection

Answer: 2
Rationale: In esophageal atresia, the esophagus terminates before it reaches the stomach, ending in a blind pouch. This condition prevents the passage of swallowed mucus and saliva into the stomach. After fluid has accumulated in the pouch, it flows from the mouth, and the infant then drools continuously. Responsiveness of the infant to stimulus would depend on the overall condition of the infant and is not considered a classic sign of esophageal atresia. Diaphragmatic breathing is not associated with this disorder. The inability to swallow amniotic fluid in utero prevents the accumulation of normal meconium, and lack of stools results.
Priority Nursing Tip: Tracheoesophageal fistula would be suspected if the child exhibits the "3 C's"—coughing, choking with feedings, and cyanosis.

Content Area: Pediatrics: Gastrointestinal
Health Problem: Pediatric-Specific: Disorders of Prenatal Development

Test-Taking Strategy: Focus on the **subject**, esophageal atresia. Review the anatomical location of the disorder to eliminate options 1 and 4 first. From the remaining options, recalling the pathophysiology associated with esophageal atresia and recalling that the word *atresia* indicates narrowing will direct you to the correct option.

---

220. Which observation by the nurse indicates a need to suction a client with an endotracheal (ET) tube attached to a mechanical ventilator? **Select all that apply.**

1 Audible crackles
2 Client notably restless
3 Visible mucus bubbling in the ET tube
4 Apical pulse rate of 72 beats per minute
5 Low peak inspiratory pressure on the ventilator
6 A high pressure alarm on the ventilator

Level of Cognitive Ability: Analyzing
Client Needs: Physiological Integrity
Clinical Judgment/Cognitive Skills: Analyze Cues
Integrated Process: Nursing Process/Data Collection
Content Area: Skills: Oxygenation
Health Problem: N/A

Answer: 1, 2, 3, 6
Rationale: Indications for suctioning include visible mucus bubbling in the ET tube, wet respirations, restlessness, rhonchi or crackles on auscultation of the lungs, increased pulse and respiratory rates, and increased peak inspiratory pressures on the ventilator and high-pressure alarms on the ventilator. A low peak inspiratory pressure indicates a leak in the mechanical ventilation system.
Priority Nursing Tip: The nurse needs to hyperoxygenate the client before and after performing respiratory suctioning.

Test-Taking Strategy: Focus on the **subject,** the need for suctioning in a client with an ET tube attached to a mechanical ventilator. Eliminate option 4 first because it is a normal finding. From the remaining options, note that a low-pressure alarm is sounded if there is an air leak.

---

221. A client is intubated and receiving mechanical ventilation. The intensivist has added 7 cm of positive end-expiratory pressure (PEEP) to the client's ventilator settings. The nurse assisting in the care of the client would check for which expected but adverse effect of PEEP?

1 Decreased peak pressure on the ventilator
2 Increased rectal temperature from 98°F to 100°F
3 Decreased heart rate from 78 to 64 beats per minute
4 Systolic blood pressure decrease from 122 to 98 mm Hg

Level of Cognitive Ability: Synthesizing
Client Needs: Physiological Integrity
Clinical Judgment/Cognitive Skills: Recognize Cues
Integrated Process: Nursing Process/Data Collection
Content Area: Complex Care: Emergency Situations/Management
Health Problem: N/A

Answer: 4
Rationale: PEEP improves oxygenation by enhancing gas exchange and preventing atelectasis. PEEP leads to increased intrathoracic pressure, which in turn leads to decreased cardiac output. This is manifested in the client by decreased systolic blood pressure and increased pulse (compensatory). Peak pressures on the ventilator would not be affected, although the pressure at the end of expiration remains positive at the level set for the PEEP. Fever indicates respiratory infection or infection from another source.
Priority Nursing Tip: The need for PEEP indicates a severe gas exchange disturbance.

Test-Taking Strategy: Focus on the **subject,** expected but adverse effect of PEEP. Knowing that PEEP increases intrathoracic pressure leads you to look for the option that reflects a consequence of this event. Fever is irrelevant, and option 2 is eliminated first. From the remaining options, think about the effects of PEEP to direct you to the correct option.

222. The nurse is checking the respiratory status of the client after a thoracentesis has been performed. The nurse would become concerned with which finding?
1 Equal bilateral chest expansion
2 Respiratory rate of 22 breaths per minute
3 Diminished breath sounds on the affected side
4 Few scattered wheezes, unchanged from baseline

Level of Cognitive Ability: Analyzing
Client Needs: Physiological Integrity
Clinical Judgment/Cognitive Skills: Recognize Cues
Integrated Process: Nursing Process/Data Collection
Content Area: Adult Health: Respiratory
Health Problem: N/A

Answer: 3
Rationale: After thoracentesis, the nurse checks vital signs and breath sounds. The nurse especially notes increased respiratory rates, dyspnea, retractions, diminished breath sounds, or cyanosis, which could indicate pneumothorax. Any of these manifestations need to be reported to the primary health care provider. Options 1 and 2 are normal findings. Option 4 indicates a finding that is unchanged from the baseline.
Priority Nursing Tip: For a thoracentesis, the client is positioned sitting upright, with the arms and shoulders supported by a bedside table. If the client cannot sit up, the client is placed lying in bed on the unaffected side, with the head of the bed elevated.

Test-Taking Strategy: Focus on the **subject,** respiratory status. Eliminate options 1 and 2 first because they are normal findings. Option 4 is an abnormality, but note that the wheezes are unchanged from the client's baseline. Option 3 is the abnormal finding.

---

223. The nurse is preparing to administer a tuberculin skin test to a client. The nurse determines that which area is to be used for injection of the medication?
1 Dorsal aspect of the upper arm near a mole
2 Inner aspect of the forearm that is close to a burn scar
3 Inner aspect of the forearm that is not heavily pigmented
4 Dorsal aspect of the upper arm that has a small amount of hair

Level of Cognitive Ability: Applying
Client Needs: Physiological Integrity
Clinical Judgment/Cognitive Skills: Take Action
Integrated Process: Nursing Process/Implementation
Content Area: Foundations of Care: Diagnostic Tests
Health Problem: Adult Health: Respiratory: Tuberculosis

Answer: 3
Rationale: Intradermal injections are most commonly given in the inner surface of the forearm. Other sites include the dorsal area of the upper arm or the upper back beneath the scapulae. The nurse finds an area that is not heavily pigmented and is clear of hairy areas or lesions that could interfere with reading the results.
Priority Nursing Tip: After administering a skin test, document the date and time of administration and the test site. Interpret the reaction at the injection site 48 to 72 hours after administration of the test antigen.

Test-Taking Strategy: Focus on the **subject,** tuberculin skin test. Note that options 1, 2, and 4 are **comparable or alike** in that they indicate areas that are not clear of lesions or hair.

---

224. Which questions would the nurse ask when collecting data from a client for possible manifestations of Ménière's disease? **Select all that apply.**

1 "Do you experience ringing in your ears?"
2 "Are you prone to vertigo that can last for days?"
3 "Can you hear better out of one ear than the other?"
4 "Is there a history of Ménière's disease in your family?"
5 "Have you ever experienced a head injury in the area of your ears?"

Level of Cognitive Ability: Analyzing
Client Needs: Physiological Integrity
Clinical Judgment/Cognitive Skills: Recognize Cues
Integrated Process: Nursing Process/Data Collection
Content Area: Adult Health: Ear
Health Problem: Adult Health: Ear: Ménière's Disease

Answer: 1, 2, 3
Rationale: Ménière's disease is characterized by dilation of the endolymphatic system by overproduction or decreased reabsorption of endolymphatic fluid. Manifestations include tinnitus, vertigo that can last for days, and one-sided sensorineural hearing loss. Although the exact cause of the disease is unknown, there does not seem to be a connection with either genetics or head trauma.
Priority Nursing Tip: Ménière's disease has characteristic manifestations that include tinnitus, unilateral hearing impairment, and severe episodes of vertigo.

Test-Taking Strategy: Focus on the **subject,** Ménière's disease. Specific knowledge regarding the manifestations of this condition will direct you to the correct options: 1, 2, and 3. Remember that tinnitus, hearing loss, and vertigo are characteristic of this disease.

---

225. A client has been diagnosed with left tension pneumothorax. Which finding observed by the nurse indicates that the pneumothorax is rapidly worsening? **Select all that apply.**

1 Hypertension
2 Flat neck veins
3 Increased cyanosis
4 Tracheal deviation to the right
5 Diminished breath sounds on the left
6 Observable asymmetry of the thorax

Level of Cognitive Ability: Analyzing
Client Needs: Physiological Integrity
Clinical Judgment/Cognitive Skills: Analyze Cues
Integrated Process: Nursing Process/Data Collection
Content Area: Complex Care: Emergency Situations/Management
Health Problem: Adult Health: Respiratory: Chest Injuries

Answer: 3, 4, 5, 6
Rationale: A tension pneumothorax is characterized by distended neck veins, displaced point of maximal impulse, tracheal deviation to the unaffected side, asymmetry of the thorax, decreased to absent breath sounds on the affected side, worsening cyanosis, and worsening dyspnea. The increased intrathoracic pressure causes the blood pressure to fall, not rise.
Priority Nursing Tip: After insertion of a central venous catheter, catheter placement must be confirmed by radiography before infusing fluids into it.

Test-Taking Strategy: Focus on the **subject,** tension pneumothorax, and note the words *rapidly worsening.* Flat neck veins and hypertension are the least specific indicators and are eliminated first. From the remaining options, remember that a tension pneumothorax causes the trachea to be pushed in the opposite direction, to the unaffected side.

---

226. A client is admitted to the hospital with a diagnosis of right lower lobe pneumonia. The nurse listens to the right lower lobe, expecting to note which type of breath sounds?

1 Absent
2 Vesicular
3 Bronchial
4 Bronchovesicular

Level of Cognitive Ability: Analyzing
Client Needs: Physiological Integrity
Clinical Judgment/Cognitive Skills: Recognize Cues
Integrated Process: Nursing Process/Data Collection
Content Area: Health Assessment/Physical Exam: Thorax and Lungs
Health Problem: Adult Health: Respiratory: Viral, Bacterial, Fungal Infections

Answer: 3

Rationale: Bronchial sounds are normally heard over the trachea. The client with pneumonia will have bronchial breath sounds over area(s) of consolidation because the consolidated tissue carries bronchial sounds to the peripheral lung fields. The client may also have crackles in the affected area resulting from fluid in the interstitium and alveoli. Absent breath sounds are unlikely to occur unless a serious complication of the pneumonia occurs. Vesicular sounds are normally heard over the lesser bronchi, bronchioles, and lobes. Bronchovesicular sounds are normally heard over the main bronchi.

Priority Nursing Tip: Pneumonia can be community acquired or hospital acquired. The sputum culture identifies organisms that may be present and assists in determining the appropriate treatment.

Test-Taking Strategy: Focus on the **subject**, breath sounds in a client with lower lobe pneumonia. Recalling that vesicular breath sounds are normal in the lung periphery and bronchovesicular sounds are normally heard over the main bronchi helps eliminate options 2 and 4. From the remaining options, recall that pneumonia transmits bronchial breath sounds, so they are heard over the area of consolidation.

---

227. The nurse checks the client diagnosed with AIDS for early signs of Kaposi's sarcoma. What characteristics would be consistent with that lesion? **Select all that apply.**

1 Flat
2 Raised
3 Resembling a blister
4 Light blue in color
5 Brownish and scaly in appearance
6 Color varies from pink to dark violet or black

Level of Cognitive Ability: Analyzing
Client Needs: Physiological Integrity
Clinical Judgment/Cognitive Skills: Recognize Cues
Integrated Process: Nursing Process/Data Collection
Content Area: Adult Health: Immune
Health Problem: Adult Health: Immune: Immunodeficiency Syndrome

Answer: 1, 6

Rationale: Kaposi's sarcoma generally starts with an area that is flat and pink that changes to a dark violet or black color. The lesions are usually present bilaterally. They may appear in many areas of the body and are treated with radiation, chemotherapy, and cryotherapy. None of the other options are associated with this type of lesion.

Priority Nursing Tip: Kaposi's sarcoma is characterized by skin lesions that occur in individuals with a compromised immune system.

Test-Taking Strategy: Focus on the **subject**, Kaposi's sarcoma. Recalling that Kaposi's sarcoma lesions are flat and have a variety of colors from pink to dark violet or black eliminates the remaining options.

---

228. When a client with a chest injury is suspected of experiencing a pleural effusion, the nurse would check for which typical manifestations of this respiratory problem? **Select all that apply.**

1 Dry cough
2 Moist cough
3 Dyspnea at rest
4 Productive cough
5 Dyspnea on exertion
6 Nonproductive cough

Level of Cognitive Ability: Analyzing
Client Needs: Physiological Integrity
Clinical Judgment/Cognitive Skills: Recognize Cues
Integrated Process: Nursing Process/Data Collection
Content Area: Adult Health: Respiratory
Health Problem: Adult Health: Respiratory: Chest Injuries

Answer: 1, 5, 6
Rationale: A pleural effusion is the collection of fluid in the pleural space. Typical findings in the client with a pleural effusion include dyspnea, which usually occurs with exertion, and a dry, nonproductive cough. The cough is caused by bronchial irritation and possible mediastinal shift.
Priority Nursing Tip: Any condition that interferes with the secretion or drainage of pleural fluid will lead to pleural effusion.

Test-Taking Strategy: Focus on the **subject,** pleural effusion. Specific knowledge that pleural effusion is in the pleural space and not the airway helps eliminate options 2 and 4 (moist productive cough does not occur). Remembering that dyspnea occurs on exertion before it occurs at rest will direct you to the correct options from the remaining options.

---

229. After a client diagnosed with pleural effusion from a chest injury had a thoracentesis, a sample of fluid was sent to the laboratory. Analysis of the fluid reveals a high red blood cell count. Based on this test result, what was the cause of this client's pleural effusion?

1 Trauma
2 Infection
3 Liver failure
4 Heart failure

Level of Cognitive Ability: Analyzing
Client Needs: Physiological Integrity
Clinical Judgment/Cognitive Skills: Analyze Cues
Integrated Process: Nursing Process/Data Collection
Content Area: Foundations of Care: Laboratory Tests
Health Problem: Adult Health: Respiratory: Chest Injuries

Answer: 1
Rationale: Pleural fluid from an effusion that has a high red blood cell count may result from trauma and may be treated with placement of a chest tube for drainage. Other causes of pleural effusion include infection, heart failure, liver or renal failure, malignancy, or inflammatory processes. Infection would be accompanied by white blood cells. The fluid portion of the serum would accumulate with liver failure and heart failure.
Priority Nursing Tip: With a pleural effusion, the client experiences pleuritic pain that is sharp and increases with inspiration.

Test-Taking Strategy: Focus on the **subject,** pleural effusion with a high red blood cell count. Recall that infection would be accompanied by white blood cells, not red, to eliminate option 2. Remember that in liver and heart failure, the fluid portion of the serum would accumulate to direct you to eliminate options 3 and 4.

230. The nurse is assisting in scheduling a client for a series of diagnostic studies of the gastrointestinal (GI) system. Which of these studies would the nurse expect to be scheduled last to avoid altering the results of the remaining tests?

1 Ultrasound
2 Colonoscopy
3 Barium enema
4 Computed tomography

Answer: 3

Rationale: When barium is instilled into the lower GI tract, it may take up to 72 hours to clear the GI tract. The presence of barium could cause interference with obtaining clear visualization and accurate results of the other tests listed if performed before the client has fully excreted the barium. For this reason, diagnostic studies that involve barium contrast are scheduled at the conclusion of other medical imaging studies.

Priority Nursing Tip: After a barium enema, the client is instructed to increase oral fluid intake to help pass the barium.

Test-Taking Strategy: Focus on the **subject,** diagnostic studies of the GI system. Note the word *last.* Recall that barium shows up on an x-ray as opaque and that this substance would impair visualization during other tests.

Level of Cognitive Ability: Analyzing
Client Needs: Physiological Integrity
Clinical Judgment/Cognitive Skills: Generate Solutions
Integrated Process: Nursing Process/Planning
Content Area: Foundations of Care: Diagnostic Tests
Health Problem: N/A

---

231. The nurse is caring for a client who is scheduled to have a liver biopsy. Before the procedure, it is important for the nurse to check which parameter to ensure client safety?

1 Tolerance for pain
2 Allergy to iodine or shellfish
3 History of nausea and vomiting
4 Ability to lie still and hold the breath

Answer: 4

Rationale: It is most important for the nurse to check the client's ability to lie still and hold the breath for the procedure. This helps the primary health care provider avoid complications, such as puncturing the lung or other organs. The client's tolerance for pain is a useful item to know. However, the area will receive a local anesthetic. Assessment of allergy to iodine or shellfish is unnecessary for this procedure because no contrast dye is used. Knowledge of the history related to nausea and vomiting is generally a part of assessment of the gastrointestinal system but has no relationship to the procedure.

Priority Nursing Tip: Bleeding is a concern after a liver biopsy. Check the results of coagulation tests (prothrombin time, partial thromboplastin time, platelet count) before a liver biopsy is performed; abnormal results need to be reported to the primary health care provider.

Test-Taking Strategy: Focus on the **subject,** a liver biopsy. Visualizing this procedure and thinking about its complications will direct you to the correct option.

Level of Cognitive Ability: Analyzing
Client Needs: Physiological Integrity
Clinical Judgment/Cognitive Skills: Recognize Cues
Integrated Process: Nursing Process/Data Collection
Content Area: Foundations of Care: Diagnostic Tests
Health Problem: N/A

---

232. The nurse is caring for a client diagnosed with pneumonia. When considering the client's safety, when will the nurse plan to take the client for a short walk?

1 After the client eats lunch
2 After the client has a brief nap
3 After the client uses the metered-dose inhaler
4 After checking the client's oxygen saturation

Level of Cognitive Ability: Analyzing
Client Needs: Physiological Integrity
Clinical Judgment/Cognitive Skills: Generate Solutions
Integrated Process: Nursing Process/Planning
Content Area: Adult Health: Respiratory
Health Problem: Adult Health: Respiratory: Viral, Bacterial, Fungal Infections

Answer: 3

Rationale: The nurse would schedule activities for the client with pneumonia after the client has received respiratory treatments or medications. After the administration of bronchodilators (often administered by metered-dose inhaler), the client has the best oxygen exchange possible and would tolerate the activity best. Still, the nurse implements activity cautiously, so as not to increase the client's dyspnea. The client would become fatigued after eating; therefore, this is not a good time to ambulate the client. Although the client may be rested somewhat after a nap, the respiratory status of the client may not be at its best. Although monitoring oxygen saturation is appropriate, the intervention itself does not affect the client's respiratory function.

Priority Nursing Tip: Clients with a respiratory disorder would be positioned with the head of the bed elevated.

Test-Taking Strategy: Focus on the **subject,** ambulation of the respiratory client. Use the **ABCs—airway, breathing, and circulation.** The use of bronchodilator medication would widen the air passages, allowing for more air to enter the client's lungs.

---

233. The nurse inserts an indwelling Foley's catheter into the bladder of a postoperative client who has not voided for 8 hours and has a distended bladder. After the tubing is secured and the collection bag is hung on the bed frame, the nurse notices that 900 mL of urine has drained into the collection bag. What is the appropriate nursing action for the safety of this client?

1 Check the specific gravity of the urine.
2 Clamp the tubing for 30 minutes and then release.
3 Provide suprapubic pressure to maintain a steady flow of urine.
4 Raise the collection bag high enough to slow the rate of drainage.

Level of Cognitive Ability: Applying
Client Needs: Physiological Integrity
Clinical Judgment/Cognitive Skills: Take Action
Integrated Process: Nursing Process/Implementation
Content Area: Skills: Elimination
Health Problem: N/A

Answer: 2

Rationale: Rapid emptying of a large volume of urine may cause engorgement of pelvic blood vessels and hypovolemic shock, prolapse of the bladder, or bladder spasms. Clamping the tubing for 30 minutes allows for equilibration to prevent complications. Option 1 is an assessment and would not affect the flow of urine or prevent possible hypovolemic shock. Option 3 would increase the flow of urine, which could lead to hypovolemic shock. Option 4 could cause backflow of urine. Infection is likely to develop if urine is allowed to flow back into the bladder.

Priority Nursing Tip: The total bladder capacity is approximately 1 L, and normal adult urine output is 1500 mL/day.

Test-Taking Strategy: Focus on the **subject,** slowing the urine drainage in a postoperative client with an indwelling Foley's catheter. Note the amount *900 mL*. Recall the physiology of the hemodynamic changes after the rapid collapse of an overdistended bladder. Eliminate option 3 because this action will increase flow rate. Eliminate option 4 because this increases pressure in the bladder and places the client at risk for infection. Note that option 1 is an assessment action rather than an action that affects the amount of urine drainage.

---

234. The licensed practical nurse (LPN) is assisting the registered nurse (RN) in monitoring a client receiving amphotericin B intravenously to treat histoplasmosis. Which would the LPN specifically plan to assist to implement during administration of the medication to minimize the client's risk for injury? **Select all that apply.**

1 Monitor for hyperthermia.
2 Monitor for an excessive urine output.
3 Check the intravenous (IV) infusion site.
4 Check the chest and back for a red, itchy rash.
5 Monitor the client's orientation to time, place, and person.

Level of Cognitive Ability: Applying
Client Needs: Physiological Integrity
Clinical Judgment/Cognitive Skills: Generate Solutions
Integrated Process: Nursing Process/Planning
Content Area: Pharmacology: Immune: Antifungals
Health Problem: Adult Health: Respiratory: Viral, Bacterial, Fungal Infections

Answer: 1, 3
Rationale: Amphotericin B is an antifungal medication and is toxic; it can produce symptoms during administration such as chills, fever (hyperthermia), headache, vomiting, and impaired renal function (decreased urine output). The medication is also very irritating to the IV site, commonly causing thrombophlebitis. The nurse administering this medication monitors for these complications. A rash or disorientation is not specific to this medication.
Priority Nursing Tip: If a medication is nephrotoxic, check kidney function before, during, and after administration. The primary health care provider may prescribe blood urea nitrogen and creatinine studies. Urine output is also monitored closely.

Test-Taking Strategy: Focus on the **subject,** amphotericin B administration. Recalling the toxic effects of this medication will help direct you to the correct options.

---

235. A client who experienced repeated pleural effusions from inoperable lung cancer is to undergo pleurodesis. What intervention would the nurse anticipate will be done after the primary health care provider injects the sclerosing agent through the chest tube to help ensure the **effectiveness** of the procedure?

1 Ambulate the client.
2 Clamp the chest tube.
3 Ask the client to cough and deep-breathe.
4 Ask the client to remain in a side-lying position.

Level of Cognitive Ability: Applying
Client Needs: Physiological Integrity
Clinical Judgment/Cognitive Skills: Generate Solutions
Integrated Process: Nursing Process/Planning
Content Area: Adult Health: Respiratory
Health Problem: Adult Health: Cancer: Laryngeal and Lung

Answer: 2
Rationale: After injection of the sclerosing agent, the chest tube is clamped to prevent the agent from draining back out of the pleural space. Depending on primary health care provider preference, a repositioning schedule is used to disperse the substance. Ambulation, coughing, and deep breathing have no specific purpose in the immediate period after injection.
Priority Nursing Tip: The agent injected during pleurodesis creates an inflammatory response that scleroses pleural tissue together.

Test-Taking Strategy: Focus on the **subject,** pleurodesis, and note the **strategic word**, *effectiveness*. Recalling the purpose of the procedure will help direct you to the correct option. It is most reasonable to clamp the chest tube so that the sclerosing agent cannot flow back out of the tube. Coughing and deep breathing have no specific purpose in this situation. Ambulation is not advised.

---

236. A client with a posterior wall bladder injury has had surgical repair and placement of a suprapubic catheter. What intervention would the nurse plan to implement to prevent complications associated with the use of this catheter?

1 Monitor urine output every shift.
2 Measure specific gravity once a shift.
3 Encourage a high intake of oral fluids.
4 Avoid kinking of the catheter tubing.

Level of Cognitive Ability: Applying
Client Needs: Physiological Integrity
Clinical Judgment/Cognitive Skills: Generate Solutions
Integrated Process: Nursing Process/Planning
Content Area: Skills: Elimination
Health Problem: N/A

Answer: 4
Rationale: A complication after surgical repair of the bladder is disruption of sutures caused by tension on them from urine buildup. The nurse prevents this from happening by ensuring that the catheter is able to drain freely. This involves basic catheter care, including keeping the tubing free from kinks, keeping the tubing below the level of the bladder, and monitoring the flow of urine frequently. Monitoring urine output every shift is insufficient to detect decreased flow from catheter kinking. Measurement of urine specific gravity and a high oral fluid intake do not prevent complications of the catheter or bladder surgery.
Priority Nursing Tip: A blunt or penetrating injury to the lower abdomen can cause bladder trauma. Monitor the client for hematuria and pain below the level of the umbilicus, which can radiate to the shoulders.

Test-Taking Strategy: Focus on the **subject,** suprapubic catheter. Eliminate option 1 first, because once-a-shift measurement is not a preventive action and is also insufficient in terms of frequency. Eliminate option 2 next because specific gravity measurement is not a preventive action. From the remaining options, knowing that a high oral fluid intake will not prevent complications with the catheter directs you to the correct option.

---

237. A client undergoes transurethral resection of the prostate (TURP). Which solution would the nurse have available postoperatively for continuous bladder irrigation (CBI)?

1 Sterile water
2 Sterile normal saline
3 Sterile Dakin's solution
4 Sterile water with 5% dextrose

Level of Cognitive Ability: Applying
Client Needs: Physiological Integrity
Clinical Judgment/Cognitive Skills: Take Action
Integrated Process: Nursing Process/Implementation
Content Area: Foundations of Care: Fluids & Electrolytes
Health Problem: Adult Health: Renal and Urinary: Obstructive Problems

Answer: 2
Rationale: CBI is done after TURP using sterile normal saline, which is isotonic. Sterile water is not used because the solution could be absorbed systemically, precipitating hemolysis and possibly kidney failure. Dakin's solution contains hypochlorite and is used only for wound irrigation in selected circumstances. Solutions containing dextrose are not introduced into the bladder.
Priority Nursing Tip: Bleeding is common after TURP, and the surgeon usually prescribes continuous or intermittent bladder irrigation. An isotonic solution is used for irrigation. Hypotonic solutions absorb into the bloodstream and place the client at risk for transurethral resection syndrome; therefore, they are not used.

Test-Taking Strategy: Note the **subject,** CBI. Recalling that normal saline is isotonic will direct you to the correct option.

---

238. A client diagnosed with acquired immunodeficiency syndrome (AIDS) is being admitted to the hospital for treatment of a *Pneumocystis jiroveci* respiratory infection. Which intervention would the nurse include in the plan of care to assist in maintaining the comfort of this client?

1 Monitoring for bloody sputum
2 Evaluating arterial blood gas results
3 Keeping the head of the bed elevated
4 Checking respiratory rate, rhythm, depth, and breath sounds

Level of Cognitive Ability: Applying
Client Needs: Physiological Integrity
Clinical Judgment/Cognitive Skills: Generate Solutions
Integrated Process: Nursing Process/Planning
Content Area: Adult Health: Respiratory
Health Problem: Adult Health: Immune: Immunodeficiency Syndrome

Answer: 3
Rationale: Clients with respiratory difficulties are often more comfortable with the head of the bed elevated. Options 1, 2, and 4 are appropriate measures to evaluate respiratory function and avoid complications. Option 3 is the only choice that addresses planning for client comfort.
Priority Nursing Tip: *Pneumocystis jiroveci* infection is a major source of mortality in the client with AIDS. The client must be monitored closely for manifestations of this respiratory infection.

Test-Taking Strategy: Focusing on the **subject,** maintaining comfort, will direct you to the correct option. Also, note that options 1, 2, and 4 are **comparable or alike** and are all measures to evaluate respiratory function.

---

239. A client with significant flail chest has arterial blood gases (ABGs) that reveal a PaO_2 of 68 and a $PaCO_2$ of 51. Two hours ago the PaO_2 was 82 and the $PaCO_2$ was 44. Based on these changes, which item would the nurse assisting in caring for the client ensure easy access to in order to help ensure client safety?

1 Intubation tray
2 Injectable lidocaine
3 Chest tube insertion set
4 Portable chest x-ray machine

Level of Cognitive Ability: Synthesizing
Client Needs: Physiological Integrity
Clinical Judgment/Cognitive Skills: Take Action
Integrated Process: Nursing Process/Implementation
Content Area: Complex Care: Emergency Situations/Management
Health Problem: Adult Health: Respiratory: Chest Injuries

Answer: 1
Rationale: Flail chest occurs from a blunt trauma to the chest. The loose segment from the chest wall becomes paradoxical to the expansion and contraction of the rest of the chest wall. The client with flail chest has painful, rapid, shallow respirations while experiencing severe dyspnea. The laboratory results indicate worsening respiratory acidosis. The effort of breathing and the paradoxical chest movement have the net effect of producing hypoxia and hypercapnia. The client develops respiratory failure and requires intubation and mechanical ventilation, usually with positive end-expiratory pressure; therefore, an intubation tray is necessary. None of the other options have a direct purpose with the client's current respiratory status.
Priority Nursing Tip: The client with a flail chest experiences paradoxical respirations (inward movement of a segment of the thorax during inspiration with outward movement during expiration).

Test-Taking Strategy: Focus on the **subject,** flail chest. Review the changes in the ABG values. Recall that a falling arterial oxygen level and a rising carbon dioxide level indicate respiratory failure. The usual treatment for respiratory failure is intubation, which will lead you to the correct option.

---

240. A client experiencing empyema is to have a bedside thoracentesis performed. The nurse plans to have which equipment available in the event that the procedure is ineffective?

1 Code cart
2 A small-bore needle
3 Extra-large drainage bottle
4 Chest tube and drainage system

Level of Cognitive Ability: Applying
Client Needs: Physiological Integrity
Clinical Judgment/Cognitive Skills: Generate Solutions
Integrated Process: Nursing Process/Planning
Content Area: Adult Health: Respiratory
Health Problem: Adult Health: Respiratory: Viral, Bacterial, Fungal Infections

Answer: 4

Rationale: Empyema is the collection of pus within the pleural cavity. If the exudate is too thick for drainage via thoracentesis, the client may require placement of a chest tube to adequately drain the purulent effusion. A small-bore needle would not effectively allow exudate to drain. Options 1 and 3 are also unnecessary.

Priority Nursing Tip: Empyema is usually caused by pulmonary infection and lung abscess after thoracic surgery or chest trauma in which bacteria are introduced directly into the pleural space.

Test-Taking Strategy: Focus on the **subject**, equipment available in the event that the procedure is ineffective. A client with empyema will have exudate that is often very thick. Recalling that the purpose of thoracentesis is to provide drainage of the pleura will direct you to the correct option.

---

241. A child is admitted to the hospital with a suspected diagnosis of idiopathic thrombocytopenic purpura (ITP), and diagnostic studies are performed. Which diagnostic result is indicative of this disorder?

1 An elevated platelet count
2 Elevated hemoglobin and hematocrit levels
3 Bone marrow exam showing increased megakaryocytes
4 Bone marrow exam indicating increased immature white blood cells

Level of Cognitive Ability: Analyzing
Client Needs: Physiological Integrity
Clinical Judgment/Cognitive Skills: Recognize Cues
Integrated Process: Nursing Process/Data Collection
Content Area: Pediatrics: Hematological
Health Problem: Pediatric Specific: Bleeding Disorders

Answer: 3

Rationale: The laboratory manifestations of ITP include the presence of a low platelet count of usually less than 20,000 mm^3. Thrombocytopenia is the only laboratory abnormality expected with ITP. If there has been significant blood loss, there is evidence of anemia in the blood cell count. If a bone marrow examination is performed, the results with ITP show a normal or increased number of megakaryocytes, which are the precursors of platelets. Option 4 indicates the bone marrow result that would be found in a child with leukemia.

Priority Nursing Tip: For the client with idiopathic thrombocytopenic purpura (ITP), platelet transfusions may be administered when platelet counts are less than 20,000 mm^3.

Test-Taking Strategy: Focus on the **subject**, ITP and associated diagnostic tests. Think about the pathophysiology of this diagnosis. Recalling that megakaryocytes are the precursors of platelets will assist with directing you to the correct option.

---

242. The nurse is assisting in planning care for a client with a chest tube attached to a chest tube drainage system. The nurse would include which interventions in the plan? **Select all that apply.**
1 Changing the client's position often
2 Clamping the chest tube intermittently
3 Maintaining the collection chamber below the client's waist
4 Adding water to the suction control chamber as it evaporates
5 Taping the connection between the chest tube and the drainage system

Level of Cognitive Ability: Analyzing
Client Needs: Physiological Integrity
Clinical Judgment/Cognitive Skills: Generate Solutions
Integrated Process: Nursing Process/Planning
Content Area: Skills: Tube Care
Health Problem: N/A

Answer: 1, 3, 4, 5
Rationale: Changing the client's position frequently is necessary to promote drainage and ventilation. Maintaining the system below waist level is indicated to prevent fluid from reentering the pleural space. Adding water to the suction control chamber is an appropriate nursing action and is done as needed to maintain the full suction level prescribed. Taping the connection between the chest tube and system is also indicated to prevent accidental disconnection. To prevent a tension pneumothorax, the nurse avoids clamping the chest tube, unless specifically prescribed. In many facilities, clamping of the chest tube is contraindicated by agency policy.
Priority Nursing Tip: Confirmation of pneumothorax is made by chest radiography.

Test-Taking Strategy: Focus on the **subject**, interventions in the care of the client with a chest tube. Recall that tension pneumothorax occurs when air is trapped in the pleural space and has no exit. Therefore, it is necessary to evaluate each of the options in terms of relative risk for air trapping in the pleural space. Clamping the chest tube could trap air in the pleural space.

---

243. The nurse is assisting a client with a chest tube to get out of bed, when the chest tubing accidentally gets caught in the bed rail and disconnects. While trying to reestablish the connection, the chest tube drainage system falls over and cracks. The nurse would take which action to minimize the client's risk for injury?
1 Clamp the chest tube.
2 Encourage the client to deep-breathe.
3 Apply a petroleum gauze over the end of the chest tube.
4 Immerse the chest tube in a bottle of sterile water or normal saline.

Level of Cognitive Ability: Analyzing
Client Needs: Physiological Integrity
Clinical Judgment/Cognitive Skills: Take Action
Integrated Process: Nursing Process/Implementation
Content Area: Complex Care: Emergency Situations/Management
Health Problem: N/A

Answer: 4
Rationale: If a chest tube accidentally disconnects from the tubing of the drainage apparatus, the nurse would first reestablish an underwater seal to prevent tension pneumothorax and mediastinal shift. This can be accomplished by reconnecting the chest tube or, in this case, immersing the end of the chest tube 1 to 2 inches below the surface of a 250-mL bottle of sterile water or normal saline until a new chest tube can be set up. Deep breathing could be harmful at this time. Clamping the chest tube could also cause tension pneumothorax. A petroleum gauze would be applied to the skin over the chest tube insertion site if the entire chest tube was accidentally removed from the chest. The primary health care provider needs to be notified but only after taking corrective action.
Priority Nursing Tip: If a closed chest tube drainage system cracks or breaks, insert the chest tube into a bottle of sterile water, remove the cracked or broken system, and replace it with a new system.

Test-Taking Strategy: Focus on the **subject,** care of a chest tube. Option 1 would create a tension pneumothorax because this action does not reestablish an underwater seal. Eliminate option 2 because it could be harmful. From the remaining options, noting that an underwater seal must be established will direct you to the correct option.

---

244. When planning care for a client diagnosed with Cushing's syndrome, the nurse would include which intervention to prevent a common complication of this disorder?

1 Monitoring glucose levels
2 Encouraging rigorous exercise
3 Monitoring epinephrine levels
4 Encouraging visits from friends

Level of Cognitive Ability: Analyzing
Client Needs: Physiological Integrity
Clinical Judgment/Cognitive Skills: Generate Solutions
Integrated Process: Nursing Process/Planning
Content Area: Adult Health: Endocrine
Health Problem: Adult Health: Endocrine: Adrenal Disorders

Answer: 1
Rationale: Cushing's syndrome is a metabolic disorder resulting from the chronic and excessive production of cortisol by the adrenal cortex or the administration of glucocorticoids in large doses for several weeks or longer. In the client with Cushing's syndrome, increased levels of glucocorticoids can result in hyperglycemia and signs and symptoms of diabetes mellitus. Clients experience activity intolerance related to muscle weakness and fatigue; therefore, option 2 is incorrect. Epinephrine levels are not affected. Visitors need to be limited because of the client's impaired immune response.
Priority Nursing Tip: Hyperglycemia, hypernatremia, hypokalemia, and hypocalcemia occur in Cushing's syndrome. The opposite effects occur in Addison's disease.

Test-Taking Strategy: Focus on the **subject,** complications of Cushing's syndrome. Recalling that increased levels of glucocorticoids can result in hyperglycemia will direct you to the correct option.

---

245. A client with a central venous catheter who is receiving total parenteral nutrition (TPN) suddenly experiences signs/symptoms associated with an air embolism. The nurse assisting in caring for the client would implement which interventions to minimize the client's risk for injury? **Select all that apply.**

1 Clamps the catheter
2 Checks the line for air
3 Notifies the registered nurse
4 Administers 500 mL normal saline
5 Places the client in Trendelenburg's position on the left side

Level of Cognitive Ability: Synthesizing
Client Needs: Physiological Integrity
Clinical Judgment/Cognitive Skills: Take Action
Integrated Process: Nursing Process/Implementation
Content Area: Complex Care: Emergency Situations/Management of Care
Health Problem: N/A

Answer: 1, 3, 5
Rationale: If the client experiences air embolus, the client is placed in the lateral Trendelenburg's position on the left side to trap the air in the right atrium. The nurse would also clamp the catheter and notify the registered nurse, who will contact the primary health care provider. Checking for air in the line will not minimize the client's risk at this time; additionally, the catheter will be clamped. A fluid bolus would cause the air embolus to travel.
Priority Nursing Tip: Air embolism can be caused by an inadequately primed intravenous (IV) line or a loose connection. Air embolism may occur during tubing change or during removal of the IV.

Test-Taking Strategy: Focus on the **subject,** suspected air embolism. Recall that air embolism is a life-threatening condition requiring immediate nursing intervention that includes notifying the primary health care provider.

---

246. The nurse is assisting in caring for a 33-week pregnant client who has experienced a premature rupture of the membranes (PROM). Which interventions would the nurse expect to be part of the plan of care? **Select all that apply.**

1 Perform frequent biophysical profiles.
2 Monitor for elevated serum creatinine.
3 Monitor for manifestations of infection.
4 Teach the client how to count fetal movements.
5 Use strict sterile technique for vaginal examinations.
6 Inform the client about the need for tocolytic therapy.

Level of Cognitive Ability: Analyzing
Client Needs: Physiological Integrity
Clinical Judgment/Cognitive Skills: Generate Solutions
Integrated Process: Nursing Process/Planning
Content Area: Maternity: Antepartum
Health Problem: Maternity: Premature Rupture of the Membranes

Answer: 1, 3, 4, 5

Rationale: PROM is membrane rupture before 37 weeks of gestation. Frequent biophysical profiles are performed to determine fetal health status and estimate amniotic fluid volume. Monitoring for signs of infection is a major part of the nursing care. The woman would also be taught how to count fetal movements daily, because slowing of fetal movement has been shown to be a precursor to severe fetal compromise. Whenever PROM is suspected, strict sterile technique would be used in any vaginal examination to prevent infection. Elevated serum creatinine does not occur in PROM but may be noted in severe preeclampsia. Tocolytic therapy is used for women in preterm labor (not for PROM).

Priority Nursing Tip: A finding in PROM is the evidence of fluid pooling in the vaginal vault. The fluid tests positive with the Nitrazine test.

Test-Taking Strategy: Focus on the **subject,** PROM. Think about the pathophysiology of this condition. Select options 3 and 5 because they relate to preventing infection. Next select options 1 and 4 because they relate to determining fetal health status. Recalling the causes of an elevated serum creatinine and the purpose of tocolytic therapy will assist in eliminating these options.

---

247. A client who has been diagnosed with carbon monoxide poisoning is asking that the oxygen mask be removed. The nurse shares with the client that the oxygen may be safely removed once the carboxyhemoglobin level decreases to less than which level?

1 5%
2 10%
3 15%
4 25%

Level of Cognitive Ability: Applying
Client Needs: Physiological Integrity
Clinical Judgment/Cognitive Skills: Generate Solutions
Integrated Process: Nursing Process/Planning
Content Area: Complex Care: Poisoning
Health Problem: Adult Health: Respiratory: Environmental

Answer: 1

Rationale: Oxygen may be removed safely from the client with carbon monoxide poisoning once carboxyhemoglobin levels are less than 5%. Normal carboxyhemoglobin (HbCO) levels are 0% to 3% for nonsmokers and 3% to 8% for smokers. Levels of 10% to 20% cause headaches, nausea, vomiting, and dyspnea. Levels of 30% to 40% cause severe headaches, syncope, and tachydysrhythmias. Levels greater than 40% cause Cheyne–Stokes respiration or respiratory failure, seizures, unconsciousness, permanent brain damage, cardiac arrest, and even death. Options 2, 3, and 4 are elevated levels.

Priority Nursing Tip: Carbon monoxide is a colorless, odorless, and tasteless gas.

Test-Taking Strategy: Focus on the **subject,** safely removing the oxygen in CO poisoning. If you are unsure, it would be best to select the lowest level as identified in the correct option.

248. The nurse is reinforcing information to a pregnant client about prenatal nutritional needs. The nurse would plan to include which information in the client's teaching plan?

1 All parents are at high risk for nutritional deficiencies.
2 Calcium intake is not necessary until the third trimester.
3 Iron supplements are not necessary unless the parent has iron-deficiency anemia.
4 The nutritional status of the parent significantly influences fetal growth and development.

Level of Cognitive Ability: Applying
Client Needs: Physiological Integrity
Clinical Judgment/Cognitive Skills: Generate Solutions
Integrated Process: Nursing Process/Implementation
Content Area: Maternity: Antepartum
Health Problem: N/A

Answer: 4
Rationale: Poor nutrition during pregnancy can negatively influence fetal growth and development. Although pregnancy poses some nutritional risk for the parent, not all clients are at high risk. Calcium intake is critical during the third trimester but must be increased from the onset of pregnancy. Intake of dietary iron is insufficient for the majority of pregnant women, and iron supplements are routinely prescribed.
Priority Nursing Tip: An increase of about 300 calories/day is needed during the last 6 months of pregnancy.

Test-Taking Strategy: Focus on the **subject**, nutrition during pregnancy. Option 1 uses the **closed-ended word** "all"; therefore, eliminate this option. Options 2 and 3 offer specific time frames or conditions for interventions; therefore, eliminate these options. Option 4 is also a general statement that is true for any stage of pregnancy.

---

249. A client is admitted to the hospital with a diagnosis of acute bacterial pericarditis. Which findings are associated with this form of heart disease? **Select all that apply.**

1 Fever
2 Leukopenia
3 Bradycardia
4 Pericardial friction rub
5 Decreased erythrocyte sedimentation rate
6 Precordial chest pain that is intensified by the supine position

Level of Cognitive Ability: Analyzing
Client Needs: Physiological Integrity
Clinical Judgment/Cognitive Skills: Recognize Cues
Integrated Process: Nursing Process/Data Collection
Content Area: Adult Health: Cardiovascular
Health Problem: Adult Health: Cardiovascular: Inflammatory and Structural Heart Disorders

Answer: 1, 4, 6
Rationale: In acute bacterial pericarditis, the membranes surrounding the heart become inflamed and rub against each other, producing the classic pericardial friction rub. Fever typically occurs and is accompanied by leukocytosis and an elevated erythrocyte sedimentation rate. The client complains of severe precordial chest pain that intensifies when lying supine and decreases in a sitting position. The pain also intensifies when the client breathes deeply. Malaise, myalgia, and tachycardia are common.
Priority Nursing Tip: Monitor the client with pericarditis for signs of heart failure or cardiac tamponade as complications.

Test-Taking Strategy: Focus on the **subject**, bacterial pericarditis. The diagnosis will assist in determining that the client has a fever (option 1); the compensatory response to fever is an increased metabolic rate and tachycardia. Also remember that when the client has an inflammatory disease, the erythrocyte sedimentation rate will increase, as will the white blood cell count (leukocytosis, not leukopenia). Lastly, focusing on the diagnosis will assist in determining that a pericardial friction rub and severe precordial chest pain are present (options 4 and 6).

250. A client is admitted to the hospital with a diagnosis of Cushing's syndrome. The nurse monitors the client for which problem that is likely to occur with this diagnosis?

1 Hypovolemia
2 Hypoglycemia
3 Mood disturbances
4 Deficient fluid volume

Level of Cognitive Ability: Applying
Client Needs: Physiological Integrity
Clinical Judgment/Cognitive Skills: Recognize Cues
Integrated Process: Nursing Process/Data Collection
Content Area: Adult Health: Endocrine
Health Problem: Adult Health: Endocrine: Adrenal Disorders

Answer: 3
Rationale: Cushing's syndrome is a metabolic disorder resulting from the chronic and excessive production of cortisol. When Cushing's syndrome develops, the normal function of the glucocorticoids becomes exaggerated and the classic picture of the syndrome emerges. This exaggerated physiological action can cause mood disturbances, including memory loss, poor concentration and cognition, euphoria, and depression. It can also cause persistent hyperglycemia, along with sodium and water retention (hypernatremia), producing edema (hypervolemia; fluid volume excess) and hypertension.
Priority Nursing Tip: Cushing's disease is characterized by the hypersecretion of glucocorticoids, whereas Addison's disease is characterized by a hyposecretion of adrenal cortex hormones (glucocorticoids and mineralocorticoids).

Test-Taking Strategy: Focus on the **subject,** Cushing's syndrome. Eliminate options 1 and 4 first because they are **comparable or alike;** both involve a deficit in blood volume. Recalling that hyperglycemia rather than hypoglycemia occurs in this condition will direct you to the correct option.

---

251. An assessment of a client's vocal cords requires indirect visualization of the larynx. Which instruction would the nurse assisting in the procedure give the client to facilitate this procedure?

1 Try to swallow.
2 Hold your breath.
3 Breathe normally.
4 Roll the tongue to the back of the mouth.

Level of Cognitive Ability: Applying
Client Needs: Physiological Integrity
Clinical Judgment/Cognitive Skills: Take Action
Integrated Process: Nursing Process/Implementation
Content Area: Foundations of Care: Diagnostic Tests
Health Problem: N/A

Answer: 3
Rationale: Indirect laryngoscopy is done to assess the function of the vocal cords or obtain tissue for biopsy. Observations are made during rest and phonation by using a laryngeal mirror, head mirror, and light source. The client is placed in an upright position to facilitate passage of the laryngeal mirror into the mouth and is instructed to breathe normally. Swallowing cannot be done with the mirror in place. The procedure takes longer than the time the client would be able to hold the breath, and this action is ineffective anyway. The tongue cannot be moved back because it would occlude the airway.
Priority Nursing Tip: After laryngoscopy, maintain an NPO status until the gag reflex returns.

Test-Taking Strategy: Focus on the **subject,** indirect laryngoscopy. Option 4 is eliminated first because it is not possible to move the tongue back with the mirror in place. It would also cause the airway to become occluded. Given the length of time needed to do the procedure, the client could not realistically hold the breath, so option 2 is eliminated next. Trying to swallow would actually cause the larynx to move against the mirror and could cause gagging; therefore, eliminate option 1.

---

252. The nurse is assisting in caring for a client scheduled for a bilateral adrenalectomy for treatment of an adrenal tumor. What information would the nurse give the client about the postsurgical needs?

1 "You will need to undergo chemotherapy after surgery."
2 "You will need to wear an abdominal binder after surgery."
3 "You will not need any special long-term treatment after surgery."
4 "You will need to take daily hormone replacements beginning after the surgery."

Level of Cognitive Ability: Applying
Client Needs: Physiological Integrity
Clinical Judgment/Cognitive Skills: Take Action
Integrated Process: Nursing Process/Implementation
Content Area: Adult Health: Endocrine
Health Problem: Adult Health: Endocrine: Adrenal Disorders

Answer: 4
Rationale: The major cause of primary hyperaldosteronism is an aldosterone-secreting tumor called an *aldosteronoma*. Surgery is the treatment of choice. Clients undergoing a bilateral adrenalectomy require permanent replacement of adrenal hormones. Options 1, 2, and 3 are inaccurate statements regarding this surgery.
Priority Nursing Tip: After adrenalectomy, monitor for signs of acute adrenal insufficiency, which is also known as *addisonian crisis*.

Test-Taking Strategy: Focus on the **subject**, bilateral adrenalectomy. Recalling the function of the adrenal glands and that glucocorticoids and mineralocorticoids are essential to sustain life will direct you to the correct option.

---

253. The nurse is assisting in caring for a client who is scheduled for an adrenalectomy. The nurse expects that which medication will be prescribed in the preoperative period to prevent addisonian crisis?

1 Prednisone orally
2 Fludrocortisone orally
3 Spironolactone intramuscularly
4 Methylprednisolone sodium succinate intravenously

Level of Cognitive Ability: Analyzing
Client Needs: Physiological Integrity
Clinical Judgment/Cognitive Skills: Generate Solutions
Integrated Process: Nursing Process/Planning
Content Area: Adult Health: Endocrine
Health Problem: Adult Health: Endocrine: Adrenal Disorders

Answer: 4
Rationale: A glucocorticoid preparation will be administered intravenously or intramuscularly in the immediate preoperative period to a client scheduled for an adrenalectomy. Methylprednisolone sodium succinate protects the client from developing acute adrenal insufficiency (addisonian crisis) that can occur as a result of the adrenalectomy. Prednisone is an oral corticosteroid. Fludrocortisone is a mineralocorticoid. Spironolactone is a potassium-sparing diuretic.
Priority Nursing Tip: Emergency care of the client with addisonian crisis includes hormone replacement and hyperkalemia and hypoglycemia management.

Test-Taking Strategy: Focus on the **subject**, preventing addisonian crisis in a client scheduled for adrenalectomy. Recalling the function of the adrenals will assist in eliminating options 2 and 3. From the remaining options, select option 4 because the client is preoperative and would receive medications via routes other than orally.

---

254. A client diagnosed with Graves' disease is to receive radioactive iodine therapy. What information would the nurse share with the client about the therapy?

1. After the initial dose, subsequent treatments must continue for the rest of the client's life.
2. The radioactive iodine is designed to destroy the entire thyroid gland with just one dose.
3. It takes 6 to 8 weeks after treatment to experience relief from the symptoms of the disease.
4. High radioactivity levels prohibit contact with family for 4 weeks after the initial treatment.

Level of Cognitive Ability: Applying
Client Needs: Physiological Integrity
Clinical Judgment/Cognitive Skills: Take Action
Integrated Process: Nursing Process/Implementation
Content Area: Adult Health: Endocrine
Health Problem: Adult Health: Endocrine: Thyroid Disorders

Answer: 3

Rationale: Graves' disease is also known as *toxic diffuse goiter* and is characterized by a hyperthyroid state resulting from hypersecretion of thyroid hormones. After treatment with radioactive iodine therapy, a decrease in the thyroid hormone level would be noted, which helps alleviate symptoms. Relief of symptoms does not occur until 6 to 8 weeks after initial treatment. Occasionally, a client may require a second or third dose, but treatments are not lifelong. This form of therapy is not designed to destroy the entire gland; rather, some of the cells that synthesize thyroid hormone will be destroyed by the local radiation. The nurse must reassure the client and family that unless the dosage is extremely high, clients are not required to observe radiation precautions. The rationale for this is that the radioactivity quickly dissipates.

Priority Nursing Tip: The consumption or administration of any substance that contains a stimulant needs to be avoided in the client with hyperthyroidism.

Test-Taking Strategy: Focus on the **subject,** Graves' disease. Recall knowledge regarding this treatment. Note the **closed-ended words** "must," "entire," and "prohibit" in the incorrect options.

---

255. A client arrives at the emergency department with upper gastrointestinal (GI) bleeding that began 3 hours ago. The nurse assisting in caring for the client plans for which **priority** action?

1. Obtaining vital signs
2. Inserting a nasogastric (NG) tube
3. Asking the client about the precipitating events
4. Completing an abdominal physical assessment

Level of Cognitive Ability: Analyzing
Client Needs: Physiological Integrity
Clinical Judgment/Cognitive Skills: Generate Solutions
Integrated Process: Nursing Process/Implementation
Content Area: Complex Care: Emergency Situations/Management
Health Problem: Adult Health: Gastrointestinal: Upper GI Disorders

Answer: 1

Rationale: The priority action for the client with GI bleeding is to obtain vital signs to determine whether the client is in shock from blood loss and obtain a baseline by which to monitor the progress of treatment. The client may be unable to provide subjective data until the immediate physical needs are met. A complete abdominal physical assessment must be performed but is not the priority. Insertion of an NG tube may be prescribed but is not the priority action.

Priority Nursing Tip: For the client experiencing active GI bleeding, check for signs of dehydration and hypovolemic shock.

Test-Taking Strategy: Note the **strategic word,** *priority.* Recall that the client with a GI bleed is at risk for shock. Also, the correct option addresses the **ABCs—airway, breathing, and circulation.**

---

256. A client who has experienced an acute kidney injury is prescribed a fluid restriction of 1500 mL per day. Which interventions will the nurse implement to assist the client in maintaining this restriction? **Select all that apply.**

1 Removing the water pitcher from the bedside
2 Using mouthwash with alcohol for mouth care
3 Prohibiting beverages with sugar to minimize thirst
4 Providing the client with lip balm to keep lips moist
5 Offering the client ice chips at intervals during the day

Level of Cognitive Ability: Applying
Client Needs: Physiological Integrity
Clinical Judgment/Cognitive Skills: Take Action
Integrated Process: Nursing Process/Implementation
Content Area: Foundations of Care: Fluids and Electrolytes
Health Problem: Adult Health: Renal and Urinary: Acute Kidney Injury

Answer: 1, 4, 5
Rationale: The nurse can help the client maintain fluid restriction through a variety of means. The water pitcher needs to be removed from the bedside to aid in adherence to fluid restriction. The use of ice chips and lip ointments is another intervention that may be helpful to the client on fluid restriction. Frequent mouth care is important; however, alcohol-based products need to be avoided because they are drying to mucous membranes. Beverages that the client enjoys are provided and are not restricted based on sugar content.
Priority Nursing Tip: As long as the beverage is not contraindicated, allow the client on fluid restriction to select preferred beverages.

Test-Taking Strategy: Focus on the **subject,** a client with acute kidney injury who is on fluid restriction. Eliminate options 2 and 3 because they are ineffective or unnecessary.

---

257. The nurse has administered approximately half of a high-cleansing enema when the client reports pain and cramping. Which nursing action is appropriate?

1 Reassuring the client that those sensations will subside
2 Raising the enema bag so that the solution can be introduced quickly
3 Discontinuing the enema and notifying the primary health care provider
4 Clamping the tubing for 30 seconds and restarting the flow at a slower rate

Level of Cognitive Ability: Applying
Client Needs: Physiological Integrity
Clinical Judgment/Cognitive Skills: Take Action
Integrated Process: Nursing Process/Implementation
Content Area: Skills: Elimination
Health Problem: N/A

Answer: 4
Rationale: The enema fluid would be administered slowly. If the client complains of pain or cramping, the flow is stopped for 30 seconds and restarted at a slower rate. Slow enema administration and stopping the flow temporarily, if necessary, will decrease the likelihood of intestinal spasm and premature ejection of the solution. The client's report of pain and cramping would not be ignored. The higher the solution container is held above the rectum, the faster the flow and the greater the force in the rectum. There is no need to discontinue the enema and notify the primary health care provider at this time.
Priority Nursing Tip: During enema administration, ask the client to breathe slowly in through the nose and out through the mouth. This will assist the client in tolerating the instillation of the solution.

Test-Taking Strategy: Focus on the **subject,** alleviating pain and cramping with enema instillation. Noting that there is no need to notify the primary health care provider will allow you to eliminate that option.

---

258. The client diagnosed with chronic kidney disease is scheduled for hemodialysis. When would the nurse plan to administer the client's daily dose of enalapril to ensure its **effectiveness**?

1 During dialysis
2 Just before dialysis
3 The day after dialysis
4 Upon return from dialysis

Level of Cognitive Ability: Applying
Client Needs: Physiological Integrity
Clinical Judgment/Cognitive Skills: Generate Solutions
Integrated Process: Nursing Process/Planning
Content Area: Pharmacology: Cardiovascular: Angiotensin Converting Enzyme Inhibitors
Health Problem: Adult Health: Renal and Urinary: Chronic Kidney Disease

Answer: 4

Rationale: Antihypertensive medications, such as enalapril, are administered to the client after hemodialysis. This prevents the client from becoming hypotensive during dialysis and also from having the medication removed from the bloodstream by dialysis. There is no rationale for waiting a full day to resume the medication. This would lead to ineffective control of the blood pressure.

Priority Nursing Tip: In addition to antihypertensive medications, water-soluble vitamins, certain antibiotics, and digoxin are withheld before a hemodialysis treatment because they can be removed by dialysis.

Test-Taking Strategy: Note the **strategic word,** *effectiveness*. Focus on the **subject,** medication administration with hemodialysis. Think about the effects of an antihypertensive medication on the blood pressure when fluid is being removed from the body. Because hypotension is much more likely to occur in this circumstance, eliminate options 1 and 2. Most clients are hemodialyzed 3 times a week, so if the medication were held for dialysis until the following day, the client would miss three of the seven doses that would usually be given in a week. This would lead to ineffective blood pressure control; therefore, eliminate option 3.

---

259. The client reports a smoking pattern of three-fourths of a pack of cigarettes per day over the last 10 years. The nurse calculates that the client has a smoking history of how many pack-years? **Fill in the blank.**

Answer: _____ pack-years

Level of Cognitive Ability: Applying
Client Needs: Physiological Integrity
Clinical Judgment/Cognitive Skills: Generate Solutions
Integrated Process: Nursing Process/Data Collection
Content Area: Health Assessment/Physical Exam: Respiratory
Health Problem: N/A

Answer: 7.5

Rationale: The standard method for quantifying smoking history is to multiply the number of packs smoked per day by the number of years of smoking. The number is recorded as the number of pack-years. The calculation for the number of pack-years for the client who has smoked three-fourths of a pack per day for 10 years is 0.75 pack × 10 years = 7.5 pack-years.

Priority Nursing Tip: When obtaining a smoking history, ask the client about possible exposure to passive smoke.

Test-Taking Strategy: Focus on the **subject,** number of pack-years. Review the information in the question, and multiply the number of packs of cigarettes smoked per day by the number of years of smoking.

---

260. The nurse is preparing to assist in providing postsurgical care for a client after a subtotal thyroidectomy. The nurse anticipates the need for which item to be placed at the bedside to minimize the client's risk for injury?

1 Hypothermia blanket
2 Emergency tracheostomy kit
3 Magnesium sulfate in a ready-to-inject vial
4 Ampule of saturated solution of potassium iodide

Answer: 2

Rationale: Respiratory distress can occur after thyroidectomy as a result of swelling in the tracheal area. The nurse would ensure that an emergency tracheostomy kit is available. Surgery on the thyroid does not alter the heat control mechanism of the body. Magnesium sulfate would not be indicated because the incidence of hypomagnesemia is not a common problem after thyroidectomy. Saturated solution of potassium iodide is typically administered preoperatively to block thyroid hormone synthesis and release and to place the client in a euthyroid state.

Priority Nursing Tip: After thyroidectomy, maintain the client in a semi-Fowler's position to assist in preventing edema at the operative site.

Level of Cognitive Ability: Applying
Client Needs: Physiological Integrity
Clinical Judgment/Cognitive Skills: Generate Solutions
Integrated Process: Nursing Process/Planning
Content Area: Adult Health: Endocrine
Health Problem: Adult Health: Endocrine: Thyroid Disorders

Test-Taking Strategy: Focus on the **subject,** postoperative thyroidectomy. Recall the anatomical location of the thyroid gland to direct you to the correct option. Also, use the **ABCs—airway, breathing, and circulation.** Maintaining a patent airway is critical.

---

261. When caring for a client diagnosed with myasthenia gravis, the nurse needs to be alert for which manifestations of myasthenic crisis? **Select all that apply.**

1 Bradycardia
2 Increased diaphoresis
3 Decreased lacrimation
4 Bowel and bladder incontinence
5 Absent cough and swallow reflex
6 Sudden marked rise in blood pressure

Level of Cognitive Ability: Analyzing
Client Needs: Physiological Integrity
Clinical Judgment/Cognitive Skills: Recognize Cues
Integrated Process: Nursing Process/Data Collection
Content Area: Adult Health: Neurological
Health Problem: Adult Health: Neurological: Myasthenia Gravis

Answer: 2, 4, 5, 6
Rationale: Myasthenic crisis is caused by undermedication or can be precipitated by an infection or sudden withdrawal of anticholinesterase medications. It may also occur spontaneously. Clinical manifestations include increased diaphoresis, bowel and bladder incontinence, absent cough and swallow reflex, sudden marked rise in blood pressure because of hypoxia, increased heart rate, severe respiratory distress and cyanosis, increased secretions, increased lacrimation, restlessness, and dysarthria.
Priority Nursing Tip: Myasthenic crisis is an acute exacerbation of myasthenia gravis; one cause is undermedication. Cholinergic crisis is caused by overmedication with an anticholinesterase. It is imperative that the nurse documents the time of medication administration, as well as the time of any change in client condition.

Test-Taking Strategy: Focus on the **subject,** myasthenia gravis. Specific knowledge regarding the manifestations of myasthenic crisis is needed to answer this question. Recall that myasthenic crisis is caused by undermedication. With this in mind, think about the manifestations of myasthenia gravis to assist in selecting the correct options.

---

262. The nurse is encouraging the client to cough and deep-breathe after cardiac surgery. The nurse ensures that which item is available to maximize the **effectiveness** of this procedure?

1 Nebulizer
2 Ambu bag
3 Suction equipment
4 Incisional splinting pillow

Level of Cognitive Ability: Applying
Client Needs: Physiological Integrity
Clinical Judgment/Cognitive Skills: Take Action
Integrated Process: Nursing Process/Implementation
Content Area: Foundations of Care: Perioperative Care
Health Problem: N/A

Answer: 4
Rationale: The use of an incisional splint such as a "cough pillow" can ease discomfort during coughing and deep breathing. The client who is comfortable will do more effective deep breathing and coughing exercises. Use of an incentive spirometer is also indicated. Options 1, 2, and 3 will not encourage the client to cough and deep-breathe.
Priority Nursing Tip: If a surgical incision is located in the abdominal or thoracic area, instruct the client to place a folded towel or pillow, or one hand with the other on top, over the incisional area to splint it during coughing and deep breathing.

Test-Taking Strategy: Focus on the **subject,** coughing and deep breathing after cardiac surgery. Note the **strategic word,** *effectiveness.* The cough pillow is an item that will maximize effectiveness. Eliminate options 2 and 3, which are items used by the nurse. A nebulizer (option 1) is used to deliver medication.

---

263. The nurse preparing to administer an intermittent tube feeding through a nasogastric (NG) tube checks for residual volume. How do the resulting data assist in ensuring the client's safety?

1 Confirms proper NG tube placement
2 Determines the client's nutritional status
3 Evaluates the adequacy of gastric emptying
4 Checks the client's fluid and electrolyte status

Level of Cognitive Ability: Analyzing
Client Needs: Physiological Integrity
Clinical Judgment/Cognitive Skills: Analyze Cues
Integrated Process: Nursing Process/Implementation
Content Area: Skills: Tube Care
Health Problem: N/A

Answer: 3

Rationale: All stomach contents are aspirated and measured before administering a tube feeding to determine the gastric residual volume. If the stomach fails to empty and propel its contents forward, the tube feeding accumulates in the stomach and increases the client's risk of aspiration. If the aspirated gastric contents exceed the predetermined limit, the nurse withholds the tube feeding and collaborates with the primary health care provider on a plan of care. Checking gastric residual volume does not confirm placement or assess fluid and electrolyte status. The nurse uses clinical indicators, including serum albumin levels, to determine the client's nutritional status.

Priority Nursing Tip: When administering an NG tube feeding, warm the feeding to room temperature to prevent stomach cramps and diarrhea.

Test-Taking Strategy: Focus on the **subject,** the purpose for checking the gastric residual volume. Eliminate options 1 and 4 because checking gastric residual volume does not confirm proper tube placement or assess fluid and electrolyte status. Other clinical indicators will determine client nutritional status, so eliminate option 2. Note the relationship between the subject and option 3 to direct you to this option.

---

264. A licensed practical nurse (LPN) is caring for a client scheduled to undergo a renal biopsy. To minimize the risk of postprocedure complications, the LPN reports which laboratory results to the registered nurse (RN) before the procedure?

1 Prothrombin time: 15 seconds
2 Potassium: 3.8 mEq/L
3 Serum creatinine: 1.2 mg/dL
4 Blood urea nitrogen (BUN): 18 mg/dL

Level of Cognitive Ability: Applying
Client Needs: Physiological Integrity
Clinical Judgment/Cognitive Skills: Take Action
Integrated Process: Nursing Process/Implementation
Content Area: Foundations of Care: Laboratory Tests
Health Problem: N/A

Answer: 1

Rationale: Postprocedure hemorrhage is a complication after renal biopsy. Because of this, prothrombin time is checked before the procedure. The normal prothrombin time range is 11 to 12.5 seconds. The nurse ensures that these results are available and reports abnormalities promptly. Options 2, 3, and 4 identify normal values. The normal potassium is 3.5 to 5.0 mEq/L; the normal serum creatinine is 0.5 to 1.2 mg/dL; and the normal BUN is 10 to 20 mg/dL.

Priority Nursing Tip: After renal biopsy, monitor for bleeding. Provide pressure to the site and check the biopsy site and under the client for bleeding.

Test-Taking Strategy: Focus on the **subject,** renal biopsy. When a client is to have a biopsy, remember that bleeding is a concern. This will direct you to the correct option. Also note that options 2, 3, and 4 identify normal values.

---

265. A client who survived a house fire is experiencing respiratory distress, and an inhalation injury is suspected. What would the nurse expect will be monitored to determine the presence of carbon monoxide poisoning?

1 Pulse oximetry
2 Urine myoglobin
3 Sputum carbon levels
4 Serum carboxyhemoglobin levels

Answer: 4

Rationale: Serum carboxyhemoglobin levels are the most direct measure of carbon monoxide poisoning, provide the level of poisoning, and thus determine the appropriate treatment measures. The carbon monoxide molecule has a 200 times greater affinity for binding with hemoglobin than an oxygen molecule, causing decreased availability of oxygen to the cells. Clients are treated with 100% oxygen under pressure (hyperbaric oxygen therapy). Options 1, 2, and 3 would not identify carbon monoxide poisoning.

Priority Nursing Tip: The reference range for carboxyhemoglobin in nonsmokers is up to 3% and up to 10% to 15% in smokers.

Test-Taking Strategy: Focus on the **subject,** carbon monoxide poisoning. Note the relationship between *carbon monoxide* and the correct option.

Level of Cognitive Ability: Applying
Client Needs: Physiological Integrity
Clinical Judgment/Cognitive Skills: Recognize Cues
Integrated Process: Nursing Process/Data Collection
Content Area: Complex Care: Poisoning
Health Problem: Adult Health: Integumentary: Burns

---

266. The nurse is assigned to assist in care for a client experiencing hypertonic labor contractions. The nurse plans to conserve the client's energy and promote rest by performing which intervention?

1 Keeping the TV or radio on to provide distraction
2 Assisting the client with breathing and relaxation techniques
3 Keeping the room brightly lit so the client can watch the monitor
4 Avoiding uncomfortable procedures such as intravenous infusions or epidural anesthesia

Answer: 2

Rationale: Breathing and relaxation techniques aid the client in coping with the discomfort of labor and in conserving energy. A brightly lit room and noise from a TV or radio do not promote rest. A quiet, dim environment would be more advantageous. Intravenous or epidural pain relief can be useful. Intravenous hydration can increase perfusion and oxygenation of maternal and fetal tissues and provide glucose for energy needs.

Priority Nursing Tip: In hypertonic labor contractions, the uterine resting tone between contractions is high, reducing uterine blood flow and decreasing fetal oxygen supply.

Test-Taking Strategy: Focus on the **subject,** hypertonic labor contractions. Review methods to help conserve energy and promote rest for the client. Noting the word *assisting* in option 2 will direct you to the correct option.

Level of Cognitive Ability: Applying
Client Needs: Physiological Integrity
Clinical Judgment/Cognitive Skills: Generate Solutions
Integrated Process: Nursing Process/Planning
Content Area: Maternity: Intrapartum
Health Problem: Maternity: Dystocia

---

267. A client diagnosed with acute pyelonephritis is scheduled for an intravenous pyelogram (IVP) this morning. During report the nurse learns that the client vomited several times during the night and continues to report being nauseated. What intervention would the nurse expect to be implemented to ensure the client's safety regarding the scheduled procedure?

1 Canceling the pyelogram
2 Monitoring the client closely for any additional vomiting
3 Medicating the client with a standing prescription for metoclopramide
4 Carrying out a prescription for a 0.9% saline intravenous infusion

Level of Cognitive Ability: Applying
Client Needs: Physiological Integrity
Clinical Judgment/Cognitive Skills: Take Action
Integrated Process: Nursing Process/Implementation
Content Area: Foundations of Care: Diagnostic Tests
Health Problem: Adult Health: Renal and Urinary: Inflammation/Infections

Answer: 4
Rationale: The highest priority of the nurse would be to request a prescription for an intravenous infusion. This is needed to replace fluid lost with vomiting, will be necessary for dye injection for the procedure, and will assist with the elimination of the dye after the procedure. The cancellation of the procedure is premature. Neither monitoring nor medicating the client with an antiemetic will address the fluid loss problem.
Priority Nursing Tip: Inform the client who will undergo an IVP about the possibility of experiencing throat irritation, flushing of the face, warmth, or a salty or metallic taste during the test.

Test-Taking Strategy: Focus on the **subject,** the effect of vomiting on an intravenous pyelogram. Using **Maslow's Hierarchy of Needs theory** will assist in directing you to the correct option.

---

268. The nurse is assisting in planning care for a client who has experienced a T3 spinal cord injury. The nurse would include which intervention in the plan to prevent autonomic dysreflexia (hyperreflexia)?

1 Assist the client to develop a daily bowel routine to prevent constipation.
2 Teach the client to manage emotional stressors by using mental imaging.
3 Check vital signs and observe for hypotension, tachycardia, and tachypnea.
4 Administer dexamethasone orally per the primary health care provider's prescription.

Level of Cognitive Ability: Applying
Client Needs: Physiological Integrity
Clinical Judgment/Cognitive Skills: Generate Solutions
Integrated Process: Nursing Process/Planning
Content Area: Adult Health: Neurological
Health Problem: Adult Health: Neurological: Spinal Cord Injury

Answer: 1
Rationale: Autonomic dysreflexia is a potentially life-threatening condition and may be triggered by bladder distention, bowel distention, visceral distention, or stimulation of pain receptors in the skin. A daily bowel program eliminates this trigger. Options 3 and 4 are unrelated to this specific condition. A client with autonomic hyperreflexia would be severely hypertensive and bradycardic. Removal of the stimuli results in prompt resolution of the signs and symptoms.
Priority Nursing Tip: Autonomic dysreflexia is a neurological emergency and must be treated immediately to prevent a hypertensive stroke.

Test-Taking Strategy: Focus on the **subject,** autonomic dysreflexia. Focus on the word *prevent* to eliminate options 2 and 3. From the remaining options, remembering that this condition may be triggered by bowel distention will direct you to the correct option.

---

269. The nurse monitors a client prescribed a thiazide diuretic for which clinical manifestations of hypokalemia? **Select all that apply.**

1 Muscle twitches
2 Deep tendon hyporeflexia
3 Prominent U wave on electrocardiogram (ECG)
4 General skeletal muscle weakness
5 Hypoactive to absent bowel sounds
6 Tall T waves on ECG

Level of Cognitive Ability: Applying
Client Needs: Physiological Integrity
Clinical Judgment/Cognitive Skills: Recognize Cues
Integrated Process: Nursing Process/Data Collection
Content Area: Pharmacology: Fluid and Electrolyte Balance: Diuretics
Health Problem: N/A

Answer: 2, 3, 4, 5
Rationale: Hypokalemia is a serum potassium level of less than 3.5 mEq/L. Clinical manifestations include ECG abnormalities such as ST depression, inverted T wave, prominent U wave, and heart block. Other manifestations include deep tendon hyporeflexia, general skeletal muscle weakness, decreased bowel motility and hypoactive to absent bowel sounds, shallow ineffective respirations and diminished breath sounds, polyuria, decreased ability to concentrate urine, and decreased urine specific gravity. Tall T waves and muscle twitches are manifestations of hyperkalemia.
Priority Nursing Tip: A potassium deficit is potentially life threatening because every body system is affected.

Test-Taking Strategy: Focus on the **subject**, the manifestations of hypokalemia. Note that options 2, 4, and 5 are **comparable or alike** in that they identify a decreased, or *hypo-*, response; these are manifestations of hypokalemia. Next remember that a prominent U wave on ECG is a manifestation of hypokalemia.

---

270. A client diagnosed with left pleural effusion has just been admitted for treatment. The licensed practical nurse (LPN) is assisting the registered nurse in preparing the client. What would the LPN plan to have available for use at the bedside for treatment?

1 Intubation equipment
2 Paracentesis tray
3 Thoracentesis tray
4 Central venous line insertion set

Level of Cognitive Ability: Applying
Client Needs: Physiological Integrity
Clinical Judgment/Cognitive Skills: Generate Solutions
Integrated Process: Nursing Process/Planning
Content Area: Foundations of Care: Diagnostic Tests
Health Problem: N/A

Answer: 3
Rationale: The client with a significant pleural effusion is usually treated by thoracentesis. This procedure allows drainage of the fluid from the pleural space, which may then be analyzed to determine the precise cause of the effusion. The nurse ensures that a thoracentesis tray is readily available in case the client's symptoms rapidly become more severe. A paracentesis tray is needed for the removal of abdominal effusion. Options 1 and 4 are not specifically indicated for this procedure.
Priority Nursing Tip: Instruct the client undergoing thoracentesis not to cough, breathe deeply, or move during the procedure.

Test-Taking Strategy: Focus on the **subject**, pleural effusion and thoracentesis. Recall knowledge regarding the usual treatment for pleural effusion. Note the relationship between the words *pleural* in the question and *thoracentesis* in the correct option.

---

271. A client has been prescribed oral procainamide. The nurse implements which intervention before administering the medication to minimize the client's risk for injury?

1 Obtaining a chest x-ray
2 Checking blood pressure and pulse
3 Obtaining a complete blood cell count and liver function studies
4 Scheduling a medication level to be drawn 1 hour after the dose is administered

Level of Cognitive Ability: Applying
Client Needs: Physiological Integrity
Clinical Judgment/Cognitive Skills: Take Action
Integrated Process: Nursing Process/Implementation
Content Area: Pharmacology: Cardiovascular: Antidysrhythmics
Health Problem: Adult Health: Cardiovascular: Dysrhythmias

Answer: 2
Rationale: Procainamide is an antidysrhythmic medication. Before the medication is administered, the client's blood pressure and pulse are checked. This medication can cause toxic effects, and serum blood levels would be checked before administering the medication (therapeutic serum level is 4 to 10 mcg/mL). A chest x-ray and obtaining a complete blood cell count and liver function studies are unnecessary.
Priority Nursing Tip: Antidysrhythmic medications suppress dysrhythmias by inhibiting abnormal pathways of electrical conduction through the heart.

Test-Taking Strategy: Focus on the **subject,** the medication procainamide. Use the **steps of the nursing process.** This will direct you to option 2 because it is the only data collection action. Also recalling that this medication is an antidysrhythmic will direct you to the correct option.

---

272. A client diagnosed with urolithiasis is being evaluated to determine the type of calculi that are present. The nurse would plan to keep which item available in the client's room to assist in this process?

1 A urine strainer
2 A calorie count sheet
3 A vital signs graphic sheet
4 An intake and output record

Level of Cognitive Ability: Applying
Client Needs: Physiological Integrity
Clinical Judgment/Cognitive Skills: Generate Solutions
Integrated Process: Nursing Process/Planning
Content Area: Adult Health: Renal and Urinary
Health Problem: Adult Health: Renal and Urinary: Obstructive Problems

Answer: 1
Rationale: The urine is strained until the stone is passed, obtained, and analyzed. Straining the urine will catch small stones that need to be sent to the laboratory for analysis. Once the type of stone is determined, an individualized plan of care for prevention and treatment is developed. Options 2, 3, and 4 are unrelated to the question.
Priority Nursing Tip: Urolithiasis refers to the formation of urinary calculi, and these calculi form in the ureters.

Test-Taking Strategy: Focus on the **subject,** urolithiasis. You will need an item that will help determine the type of stone. Eliminate options 2, 3, and 4 because these items give information about food intake, vital signs, and fluid balance, but they will not provide data that will help determine the type of stone.

---

273. The nurse provides dietary instructions to a client who needs to limit intake of sodium. The nurse instructs the client that which food items must be avoided because of their high sodium content? **Select all that apply.**

1 Ham
2 Apples
3 Broccoli
4 Soy sauce
5 Asparagus
6 Cantaloupe

Level of Cognitive Ability: Applying
Client Needs: Physiological Integrity
Clinical Judgment/Cognitive Skills: Take Action
Integrated Process: Teaching and Learning
Content Area: Foundations of Care: Therapeutic Diets
Health Problem: N/A

Answer: 1, 4
Rationale: Foods highest in sodium include table salt, some cheeses, soy sauce, cured pork, canned foods because of the preservatives, and foods such as cold cuts. Fruits and vegetables contain minimal amounts of sodium.
Priority Nursing Tip: Sodium causes the retention of fluid, and the primary health care provider may prescribe limited sodium intake for clients with hypertension, heart disease, respiratory disease, and certain gastrointestinal and neurological disorders.

Test-Taking Strategy: Focus on the **subject,** foods high in sodium. Eliminate options 2, 3, 5, and 6 because they are **comparable or alike** in that they are fruits and vegetables and are low in sodium.

---

274. The nurse is preparing to assist in caring for a client postureterolithotomy who has a ureteral catheter in place. The nurse would plan to implement which action in the management of this catheter when the client arrives from the recovery room?

1 Clamp the catheter.
2 Place tension on the catheter.
3 Check the drainage from the catheter.
4 Irrigate the catheter using 10 mL sterile normal saline.

Level of Cognitive Ability: Applying
Client Needs: Physiological Integrity
Clinical Judgment/Cognitive Skills: Generate Solutions
Integrated Process: Nursing Process/Implementation
Content Area: Skills: Elimination
Health Problem: Adult Health: Renal and Urinary: Obstructive Problems

Answer: 3
Rationale: Drainage from the ureteral catheter needs to be checked when the client returns from the recovery room and at least every 1 to 2 hours thereafter. The catheter drains urine from the renal pelvis, which has a capacity of 3 to 5 mL. If the volume of urine or fluid in the renal pelvis increases, tissue damage to the pelvis will result from pressure. Therefore, the ureteral tube is never clamped. Additionally, irrigation is not performed unless there is a specific primary health care provider's prescription to do so.
Priority Nursing Tip: If the client has a ureteral catheter, monitor urine output closely. If the urine output is less than 30 mL/hr or there is a lack of urine output for more than 15 minutes, the primary health care provider needs to be notified immediately.

Test-Taking Strategy: Focus on the **subject,** a ureteral catheter, and think about the anatomy of the kidney. Recalling both that the ureteral catheter is placed in the renal pelvis and the structure of this anatomical location will assist in eliminating options 1, 2, and 4.

---

275. In preparation to administer an intermittent tube feeding, the nurse aspirates 40 mL of undigested formula from the client's nasogastric tube. Which intervention would the nurse implement as a result of this finding?

1 Discard the aspirate and record as client output.
2 Mix with new formula to administer the feeding.
3 Dilute with water and inject into the nasogastric tube.
4 Reinstill the aspirate through the nasogastric tube via gravity and syringe.

Level of Cognitive Ability: Applying
Client Needs: Physiological Integrity
Clinical Judgment/Cognitive Skills: Take Action
Integrated Process: Nursing Process/Implementation
Content Area: Skills: Tube Care
Health Problem: N/A

Answer: 4

Rationale: After checking residual feeding contents, the nurse reinstills the gastric contents into the stomach by removing the syringe bulb or plunger and pouring the gastric contents via the syringe into the nasogastric tube. Gastric contents would be reinstilled (unless they exceed an amount of 100 mL or as defined by agency policy) to maintain the client's fluid and electrolyte balance. The nurse avoids mixing gastric aspirate with fresh formula to prevent contamination. Because the gastric aspirate is a small volume, it would be reinstilled; however, mixing the formula with water can also disrupt the client's fluid and electrolyte balance unless the client is dehydrated.

Priority Nursing Tip: If the client is receiving nasogastric tube feedings, check the gastric residual volume before each feeding if the client is receiving intermittent feedings, and every 4 to 6 hours if the client is receiving continuous feedings.

Test-Taking Strategy: Focus on the **subject,** residual tube feeding. Eliminate option 1 because it increases the risk of dehydration and disrupts the client's fluid and electrolyte balance. Also, recalling that aspirated gastric contents are not mixed with formula will assist in directing you to the correct option.

---

276. To ensure the desired results, how would the nurse instruct the client prescribed oral bisacodyl to take the medication?

1 At bedtime
2 With a large meal
3 With a glass of milk
4 On an empty stomach

Level of Cognitive Ability: Applying
Client Needs: Physiological Integrity
Clinical Judgment/Cognitive Skills: Take Action
Integrated Process: Nursing Process/Implementation
Content Area: Pharmacology: Gastrointestinal: Laxatives
Health Problem: N/A

Answer: 4

Rationale: Bisacodyl is a laxative. The most rapid effect from bisacodyl occurs when it is taken on an empty stomach. If it is taken at bedtime, the client will have a bowel movement in the morning. It will not have a rapid effect if taken with a large meal. Taking the medication with a glass of milk will not speed up its effect.

Priority Nursing Tip: The client taking a laxative needs to increase fluid intake to prevent dehydration.

Test-Taking Strategy: Focus on the **subject,** bisacodyl. Recalling that medications generally are more effective if taken on an empty stomach will direct you to the correct option.

---

277. A client diagnosed with acute respiratory distress syndrome has a prescription to be placed on a continuous positive airway pressure (CPAP) face mask. What intervention would the nurse assisting in caring for the client implement for this procedure to be beneficial?

1 Obtain baseline arterial blood gases.
2 Obtain baseline pulse oximetry levels.
3 Apply the mask to the face with a snug fit.
4 Remove the mask for deep breathing exercises.

Level of Cognitive Ability: Applying
Client Needs: Physiological Integrity
Clinical Judgment/Cognitive Skills: Take Action
Integrated Process: Nursing Process/ Implementation
Content Area: Complex Care: Acute Respiratory Failure
Health Problem: Adult Health: Respiratory: Acute Respiratory Distress Syndrome

Answer: 3
Rationale: The CPAP face mask must be applied over the nose and mouth with a snug fit, which is necessary to maintain positive pressure in the client's airways. The nurse obtains baseline respiratory assessments and arterial blood gases to evaluate the effectiveness of therapy, but these are not done to increase the effectiveness of the procedure. A disadvantage of the CPAP face mask is that the client must remove it for coughing, eating, or drinking. This removes the benefit of positive pressure in the airway each time it is removed.
Priority Nursing Tip: In acute respiratory distress syndrome, the major site of injury is the alveolar capillary membrane.

Test-Taking Strategy: Focus on the **subject,** CPAP. Options 1 and 2 do not make the therapy more effective and are eliminated. From the remaining options, knowing that positive pressure must be maintained to be effective will direct you to the correct option.

---

278. The nurse is assisting in caring for a client scheduled to undergo a cardiac catheterization for the first time. Which information would the nurse share with the client regarding the procedure?

1 "The procedure is performed in the operating room."
2 "The initial catheter insertion is quite painful; after that, there is little or no pain."
3 "You may feel fatigue and have various aches because it is necessary to lie quietly on a stationary x-ray table for about 4 hours."
4 "You may feel certain sensations at various points during the procedure, such as a fluttery feeling, flushed warm feeling, desire to cough, or palpitations."

Level of Cognitive Ability: Applying
Client Needs: Physiological Integrity
Clinical Judgment/Cognitive Skills: Take Action
Integrated Process: Nursing Process/ Implementation
Content Area: Foundations of Care: Diagnostic Tests
Health Problem: N/A

Answer: 4
Rationale: Cardiac catheterization is an invasive test that involves the insertion of a catheter and the injection of dye into the heart and surrounding vessels to obtain information about the structure and function of the heart chambers and valves and the coronary circulation. Access is made by the insertion of a needle in either side of the groin into an artery and the catheter is advanced up to the heart through the abdomen and chest. Preprocedure teaching points include that the procedure is done in a darkened cardiac catheterization room and that electrocardiogram (ECG) leads are attached to the client. A local anesthetic is used so that there is little to no pain with catheter insertion. The x-ray table is hard but can be tilted periodically. The procedure may take up to 2 hours, and the client may feel various sensations with catheter passage and dye injection.
Priority Nursing Tip: Monitor the postcardiac catheterization client closely. Notify the primary health care provider immediately if the client complains of numbness or tingling of the affected extremity; the extremity becomes cool, pale, or cyanotic; or if loss of peripheral pulses occurs.

Test-Taking Strategy: Focus on the **subject,** cardiac catheterization. The location (operating room) eliminates option 1. The duration of the procedure, 4 hours, eliminates option 3. From the remaining options, noting the words *quite painful* in option 2 will assist in eliminating this option.

---

279. The nurse hangs an intravenous (IV) bag of 1000 mL of 5% dextrose in water (D_5W) at 3 PM and sets the flow rate to infuse at 75 mL/hr. At 11 PM, the nurse would expect the fluid remaining in the IV bag to be at approximately which level? **Fill in the blank.**

Answer: ______ mL

Level of Cognitive Ability: Applying
Client Needs: Physiological Integrity
Clinical Judgment/Cognitive Skills: Generate Solutions
Integrated Process: Nursing Process/Data Collection
Content Area: Skills: Dosage Calculations
Health Problem: N/A

Answer: 400
Rationale: In an 8-hour period, 600 mL would infuse if an IV is set to infuse at 75 mL/hr. Therefore, 400 mL would remain in the IV bag.
Priority Nursing Tip: If a solution of D_5W is prescribed for a client with diabetes mellitus, confirm the prescription because the solution can increase the client's blood glucose level.

Test-Taking Strategy: Focus on the **subject,** IV calculations. Review the data in the question and use simple math to determine that in an 8-hour period (3 PM to 11 PM), 600 mL would infuse (8 hours × 75 mL/hr = 600 mL). This means that 400 mL would remain. Perform the calculation and then verify your answer using a calculator.

---

280. The licensed practical nurse (LPN) is assisting the registered nurse in admitting a client diagnosed with myocardial infarction (MI) to the coronary care unit (CCU). The LPN would plan care by implementing which intervention?

1 Beginning thrombolytic therapy
2 Placing the client on continuous cardiac monitoring
3 Infusing intravenous (IV) fluid at a rate of 150 mL/hr
4 Administering oxygen at a rate of 6 L/min by nasal cannula

Level of Cognitive Ability: Applying
Client Needs: Physiological Integrity
Clinical Judgment/Cognitive Skills: Generate Solutions
Integrated Process: Nursing Process/Planning
Content Area: Complex Care: Emergency Situations/Management
Health Problem: Adult Health: Cardiovascular: Myocardial Infarction

Answer: 2
Rationale: Standard interventions upon admittance to the CCU as they relate to this question include continuous cardiac monitoring. Thrombolytic therapy may or may not be prescribed by the primary health care provider. Thrombolytic agents are most effective if administered within the first 6 hours of the coronary event. The nurse needs to ensure that there is an adequate IV line insertion of an intermittent lock. If an IV infusion is administered, it is maintained at a keep-vein-open rate to prevent fluid overload and heart failure. Oxygen needs to be administered at a rate of 2 to 4 L/min unless otherwise prescribed.
Priority Nursing Tip: Not all clients experience the classic symptoms of MI. Women may experience atypical discomfort, shortness of breath, or fatigue, and often present with non–ST elevation myocardial infarction or T-wave inversion.

Test-Taking Strategy: Focus on the **subject,** MI care. Eliminate options 3 and 4 because the values related to the rates of IV fluid and oxygen are high. From the remaining options, note the relationship between the client's diagnosis and option 2.

---

281. The licensed practical nurse (LPN) is looking at an electrocardiogram (ECG) rhythm strip with the registered nurse. The LPN understands that which is a normal PR interval? **Refer to the figure.**

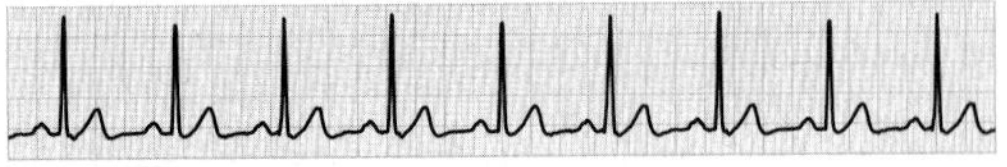

1 0.12 second
2 0.20 second
3 0.24 second
4 0.40 second

Level of Cognitive Ability: Applying
Client Needs: Physiological Integrity
Clinical Judgment/Cognitive Skills: Recognize Cues
Integrated Process: Nursing Process/Data Collection
Content Area: Foundations of Care: Diagnostic Tests
Health Problem: N/A

Answer: 1
Rationale: Standard ECG graph paper measurements are 0.04 second for each small box on the horizontal axis (measuring time) and 1 mm (measuring voltage) for each small box on the vertical axis. The normal PR interval is 0.12 second.
Priority Nursing Tip: Inform the client that an electrical shock will not occur when performing an electrocardiogram test.

Test-Taking Strategy: Focus on the **subject,** ECG. Knowledge regarding ECG basics is necessary to answer this question. Knowing that each small box is equal to 0.04 second and that there are three small boxes will direct you to the correct option.

---

282. The nurse is applying electrocardiogram (ECG) electrodes to a diaphoretic client. Which intervention would the nurse take to keep the electrodes securely in place?
1 Secure the electrodes with adhesive tape.
2 Place clear, transparent dressings over the electrodes.
3 Apply lanolin to the skin before applying the electrodes.
4 Cleanse the skin with alcohol before applying the electrodes.

Level of Cognitive Ability: Applying
Client Needs: Physiological Integrity
Clinical Judgment/Cognitive Skills: Take Action
Integrated Process: Nursing Process/Implementation
Content Area: Foundations of Care: Diagnostic Tests
Health Problem: N/A

Answer: 4
Rationale: Alcohol defats the skin and helps the electrodes adhere to it. Placing adhesive tape or a clear dressing over the electrodes will not help the adhesive gel of the actual electrode make better contact with the diaphoretic skin. Lanolin or any other lotion makes the skin slippery and prevents good initial adherence.
Priority Nursing Tip: To obtain an accurate reading when performing an ECG, instruct the client to lie still, breathe normally, and refrain from talking during the test.

Test-Taking Strategy: Focus on the **subject,** ECG. Note that options 1 and 2 are **comparable or alike** in that they both provide an external form of providing security of the electrodes. From the remaining options, note that option 4 addresses cleansing the skin.

---

283. The nurse has assisted in creating a plan of care for a client with a diagnosis of anterior cord syndrome. Which intervention would the nurse include in the plan of care to minimize the client's long-term risk for injury?

1 Change the client's positions slowly.
2 Check the client for decreased sensation to touch.
3 Check the client for decreased sensation to vibration.
4 Teach the client about loss of motor function and decreased pain sensation.

Level of Cognitive Ability: Creating
Client Needs: Physiological Integrity
Clinical Judgment/Cognitive Skills: Generate Solutions
Integrated Process: Nursing Process/Planning
Content Area: Adult Health: Neurological
Health Problem: Adult Health: Neurological: Spinal Cord Injury

Answer: 4

Rationale: Anterior cord syndrome is caused by damage to the anterior portion of the gray and white matter. Clinical findings related to anterior cord syndrome include loss of motor function, temperature sensation, and pain sensation below the level of injury. The syndrome does not affect sensations of fine touch, position, and vibration.

Priority Nursing Tip: The level of the spinal cord injury is determined by checking for the lowest spinal cord segment with intact motor and sensory function.

Test-Taking Strategy: Focus on the **subject,** anterior cord syndrome. Specific knowledge of anterior cord syndrome is necessary to answer this question. Eliminate option 1 first, knowing that position is not affected below the level of injury. Eliminate options 2 and 3, knowing that in anterior cord syndrome sensations of touch and vibration remain intact. Remember that this type of injury involves complete motor function loss and decreased temperature and pain sensation, directing you to the correct option.

---

284. The nurse is caring for a client who has experienced a thoracic spinal cord injury. In the event that spinal shock occurs, which intravenous (IV) fluid would the nurse anticipate being prescribed for the client?

1 Dextran
2 0.9% normal saline
3 5% dextrose in water
4 5% dextrose in 0.9% normal saline

Level of Cognitive Ability: Analyzing
Client Needs: Physiological Integrity
Clinical Judgment/Cognitive Skills: Generate Solutions
Integrated Process: Nursing Process/Planning
Content Area: Complex Care: Shock
Health Problem: Adult Health: Neurological: Spinal Cord Injury

Answer: 2

Rationale: Normal saline 0.9% is an isotonic solution that primarily remains in the intravascular space, increasing intravascular volume. This IV fluid would increase the client's blood pressure. Dextran is rarely used in spinal shock because isotonic fluid administration is usually sufficient. Additionally, Dextran has potential adverse effects. Dextrose 5% in water is a hypotonic solution that pulls fluid out of the intravascular space and is not indicated for shock. Dextrose 5% in normal saline 0.9% is hypertonic and may be indicated for shock resulting from hemorrhage or burns.

Priority Nursing Tip: Spinal shock occurs within the first hour of spinal cord injury and can last days to months.

Test-Taking Strategy: Focus on the **subject,** spinal shock. Thinking about the manifestations of shock and using knowledge of the treatment for spinal shock and the purpose of the various IV fluids will direct you to the correct option. Also, remember that normal saline 0.9% is an isotonic solution that primarily remains in the intravascular space, increasing intravascular volume.

---

285. The nurse is caring for a client who will be taught to ambulate with a cane. Before cane-assisted ambulation instructions begin, what would the nurse check for as the **priority** to ensure client safety?

1 A high level of stamina and energy
2 Self-consciousness about using a cane
3 Full range of motion in lower extremities
4 Balance, muscle strength, and confidence

Level of Cognitive Ability: Applying
Client Needs: Physiological Integrity
Clinical Judgment/Cognitive Skills: Recognize Cues
Integrated Process: Nursing Process/Data Collection
Content Area: Skills: Activity/Mobility
Health Problem: N/A

Answer: 4

Rationale: Checking the client's balance, strength, and confidence helps determine whether the cane is a suitable assistive device for the client. A high level of stamina and full range of motion are not needed for walking with a cane. Although body image (self-consciousness) is a component of the assessment, it is not the priority.

Priority Nursing Tip: Safety is a priority concern when the client uses an assistive device such as a cane.

Test-Taking Strategy: Note the **strategic word,** *priority,* and focus on the **subject,** cane-assisted ambulation. Eliminate options 1 and 2 first because they are not required for the use of a cane. Use **Maslow's Hierarchy of Needs theory** to assist in directing you to the correct option.

---

286. A primary health care provider prescribes 1000 mL of normal saline to infuse at 100 mL/hr. The drop factor is 10 drops/mL. The nurse would set the flow rate at how many drops per minute? **Fill in the blank and round your answer to the nearest whole number.**

Answer: _____ drops per minute

Level of Cognitive Ability: Applying
Client Needs: Physiological Integrity
Clinical Judgment/Cognitive Skills: Generate Solutions
Integrated Process: Nursing Process/Implementation
Content Area: Skills: Dosage Calculations
Health Problem: N/A

Answer: 17

Rationale: It will take 10 hours for 1000 mL to infuse at 100 mL/hr (1000 mL ÷ 100 mL = 10 hour × 60 min = 600 min). Next, use the intravenous (IV) flow rate formula.

Formula:

$$\frac{\text{Total volume} \times \text{drop factor}}{\text{Time in minutes}} = \text{drops/minute}$$

$$\frac{1000 \text{ mL} \times 10 \text{ drops/mL}}{600 \text{ min}} = \frac{10{,}000}{600} = 16.6, \text{ or } 17 \text{ drops/minute}$$

Priority Nursing Tip: The nurse would never increase the rate of an IV solution to catch up if the infusion is running behind schedule.

Test-Taking Strategy: Focus on the **subject,** IV calculations. First, determine how many hours that it will take for 1000 mL to infuse at 100 mL/hr. Next use the formula for calculating IV flow rates and verify the answer using a calculator. Remember to round the answer to the nearest whole number.

---

287. The nurse is collecting data on a pregnant client who has cardiac disease at the 30 weeks' gestation antenatal visit. The nurse checks lung sounds in the lower lobes after a routine blood pressure screening. The nurse performs this assessment to elicit what information?

1 Identify mitral valve prolapse
2 Identify cardiac dysrhythmias
3 Rule out the possibility of pneumonia
4 Identify early signs of heart failure (HF)

Level of Cognitive Ability: Analyzing
Client Needs: Physiological Integrity
Clinical Judgment/Cognitive Skills: Recognize Cues
Integrated Process: Nursing Process/Data Collection
Content Area: Maternity: Antepartum
Health Problem: Maternity: Cardiac Disease

Answer: 4
Rationale: Fluid volume during pregnancy peaks between 18 and 32 weeks' gestation. During this period, it is essential to observe and record maternal data that would indicate further signs of cardiac decompensation or HF in the pregnant client with cardiac disease. By checking lung sounds, the nurse may identify early symptoms of diminished oxygen exchange and potential HF. Options 1, 2, and 3 are unrelated to the data in the question.
Priority Nursing Tip: Monitor the pregnant client with cardiac disease for manifestations of cardiac stress and decompensation, such as cough, fatigue, dyspnea, chest pain, and tachycardia.

Test-Taking Strategy: Focus on the **subject**, a pregnant client with cardiac disease. Note the relationship between cardiac disease and lung sounds in the question and the words *heart failure* in the correct option.

---

288. The nurse is caring for a client prescribed digoxin. Which manifestations correlate with a digoxin level of 2.3 ng/dL? **Select all that apply.**

1 Nausea
2 Drowsiness
3 Photophobia
4 Increased appetite
5 Increased energy level
6 Seeing halos around bright objects

Level of Cognitive Ability: Analyzing
Client Needs: Physiological Integrity
Clinical Judgment/Cognitive Skills: Recognize Cues
Integrated Process: Nursing Process/Data Collection
Content Area: Pharmacology: Cardiovascular: Antidysrhythmics
Health Problem: N/A

Answer: 1, 2, 3, 6
Rationale: Digoxin is a cardiac glycoside used to manage and treat heart failure, control ventricular rate in clients with atrial fibrillation, and treat and prevent recurrent paroxysmal atrial tachycardia. The therapeutic range is 0.8 to 2.0 ng/mL (1.02 to 2.56 nmol/L). Signs of toxicity include gastrointestinal disturbances including anorexia, nausea, and vomiting; neurological abnormalities such as fatigue, headache, depression, weakness, drowsiness, confusion, and nightmares; facial pain; personality changes; and ocular disturbances such as photophobia, halos around bright lights, and yellow or green color perception.
Priority Nursing Tip: The nurse needs to check the client's apical pulse rate for 1 full minute before administering digoxin. If it is lower than 60 beats per minute, the medication is withheld and the primary health care provider is notified.

Test-Taking Strategy: Focus on the **subject**, a digoxin level of 2.3 ng/dL. Recalling that signs of digoxin toxicity include gastrointestinal disturbances, neurological abnormalities, and ocular disturbances will assist in answering the question correctly.

---

289. Which interventions would the emergency department nurse prepare for in the care of a child with croup and epiglottitis? **Select all that apply.**

1 Obtaining a chest x-ray
2 Obtaining a throat culture
3 Monitoring pulse oximetry
4 Maintaining a patent airway
5 Providing humidified oxygen
6 Administering antipyretics and antibiotics

Level of Cognitive Ability: Analyzing
Client Needs: Physiological Integrity
Clinical Judgment/Cognitive Skills: Take Action
Integrated Process: Nursing Process/Implementation
Content Area: Complex Care: Emergency Situations/Management
Health Problem: Pediatric-Specific: Croup

Answer: 1, 3, 4, 5, 6

Rationale: Epiglottitis is an acute inflammation and swelling of the epiglottis and surrounding tissue. It is a life-threatening, rapidly progressive condition that may cause complete airway obstruction within a few hours of onset. The most reliable diagnostic sign is an edematous, cherry-red epiglottis. Some interventions include obtaining a chest x-ray film, monitoring pulse oximetry, maintaining a patent airway, providing humidified oxygen, and administering antipyretics and antibiotics. The child may also require intubation and mechanical ventilation. The primary concern in a child with epiglottitis is the development of complete airway obstruction. Therefore, the child's throat is not examined or cultured because any stimulation with a tongue depressor or culture swab could trigger complete airway obstruction.

Priority Nursing Tip: Epiglottitis is considered an emergency situation because it can progress rapidly to severe respiratory distress.

Test-Taking Strategy: Focus on the **subject,** epiglottitis. Focus on the **ABCs—airway, breathing, and circulation.** Remember that the primary concern is the development of complete airway obstruction and that any stimulation with a tongue depressor or culture swab could trigger complete airway obstruction. This will assist in eliminating the only incorrect option, option 2.

---

290. A child diagnosed with rheumatic fever is admitted to the hospital. The nurse assisting in the care of the child prepares to manage which clinical manifestations of this disorder? **Select all that apply.**

1 Cardiac murmur
2 Cardiac enlargement
3 Cool, pale skin over the joints
4 White, painful skin lesions on the trunk
5 Small, nontender lumps on bony prominences
6 Purposeless, jerky movements of the extremities and face

Level of Cognitive Ability: Analyzing
Client Needs: Physiological Integrity
Clinical Judgment/Cognitive Skills: Recognize Cues
Integrated Process: Nursing Process/Data Collection
Content Area: Pediatrics: Cardiovascular
Health Problem: Pediatric-Specific: Rheumatic Fever

Answer: 1, 2, 5, 6

Rationale: Rheumatic fever is a systemic inflammatory disease that may develop as a delayed reaction to an inadequately treated infection of the upper respiratory tract by group A beta-hemolytic streptococci. Clinical manifestations of rheumatic fever are related to the inflammatory response. Major manifestations include carditis, manifested as inflammation of the endocardium, including the valves, myocardium, and pericardium; cardiac murmur and cardiac enlargement; subcutaneous nodules, manifested as small, nontender lumps on joints and bony prominences; chorea, manifested as involuntary, purposeless, jerky movements of the legs, arms, and face with speech impairment; arthritis manifested as tender, warm, erythematous skin over the joints; and erythema marginatum, manifested as red, painless skin lesions usually over the trunk.

Priority Nursing Tip: Initiate seizure precautions if the child with rheumatic fever exhibits manifestations of chorea (involuntary, purposeless, jerky movements of the legs, arms, and face with speech impairment).

Test-Taking Strategy: Focus on the **subject**, rheumatic fever. Recalling that rheumatic fever is a systemic inflammatory disease and noting the words *cool* in option 3 and *white* in option 4 will assist in answering this question. Remember that the client will exhibit tender, warm, erythematous skin over the joints and red, painless skin lesions, usually over the trunk.

---

291. A client hospitalized with a diagnosis of thrombophlebitis is being treated with heparin infusion therapy. About 24 hours after the infusion has begun, the nurse notes that the client's partial thromboplastin time (PTT) is 65 seconds with a control of 30 seconds. What nursing action would the nurse expect will be done?

1 Repeating the laboratory test
2 Administering protamine sulfate
3 Discontinuing the heparin infusion
4 Documenting that the client is adequately anticoagulated

Level of Cognitive Ability: Applying
Client Needs: Physiological Integrity
Clinical Judgment/Cognitive Skills: Take Action
Integrated Process: Nursing Process/Implementation
Content Area: Pharmacology: Cardiovascular: Anticoagulants
Health Problem: Adult Health: Cardiovascular: Vascular Disorders

Answer: 4

Rationale: The effectiveness of heparin therapy is monitored by the results of the PTT. Desired range for therapeutic anticoagulation is 1.5 to 2.5 times the control. A PTT of 65 seconds is within the therapeutic range. Therefore, options 1, 2, and 3 are incorrect actions.

Priority Nursing Tip: Heparin is an anticoagulant, and the priority concern when a client is receiving an anticoagulant is bleeding.

Test-Taking Strategy: Focus on the **subject**, heparin infusion therapy. Remember that the desired range for therapeutic anticoagulation is 1.5 to 2.5 times the control. Noting that the control is 30 and that 1.5 to 2.5 times the control is a range of 45 to 75 will direct you to the correct option.

---

292. A client is brought to the emergency department reporting chest pain. Vital sign findings include a blood pressure (BP) of 150/90 mm Hg, pulse (P) 88 beats per minute (BPM), and respirations (R) 20 breaths per minute. As prescribed, the nurse administers nitroglycerin 0.4 mg sublingually. The treatment is found to be **effective** when the reassessment of vital signs shows which data?

1 BP 150/90 mm Hg, P 70 BPM, R 24 breaths per minute
2 BP 100/60 mm Hg, P 96 BPM, R 20 breaths per minute
3 BP 100/60 mm Hg, P 70 BPM, R 24 breaths per minute
4 BP 160/100 mm Hg, P 120 BPM, R 16 breaths per minute

Level of Cognitive Ability: Evaluating
Client Needs: Physiological Integrity
Clinical Judgment/Cognitive Skills: Evaluate Outcomes
Integrated Process: Nursing Process/Evaluation
Content Area: Pharmacology: Cardiovascular: Vasodilators
Health Problem: Adult Health: Cardiovascular: Coronary Artery Disease

Answer: 2

Rationale: Nitroglycerin dilates both arteries and veins, causing blood to pool in the periphery. This causes a reduced preload and therefore a drop in cardiac output. This vasodilation causes the blood pressure to fall. The drop in cardiac output causes the sympathetic nervous system to respond and attempt to maintain cardiac output by increasing the pulse. Beta blockers, such as propranolol, are often used in conjunction with nitroglycerin to prevent this rise in heart rate. If chest pain is reduced and cardiac workload is reduced, the client will be more comfortable; therefore, a rise in respirations would not be seen.

Priority Nursing Tip: Check the client's blood pressure before administering each dose of nitroglycerin. Nitroglycerin dilates the blood vessels and causes a drop in blood pressure.

Test-Taking Strategy: Focus on the **subject**, nitroglycerin administration. Note the **strategic word,** *effective.* Knowing that nitroglycerin is a vasodilator and that it causes the BP to drop will assist in eliminating options 1 and 4. Next, recall that if chest pain is reduced and cardiac workload is reduced, the client will be more comfortable; therefore, a rise in respirations would not be seen. This assists in eliminating option 3.

---

293. A client who underwent surgical repair of an abdominal aortic aneurysm is 1 day postoperative. The nurse assisting in caring for the client performs an abdominal assessment and notes the absence of bowel sounds. What action would the nurse take?

1 Start the client on sips of water.
2 Remove the nasogastric (NG) tube.
3 Document the finding and continue to check for bowel sounds.
4 Ask the registered nurse to call the primary health care provider immediately.

Level of Cognitive Ability: Applying
Client Needs: Physiological Integrity
Clinical Judgment/Cognitive Skills: Take Action
Integrated Process: Nursing Process/Implementation
Content Area: Foundations of Care: Perioperative Care
Health Problem: Adult Health: Cardiovascular: Vascular Disorders

Answer: 3

Rationale: Bowel sounds may be absent for 3 to 4 postoperative days because of bowel manipulation during surgery. The nurse would document the finding and continue to monitor the client. The NG tube would stay in place if present, and the client is kept NPO until after the onset of bowel sounds. Additionally, the nurse does not remove the tube without a prescription to do so. The nurse would report the findings to the registered nurse, but there is no need to call the primary health care provider immediately at this time.

Priority Nursing Tip: In the postoperative period, ask the client about the passage of flatus. This is the best initial indicator of the return of intestinal activity.

Test-Taking Strategy: Focus on the **subject,** postoperative care. Note the words *1 day postoperative*. Eliminate option 2 because there are no data in the question regarding the presence of an NG tube. Additionally, an NG tube would not be removed and the client would not be fed (option 1) if bowel sounds were absent. Recalling that bowel sounds may not return for 3 to 4 postoperative days will direct you to the correct option from the remaining options.

---

294. The nurse has assisted to admit a client diagnosed with gestational hypertension who is in labor. The nurse monitors the client closely for which complication of gestational hypertension?

1 Seizures
2 Hallucinations
3 Placenta previa
4 Altered respiratory status

Level of Cognitive Ability: Applying
Client Needs: Physiological Integrity
Clinical Judgment/Cognitive Skills: Recognize Cues
Integrated Process: Nursing Process/Data Collection
Content Area: Maternity: Intrapartum
Health Problem: Maternity: Gestational Hypertension/Preeclampsia and Eclampsia

Answer: 1

Rationale: Gestational hypertension can lead to preeclampsia and eclampsia; therefore, a major complication of gestational hypertension is seizures. Hallucinations, placenta previa, and altered respiratory status are not directly associated with gestational hypertension.

Priority Nursing Tip: Gestational hypertension refers to a condition in which blood pressure elevation is first detected after midpregnancy. Proteinuria is absent.

Test-Taking Strategy: Focus on the **subject,** complications of gestational hypertension. Remember that seizures are a concern with gestational hypertension to direct you to the correct option.

---

295. Which medication instructions would the nurse reinforce to a client who has been prescribed levothyroxine? **Select all that apply.**

1 Monitor your own pulse rate.
2 Take the medication in the morning.
3 Take the medication at the same time each day.
4 Notify the primary health care provider if chest pain occurs.
5 Expect the pulse rate to be greater than 100 beats per minute.
6 It may take 1 to 3 weeks for a full therapeutic effect to occur.

Level of Cognitive Ability: Applying
Client Needs: Physiological Integrity
Clinical Judgment/Cognitive Skills: Take Action
Integrated Process: Teaching and Learning
Content Area: Pharmacology: Endocrine: Thyroid Hormones
Health Problem: Adult Health: Endocrine: Thyroid Disorders

Answer: 1, 2, 3, 4, 6

Rationale: Levothyroxine is a thyroid hormone. The client is instructed to monitor her or his own pulse rate. The client is also instructed to take the medication in the morning before breakfast to prevent insomnia and to take the medication at the same time each day to maintain hormone levels. The client is told not to discontinue the medication and that thyroid replacement is lifelong. Additional instructions include contacting the primary health care provider if the rate is more than 100 beats per minute and notifying the primary health care provider if chest pain occurs, or if weight loss, nervousness and tremors, or insomnia develops. The client is also told that full therapeutic effect may take 1 to 3 weeks and that he or she needs to have follow-up thyroid blood studies to monitor therapy.

Priority Nursing Tip: Foods that can inhibit thyroid secretion include strawberries, peaches, pears, cabbage, turnips, spinach, kale, brussels sprouts, cauliflower, radishes, and peas.

Test-Taking Strategy: Focus on the **subject,** levothyroxine. Think about the effects of the medication as you read each option. Noting the words *more than 100 beats per minute* in option 5 will assist in eliminating this option.

---

296. The hemoglobin levels of a client in the first trimester of pregnancy are indicative of iron-deficiency anemia. Which findings support the diagnosis of this type of anemia? **Select all that apply.**

1 Yellowish sclera
2 Reports of severe fatigue
3 Pink mucous membranes
4 Increased vaginal secretions
5 Reports of frequent headaches
6 Reports of increased frequency of voiding

Level of Cognitive Ability: Applying
Client Needs: Physiological Integrity
Clinical Judgment/Cognitive Skills: Recognize Cues
Integrated Process: Nursing Process/Data Collection
Content Area: Maternity: Antepartum
Health Problem: Adult Health: Hematological: Anemias

Answer: 2, 5

Rationale: Iron-deficiency anemia is described as a hemoglobin blood concentration of less than 10.5 to 11.0 g/dL. Complaints of headaches and severe fatigue are abnormal findings and may reflect complications of this type of anemia caused by the decreased oxygen supply to vital organs. Options 3, 4, and 6 are normal findings in the first trimester of pregnancy. Yellow sclera (whites of the eyes) is associated with jaundice.

Priority Nursing Tip: The hemoglobin and hematocrit levels decline during pregnancy as a result of increased plasma volume.

Test-Taking Strategy: Focus on the **subject,** iron-deficiency anemia, and note that the client is in the first trimester of pregnancy. Options 2 and 5 are abnormal and may reflect complications caused by the decreased oxygen supply to vital organs. Options 3, 4, and 6 are normal occurrences of pregnancy, whereas option 1, yellowish sclera, is not associated with either pregnancy or iron-deficiency anemia.

---

297. A client diagnosed with multiple myeloma is receiving intravenous hydration at 100 mL/hr. Which finding indicates to the nurse that the client is experiencing a positive response to the treatment plan?

1 Creatinine of 1.0 mg/dL
2 Weight increase of 1 kilogram
3 Respirations of 18 breaths per minute
4 White blood cell count of 6000 mm^3

Level of Cognitive Ability: Evaluating
Client Needs: Physiological Integrity
Clinical Judgment/Cognitive Skills: Evaluate Outcomes
Integrated Process: Nursing Process/Evaluation
Content Area: Adult Health: Oncology
Health Problem: Adult Health: Cancer: Multiple Myeloma

Answer: 1
Rationale: Multiple myeloma is a malignant proliferation of plasma cells within the bone. Renal failure is a concern in the client with this condition. In multiple myeloma, hydration is essential to prevent renal damage resulting from precipitation of protein in the renal tubules and excessive calcium and uric acid in the blood. Creatinine is the most accurate measure of renal function. Options 3 and 4 are unrelated to the subject of hydration. Weight gain is not a positive sign when concerned with renal status.
Priority Nursing Tip: The client with multiple myeloma is at risk for pathological fractures.

Test-Taking Strategy: Focus on the **subject,** hydration and multiple myeloma. Recalling that kidney failure is a concern in multiple myeloma will direct you to the correct option. Additionally, option 1 is the only choice that is related to hydration status.

---

298. The nurse reinforces discharge instructions to a client who is recovering from testicular cancer surgery. Which instruction would the nurse include?

1 To avoid driving a car for at least 2 weeks
2 Not to be fitted for a prosthesis for at least 3 months
3 To avoid sitting for long periods for at least 2 weeks
4 To report any elevation in temperature to the primary health care provider

Level of Cognitive Ability: Applying
Client Needs: Physiological Integrity
Clinical Judgment/Cognitive Skills: Take Action
Integrated Process: Teaching and Learning
Content Area: Adult Health: Oncology
Health Problem: Adult Health: Cancer: Testicular

Answer: 4
Rationale: For the client who has had testicular surgery, the nurse would emphasize the importance of notifying the primary health care provider if chills, fever, drainage, redness, or discharge occurs. These symptoms may indicate the presence of an infection. One week after testicular surgery, the client may drive. Often, a prosthesis is inserted during surgery. Sitting needs to be avoided with prostate surgery because of the risk of hemorrhage, but this risk is not as high with testicular surgery.
Priority Nursing Tip: Testicular self-examination needs to be performed monthly. A day of the month is selected, and the examination is performed on the same day each month.

Test-Taking Strategy: Focus on the **subject,** post-testicular surgery care. Use **Maslow's Hierarchy of Needs theory** and principles related to prioritizing. Infection is a priority. After any surgical procedure, elevation of temperature could signal an infection and needs to be reported. Also note the lengthy time periods in options 1, 2, and 3. These will assist in eliminating these options.

---

299. An interprofessional team working with the spouse of a home-care client who has end-stage liver failure is teaching the spouse about pain management. Which statement by the spouse indicates the **need for further teaching?**

1 "My husband can use breathing exercises to control pain."
2 "I will help prevent constipation with increased fluids."
3 "If the pain increases, I will report it to the nurse promptly."
4 "The medication causes very deep sleep that my husband needs."

Level of Cognitive Ability: Evaluating
Client Needs: Physiological Integrity
Clinical Judgment/Cognitive Skills: Evaluate Outcomes
Integrated Process: Teaching and Learning
Content Area: Skills: Client Teaching
Health Problem: Adult Health: Gastrointestinal: Accessory Organs

Answer: 4

Rationale: In the client with liver disease, the ability to metabolize medication is affected. A decreased level of consciousness is a potential clinical indicator of medication overdose, as well as fluid, electrolyte, and oxygenation deficiencies; thus, the nurse teaches the client's spouse about the differences between sleep related to pain relief and a deteriorating change in neurological status. Options 1, 2, and 3 all indicate an understanding of suitable steps to be taken in pain management.

Priority Nursing Tip: The administration of opioids, sedatives, barbiturates, and any hepatotoxic medications is avoided in the client with liver disease.

Test-Taking Strategy: Note the **strategic words,** *need for further teaching.* These words indicate a **negative event query** and the need to select the option that is an incorrect statement. Note that the client has end-stage liver disease, meaning that analgesics take longer to metabolize, so the dosage is likely to have a greater and longer effect than in a client without liver disease. Focusing on the **subject,** pain management in a client who has end-stage liver failure, will direct you to the correct option.

---

300. The nurse is reviewing the antenatal history of several clients in early labor. The nurse recognizes which factor documented in the history as having the potential for causing neonatal sepsis after delivery? **Select all that apply.**

1 Of non-American heritage
2 Two previous miscarriages
3 Prenatal care began during the third trimester
4 History of substance abuse during pregnancy
5 Dietary information identified poor eating habits
6 Spontaneous rupture of membranes 24 hours ago

Level of Cognitive Ability: Analyzing
Client Needs: Physiological Integrity
Clinical Judgment/Cognitive Skills: Recognize Cues
Integrated Process: Nursing Process/Data Collection
Content Area: Maternity: Intrapartum
Health Problem: Maternity: Infections/Inflammations

Answer: 3, 4, 5, 6

Rationale: Risk factors for neonatal sepsis can arise from maternal, intrapartal, or neonatal conditions. Maternal risk factors before delivery include a history of substance abuse during pregnancy, low socioeconomic status, and poor prenatal care and nutrition. Premature rupture of the membranes or prolonged rupture of membranes longer than 18 hours before birth is also a risk factor for neonatal acquisition of infection. There is no research to associate heritage or previous miscarriages to the development of neonatal sepsis.

Priority Nursing Tip: If antibiotics are prescribed for a newborn, monitor the newborn carefully for toxicity because a newborn's liver and kidneys are immature.

Test-Taking Strategy: Focus on the **subject,** risk factor for neonatal sepsis. Eliminate options that have no connection to the risk of infection.

---

301. The nurse collecting data on a prenatal client in the first trimester of pregnancy discovers that the client frequently consumes beverages containing alcohol. Why would the nurse initiate interventions **immediately** to assist the client in avoiding alcohol consumption?

1 To reduce the potential for fetal growth restriction in utero
2 To promote the normal psychosocial adaptation of the parent to pregnancy
3 To minimize the potential for placental abruptions during the intrapartum period
4 To reduce the risk of teratogenic effects to the embryo's developing fetal organs and tissue

Level of Cognitive Ability: Analyzing
Client Needs: Physiological Integrity
Clinical Judgment/Cognitive Skills: Take Action
Integrated Process: Nursing Process/Implementation
Content Area: Maternity: Antepartum
Health Problem: N/A

Answer: 4

Rationale: In the first trimester, organogenesis is characterized by the differentiation and development of fetal organs, systems, and structures. The effects of alcohol on the developing fetus during this critical period depend not only on the amount of alcohol consumed but also on the interaction of quantity, frequency, type of alcohol, and other medications that may be abused during this period by the pregnant woman. Eliminating consumption of alcohol during this time may promote normal fetal organ development. Although options 1, 2, and 3 may be concerns, they are not specifically associated with the first trimester of pregnancy.

Priority Nursing Tip: Fetal alcohol syndrome is caused by maternal alcohol use during pregnancy and causes physical and intellectual disabilities.

Test-Taking Strategy: Focus on the **subject,** effects of alcohol on the fetus, and note the **strategic word,** *immediately.* Recall that during the first trimester, development of fetal organs, tissues, and structures takes place.

---

302. The nurse is assisting in admitting a client with a diagnosis of hypothyroidism. Which would the nurse perform to obtain data related to this diagnosis?

1 Inspect facial features.
2 Auscultate lung sounds.
3 Percuss the thyroid gland.
4 Inspect ability to ambulate safely.

Level of Cognitive Ability: Applying
Client Needs: Physiological Integrity
Clinical Judgment/Cognitive Skills: Recognize Cues
Integrated Process: Nursing Process/Data Collection
Content Area: Adult Health: Endocrine
Health Problem: Adult Health: Endocrine: Thyroid Disorders

Answer: 1

Rationale: Inspection of facial features will reveal the characteristic coarse features, presence of edema around the eyes and face, and the blank expression that are characteristics of hypothyroidism. The techniques in options 2, 3, and 4 will not reveal information related to the diagnosis of hypothyroidism.

Priority Nursing Tip: Hypothyroidism is characterized by a decreased rate of metabolism. Clinical manifestations relate to this characteristic.

Test-Taking Strategy: Focus on the **subject,** hypothyroidism. Eliminate options 2 and 4 because they do not relate to the thyroid gland. From the remaining options, recall that palpation, rather than percussion, of the thyroid is the assessment technique used to evaluate the thyroid gland.

---

303. The nurse is teaching a client diagnosed with chronic obstructive pulmonary disease (COPD) how to do pursed-lip breathing. Evaluation of understanding is evident if the client performs which action?

1 Breathes in and then holds the breath for 30 seconds
2 Loosens the abdominal muscles while breathing out
3 Inhales with puckered lips and exhales with the mouth open wide
4 Breathes so that expiration is 2 to 3 times as long as inspiration

Level of Cognitive Ability: Evaluating
Client Needs: Physiological Integrity
Clinical Judgment/Cognitive Skills: Evaluate Outcomes
Integrated Process: Nursing Process/Evaluation
Content Area: Adult Health: Respiratory
Health Problem: Adult Health: Respiratory: Obstructive Pulmonary Disease

Answer: 4
Rationale: COPD is a disease state characterized by airflow obstruction. Prolonging expiration time reduces air trapping caused by airway narrowing that occurs in COPD. The client is not instructed to breathe in and hold the breath for 30 seconds; this action has no useful purpose for the client with COPD. Tightening (not loosening) the abdominal muscles aids in expelling air. Exhaling through pursed lips (not with the mouth wide open) increases the intraluminal pressure and prevents the airways from collapsing.
Priority Nursing Tip: For the client with COPD, the stimulus to breathe is a low arterial Po_2 instead of an increased Pco_2.

Test-Taking Strategy: Focus on the **subject**, pursed-lip breathing in a client with COPD. Visualize each of the actions in the options. Recalling that a major purpose of pursed-lip breathing is to prevent air trapping during exhalation will direct you to the correct option.

---

304. While providing care to a client with a head injury, the nurse notes that a client exhibits this posture. What would the nurse document that the client is exhibiting? **Refer to the figure.**

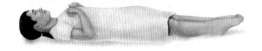

1 Flaccidity
2 Decorticate posturing
3 Decerebrate posturing
4 Rigidity in the upper extremities

Level of Cognitive Ability: Analyzing
Client Needs: Physiological Integrity
Clinical Judgment/Cognitive Skills: Recognize Cues
Integrated Process: Nursing Process/Data Collection
Content Area: Adult Health: Neurological
Health Problem: Adult Health: Neurological: Head Injury/Trauma

Answer: 2
Rationale: Decortication is abnormal posturing seen in the client with lesions that interrupt the corticospinal pathways. In this posturing, the client's arms, wrists, and fingers are flexed with internal rotation and plantar flexion of the feet and legs extended. Flaccidity indicates weak, soft, and flabby muscles that lack normal muscle tone. Decerebration is abnormal posturing and rigidity characterized by extension of the arms and legs, pronation of the arms, plantar flexion, and opisthotonos. Decerebration is usually associated with dysfunction in the brainstem area. Rigidity indicates hardness, stiffness, or inflexibility. Decerebrate posturing is associated with rigidity.
Priority Nursing Tip: Decorticate posturing is also known as *flexor posturing,* and decerebrate posturing is also known as *extensor posturing.*

Test-Taking Strategy: Focus on the **subject**, posturing. Review the figure and use knowledge regarding the characteristics of posturing to answer the question. First eliminate options 3 and 4 because they are **comparable or alike** in that decerebrate posturing is associated with rigidity. Next, recalling that flaccidity indicates weak, soft, and flabby muscles that lack normal muscle tone will assist in eliminating option 1.

---

305. A client prescribed lithium carbonate for the treatment of bipolar disorder has a medication blood level of 1.6 mEq/L. Which question would the nurse ask to determine whether the client is experiencing signs of lithium toxicity associated with this level?

1 "Do you hear ringing in your ears?"
2 "Have you noted that your vision is blurred?"
3 "Have you fallen recently because you are dizzy?"
4 "Have you been experiencing any nausea, vomiting, or diarrhea?"

Level of Cognitive Ability: Analyzing
Client Needs: Physiological Integrity
Clinical Judgment/Cognitive Skills: Recognize Cues
Integrated Process: Nursing Process/Data Collection
Content Area: Pharmacology: Psychotherapeutic: Mood Stabilizers
Health Problem: Mental Health: Mood Disorders

Answer: 4
Rationale: Normal lithium levels are between 0.8 and 1.2 mEq/L. One of the most common early signs of lower-level lithium toxicity is gastrointestinal (GI) disturbances such as nausea, vomiting, or diarrhea. The questions in options 1, 2, and 3 are related to the findings in lithium toxicity at higher levels.
Priority Nursing Tip: Instruct the client taking lithium carbonate to drink 6 to 8 glasses of water daily and to maintain an adequate intake of salt to prevent lithium toxicity.

Test-Taking Strategy: Focus on the **subject,** signs of lithium toxicity and toxic lithium levels. Recalling that GI disturbances are early manifestations will direct you to the correct option.

---

306. A postpartum nurse caring for a client who delivered vaginally 2 hours ago palpates the fundus and notes the character of the lochia. Which characteristic of the lochia would indicate to the nurse that the client's recovery is normal?

1 Pink-colored lochia
2 White-colored lochia
3 Serosanguineous lochia
4 Dark red-colored lochia

Level of Cognitive Ability: Evaluating
Client Needs: Physiological Integrity
Clinical Judgment/Cognitive Skills: Evaluate Outcomes
Integrated Process: Nursing Process/Data Collection
Content Area: Maternity: Postpartum
Health Problem: N/A

Answer: 4
Rationale: When checking the perineum, the lochia is monitored for amount, color, and the presence of clots. The color of the lochia during the fourth stage of labor (the first 1 to 4 hours after birth) is dark red. Options 1, 2, and 3 are not the expected characteristics of lochia at this time period.
Priority Nursing Tip: Lochia discharge should smell like normal menstrual flow. If it has a foul-smelling odor, infection would be suspected.

Test-Taking Strategy: Focus on the **subject,** lochia assessment postpartum. Noting that the question refers to a client who delivered 2 hours ago will direct you to the correct option.

---

307. The licensed practical nurse (LPN) is assisting a registered nurse (RN) in performing a prenatal examination on a client in the third trimester. The RN begins an abdominal examination that includes Leopold's maneuvers. The LPN understands that which information will be obtained after performing the first maneuver?

1 Fetal descent
2 Placenta previa
3 Fetal lie and presentation
4 Strength of uterine contractions

Level of Cognitive Ability: Analyzing
Client Needs: Physiological Integrity
Clinical Judgment/Cognitive Skills: Recognize Cues
Integrated Process: Nursing Process/Data Collection
Content Area: Maternity: Antepartum
Health Problem: N/A

Answer: 3
Rationale: The first maneuver, the fundal grip, determines the contents (size, consistency, shape, and mobility) of the fundus (either the fetal head or breech) and thereby the fetal lie. Fetal descent is determined with the fourth maneuver. Placenta previa is diagnosed by ultrasound and not by palpation. Leopold's maneuvers are not performed during a contraction.
Priority Nursing Tip: Before performing Leopold's maneuvers, the nurse would assist the client in emptying their bladder.

Test-Taking Strategy: Focus on the **subject,** Leopold's maneuvers; this will assist in eliminating options 2 and 4. From the remaining options, it is necessary to know that the first maneuver determines fetal lie.

---

308. The nurse is assisting in caring for a client who sustained a spinal cord injury that has resulted in spinal shock. Which assessment will provide relevant information about recovery from spinal shock?

1 Reflexes
2 Pulse rate
3 Temperature
4 Blood pressure

Level of Cognitive Ability: Analyzing
Client Needs: Physiological Integrity
Clinical Judgment/Cognitive Skills: Recognize Cues
Integrated Process: Nursing Process/Data Collection
Content Area: Complex Care: Shock
Health Problem: Adult Health: Neurological: Spinal Cord Injury

Answer: 1
Rationale: Areflexia characterizes spinal shock; therefore, reflexes would provide the best information about recovery. Vital sign changes (options 2, 3, and 4) are not consistently affected by spinal shock. Because vital signs are affected by many factors, they do not give reliable information about spinal shock recovery. Blood pressure would provide good information about recovery from other types of shock, but not spinal shock.
Priority Nursing Tip: Spinal shock can occur after a spinal cord injury and ends when the reflexes are regained.

Test-Taking Strategy: Focus on the **subject,** recovery from spinal shock. Note that options 2, 3, and 4 are **comparable or alike** and are all vital signs. Therefore, eliminate these options.

---

309. A hospitalized client awaiting repair of an unruptured cerebral aneurysm is frequently checked by the nurse. Which finding would the nurse identify as an **early** indication that the aneurysm has ruptured?

1 Widened pulse pressure
2 Unilateral motor weakness
3 Unilateral slowing of pupil response
4 A decline in the level of consciousness

Level of Cognitive Ability: Analyzing
Client Needs: Physiological Integrity
Clinical Judgment/Cognitive Skills: Recognize Cues
Integrated Process: Nursing Process/Data Collection
Content Area: Complex Care: Emergency Situations/Management
Health Problem: Adult Health: Neurological: Aneurysm

Answer: 4
Rationale: Rupture of a cerebral aneurysm usually results in increased intracranial pressure (ICP). The first sign of pressure in the brain is a change in the level of consciousness. This change in consciousness can be as subtle as drowsiness or restlessness. Because centers that control blood pressure are located lower in the brain than those that control consciousness, blood pressure alteration is a later sign. Slowing of pupil response and motor weakness are also late signs.
Priority Nursing Tip: The level of consciousness is the most sensitive and earliest indicator of a change in the neurological status.

Test-Taking Strategy: Focus on the **subject,** signs of a ruptured cerebral aneurysm. Note the **strategic word,** *early.* Remember that changes in level of consciousness are the first indication of increased ICP.

---

310. The nurse working in the mental health unit is preparing to care for a severely depressed client. Which findings support the diagnosis of this client? **Select all that apply.**

1 Insomnia
2 Flat affect
3 Hypersomnia
4 Substantial weight loss
5 Weight gain since onset of depression
6 Reports, "I don't have any more tears to cry."

Level of Cognitive Ability: Analyzing
Client Needs: Physiological Integrity
Clinical Judgment/Cognitive Skills: Recognize Cues
Integrated Process: Nursing Process/Data Collection
Content Area: Mental Health
Health Problem: Mental Health: Mood Disorders

Answer: 1, 2, 4, 6
Rationale: In the severely depressed client, loss of weight is typical, whereas the mildly depressed client may experience a gain in weight. Sleep is generally affected in a similar way, with hypersomnia in the mildly depressed client and insomnia in the severely depressed client. The severely depressed client may report that no tears are left for crying. A flat affect may be associated with depression.
Priority Nursing Tip: If the client has depression, always check the client's risk of harm to self or others.

Test-Taking Strategy: Focus on the **subject,** a severely depressed client. Recall that there are varying degrees of depression that can present with different physical signs and symptoms. Focusing on severe depression will direct you to the correct option.

---

311. A client admitted to the hospital is suspected of having Guillain–Barré syndrome. Which findings would the nurse identify as manifestations of this disorder? **Select all that apply.**

1 Dysphagia
2 Paresthesia
3 Facial weakness
4 Difficulty speaking
5 Hyperactive deep tendon reflexes
6 Descending symmetrical muscle weakness

Level of Cognitive Ability: Analyzing
Client Needs: Physiological Integrity
Clinical Judgment/Cognitive Skills: Recognize Cues
Integrated Process: Nursing Process/Data Collection
Content Area: Adult Health: Neurological
Health Problem: Adult Health: Neurological: Guillain–Barré Syndrome

Answer: 1, 2, 3, 4
Rationale: Guillain–Barré syndrome is an acute autoimmune disorder characterized by varying degrees of motor weakness and paralysis. Motor manifestations include ascending symmetrical muscle weakness that leads to flaccid paralysis without muscle atrophy, decreased or absent deep tendon reflexes, respiratory compromise and respiratory failure, and loss of bladder and bowel control. Sensory manifestations include pain (cramping) and paresthesia. Cranial nerve manifestations include facial weakness, dysphagia, diplopia, and difficulty speaking. Autonomic manifestations include labile blood pressure, dysrhythmias, and tachycardia.
Priority Nursing Tip: To remember that an ascending progression of paralysis occurs in Guillain–Barré syndrome, think about G to B (Guillain–Barré), from the Ground to the Brain.

Test-Taking Strategy: Focus on the **subject,** Guillain–Barré syndrome, and note that it is an acute autoimmune disorder characterized by varying degrees of motor weakness and paralysis. This will assist in determining that options 1, 2, 3, and 4 are correct.

---

312. A visiting home-care nurse finds a client unconscious in the bedroom. The client has a history of abusing the selective serotonin reuptake inhibitor (SSRI) sertraline. The nurse would **immediately** conduct which assessment?

1 Pulse
2 Respirations
3 Blood pressure
4 Urinary output

Level of Cognitive Ability: Analyzing
Client Needs: Physiological Integrity
Clinical Judgment/Cognitive Skills: Recognize Cues
Integrated Process: Nursing Process/Data Collection
Content Area: Complex Care: Emergency Situations/Management
Health Problem: N/A

Answer: 2
Rationale: In an emergency situation, the nurse would determine breathlessness first and then check for a pulse. Blood pressure would be checked after these assessments are performed. Urinary output is also important but is not the priority at this time.
Priority Nursing Tip: SSRIs can interact with numerous medications. Therefore, it is important to check the client's prescribed medications to determine the potential for an adverse interaction.

Test-Taking Strategy: Note the **strategic word,** ***immediately.*** Use the **ABCs—airway, breathing, and circulation**—as the guide for answering this question. Respirations specifically relate to airway and breathing.

---

313. The licensed practical nurse (LPN) prepares to assist the registered nurse (RN) to check a unit of blood received from the blood bank and notes the presence of gas bubbles in the bag. What action would the nurse plan to take?

1 Return the bag to the blood bank.
2 Infuse the blood using filter tubing.
3 Add 10 mL normal saline to the bag.
4 Agitate the bag to mix contents gently.

Level of Cognitive Ability: Applying
Client Needs: Physiological Integrity
Clinical Judgment/Cognitive Skills: Take Action
Integrated Process: Nursing Process/Implementation
Content Area: Complex Care: Blood Administration
Health Problem: N/A

Answer: 1
Rationale: The nurse would return the unit of blood to the blood bank because the gas bubbles in the bag indicate possible contamination. Whenever administering blood, the nurse would use filter tubing to trap particulate matter. Although normal saline can be infused concurrently with the blood, normal saline or any other substance would never be added to the blood in a blood bag. The bag would not be agitated because this can harm red blood cells.
Priority Nursing Tip: The blood for infusion is always checked for leaks, abnormal color, clots, and bubbles before administration. If any of these are noted, it is not administered and is returned to the blood bank.

Test-Taking Strategy: Focus on the **subject**, blood administration. Recalling that the presence of gas bubbles indicates potential bacterial growth directs you to the correct option. When in doubt, remember to consult with the blood bank.

---

314. The licensed practical nurse (LPN) prepares to assist the registered nurse (RN) to insert an intravenous catheter for the administration of blood. The LPN understands that the smallest-gauge catheter that the RN can use to administer blood is which gauge?

1 12 gauge
2 20 gauge
3 22 gauge
4 24 gauge

Level of Cognitive Ability: Applying
Client Needs: Physiological Integrity
Clinical Judgment/Cognitive Skills: Take Action
Integrated Process: Nursing Process/Implementation
Content Area: Complex Care: Blood Administration
Health Problem: N/A

Answer: 2
Rationale: An intravenous catheter used to infuse blood needs to be at least 20 gauge or larger to help prevent additional hemolysis of red blood cells and to allow infusion of the blood without occluding the IV catheter.
Priority Nursing Tip: Ensure that the client has an adequate and functioning intravenous catheter inserted before obtaining the blood for administration from the blood bank.

Test-Taking Strategy: Focus on the **subject**, the smallest-gauge catheter that the nurse can use for infusion of blood. This focus will assist in eliminating options 3 and 4. From the remaining options, think about the gauge of IV catheters to direct you to the correct option.

---

315. A client began receiving an intravenous (IV) infusion of packed red blood cells 30 minutes ago. What is the **initial** nursing action when the client reports itching and a tight sensation in the chest?

1 Stop the transfusion.
2 Check the client's temperature.
3 Call the registered nurse.
4 Recheck the unit of blood for compatibility.

Answer: 1
Rationale: The symptoms reported by the client indicate that the client is experiencing a transfusion reaction. The first action of the nurse when a transfusion reaction is observed is to stop the transfusion. The nurse then calls the registered nurse. An IV of normal saline with new IV tubing is started, and the primary health care provider is notified. The nurse then checks the client's vital signs— temperature, pulse, and respirations—and rechecks the unit of blood as appropriate for infusion into the client. Depending on agency protocol, the nurse may also obtain a urinalysis, draw a sample of blood, and return the unit of blood and tubing to the blood bank. The nurse also institutes supportive

Level of Cognitive Ability: Analyzing
Client Needs: Physiological Integrity
Clinical Judgment/Cognitive Skills: Take Action
Integrated Process: Nursing Process/Implementation
Content Area: Complex Care: Blood Administration
Health Problem: Adult Health: Immune: Hypersensitivity Reactions

care for the client, which may include administration of antihistamines, crystalloids, epinephrine steroids, or vasopressors as prescribed.
Priority Nursing Tip: If a blood transfusion reaction occurs, do not leave the client alone, and continuously monitor the client for any life-threatening symptoms.

Test-Taking Strategy: Focus on the **subject,** the action to take if a transfusion reaction occurs. Noting the **strategic word,** *initial,* will direct you to the correct option. Remember that the first action of the nurse when a transfusion reaction is observed is to stop the transfusion.

---

316. A client has not ingested any food or liquids for 4 hours after two episodes of nausea and vomiting. What will the nurse offer the client **initially** now that she or he is no longer nauseated?
1 Toast
2 Gelatin
3 Dry cereal
4 Ginger ale

Level of Cognitive Ability: Applying
Client Needs: Physiological Integrity
Clinical Judgment/Cognitive Skills: Take Action
Integrated Process: Nursing Process/Implementation
Content Area: Skills: Nutrition
Health Problem: Adult Health: Gastrointestinal: Nutrition Problems

Answer: 4
Rationale: Clear liquids are best tolerated first after episodes of nausea and vomiting. If the client tolerates sips (20 to 30 mL at a time) of clear liquids, such as water or ginger ale (with the carbonation removed if better tolerated), then the amounts may be increased and gelatin, tea, and broth may be added. Once these are tolerated, solid foods such as toast, cereal, chicken, and other easily digested foods may be tried.
Priority Nursing Tip: Vomiting places the client at risk for dehydration and metabolic alkalosis.

Test-Taking Strategy: Focus on the **subject,** nausea and vomiting, and the **strategic word,** *initially.* Begin to answer this question by eliminating options 1 and 3, which identify solid foods and are less well tolerated than liquids. Choose ginger ale over gelatin because it is a liquid at all temperatures.

---

317. A client has just undergone an upper gastrointestinal (GI) series. Upon the client's return to the unit, what primary health care provider's prescription does the nurse expect to note as a part of routine postprocedure care?
1 Bland diet
2 NPO status
3 Mild laxative
4 Decreased fluids

Level of Cognitive Ability: Applying
Client Needs: Physiological Integrity
Clinical Judgment/Cognitive Skills: Recognize Cues
Integrated Process: Nursing Process/Implementation
Content Area: Foundations of Care: Diagnostic Tests
Health Problem: N/A

Answer: 3
Rationale: Barium sulfate, which is used as a contrast material during an upper GI series, is constipating. If it is not eliminated from the GI tract, it can cause obstruction. Therefore, laxatives or cathartics are administered as part of routine postprocedure care. Increased (not decreased) fluids are also helpful but do not act in the same way as a laxative to eliminate the barium. Options 1 and 2 are not routine postprocedure measures.
Priority Nursing Tip: After an upper GI series, instruct the client to increase oral fluid intake to help pass the barium.

Test-Taking Strategy: Focus on the **subject,** upper GI series, and the words *routine postprocedure.* Recalling that barium is used in this diagnostic test will direct you to the correct option.

---

318. The nurse prepares the client for the removal of a nasogastric tube. During the tube removal, the nurse instructs the client to take which action?

1 Inhale deeply.
2 Exhale slowly.
3 Hold in a deep breath.
4 Pause between breaths.

Level of Cognitive Ability: Applying
Client Needs: Physiological Integrity
Clinical Judgment/Cognitive Skills: Take Action
Integrated Process: Nursing Process/Implementation
Content Area: Skills: Tube Care
Health Problem: N/A

Answer: 3

Rationale: Just before removing the tube, the client is asked to take a deep breath and hold it because breath-holding minimizes the risk of aspirating gastric contents spilled from the tube during removal. The maneuver partially occludes the airway during tube removal; afterward, the client exhales as soon as the tube is out and thus avoids drawing the gastric contents into the trachea. The nurse pulls the tube out steadily and smoothly while the client holds the breath. The remaining options are incorrect because options 1 and 2 increase the risk of aspiration, and option 4 is ineffective.

Priority Nursing Tip: After removal of a nasogastric tube, monitor the client for abdominal distention and signs of aspiration.

Test-Taking Strategy: Focus on the **subject,** nasogastric tube removal. Visualize this procedure. Recalling that the airway is partially occluded during tube removal and that the risk of aspiration is present will direct you to the correct option.

---

319. The licensed practical nurse (LPN) is assisting in caring for a client who is receiving total parenteral nutrition and has a prescription for an intravenous intralipid infusion. What action would the LPN take before assisting the registered nurse to hang the intralipid infusion?

1 Refrigerate the bottle of solution.
2 Add 100 mL normal saline to the infusion bottle.
3 Place an inline filter on the administration tubing.
4 Check the solution for separation or an oily residue.

Level of Cognitive Ability: Applying
Client Needs: Physiological Integrity
Clinical Judgment/Cognitive Skills: Take Action
Integrated Process: Nursing Process/Implementation
Content Area: Skills: Nutrition
Health Problem: N/A

Answer: 4

Rationale: Intralipids provide nonprotein calories and prevent or correct fatty acid deficiency. The nurse checks the solution for separation or an oily appearance because this can indicate a spoiled or contaminated solution. Refrigeration renders the intralipid solution too thick to administer. Because any additive can affect the stability of the solution, the nurse avoids injecting normal saline into the intralipid infusion. Furthermore, an inline filter is not used because it can disrupt the flow of solution by becoming clogged.

Priority Nursing Tip: Fat emulsions (lipids) would not be given to a client with an egg allergy because lipids contain egg yolk phospholipids.

Test-Taking Strategy: Focus on the **subject,** actions to take before administering intralipids. Think about the consistency of this solution to direct you to the correct option.

---

320. The nurse assists to create a discharge plan for a client with diabetes mellitus diagnosed with peripheral neuropathy of the lower extremities. Which instructions would the nurse include in the plan? **Select all that apply.**

1 Wear support or elastic stockings.
2 Wear well-fitted shoes and walk barefoot when at home.
3 Wear dark-colored stockings or socks and change them daily.
4 Use a heating pad set at low setting on the feet if they feel cold.
5 Apply lanolin or lubricating lotion to the legs and feet once or twice daily.
6 Wash the feet and legs with mild soap and water and rinse and dry them well.

Level of Cognitive Ability: Creating
Client Needs: Physiological Integrity
Clinical Judgment/Cognitive Skills: Generate Solutions
Integrated Process: Teaching and Learning
Content Area: Adult Health: Endocrine
Health Problem: Adult Health: Endocrine: Diabetes Mellitus

Answer: 1, 5, 6
Rationale: Peripheral neuropathy is any functional or organic disorder of the peripheral nervous system. Clinical manifestations can include muscle weakness, stabbing pain, paresthesia or loss of sensation, impaired reflexes, and autonomic manifestations. Home-care instructions include wearing support or elastic stockings for dependent edema, applying lanolin or lubricating lotion to the legs and feet once or twice daily, washing the feet and legs with mild soap and water and rinsing and drying them well, inspecting the legs and feet daily and reporting any skin changes or open areas to the primary health care provider, wearing white or colorfast stockings or socks and changing them daily, checking the temperature of the bathwater with a thermometer before putting the feet into the water, avoiding the use of heat (hot foot soaks, heating pad, hot water bottle) on the feet because of the risk of burning, avoiding the use of sharp devices to cut nails, and wearing well-fitted shoes and avoiding going barefoot.
Priority Nursing Tip: A complication of diabetes mellitus is peripheral neuropathy. The client experiences decreased sensation and must be cautious about exposure to extreme temperatures and potential injuries.

Test-Taking Strategy: Focus on the **subject,** peripheral neuropathy. This client will experience paresthesia or loss of sensation. This will assist in eliminating option 4. Finally eliminate options 2 and 3 because the client should not walk barefoot and needs to wear white or colorfast stockings or socks.

---

321. A primary health care provider is inserting a chest tube. Which materials would the nurse have available to be used as the first layer of the dressing at the chest tube insertion site?

1 Petrolatum jelly gauze
2 Sterile 4 × 4 gauze pad
3 Absorbent gauze dressing
4 Gauze impregnated with povidone–iodine

Level of Cognitive Ability: Applying
Client Needs: Physiological Integrity
Clinical Judgment/Cognitive Skills: Take Action
Integrated Process: Nursing Process/Implementation
Content Area: Skills: Wound Care
Health Problem: Adult Health: Integumentary: Wounds

Answer: 1
Rationale: The first layer of the chest tube dressing is petrolatum gauze, which allows for an occlusive seal at the chest tube insertion site. Additional layers of gauze cover this layer, and the dressing is secured with a strong adhesive tape or Elastoplast tape. The items in the remaining options would not be selected as the first protective layer.
Priority Nursing Tip: An occlusive sterile dressing is maintained at the chest tube insertion site to prevent an air leak.

Test-Taking Strategy: Focus on the **subject,** the first layer of the dressing at the chest tube insertion site. Recall that an occlusive seal at the site is needed, and think about which dressing material will help achieve this seal.

---

322. During a follow-up visit 2 weeks after pneumonectomy, the client reports numbness and tenderness at the surgical site. Which statement would the nurse make to accurately address the client's concerns?

1. "This is not likely to be permanent but may last for some months."
2. "You are having a severe problem and will probably be rehospitalized."
3. "This is probably caused by permanent nerve damage as a result of surgery."
4. "This is often the first sign of a wound infection; I will check your temperature."

Level of Cognitive Ability: Applying
Client Needs: Physiological Integrity
Clinical Judgment/Cognitive Skills: Take Action
Integrated Process: Nursing Process/Implementation
Content Area: Foundations of Care: Perioperative Care
Health Problem: N/A

Answer: 1

Rationale: Clients who undergo pneumonectomy or other surgical procedures may experience numbness, altered sensation, or tenderness in the area that surrounds the incision. These sensations may last for months. It is not considered to be a severe problem and is not indicative of a wound infection.

Priority Nursing Tip: After pneumonectomy, check the primary health care provider's prescription regarding client positioning. Avoid complete lateral turning of the client.

Test-Taking Strategy: Focus on the **subject,** numbness and tenderness at the surgical site after pneumonectomy. Eliminate option 2 because of the word *severe.* Eliminate option 3 because of the word *permanent.* Eliminate option 4 because numbness and tenderness are not signs of infection.

---

323. A client scheduled for pneumonectomy tells the nurse that a friend had lung surgery that required chest tubes. The client asks how long to expect chest tubes to be in place. Which statement by the nurse appropriately educates the client about the presence of a chest tube postpneumonectomy?

1. "They are generally removed after 36 to 48 hours."
2. "Not every lung surgery requires chest tubes to be used."
3. "They usually remain in place for a full week after surgery."
4. "Your type of surgery rarely requires chest tubes to be inserted after surgery."

Level of Cognitive Ability: Applying
Client Needs: Physiological Integrity
Clinical Judgment/Cognitive Skills: Take Action
Integrated Process: Nursing Process/Implementation
Content Area: Foundations of Care: Perioperative Care
Health Problem: N/A

Answer: 4

Rationale: Pneumonectomy involves removal of the entire lung, usually caused by extensive disease such as bronchogenic carcinoma, unilateral tuberculosis, or lung abscess. Chest tubes are not inserted because the cavity is left to fill with serosanguineous fluid, which later solidifies. Therefore, options 1, 2, and 3 are incorrect.

Priority Nursing Tip: After pneumonectomy, serous fluid accumulates in the empty thoracic cavity and eventually consolidates, preventing shifts of the mediastinum, heart, and remaining lung.

Test-Taking Strategy: Focus on the **subject,** postoperative expectations after pneumonectomy. Recall that the entire lung is removed with this procedure. This would guide you to reason that chest tubes are unnecessary because there is no lung remaining to reinflate to fill the pleural space (option 4).

---

324. The nurse is assisting in creating a plan of care for a client diagnosed with a dissecting abdominal aortic aneurysm. Which interventions would be included in the plan of care? **Select all that apply.**

1 Check peripheral circulation.
2 Monitor for abdominal distention.
3 Educate the client that abdominal pain is to be expected.
4 Check the client for observable ecchymoses on the lower back.
5 Perform deep palpation of the abdomen to check the size of the aneurysm.

Level of Cognitive Ability: Creating
Client Needs: Physiological Integrity
Clinical Judgment/Cognitive Skills: Generate Solutions
Integrated Process: Nursing Process/Planning
Content Area: Complex Care: Emergency Situations/Management
Health Problem: Adult Health: Cardiovascular: Vascular Disorders

Answer: 1, 2, 4

Rationale: If the client has an abdominal aortic aneurysm, the nurse is concerned about rupture and monitors the client closely. The nurse would check peripheral circulation and monitor for abdominal distention. The nurse also looks for ecchymoses on the lower back to determine whether the aneurysm is leaking. The nurse tells the client to report abdominal pain or back pain, which may radiate to the groin, buttocks, or legs, because this is a sign of rupture. The nurse also avoids deep palpation in the client in whom a dissecting abdominal aortic aneurysm is known or suspected. Doing so could place the client at risk for rupture.

Priority Nursing Tip: Systolic bruit heard over the abdominal aorta is a manifestation of an abdominal aortic aneurysm.

Test-Taking Strategy: Focus on the **subject**, care for a client with a dissecting abdominal aortic aneurysm. Eliminate options 3 and 5 because the presence of abdominal pain is a sign of rupture, and deep palpation places the aneurysm at risk for rupture.

---

325. A client has undergone angioplasty of the iliac artery. Which technique would the nurse perform to **best** detect bleeding from the angioplasty in the region of the iliac artery?

1 Palpate the pedal pulses.
2 Measure the abdominal girth.
3 Check the client about the level of pain in the area.
4 Auscultate over the iliac area with a Doppler device.

Level of Cognitive Ability: Analyzing
Client Needs: Physiological Integrity
Clinical Judgment/Cognitive Skills: Recognize Cues
Integrated Process: Nursing Process/Data Collection
Content Area: Adult Health: Cardiovascular
Health Problem: Adult Health: Cardiovascular: Vascular Disorders

Answer: 2

Rationale: Bleeding after iliac artery angioplasty causes blood to accumulate in the retroperitoneal area. This can most directly be detected by measuring abdominal girth. Palpation and auscultation of pulses determine patency. Assessment of pain is routinely done, and mild regional discomfort is expected.

Priority Nursing Tip: After angioplasty, check the insertion site frequently for the presence of bloody drainage or hematoma formation.

Test-Taking Strategy: Note the **strategic word,** *best.* Focus on the **subject,** bleeding from the angioplasty in the region of the iliac artery. Select the option that addresses an abdominal assessment because the iliac arteries are located in the peritoneal cavity. This will direct you to the correct option.

---

326. A client states, "I'm sure I have restless legs syndrome." The nurse determines that the client is in **need of further teaching** on the condition when the client identifies the presence of which characteristics? **Select all that apply.**

1 A heavy feeling in the legs
2 Burning sensations in the limbs
3 Symptom relief when lying down
4 Decreased ability to move the legs
5 Symptoms that are worse in the morning
6 Feeling the need to move the limbs repeatedly

Level of Cognitive Ability: Analyzing
Client Needs: Physiological Integrity
Clinical Judgment/Cognitive Skills: Evaluate Outcomes
Integrated Process: Nursing Process/Data Collection
Content Area: Adult Health: Neurological
Health Problem: Adult Health: Neurological: Restless Legs Syndrome

Answer: 1, 3, 4, 5

Rationale: Restless legs syndrome is characterized by leg paresthesia associated with an irresistible urge to move. The client complains of intense burning or "crawling-type" sensations in the limbs and subsequently feels the need to move the limbs repeatedly to relieve the symptoms. The symptoms are worse in the evening and night when the client is still.

Priority Nursing Tip: Some nonpharmacological measures to relieve the symptoms of restless legs syndrome include walking, stretching, moderate exercise, or a warm bath.

Test-Taking Strategy: Focus on the **subject,** manifestations of restless legs syndrome. Note the **strategic words,** *need of further teaching.* These words indicate a **negative event query** and the need to select incorrect characteristics. This will assist in eliminating options 2 and 6, which are characteristics of restless legs syndrome.

---

327. A client who underwent peripheral arterial bypass surgery 16 hours ago reports that there is increasing pain in the leg that worsens with movement and is accompanied by paresthesias. Based on these data, which action would the nurse take?

1 Notify the registered nurse.
2 Administer an opioid analgesic.
3 Apply warm, moist heat for comfort.
4 Apply ice to minimize any developing swelling.

Level of Cognitive Ability: Analyzing
Client Needs: Physiological Integrity
Clinical Judgment/Cognitive Skills: Take Action
Integrated Process: Nursing Process/Implementation
Content Area: Adult Health: Cardiovascular
Health Problem: Adult Health: Cardiovascular: Vascular Disorders

Answer: 1

Rationale: Compartment syndrome is characterized by increased pressure within a muscle compartment caused by bleeding or excessive edema. It compresses the nerves in the area and can cause vascular compromise. The classic signs of compartment syndrome are pain at rest that intensifies with movement and the development of paresthesias. Compartment syndrome is an emergency, and the registered nurse is notified immediately and contacts the surgeon, because the client could require an emergency fasciotomy to relieve the pressure and restore perfusion. Options 2, 3, and 4 are incorrect actions.

Priority Nursing Tip: After arterial bypass surgery, warmth, redness, and edema of the affected extremity are expected occurrences because of the increased blood flow to the area.

Test-Taking Strategy: Focus on the **subject,** a postoperative client who had peripheral arterial bypass surgery. Note the words *increasing pain.* Also note that the surgery was 16 hours ago. The signs and symptoms described indicate a new problem. These factors would indicate that the registered nurse and surgeon need to be notified.

---

328. The nurse in an ambulatory care clinic takes a client's blood pressure (BP) in the left arm; it is 200/118 mm Hg. Which action would the nurse implement **next**?

1 Notify the registered nurse.
2 Inquire about the presence of kidney disorders.
3 Check the client's blood pressure in the right arm.
4 Recheck the pressure in the same arm within 30 seconds.

Level of Cognitive Ability: Analyzing
Client Needs: Physiological Integrity
Clinical Judgment/Cognitive Skills: Take Action
Integrated Process: Nursing Process/Implementation
Content Area: Skills: Vital Signs
Health Problem: N/A

Answer: 3
Rationale: When a high BP reading is noted, the nurse takes the pressure in the opposite arm to see if the blood pressure is elevated in one extremity only. The nurse would also recheck the blood pressure in the same arm but would wait at least 2 minutes between readings. The nurse would inquire about the presence of kidney disorders that could contribute to the elevated blood pressure. The nurse would notify the registered nurse, who would then contact the primary health care provider because immediate treatment may be required, but this would not be done without obtaining verification of the elevation.
Priority Nursing Tip: Hypertension is a major risk factor for coronary, cerebral, renal, and peripheral vascular disease.

Test-Taking Strategy: Focus on the **subject,** hypertension. Note the **strategic word,** *next.* Eliminate option 4 first because of the time frame, 30 seconds. From the remaining options, select the correct option because it provides verification of the initial reading.

---

329. A prenatal client is being evaluated for possible gestational diabetes. Which data identified and documented after the client's initial assessment would support that diagnosis?

1 22 years old
2 A gravida 4, para 0, abortus 3
3 5′6″ tall, weighs 130 pounds
4 Stated, "I get really tired after working all day."

Level of Cognitive Ability: Analyzing
Client Needs: Physiological Integrity
Clinical Judgment/Cognitive Skills: Recognize Cues
Integrated Process: Nursing Process/Data Collection
Content Area: Maternity: Antepartum
Health Problem: Maternity: Diabetes

Answer: 2
Rationale: A history of unexplained stillbirths or miscarriages puts the client at high risk for gestational diabetes. Fatigue is a normal occurrence during pregnancy. The client's height (5′6″ tall) and weight (130 pounds) do not meet the criteria of 20% over ideal weight. Therefore, the client is not obese, a possible factor related to gestational diabetes. To be at high risk for gestational diabetes, the maternal age would be greater than 25 years.
Priority Nursing Tip: Pregnant women need to be screened for gestational diabetes between 24 and 28 weeks of pregnancy.

Test-Taking Strategy: Focus on the **subject,** gestational diabetes. Option 4 can be eliminated because fatigue is a normal occurrence during pregnancy. Recalling the risk factors associated with gestational diabetes will indicate that options 1 and 3 do not apply to this client.

---

330. The nurse is assisting in caring for a client diagnosed with preeclampsia. When the client's condition progresses from preeclampsia to eclampsia, what would the nurse's **first** action be?

1 Maintain an open airway.
2 Administer oxygen by face mask.
3 Check the maternal blood pressure and fetal heart tones.
4 Administer an intravenous infusion of magnesium sulfate.

Answer: 1
Rationale: Eclampsia is characterized by the occurrence of seizures. If the client experiences seizures, it is important as a first action to establish and maintain an open airway and prevent injuries to the client. Options 2, 3, and 4 are all interventions that need to be done, but not initially.
Priority Nursing Tip: The nurse would never leave the client who is having a seizure. The nurse stays with the client, maintaining an open airway and calling for help.

Level of Cognitive Ability: Analyzing
Client Needs: Physiological Integrity
Clinical Judgment/Cognitive Skills: Take Action
Integrated Process: Nursing Process/Implementation
Content Area: Complex Care: Emergency Situations/Management
Health Problem: Maternity: Gestational Hypertension/Preeclampsia and Eclampsia

Test-Taking Strategy: Note the **strategic word,** ***first.*** Use the **ABCs—airway, breathing, and circulation**—to direct you to the correct option.

---

331. The nurse assists to admit a client who is bleeding freely from a scalp laceration that resulted from a fall. The nurse would take which action **first** in the care of this wound?

1 Prepare for suturing the area.
2 Determine when the client last had a tetanus vaccine.
3 Cleanse the wound by flushing with sterile normal saline.
4 Apply direct pressure to the laceration to stop the bleeding.

Level of Cognitive Ability: Analyzing
Client Needs: Physiological Integrity
Clinical Judgment/Cognitive Skills: Prioritize Hypotheses
Integrated Process: Nursing Process/Implementation
Content Area: Complex Care: Emergency Situations/Management
Health Problem: Adult Health: Neurological: Head Injury/Trauma

Answer: 4
Rationale: The initial nursing action is to stop the bleeding, and direct pressure is applied. The nurse will then cleanse the wound thoroughly with sterile normal saline. This action removes dirt or foreign matter in the wound and allows visualization of the size of the wound. If suturing is necessary, the surrounding hair may be shaved. The date of the client's last tetanus shot is determined, and prophylaxis is given if needed.
Priority Nursing Tip: The nurse must ask the client who sustains a laceration about the date of the last tetanus immunization because the client may need a tetanus injection.

Test-Taking Strategy: Note the **strategic word,** ***first,*** which implies that more than one or all of the options may be partially or totally correct. Focus on the **ABCs—airway, breathing, circulation.** This will direct you to the correct option.

---

332. A client admitted to the nursing unit with a closed head injury 6 hours ago has begun to vomit and reports being dizzy and having a headache. Based on these data, which is the **most important** nursing action?

1 Administering a prescribed antiemetic
2 Having the client rate the headache pain on a scale of 1 to 10
3 Notifying the primary health care provider of the client's condition
4 Reminding the client to use the call bell when needing help to the bathroom

Answer: 3
Rationale: The client with a closed head injury is at risk of developing increased intracranial pressure (ICP). Increased ICP is evidenced by signs and symptoms such as headache, dizziness, confusion, weakness, and vomiting. Because of the implications of the client's manifestations, the most important nursing action is to notify the primary health care provider. Although the other nursing actions are not inappropriate, none of them address the critical issue of the potential of the client developing ICP.
Priority Nursing Tip: The head of the bed of the client with increased intracranial pressure needs to be elevated 30 to 40 degrees.

Level of Cognitive Ability: Analyzing
Client Needs: Physiological Integrity
Clinical Judgment/Cognitive Skills: Prioritize Hypotheses
Integrated Process: Nursing Process/ Implementation
Content Area: Complex Care: Emergency Situations/Management
Health Problem: Adult Health: Neurological: Head Injury/Trauma

Test-Taking Strategy: Note the **strategic words,** *most important.* This directs you to prioritize the possible nursing actions. Considering the client's diagnosis, a closed head injury, and the signs and symptoms, the nurse would suspect increased ICP. The primary health care provider needs to be notified.

---

333. A client is brought into the emergency department after sustaining a possible closed head injury. Which assessment will the nurse perform **first**?

1 Level of consciousness
2 Pulse and blood pressure
3 Respiratory rate and depth
4 Ability to move extremities

Answer: 3

Rationale: The first action of the nurse is to ensure that the client has an adequate airway and respiratory status. In rapid sequence, the client's circulatory status is evaluated (option 2), followed by evaluation of the status of the cardiovascular and neurological systems.

Priority Nursing Tip: Complications of a head injury include cerebral bleeding, hematomas, uncontrolled increased ICP, infections, and seizures.

Level of Cognitive Ability: Applying
Client Needs: Physiological Integrity
Clinical Judgment/Cognitive Skills: Prioritize Hypotheses
Integrated Process: Nursing Process/ Implementation
Content Area: Complex Care: Emergency Situations/Management
Health Problem: Adult Health: Neurological: Head Injury/Trauma

Test-Taking Strategy: Note the **strategic word,** *first.* Use the **ABCs—airway, breathing, and circulation.** The correct option will most often be the one that deals with the client's airway. Respiratory rate and depth support this action.

---

334. A client with a spinal cord injury is at risk of developing footdrop. What intervention would the nurse use as a preventive measure?

1 Mole skin–lined heel protectors
2 Regular use of posterior splints
3 Application of pneumatic boots
4 Avoiding dorsal flexion of the foot

Answer: 2

Rationale: The effective means of preventing footdrop (plantar flexion) is the use of posterior splints or high-top sneakers. Dorsal flexing of the foot would help counteract the effects of footdrop. Heel protectors protect the skin but do not prevent footdrop. Pneumatic boots prevent deep vein thrombosis but not footdrop.

Priority Nursing Tip: Footdrop is preventable, and the nurse needs to be alert to clients at risk for developing footdrop, such as immobile and bedridden clients, and initiate measures to prevent it.

Level of Cognitive Ability: Applying
Client Needs: Physiological Integrity
Clinical Judgment/Cognitive Skills: Take Action
Integrated Process: Nursing Process/ Implementation
Content Area: Adult Health: Neurological
Health Problem: Adult Health: Neurological: Spinal Cord Injury

Test-Taking Strategy: Focus on the **subject,** preventing footdrop. This guides you to select the option that immobilizes the foot in a functional position while protecting the skin of the extremities.

---

335. After a cervical spine fracture, this device is placed on the client. The nurse assists to create a discharge plan for the client to ensure safety and includes which measures? **Refer to the figure. Select all that apply.**

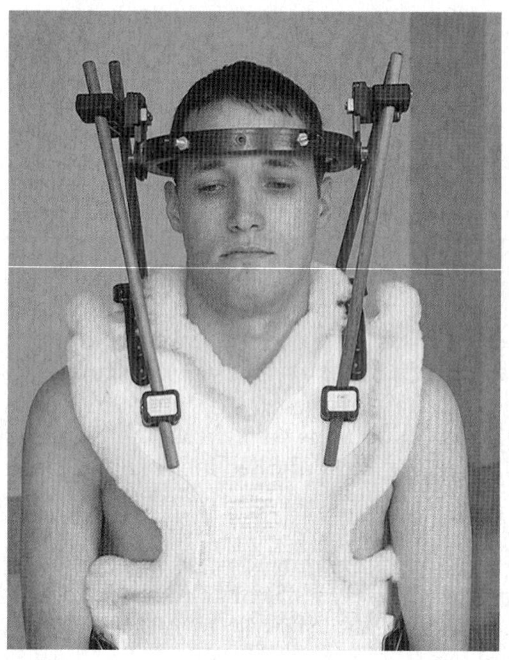

(From Ignatavicius D, Workman M: Medical-surgical nursing: patient-centered collaborative care, ed 7, Philadelphia, 2013, Saunders.)

1 Teach the client how to ambulate with a walker.
2 Instruct the client to bend at the waist to pick up needed items.
3 Demonstrate the procedure for scanning the environment for vision.
4 Inform the client about the importance of wearing rubber-soled shoes.
5 Teach the spouse to use the metal frame to assist the client to turn in bed.

Level of Cognitive Ability: Creating
Client Needs: Physiological Integrity
Clinical Judgment/Cognitive Skills: Generate Solutions
Integrated Process: Nursing Process/Planning
Content Area: Adult Health: Neurological
Health Problem: Adult Health: Neurological: Spinal Cord Injury

Answer: 1, 3, 4

Rationale: The client with a halo fixation device needs to be taught that the use of a walker and rubber-soled shoes may help prevent falls and injury and are therefore helpful. It is also helpful for the client to scan the environment visually because the client's peripheral vision is diminished from keeping the neck in a stationary position. The client with a halo fixation device needs to avoid bending at the waist because the halo vest is heavy, and the client's trunk is limited in flexibility. The nurse instructs the client and family that the metal frame on the device is never used to move or lift the client because this will disrupt the attachment to the client's skull, which is stabilizing the fracture.

Priority Nursing Tip: The weight of the halo fixation device can alter the client's balance, and the nurse must teach the client measures that will ensure safety.

Test-Taking Strategy: Focus on the **subject,** client instructions for a halo fixation device. Visualize the actions in the options to assist in identifying how injury could be prevented. This will assist in eliminating options 2 and 5.

336. To monitor for a temporary but common postsurgical complication of a transsphenoidal resection of the pituitary gland, the nurse would regularly perform which assessment?

1 Pulse rate
2 Temperature
3 Urine output
4 Oxygen saturation

Level of Cognitive Ability: Analyzing
Client Needs: Physiological Integrity
Clinical Judgment/Cognitive Skills: Recognize Cues
Integrated Process: Nursing Process/Data Collection
Content Area: Adult Health: Endocrine
Health Problem: Adult Health: Endocrine: Pituitary Disorders

Answer: 3

Rationale: A common complication of surgery on the pituitary gland is temporary diabetes insipidus. This results from a deficiency in antidiuretic hormone (ADH) secretion as a result of surgical trauma. The nurse measures the client's urine output to determine whether this complication is occurring. Polyuria of 4 to 24 L per day is characteristic of this complication. Options 1, 2, and 4 are not specifically related to a common complication after this surgery.

Priority Nursing Tip: After transsphenoidal resection of a pituitary adenoma, monitor the client for postnasal or nasal drainage, which might indicate leakage of cerebrospinal fluid.

Test-Taking Strategy: Focus on the **subject**, transsphenoidal resection of a pituitary adenoma. Recalling that the pituitary gland is responsible for the production of ADH and a deficiency results in diabetes insipidus will direct you to the correct option.

---

337. Which piece of equipment will the nurse routinely use to check the fetal heart rate of a woman at 16 weeks' gestation?

1 Fetal heart monitor
2 An adult stethoscope
3 Bell of a stethoscope
4 Ultrasound fetoscope

Level of Cognitive Ability: Applying
Client Needs: Physiological Integrity
Clinical Judgment/Cognitive Skills: Recognize Cues
Integrated Process: Nursing Process/Data Collection
Content Area: Maternity: Antepartum
Health Problem: N/A

Answer: 4

Rationale: Toward the end of the first trimester, the fetal heart tones can be heard with an ultrasound fetoscope. Options 2 and 3 are not designed to adequately check the fetal heart rate. A fetal heart monitor is used during labor or in other situations when the fetal heart rate needs continuous monitoring.

Priority Nursing Tip: The normal fetal heart rate is 120 to 160 beats per minute.

Test-Taking Strategy: Focus on the **subject**, fetal heart assessment. Eliminate options 2 and 3 first because they are **comparable or alike.** Recalling that a fetal heart monitor is used for continuous monitoring will direct you to the correct option.

---

338. The nurse is assisting in creating a discharge plan for a postoperative client who had a unilateral adrenalectomy. What area of instruction would the nurse include in the plan to minimize the client's risk for injury?

1 Teaching the client to maintain a diabetic diet
2 Encouraging the adoption of a realistic exercise routine
3 Providing a detailed list of the early signs of a wound infection
4 Explaining the need for lifelong replacement of all adrenal hormones

Answer: 3

Rationale: A client who had a unilateral adrenalectomy (one adrenal gland was removed) will be placed on corticosteroids temporarily to avoid a cortisol deficiency; lifelong replacement is not necessary. Corticosteroids will be gradually weaned in the postoperative period until they are discontinued. Also, because of the antiinflammatory properties of corticosteroids produced by the adrenals, clients who undergo an adrenalectomy are at increased risk of developing wound infections. Because of this increased risk of infection, it is important for the client to know measures to prevent infection, early signs of infection, and what to do if an infection seems to be present. The client does not need to maintain a diabetic diet. The importance of regular exercise is not specific to this client.

Level of Cognitive Ability: Creating
Client Needs: Physiological Integrity
Clinical Judgment/Cognitive Skills: Generate Solutions
Integrated Process: Nursing Process/Planning
Content Area: Adult Health: Endocrine
Health Problem: Adult Health: Endocrine: Adrenal Disorders

Priority Nursing Tip: After adrenalectomy, monitor the client closely for bleeding because the adrenal glands are highly vascular. Instruct the client in the importance of hormone replacement therapy following surgery.

Test-Taking Strategy: Focus on the **subject,** unilateral adrenalectomy. Use knowledge about the function of the adrenal glands and the hormones secreted. The client instructions in options 1 and 2 are unrelated to the adrenal glands. From the remaining options, recalling that one gland can take over the function of two adrenal glands will direct you to the correct option.

---

339. The nurse is assisting in caring for a client who has undergone transsphenoidal surgery for a pituitary adenoma. In the postoperative period, which information would the nurse provide to the client to minimize the risk for surgery-related injury?

1 Cough and deep-breathe hourly.
2 Nasal packing will be removed after 48 hours.
3 Report frequent swallowing or postnasal drip.
4 Acetaminophen is prescribed for severe postsurgical headache.

Level of Cognitive Ability: Applying
Client Needs: Physiological Integrity
Clinical Judgment/Cognitive Skills: Take Action
Integrated Process: Teaching and Learning
Content Area: Adult Health: Neurological
Health Problem: Adult Health: Endocrine: Pituitary Disorders

Answer: 3
Rationale: The client needs to report frequent swallowing or postnasal drip or nasal drainage after transsphenoidal surgery because it could indicate cerebrospinal fluid (CSF) leakage. The client needs to deep-breathe, but coughing is contraindicated because it could cause increased intracranial pressure. The surgeon removes the nasal packing placed during surgery, usually after 24 hours. The client needs to also report severe headache because it could indicate increased intracranial pressure.
Priority Nursing Tip: After transsphenoidal surgery for a pituitary adenoma, assess nasal drainage for quantity, quality, and the presence of glucose, which indicates that the drainage is CSF.

Test-Taking Strategy: Focus on the **subject,** transsphenoidal surgery. Think about the anatomical location of this surgical procedure. Recalling that the concern is increased intracranial pressure and CSF leakage will direct you to the correct option.

---

340. A client is receiving desmopressin intranasally. Which parameter would the nurse monitor to determine the **effectiveness** of this medication?

1 Daily weight
2 Temperature
3 Apical heart rate
4 Pupillary response

Level of Cognitive Ability: Evaluating
Client Needs: Physiological Integrity
Clinical Judgment/Cognitive Skills: Evaluate Outcomes
Integrated Process: Nursing Process/Evaluation
Content Area: Pharmacology: Endocrine: Antidiuretics
Health Problem: N/A

Answer: 1
Rationale: Desmopressin is an analog of vasopressin (antidiuretic hormone). It is used in the management of diabetes insipidus. The nurse monitors the client's fluid balance to determine the effectiveness of the medication. Fluid status can be evaluated by noting intake and urine output, daily weight, and the presence of edema. The measurements in options 2, 3, and 4 are unrelated to this medication.
Priority Nursing Tip: Monitor the client taking desmopressin for signs of water intoxication (drowsiness, listlessness, shortness of breath, headache), indicating the need to decrease the dosage.

Test-Taking Strategy: Focus on the **subject,** desmopressin. Note the **strategic word,** *effectiveness.* Noting the client's diagnosis and recalling the pathophysiology associated with this diagnosis will direct you to the correct option.

---

341. As the nurse begins to administer scheduled doses of furosemide and nifedipine, the client asks for a PRN dose of aluminum hydroxide. Which action by the nurse would **best** ensure the **effectiveness** of all the medications?

1 Check the client's immediate need for the antacid.
2 Administer all three medications at the same time.
3 Administer the nifedipine and aluminum hydroxide, then the furosemide 1 hour later.
4 Administer the furosemide and aluminum hydroxide, then the nifedipine 1 hour later.

Level of Cognitive Ability: Applying
Client Needs: Physiological Integrity
Clinical Judgment/Cognitive Skills: Take Action
Integrated Process: Nursing Process/Implementation
Content Area: Skills: Medication Administration
Health Problem: N/A

Answer: 1
Rationale: Antacids such as aluminum hydroxide often interfere with the absorption of other medications. For this reason, antacids need to be separated from other medications by at least 1 hour. Because of the diuretic action of the furosemide and the antihypertensive action of the nifedipine, it is important to administer them on time if the client can tolerate waiting for the aluminum hydroxide. The nurse would check the client to determine the need for the antacid. Therefore, options 2, 3, and 4 are incorrect.
Priority Nursing Tip: Always check medication interactions before administering medications. Generally, the client would not take an antacid with medication because it will affect the absorption of the medication.

Test-Taking Strategy: Note the **strategic words,** *best* and *effectiveness.* Recalling that antacids interfere with absorption of other medications will assist in eliminating options 2, 3, and 4. Also recalling that the diuretic and antihypertensive medication would be administered on time will assist in directing you to the correct option. Additionally, option 1 addresses the first **step of the nursing process,** data collection.

---

342. The nurse monitors the client taking amitriptyline for which common side effect?

1 Diarrhea
2 Drowsiness
3 Hypertension
4 Increased salivation

Level of Cognitive Ability: Analyzing
Client Needs: Physiological Integrity
Clinical Judgment/Cognitive Skills: Recognize Cues
Integrated Process: Nursing Process/Data Collection
Content Area: Pharmacology: Psychotherapeutics: Tricyclic Antidepressants
Health Problem: N/A

Answer: 2
Rationale: Common side effects of amitriptyline (a tricyclic antidepressant) include the central nervous system effects of drowsiness, fatigue, lethargy, and sedation. Other common side effects include dry mouth or eyes, blurred vision, hypotension, and constipation. The nurse monitors the client for these side effects.
Priority Nursing Tip: If a tricyclic antidepressant is prescribed, instruct the client to avoid driving or other activities requiring alertness until the response to the medication is known.

Test-Taking Strategy: Focus on the **subject,** side effects of amitriptyline. Recalling that amitriptyline is an antidepressant will lead you to the correct option.

---

343. Which nursing question would elicit the **most** thorough data regarding the client's recent sleeping patterns?

1 "Are you sleeping well at home?"
2 "Did you get much sleep last night?"
3 "May we talk about how you've been sleeping?"
4 "Do you think you get enough sleep on a nightly basis?"

Answer: 3
Rationale: Option 3 is a question and provides the client the opportunity to express thoughts and feelings. The remaining options could lead to a one-word answer that would not provide thorough data. Additionally, one night of sleep may not tell the nurse how the pattern has been over time. Anyone may or may not sleep well for one night, and that sleep or loss of sleep does not indicate a problem.
Priority Nursing Tip: Adequate sleep is essential for the client with depression because fatigue can worsen the feelings associated with depression.

Level of Cognitive Ability: Analyzing
Client Needs: Physiological Integrity
Clinical Judgment/Cognitive Skills: Recognize Cues
Integrated Process: Nursing Process/Data Collection
Content Area: Foundations of Care: Sleep and Rest
Health Problem: N/A

Test-Taking Strategy: Focus on the **subject,** therapeutic communication during a sleeping pattern assessment. Note the **strategic word,** *most.* Use the **therapeutic communication techniques.** Select the option that is open-ended and allows the client to take the lead in the conversation. This will direct you to the correct option.

---

344. A client is admitted after attempting suicide by ingesting a prescribed antipsychotic medication. What is the **most important** piece of information the nurse would obtain **initially**?

1 Where and when the medication was ingested
2 The name and amount of ingested medication
3 Whether the client continues to have suicidal ideations
4 Whether there is a history of previous suicide attempts

Answer: 2
Rationale: In an emergency, lifesaving facts are obtained first. The name of and the amount of medication ingested is of utmost importance in treating this potentially life-threatening situation. The remaining data can be checked once the client's physical condition is stabilized.
Priority Nursing Tip: Extrapyramidal side effects can occur in the client taking an antipsychotic medication.

Test-Taking Strategy: Note the **strategic words,** *most important* and *initially.* Lifesaving treatment cannot begin until the medication and dosage amount are identified.

Level of Cognitive Ability: Analyzing
Client Needs: Physiological Integrity
Clinical Judgment/Cognitive Skills: Recognize Cues
Integrated Process: Nursing Process/Data Collection
Content Area: Complex Care: Emergency Situations/Management
Health Problem: Mental Health: Suicide

---

345. The nurse determines that a client understands the purpose of a phytonadione injection for their newborn when heard making which statement to the baby's other parent?

1 "The baby's liver cannot produce that vitamin."
2 "Most newborns need a supplement of this vitamin."
3 "All newborns lack intestinal bacteria to produce this vitamin."
4 "It's unusual, but our baby lacks the vitamin that helps the blood clot."

Answer: 3
Rationale: The absence of normal flora needed to synthesize vitamin K (phytonadione) in the normal newborn gut results in low levels of vitamin K and creates a transient blood coagulation deficiency between the second and fifth day of life. From a low point at about 2 to 3 days after birth, these coagulation factors rise slowly, but do not approach normal adult levels until 9 months of age or later. Increasing levels of these vitamin K–dependent factors indicate a response to dietary intake and bacterial colonization of the intestines. An injection is administered prophylactically on the day of birth to combat the deficiency. Options 1, 2, and 4 are incorrect.
Priority Nursing Tip: In the newborn, phytonadione (vitamin K) is administered in the lateral aspect of the middle third of the vastus lateralis muscle of the thigh.

Test-Taking Strategy: Focus on the **subject,** the purpose of administering a phytonadione injection to a newborn. Recalling the physiology associated with the synthesis of phytonadione in the newborn will direct you to the correct option.

Level of Cognitive Ability: Evaluating
Client Needs: Physiological Integrity
Clinical Judgment/Cognitive Skills: Evaluate Outcomes
Integrated Process: Nursing Process/Evaluation
Content Area: Pharmacology: Maternity/Newborn: Vitamin K
Health Problem: N/A

---

346. The nurse is assigned to give a child a tepid tub bath to treat hyperthermia. After the bath, which action would the nurse take?

1 Leave the child uncovered for 15 minutes.
2 Assist the child to put on a cotton sleep shirt.
3 Take the child's axillary temperature in 2 hours.
4 Place the child in bed and cover the child with a blanket.

Level of Cognitive Ability: Applying
Client Needs: Physiological Integrity
Clinical Judgment/Cognitive Skills: Take Action
Integrated Process: Nursing Process/Implementation
Content Area: Pediatrics: Metabolic/Endocrine
Health Problem: Pediatric-Specific: Fever

Answer: 2
Rationale: Cotton is a lightweight material that will protect the child from becoming chilled after the bath. Option 1 is incorrect because the child would not be left uncovered. Option 3 is incorrect because the child's temperature needs to be rechecked a half-hour after the bath. Option 4 is incorrect because a blanket is heavy and may increase the child's body temperature and further increase metabolism.
Priority Nursing Tip: Aspirin (acetylsalicylic acid) would not be administered to a child unless specifically prescribed because of the risk of Reye's syndrome.

Test-Taking Strategy: Focus on the **subject,** treating hyperthermia. Eliminate option 1 because of the word *uncovered.* Eliminate option 3 because of the time frame. Eliminate option 4 because of the word *blanket.*

---

347. The nurse caring for an infant with diarrhea needs to monitor the infant for which **early** sign of dehydration?

1 Cool extremities
2 Gray, mottled skin
3 Capillary refill of 3 seconds
4 Apical pulse rate of 200 beats per minute

Level of Cognitive Ability: Analyzing
Client Needs: Physiological Integrity
Clinical Judgment/Cognitive Skills: Recognize Cues
Integrated Process: Nursing Process/Data Collection
Content Area: Pediatrics: Metabolic/Endocrine
Health Problem: Pediatric-Specific: Dehydration

Answer: 4
Rationale: Dehydration causes interstitial fluid to shift to the vascular compartment in an attempt to maintain fluid volume. When the body is unable to compensate for fluid lost, circulatory failure occurs. The blood pressure will decrease and the pulse rate will increase. This will be followed by peripheral symptoms. Options 1, 2, and 3 are not early signs, and these findings relate to peripheral circulatory status.
Priority Nursing Tip: Acute diarrhea is a cause of dehydration, particularly in children younger than 5 years.

Test-Taking Strategy: Note the **strategic word,** *early,* and think about the physiology that occurs in dehydration. Also note that options 1, 2, and 3 are **comparable or alike** and relate directly to peripheral circulatory status.

---

348. Acetylsalicylic acid (aspirin) is prescribed for a client diagnosed with coronary artery disease before a percutaneous transluminal coronary angioplasty (PTCA). The nurse administers the medication understanding that it is prescribed for what purpose?

1 Relieve postprocedure pain
2 Prevent thrombus formation
3 Prevent postprocedure hyperthermia
4 Prevent inflammation of the puncture site

Answer: 2
Rationale: Before PTCA, the client is usually given an anticoagulant, commonly aspirin, to help reduce the risk of occlusion of the artery during the procedure because the aspirin inhibits platelet aggregation. Options 1, 3, and 4 are unrelated to the purpose of administering aspirin to this client.
Priority Nursing Tip: A daily dose of acetylsalicylic acid (aspirin) may be prescribed after PTCA because of its antiplatelet aggregation properties.

Level of Cognitive Ability: Applying
Client Needs: Physiological Integrity
Clinical Judgment/Cognitive Skills: Take Action
Integrated Process: Nursing Process/Implementation
Content Area: Pharmacology: Cardiovascular: Antiplatelets
Health Problem: Adult Health: Cardiovascular: Coronary Artery Disease

Test-Taking Strategy: Focus on the **subject,** aspirin prescribed to a client before PTCA. Think about the potential complications of a PTCA and the action and properties of aspirin to direct you to the correct option.

---

349. The nurse reviews a primary health care provider's prescriptions and notes that a topical nitrate is prescribed. The nurse notes that acetaminophen is prescribed to be administered before the nitrate. The nurse implements the prescription with which understanding about why acetaminophen is prescribed?

1 Headache is a common side effect of nitrates.
2 Fever usually accompanies myocardial infarction.
3 Acetaminophen potentiates the therapeutic effect of nitrates.
4 Acetaminophen does not interfere with platelet action as acetylsalicylic acid (aspirin) does.

Answer: 1
Rationale: Headache occurs as a side effect of nitrates in many clients. Acetaminophen may be administered before nitrates to prevent headaches or minimize the discomfort from the headaches. Options 2, 3, and 4 are incorrect.
Priority Nursing Tip: Nitrates produce vasodilation, which can cause a headache. Although headaches are a common side effect of nitrates, they may become less frequent with continued use.

Test-Taking Strategy: Focus on the **subject,** nitrate administration. Eliminate option 3 first because this is an incorrect statement. Next eliminate options 2 and 4 because although they are true statements, they do not address the subject of the question. Also recalling that headache is a common side effect of nitrates will direct you to the correct option.

Level of Cognitive Ability: Applying
Client Needs: Physiological Integrity
Clinical Judgment/Cognitive Skills: Take Action
Integrated Process: Nursing Process/Implementation
Content Area: Pharmacology: Cardiovascular: Vasodilators
Health Problem: Adult Health: Cardiovascular: Coronary Artery Disease

---

350. The nurse collects data on a client newly diagnosed with rheumatoid arthritis. The nurse expects to note which **early** manifestations of the disease? **Select all that apply.**

1 Fatigue
2 Anorexia
3 Weakness
4 Low-grade fever
5 Joint deformities
6 Joint inflammation

Answer: 1, 2, 3, 4, 6
Rationale: Rheumatoid arthritis is a chronic, progressive, systemic inflammatory autoimmune disease process that primarily affects the synovial joints. It also affects other joints and body tissues. Early manifestations include fatigue, anorexia, weakness, joint inflammation, low-grade fever, and paresthesia. Joint deformities are late manifestations.
Priority Nursing Tip: For rheumatoid arthritis, the earlier the treatment is begun, the slower the progression of the disease. Treatment includes exercise, physical therapy, medications, and possibly surgery.

Level of Cognitive Ability: Analyzing
Client Needs: Physiological Integrity
Clinical Judgment/Cognitive Skills: Recognize Cues
Integrated Process: Nursing Process/Data Collection
Content Area: Adult Health: Musculoskeletal
Health Problem: Adult Health: Musculoskeletal: Rheumatoid Arthritis

Test-Taking Strategy: Focus on the **subject,** manifestations of rheumatoid arthritis, and note the **strategic word,** *early.* Keeping this word in mind will assist in eliminating option 5, because joint deformities are late manifestations.

---

351. A client prescribed warfarin sodium has been instructed to limit the intake of foods high in vitamin K. The nurse determines that the client understands the instructions if the client indicates that which food items need to be avoided? **Select all that apply.**

1 Tea
2 Turnips
3 Oranges
4 Cabbage
5 Broccoli
6 Strawberries

Level of Cognitive Ability: Evaluating
Client Needs: Physiological Integrity
Clinical Judgment/Cognitive Skills: Evaluate Outcomes
Integrated Process: Nursing Process/Evaluation
Content Area: Pharmacology: Cardiovascular: Anticoagulants
Health Problem: N/A

Answer: 1, 2, 4, 5
Rationale: Warfarin sodium is an anticoagulant that interferes with the hepatic synthesis of vitamin K–dependent clotting factors. The client is instructed to limit the intake of foods high in vitamin K while taking this medication. These foods include coffee or tea (caffeine), turnips, cabbage, broccoli, greens, fish, and liver. Oranges and strawberries are high in vitamin C.
Priority Nursing Tip: Warfarin sodium is an anticoagulant, and bleeding is a concern when this medication is administered.

Test-Taking Strategy: Focus on the **subject,** foods high in vitamin K that need to be avoided. Knowledge regarding the foods high in vitamin K is needed to answer correctly. However, note that options 3 and 6 are **comparable or alike** in that they are both fruits.

---

352. The nurse is caring for a newly delivered breast-feeding infant. Which intervention performed by the nurse would **best** prevent jaundice in this infant?

1 Placing the infant under phototherapy
2 Keeping the infant NPO until the second period of reactivity
3 Encouraging the parent to breast-feed the infant every 2 to 3 hours
4 Encouraging the parent to supplement breast-feeding with formula

Level of Cognitive Ability: Applying
Client Needs: Physiological Integrity
Clinical Judgment/Cognitive Skills: Take Action
Integrated Process: Nursing Process/Implementation
Content Area: Maternity: Newborn
Health Problem: Newborn: Newborn Feeding

Answer: 3
Rationale: To help prevent jaundice, the parent needs to feed the infant frequently in the immediate birth period because colostrum is a natural laxative and helps promote the passage of meconium. Breast-feeding needs to begin as soon as possible after birth while the infant is in the first period of reactivity. Delaying breast-feeding decreases the production of prolactin, which decreases the parent's milk production. Phototherapy requires a prescription and is not implemented until bilirubin levels are 12 mg/dL or higher in the healthy term infant. Offering the infant a formula supplement will cause nipple confusion and decrease the amount of milk produced by the parent.
Priority Nursing Tip: The appearance of jaundice in the first 24 hours of life is abnormal and must be reported to the pediatrician.

Test-Taking Strategy: Focus on the **subject,** newborn jaundice. Recalling the physiology associated with jaundice and noting the **strategic word,** *best,* will assist in eliminating options 1 and 2. From the remaining options, select the correct option based on the fact that offering a formula supplement will cause nipple confusion.

---

353. The nurse assists to create a postoperative plan of care for a client undergoing an arthroscopy. The nurse would include which **priority** action in the plan?
1 Monitor intake and output.
2 Check the tissue at the surgical site.
3 Monitor the area for numbness or tingling.
4 Check the complete blood cell count results.

Level of Cognitive Ability: Creating
Client Needs: Physiological Integrity
Clinical Judgment/Cognitive Skills: Generate Solutions
Integrated Process: Nursing Process/Planning
Content Area: Foundations of Care: Diagnostic Tests
Health Problem: N/A

Answer: 3
Rationale: Arthroscopy provides an endoscopic examination of the joint and is used to diagnose and treat acute and chronic disorders of the joint. The priority nursing action is to monitor the affected area for numbness or tingling. Options 1, 2, and 4 are also components of postoperative care, but from the options presented, they are not the initial priorities.
Priority Nursing Tip: Assessment of neurovascular status of an extremity includes checking distal pulses, capillary refill, warmth, presence of pain, color, movement, and sensation.

Test-Taking Strategy: Note the **strategic word,** *priority.* Use the **ABCs—airway, breathing, and circulation**—to answer the question. The correct option relates to circulation.

---

354. The nurse is caring for a client diagnosed with active tuberculosis who is prescribed rifampin therapy. The nurse instructs the client to expect which side effect of this medication?
1 Green urine
2 Yellow sclera
3 Orange secretions
4 Clay-colored stools

Level of Cognitive Ability: Applying
Client Needs: Physiological Integrity
Clinical Judgment/Cognitive Skills: Take Action
Integrated Process: Teaching and Learning
Content Area: Pharmacology: Respiratory: Tuberculosis Medications
Health Problem: Adult Health: Respiratory: Tuberculosis

Answer: 3
Rationale: Rifampin is an antituberculosis medication. Secretions will become orange in color as a result of the rifampin. The client would be instructed that this side effect will likely occur and would be told that soft contact lenses, if used by the client, will become permanently discolored. Options 1, 2, and 4 are not expected effects.
Priority Nursing Tip: Rifampin is hepatotoxic, and the client needs to notify the primary health care provider if jaundice (yellow eyes or skin) occurs.

Test-Taking Strategy: Focus on the **subject,** an expected side effect of rifampin. Eliminate options 1, 2, and 4 because they are **comparable or alike** in that they are all symptoms of intrahepatic obstruction as seen in viral hepatitis.

---

355. The nurse sends a sputum specimen to the laboratory for culture from a client with suspected active tuberculosis (TB). The results report that *Mycobacterium tuberculosis* is cultured. How would the nurse correctly analyze these results?
1 The results are positive for active TB.
2 The results indicate a less virulent strain of TB.
3 The results are inconclusive until a repeat sputum specimen is sent.
4 The results are unreliable unless the client has also had a positive tuberculin skin test (TST).

Answer: 1
Rationale: Culture of *M. tuberculosis* from sputum or other body secretions or tissue confirms the diagnosis of active TB. Options 2 and 3 are incorrect statements. The TST is performed to assist in diagnosing TB but does not confirm active disease.
Priority Nursing Tip: The client with active TB is placed in respiratory isolation precautions in a negative-pressure room.

Level of Cognitive Ability: Analyzing
Client Needs: Physiological Integrity
Clinical Judgment/Cognitive Skills: Analyze Cues
Integrated Process: Nursing Process/Data Collection
Content Area: Adult Health: Respiratory
Health Problem: Adult Health: Respiratory: Tuberculosis

Test-Taking Strategy: Focus on the **subject,** diagnosing TB. Recall that culture of the bacteria from sputum confirms the diagnosis. Because TB affects the respiratory system, it would make sense that the bacteria would be found in the sputum if the client had active disease, thereby confirming the diagnosis.

---

356. The licensed practical nurse (LPN) assists the registered nurse (RN) to care for a client admitted with acute myocardial infarction (MI). The LPN would monitor the client for which **most** common complication of MI?

1 Heart failure
2 Cardiogenic shock
3 Cardiac dysrhythmias
4 Recurrent MI

Level of Cognitive Ability: Analyzing
Client Needs: Physiological Integrity
Clinical Judgment/Cognitive Skills: Recognize Cues
Integrated Process: Nursing Process/Data Collection
Content Area: Complex Care: Emergency Situations/Management
Health Problem: Adult Health: Cardiovascular: Myocardial Infarction

Answer: 3

Rationale: Dysrhythmias are the most common complication and cause of death after an MI. Heart failure, cardiogenic shock, and recurrent MI are also complications but occur less frequently.

Priority Nursing Tip: Administering morphine sulfate as prescribed is a priority in managing pain in the client having an MI. Pain relief increases oxygen supply to the myocardium.

Test-Taking Strategy: Note the **strategic word,** *most.* Think about the pathophysiology associated with MI and the complications of MI to direct you to the correct option.

---

357. The nurse in the newborn nursery is planning to assist with the admission of a large-for-gestational-age (LGA) infant. In preparing to care for this infant, the nurse would obtain equipment to perform which diagnostic test?

1 Serum insulin level
2 Heel-stick blood glucose
3 Rh and ABO blood typing
4 Indirect and direct bilirubin levels

Level of Cognitive Ability: Applying
Client Needs: Physiological Integrity
Clinical Judgment/Cognitive Skills: Generate Solutions
Integrated Process: Nursing Process/Planning
Content Area: Maternity: Newborn
Health Problem: Newborn: Gestational Age Problems

Answer: 2

Rationale: After birth, the most common problem in the LGA infant is hypoglycemia, especially if the parent is diabetic. At delivery, when the umbilical cord is clamped and cut, maternal blood glucose supply is lost. The newborn continues to produce large amounts of insulin, which depletes the infant's blood glucose within the first hours after birth. If immediate identification and treatment of hypoglycemia are not performed, the newborn may suffer central nervous system damage caused by inadequate circulation of glucose to the brain. Serum insulin levels are not helpful because there is no intervention to decrease these levels to prevent hypoglycemia. There is no rationale for prescribing an Rh and ABO blood type unless the maternal blood type is O or Rh negative. Indirect and direct bilirubin levels are usually prescribed after the first 24 hours because jaundice is usually seen at 48 to 72 hours after birth.

Priority Nursing Tip: Feedings need to be provided to the LGA newborn soon after birth because of the risk for hypoglycemia in the infant.

Test-Taking Strategy: Focus on the **subject,** an LGA infant. Recalling that hypoglycemia is the concern will direct you to the correct option.

---

358. The nurse caring for a client receiving intravenous (IV) therapy monitors for which signs of infiltration of an IV infusion? **Select all that apply.**
1 Slowing of the IV rate
2 Tenderness at the insertion site
3 Edema around the insertion site
4 Skin tightness at the insertion site
5 Warmth of skin at the insertion site
6 Fluid leaking from the insertion site

Level of Cognitive Ability: Analyzing
Client Needs: Physiological Integrity
Clinical Judgment/Cognitive Skills: Recognize Cues
Integrated Process: Nursing Process/Data Collection
Content Area: Complex Care: Intravenous Therapy
Health Problem: N/A

Answer: 1, 2, 3, 4, 6
Rationale: Infiltration is the leakage of an IV solution into the extravascular tissue. Manifestations include slowing of the IV rate; burning, tenderness, or general discomfort at the insertion site; increasing edema in or around the catheter insertion site; complaints of skin tightness; blanching or coolness of the skin; and fluid leaking from the insertion site.
Priority Nursing Tip: Infiltration at an IV site produces coolness of the skin, whereas phlebitis at an IV site produces warmth of the skin.

Test-Taking Strategy: Focus on the **subject,** IV infiltration. Read each option, thinking about the characteristics of infiltration. Recalling that infiltration is the leakage of an IV solution into the extravascular tissue will assist in eliminating option 5. Remember that fluid infusing into tissue will result in coolness, not warmth.

---

359. A client receiving total parenteral nutrition through a subclavian catheter suddenly develops dyspnea, tachycardia, cyanosis, and decreased level of consciousness. Based on these findings, which is the **best** intervention for the nurse to implement for the client?
1 Obtain a stat oxygen saturation level.
2 Examine the insertion site for redness.
3 Perform a stat finger-stick glucose level.
4 Turn the client to the left side in Trendelenburg's position.

Level of Cognitive Ability: Applying
Client Needs: Physiological Integrity
Clinical Judgment/Cognitive Skills: Take Action
Integrated Process: Nursing Process/Implementation
Content Area: Complex Care: Emergency Situations/Management
Health Problem: N/A

Answer: 4
Rationale: Clinical indicators of air embolism include chest pain, tachycardia, dyspnea, anxiety, feelings of impending doom, cyanosis, and hypotension. Positioning the client in Trendelenburg's and on the left side helps isolate the air embolism in the right atrium and prevents a thromboembolic event in a vital organ. Monitoring the oxygen saturation is a reasonable nursing response to the client's condition; however, acting to prevent deterioration in the client's condition is more important than obtaining additional client data. Options 2 and 3 are unrelated to the symptoms identified in the question.
Priority Nursing Tip: Measures that prevent air embolism from an intravenous (IV) infusion include priming the tubing with fluid before use, securing all connections, and replacing the IV fluid before the container is empty.

Test-Taking Strategy: Focus on the **subject,** air embolism, and note the **strategic word,** *best.* Note the findings in the question and recall that the signs of air embolism are similar to those experienced with pulmonary embolism. Then analyze the options to determine the one that is the best in this situation, which will direct you to the correct option.

---

360. A client has a total serum calcium level of 7.5 mg/dL. Which clinical manifestations would the nurse expect to note on data collection of the client? **Select all that apply.**

1 Constipation
2 Muscle twitches
3 Negative Chvostek's sign
4 Positive Trousseau's sign
5 Hyperactive deep tendon reflexes
6 Prolonged ST interval on electrocardiogram (ECG)

Level of Cognitive Ability: Analyzing
Client Needs: Physiological Integrity
Clinical Judgment/Cognitive Skills: Recognize Cues
Integrated Process: Nursing Process/Data Collection
Content Area: Foundations of Care: Fluids & Electrolytes
Health Problem: N/A

Answer: 2, 4, 5, 6

Rationale: Hypocalcemia is a total serum calcium level less than 9 mg/dL. Clinical manifestations of hypocalcemia include decreased heart rate, diminished peripheral pulses, hypotension, and prolonged ST interval and QT interval on ECG. Neuromuscular manifestations include anxiety and irritability; paresthesia followed by numbness; muscle twitches, cramps, tetany, and seizures; hyperactive deep tendon reflexes; and positive Trousseau's and Chvostek's signs. Gastrointestinal manifestations include increased gastric motility, hyperactive bowel sounds, abdominal cramping, and diarrhea.

Priority Nursing Tip: Calcium gluconate 10% may be prescribed to treat acute calcium deficit.

Test-Taking Strategy: Focus on the **subject,** hypocalcemia. Note the **data in the question** and the calcium level. First determine that the level is low and the client is experiencing hypocalcemia. Next think about the manifestations associated with hypocalcemia. Remember that hyperactive bowel sounds and diarrhea occur in hypocalcemia.

---

361. A client is experiencing acute cardiac and cerebral symptoms as a result of an excess fluid volume. Which nursing measure would the nurse plan to implement to increase the client's comfort until specific therapy is prescribed by the primary health care provider?

1 Cover the client with warm blankets.
2 Minimize the visual and auditory stimuli present.
3 Elevate the client's head to at least 45 degrees.
4 Administer oxygen at 4 L/min by nasal cannula.

Level of Cognitive Ability: Applying
Client Needs: Physiological Integrity
Clinical Judgment/Cognitive Skills: Take Action
Integrated Process: Nursing Process/Implementation
Content Area: Complex Care: Emergency Situations/Management
Health Problem: N/A

Answer: 3

Rationale: Elevating the head of the bed to 45 degrees decreases venous return to the heart from the lower body, thus reducing the volume of blood that has to be pumped by the heart. It also promotes venous drainage from the brain, reducing cerebral symptoms. Oxygen is a medication and is not administered at 4 L without a prescription to do so. Options 1 and 2 are unrelated to this scenario.

Priority Nursing Tip: A client with kidney failure is at high risk for fluid volume excess.

Test-Taking Strategy: Focus on the **subject,** nursing measures to increase the client's comfort. This tells you that the correct option is one that directly involves care delivery to the client. With this in mind, eliminate options 1 and 2 because they are not associated with the condition of the client. From the remaining options, note that the correct option identifies a nursing measure.

---

362. The nurse assists to create a discharge plan for a client who had an abdominal hysterectomy. Which activity instructions would the nurse include in the plan? **Select all that apply.**

1 Avoid heavy lifting.
2 Sit as much as possible.
3 Take baths rather than showers.
4 Limit stair climbing to 5 times a day.
5 Gradually increase walking as exercise but stop before becoming fatigued.
6 Avoid jogging, aerobic exercises, sports, or any strenuous exercise for 6 weeks.

Level of Cognitive Ability: Creating
Client Needs: Physiological Integrity
Clinical Judgment/Cognitive Skills: Generate Solutions
Integrated Process: Nursing Process/Planning
Content Area: Foundations of Care: Perioperative Care
Health Problem: N/A

Answer: 1, 4, 5, 6

Rationale: After abdominal hysterectomy, the client needs to avoid lifting anything that is heavy and limit stair climbing to 5 times a day. The client needs to walk indoors for the first week and then gradually increase walking as exercise but stop before becoming fatigued. The client needs to avoid jogging, aerobic exercises, sports, or any strenuous exercise for 6 weeks. The client is also told to avoid the sitting position for extended periods, to take showers rather than tub baths, avoid crossing the legs at the knees, and avoid driving for at least 4 weeks or until the surgeon has given permission to do so.

Priority Nursing Tip: Monitor vaginal bleeding after hysterectomy. More than one saturated pad per hour may indicate excessive bleeding.

Test-Taking Strategy: Focus on the **subject**, activity instructions after abdominal hysterectomy. Read each option carefully, focusing on the type and location of the surgery and the importance of protecting the surgical area. This will assist in eliminating options 2 and 3.

---

363. The nurse has a prescription to ambulate a client with a nephrostomy tube 4 times a day. The nurse determines that the safest way to ambulate the client while maintaining the integrity of the nephrostomy tube is to implement which intervention?

1 Change the drainage bag to a leg collection bag.
2 Tie the drainage bag to the client's waist while ambulating.
3 Use a walker to hang the drainage bag from while ambulating.
4 Tell the client to hold the drainage bag higher than the level of the bladder.

Level of Cognitive Ability: Analyzing
Client Needs: Physiological Integrity
Clinical Judgment/Cognitive Skills: Generate Solutions
Integrated Process: Nursing Process/Planning
Content Area: Skills: Tube Care
Health Problem: N/A

Answer: 1

Rationale: The safest approach to protect the integrity and safety of the nephrostomy tube with a mobile client is to attach the tube to a leg collection bag. This allows for greater freedom of movement while preventing accidental disconnection or dislodgment. The drainage bag is kept below the level of the bladder. Option 3 presents the risk of tension or pulling on the nephrostomy tube by the client during ambulation.

Priority Nursing Tip: The total bladder capacity for an adult is 600 to 800 mL, and the normal urine output is 1500 to 2000 mL a day.

Test-Taking Strategy: Focus on the **subject**, safety in regard to a nephrostomy tube. Note that options 2, 3, and 4 are **comparable or alike** because they all indicate placing the drainage bag above the level of the bladder.

---

364. A client newly diagnosed with polycystic kidney disease asks the nurse to explain again what the **most** serious complication of the disorder might be. The nurse will provide the client with information concerning which condition?

1 Diabetes insipidus
2 End-stage renal disease (ESRD)
3 Chronic urinary tract infection (UTI)
4 Syndrome of inappropriate antidiuretic hormone (SIADH) secretion

Level of Cognitive Ability: Applying
Client Needs: Physiological Integrity
Clinical Judgment/Cognitive Skills: Take Action
Integrated Process: Nursing Process/Implementation
Content Area: Adult Health: Renal and Urinary
Health Problem: Adult Health: Renal and Urinary: Hereditary Diseases

Answer: 2

Rationale: In polycystic kidney disease, cystic formation and hypertrophy of the kidneys occur. The most serious complication of polycystic kidney disease is ESRD, which is managed with dialysis or transplant. There is no reliable way to predict who will ultimately progress to ESRD. Chronic UTIs are the most common complication because of the altered anatomy of the kidney and from development of resistant strains of bacteria. Diabetes insipidus and SIADH secretion are unrelated disorders.

Priority Nursing Tip: The nurse would discuss the importance of seeking genetic counseling with the client diagnosed with polycystic kidney disease because the disease is hereditary.

Test-Taking Strategy: Note the **strategic word,** *most.* Also noting the word *end-stage* and recalling that ESRD is life threatening and requires dialysis for treatment will direct you to the correct option.

---

365. The nurse is assisting in creating a plan of care for a client who has returned to the nursing unit after left nephrectomy. Which assessments would the nurse include in the plan of care? **Select all that apply.**

1 Pain level
2 Vital signs
3 Hourly urine output
4 Tolerance for sips of clear liquids
5 Ability to cough and deep-breathe

Level of Cognitive Ability: Creating
Client Needs: Physiological Integrity
Clinical Judgment/Cognitive Skills: Generate Solutions
Integrated Process: Nursing Process/Data Collection
Content Area: Adult Health: Renal and Urinary
Health Problem: N/A

Answer: 1, 2, 3, 5

Rationale: After nephrectomy, it is imperative to measure the urine output on an hourly basis. This is done to monitor the effectiveness of the remaining kidney and detect renal failure early, if it should occur. The client may also experience significant pain after this surgery, which could affect the client's ability to reposition, cough, and deep-breathe. Therefore, the next most important measurements are vital signs, pain level, and ability to cough and deep-breathe. Clear liquids are not given until the client has bowel sounds.

Priority Nursing Tip: After nephrectomy, monitor for a urinary output of 30 to 50 mL/hr.

Test-Taking Strategy: Focus on the **subject,** assessment after nephrectomy. Note the relationship between *nephrectomy* in the question and *urine output* in option 3. Remember that the client may also experience significant pain after surgery, which could affect the client's ability to cough and deep-breathe. Therefore, options 1, 2, and 5 (vital signs, pain level, and ability to cough and deep-breathe) are necessary assessments after nephrectomy.

---

366. The nurse instructs a parent of a child who had a plaster cast applied to the arm about measures that will help the cast dry. Which instructions would the nurse provide to the parent? **Select all that apply.**

1 Lift the cast using the fingertips.
2 Place the child on a firm mattress.
3 Direct a fan toward the cast to facilitate drying.
4 Support the cast and adjacent joints with pillows.
5 Place the extremity with the cast in a dependent position.
6 Reposition the extremity with the cast every 2 to 4 hours.

Answer: 2, 3, 4, 6

Rationale: To help the cast dry, the child needs to be placed on a firm mattress. A fan may be directed toward the cast to facilitate drying. Once the cast is dry, the cast would sound hollow and be cool to the touch. The cast and adjacent joints need to be elevated and supported with pillows. To ensure thorough drying, the extremity with the cast needs to be repositioned every 2 to 4 hours. The cast is lifted by using the palms of the hands (not the fingertips) to prevent indentation in the wet cast surface. Indentations could possibly cause pressure on the skin under the cast.

Priority Nursing Tip: Monitor the extremity with a cast for signs of circulatory impairment. If these occur, notify the primary health care provider immediately and prepare for bivalving and cutting the cast.

Test-Taking Strategy: Focus on the **subject**, measures that will help the cast dry. Eliminate option 1 because of the word *fingertips* and option 5 because of the word *dependent*.

Level of Cognitive Ability: Applying
Client Needs: Physiological Integrity
Clinical Judgment/Cognitive Skills: Take Action
Integrated Process: Teaching and Learning
Content Area: Pediatrics: Musculoskeletal
Health Problem: Pediatric-Specific: Fractures

---

367. A client is receiving cisplatin. On data collection of the client, which findings indicate that the client is experiencing an adverse effect of the medication?

1 Tinnitus
2 Increased appetite
3 Excessive urination
4 Yellow halos in front of the eyes

Answer: 1

Rationale: Cisplatin is an antineoplastic medication. An adverse effect related to the administration of cisplatin is ototoxicity with hearing loss. The nurse needs to check for this adverse reaction when administering this medication. Options 2, 3, and 4 are not adverse effects of this medication.

Priority Nursing Tip: Cisplatin, an antineoplastic medication, is a platinum compound and can cause ototoxicity, tinnitus, hypokalemia, hypocalcemia, hypomagnesemia, and nephrotoxicity.

Test-Taking Strategy: Focus on the **subject**, an adverse effect of cisplatin. Recalling that ototoxicity is an adverse effect will direct you to the correct option, the only option that relates to the ear.

Level of Cognitive Ability: Analyzing
Client Needs: Physiological Integrity
Clinical Judgment/Cognitive Skills: Recognize Cues
Integrated Process: Nursing Process/Data Collection
Content Area: Pharmacology: Pharmacology: Oncology/Alkylating
Health Problem: N/A

---

368. A child is admitted to the hospital with a diagnosis of nephrotic syndrome. The nurse expects to note documentation of which manifestations in the medical record? **Select all that apply.**

1 Edema
2 Proteinuria
3 Hypertension
4 Abdominal pain
5 Increased weight
6 Hypoalbuminemia

Level of Cognitive Ability: Analyzing
Client Needs: Physiological Integrity
Clinical Judgment/Cognitive Skills: Recognize Cues
Integrated Process: Nursing Process/Data Collection
Content Area: Pediatrics: Renal and Urinary
Health Problem: Pediatric-Specific: Nephrotic Syndrome

Answer: 1, 2, 4, 5, 6
Rationale: Nephrotic syndrome refers to a kidney disorder characterized by edema, proteinuria, and hypoalbuminemia. The child also experiences anorexia, fatigue, abdominal pain, respiratory infection, and increased weight. The child's blood pressure is usually normal or slightly below normal.
Priority Nursing Tip: For the client with nephrotic syndrome, a regular diet without added salt may be prescribed if the child is in remission; sodium and fluids may be restricted during periods of massive edema.

Test-Taking Strategy: Focus on the **subject**, nephrotic syndrome. Recalling that nephrotic syndrome is characterized by proteinuria, hypoalbuminemia, and edema will assist in determining the correct options. Also remember that the blood pressure is usually normal in this condition.

---

369. Twelve hours after delivery, the nurse checks the client for uterine involution. The nurse determines that the uterus is progressing normally toward its prepregnancy state when palpation of the client's fundus is at which level?

1 At the umbilicus
2 One fingerbreadth below the umbilicus
3 Two fingerbreadths below the umbilicus
4 Midway between the umbilicus and the symphysis pubis

Level of Cognitive Ability: Applying
Client Needs: Physiological Integrity
Clinical Judgment/Cognitive Skills: Recognize Cues
Integrated Process: Nursing Process/Data Collection
Content Area: Maternity: Postpartum
Health Problem: N/A

Answer: 1
Rationale: The term *involution* is used to describe the rapid reduction in size and the return of the uterus to a normal condition similar to its nonpregnant state. Immediately after the delivery of the placenta, the uterus contracts to the size of a large grapefruit. The fundus is situated in the midline between the symphysis pubis and the umbilicus. Within 6 to 12 hours after birth, the fundus of the uterus rises to the level of the umbilicus. The top of the fundus remains at the level of the umbilicus for about a day and then descends into the pelvis approximately 1 fingerbreadth on each succeeding day.
Priority Nursing Tip: By approximately 10 days postpartum, the uterus cannot be palpated abdominally.

Test-Taking Strategy: Focus on the **subject,** the location of the uterus 12 hours after birth. Visualize the process of data collection of involution and the expected finding at this time to answer the question.

---

370. A client is scheduled for a subtotal gastrectomy (Billroth II procedure). The nurse explains that the procedure will have which surgical results?

1 Proximal end of the distal stomach is anastomosed to the duodenum
2 Entire stomach is removed and the esophagus is anastomosed to the duodenum
3 Lower portion of the stomach is removed and the remainder is anastomosed to the jejunum
4 Antrum of the stomach is removed and the remaining portion is anastomosed to the duodenum

Level of Cognitive Ability: Applying
Client Needs: Physiological Integrity
Clinical Judgment/Cognitive Skills: Take Action
Integrated Process: Nursing Process/Implementation
Content Area: Adult Health: Gastrointestinal
Health Problem: Adult Health: Gastrointestinal: Upper GI Disorders

Answer: 3
Rationale: In the Billroth II procedure, the lower portion of the stomach is removed and the remainder is anastomosed to the jejunum. The duodenal stump is preserved to permit bile flow to the jejunum. Options 1, 2, and 4 are incorrect descriptions.
Priority Nursing Tip: Postoperative complications after gastrectomy procedures include hemorrhage, dumping syndrome, diarrhea, hypoglycemia, and vitamin B_{12} deficiency.

Test-Taking Strategy: Focus on the **subject,** gastrectomy (Billroth II procedure), which indicates removal of the stomach. This would assist in eliminating option 1. From the remaining options, note the word *subtotal* in the question, which indicates "lower and a part of." This would direct you to the correct option.

---

371. A client diagnosed with diabetes mellitus receives 8 units of regular insulin subcutaneously at 7:30 AM. The nurse needs to be **most** alert to signs of hypoglycemia at what time during the day?

1 9:30 AM to 11:30 AM
2 11:30 AM to 1:30 PM
3 1:30 PM to 3:30 PM
4 3:30 PM to 5:30 PM

Level of Cognitive Ability: Applying
Client Needs: Physiological Integrity
Clinical Judgment/Cognitive Skills: Recognize Cues
Integrated Process: Nursing Process/Data Collection
Content Area: Pharmacology: Endocrine: Insulin
Health Problem: Adult Health: Endocrine: Diabetes Mellitus

Answer: 1
Rationale: Regular insulin is a short-acting insulin. Its onset of action occurs in a half-hour and peaks in 2 to 4 hours. Its duration of action is 4 to 6 hours. A hypoglycemic reaction will most likely occur at peak time, which in this situation is between 9:30 AM and 11:30 AM.
Priority Nursing Tip: Not all types of insulin can be administered by the intravenous route. Regular insulin is one type of insulin that can be administered intravenously.

Test-Taking Strategy: Note the **strategic word,** *most.* Recall knowledge regarding the onset, peak, and duration of action of regular insulin to answer this question. Recalling that regular insulin is a short-acting insulin will direct you to the correct option.

---

372. The nurse assists to create a postoperative plan of care for a client scheduled for a hypophysectomy. Which interventions would be included in the plan of care? **Select all that apply.**

1 Obtain daily weights.
2 Monitor intake and output.
3 Elevate the head of the bed.
4 Use a soft toothbrush for mouth care.
5 Encourage coughing and deep breathing.

Level of Cognitive Ability: Creating
Client Needs: Physiological Integrity
Clinical Judgment/Cognitive Skills: Generate Solutions
Integrated Process: Nursing Process/Planning
Content Area: Adult Health: Endocrine
Health Problem: Adult Health: Endocrine: Pituitary Disorders

Answer: 1, 2, 3

Rationale: A hypophysectomy is done to remove a pituitary tumor. Because temporary diabetes insipidus or syndrome of inappropriate antidiuretic hormone can develop after this surgery, obtaining daily weights and monitoring intake and output are important interventions. The head of the bed is elevated to assist in preventing increased intracranial pressure. Tooth brushing, sneezing, coughing, nose blowing, and bending are activities that need to be avoided postoperatively in the client who underwent a hypophysectomy because of the risk of increasing intracranial pressure. These activities interfere with the healing of the incision and can disrupt the graft.

Priority Nursing Tip: Increased intracranial pressure is a complication of hypophysectomy.

Test-Taking Strategy: Focus on the **subject,** postoperative care after hypophysectomy. Consider the anatomical location of the surgical procedure and associated complications. Although coughing and deep breathing are usually a normal component of postoperative care, in this situation, coughing is contraindicated. Additionally, tooth brushing can interfere with healing.

---

373. After undergoing a thyroidectomy, a client is monitored for signs of damage to the parathyroid glands postoperatively. The nurse would determine that which finding suggests damage to the parathyroid glands?

1 Fever
2 Neck pain
3 Hoarseness
4 Tingling around the mouth

Level of Cognitive Ability: Analyzing
Client Needs: Physiological Integrity
Clinical Judgment/Cognitive Skills: Recognize Cues
Integrated Process: Nursing Process/Data Collection
Content Area: Adult Health: Endocrine
Health Problem: Adult Health: Endocrine: Parathyroid Disorders

Answer: 4

Rationale: The parathyroid glands can be damaged or their blood supply impaired during thyroid surgery. Hypocalcemia and tetany result when parathyroid hormone (PTH) levels decrease. The nurse monitors for complaints of tingling around the mouth or of the toes or fingers and muscular twitching because these are signs of calcium deficiency. Additional later signs of hypocalcemia are positive Chvostek's and Trousseau's signs. Fever may be expected in the immediate postoperative period but is not an indication of damage to the parathyroid glands. However, if a fever persists, the surgeon is notified. Neck pain and hoarseness are expected findings postoperatively.

Priority Nursing Tip: After thyroidectomy, maintain the client in a semi-Fowler's position to reduce swelling at the operative site.

Test-Taking Strategy: Focus on the **subject,** damage to the parathyroid glands, and consider the anatomical location of the surgical procedure. Recalling that neck pain and hoarseness are expected findings postoperatively will assist in eliminating options 2 and 3. From the remaining options, focusing on the subject will assist in eliminating option 1. Also, recalling that hypocalcemia results when PTH levels decrease will assist in directing you to the correct option.

---

374. The nurse is assisting in the admission assessment on a client admitted with a diagnosis of Raynaud's disease. The nurse checks for the associated symptoms by performing which actions?

1 Checking for a rash on the digits
2 Observing for softening of the nails or nail beds
3 Palpating for a rapid or irregular peripheral pulse
4 Palpating for diminished or absent peripheral pulses

Level of Cognitive Ability: Analyzing
Client Needs: Physiological Integrity
Clinical Judgment/Cognitive Skills: Recognize Cues
Integrated Process: Nursing Process/Data Collection
Content Area: Adult Health: Cardiovascular
Health Problem: Adult Health: Cardiovascular: Vascular Disorders

Answer: 4
Rationale: Raynaud's disease is vasospasm of the arterioles and arteries of the upper and lower extremities. It produces closure of the small arteries in the distal extremities in response to cold, vibration, or external stimuli. Palpation for diminished or absent peripheral pulses checks for interruption of circulation. Skin changes include hair loss, thinning or tightening of the skin, and delayed healing of cuts or injuries. A rash on the digits is not a characteristic of this disorder. The nails grow slowly, become brittle or deformed, and heal poorly around the nail beds when infected. Although palpation of peripheral pulses is correct, a rapid or irregular pulse would not be noted.
Priority Nursing Tip: Teach the client with Raynaud's disease to avoid smoking; wear warm clothing, socks, and gloves in cold weather; and avoid injuries to the fingers and hands.

Test-Taking Strategy: Focus on the **subject,** assessment for Raynaud's disease. Recall the physiological occurrences in Raynaud's disease. Palpation for diminished or absent peripheral pulses checks for interruption of circulation.

---

375. The nurse teaches a postpartum client about postdelivery lochia. The nurse determines that the education has been **effective** when the client says that on the second day postpartum, the lochia would be which color?

1 Red
2 Pink
3 White
4 Yellow

Level of Cognitive Ability: Evaluating
Client Needs: Physiological Integrity
Clinical Judgment/Cognitive Skills: Evaluate Outcomes
Integrated Process: Nursing Process/Evaluation
Content Area: Maternity: Postpartum
Health Problem: N/A

Answer: 1
Rationale: The uterus rids itself of the debris that remains after birth through a discharge called *lochia,* which is classified according to its appearance and contents. Lochia rubra is dark red in color. It occurs from delivery to 3 days postpartum and contains epithelial cells; erythrocytes; leukocytes; shreds of decidua; and occasionally fetal meconium, lanugo, and vernix caseosa. Lochia serosa is a brownish-pink discharge that occurs from days 4 to 10. Lochia alba is a white discharge that occurs from days 10 to 14. Lochia should not be yellow or contain large clots; if it does, the cause needs to be investigated without delay.
Priority Nursing Tip: The amount of lochial discharge may increase with ambulation.

Test-Taking Strategy: Focus on the **subject,** lochia. Note the **strategic word,** *effective.* Noting the words *second day postpartum* will direct you to the correct option.

---

376. The nurse assists to create a care plan for a client receiving hemodialysis through an arteriovenous (AV) fistula in the right arm. The nurse includes which interventions in the plan to protect the AV fistula from injury? **Select all that apply.**

1 Check pulses and circulation proximal to the fistula.
2 Palpate for thrills and auscultate for a bruit every 4 hours.
3 Check for bleeding and infection at hemodialysis needle insertion sites.
4 Avoid taking blood pressure or performing venipunctures in the extremity.
5 Instruct the client not to carry heavy objects or anything that compresses the extremity.
6 Instruct the client not to sleep in a position that places her or his body weight on top of the extremity.

Level of Cognitive Ability: Creating
Client Needs: Physiological Integrity
Clinical Judgment/Cognitive Skills: Generate Solutions
Integrated Process: Nursing Process/Planning
Content Area: Adult Health: Renal and Urinary
Health Problem: Adult Health: Renal and Urinary: Chronic Kidney Disease

Answer: 2, 3, 4, 5, 6

Rationale: An AV fistula is an internal anastomosis of an artery to a vein and is used as an access for hemodialysis. The nurse needs to implement the following to protect the fistula: palpate for thrills and auscultate for a bruit every 4 hours, check for bleeding and infection at hemodialysis needle insertion sites, avoid taking blood pressures or performing venipunctures in the extremity, instruct the client not to carry heavy objects or anything that compresses the extremity, instruct the client not to sleep in a position that places the body weight on top of the extremity, and the nurse needs to check pulses and circulation distal to the fistula.

Priority Nursing Tip: Arterial steal syndrome can develop in a client with an AV fistula. In this condition, too much blood is diverted to the vein and arterial perfusion to the hand is compromised.

Test-Taking Strategy: Focus on the **subject,** protecting the AV fistula. Visualize this vascular access device, and read each option carefully. Noting the word *proximal* in option 1 will assist in eliminating this option.

---

377. The newborn nursery nurse is assisting with the admission assessment on a newborn with the diagnosis of subdural hematoma. Which intervention would the nurse implement to check for the **primary** symptom associated with subdural hematoma?

1 Monitor the urine for blood.
2 Monitor the urinary output pattern.
3 Test for contractures of the extremities.
4 Test for equality of extremity reflexes.

Level of Cognitive Ability: Analyzing
Client Needs: Physiological Integrity
Clinical Judgment/Cognitive Skills: Recognize Cues
Integrated Process: Nursing Process/Data Collection
Content Area: Maternity: Newborn
Health Problem: Newborn: Intraventricular Hemorrhage

Answer: 4

Rationale: A subdural hematoma can cause pressure on a specific area of the cerebral tissue. This can cause changes in the stimuli responses in the extremities on the opposite side of the body, especially if the newborn is actively bleeding. Options 1 and 2 are incorrect. After delivery, a newborn would normally be incontinent of urine. Blood in the urine would indicate abdominal trauma and would not be a result of the hematoma. Option 3 is incorrect because contractures would not occur this soon after delivery.

Priority Nursing Tip: A subdural hematoma results from a venous bleed. An epidural hematoma results from arterial bleeding.

Test-Taking Strategy: Note the **strategic word,** *primary.* Eliminate options 1 and 2 because they are **comparable or alike** and are similar assessments. Remember that the method of checking for complications and active bleeding into the cranial cavity is a neurological assessment. Checking newborn reflexes is a neurological assessment. Although contractures of extremities could occur as residual effects, this would not occur immediately.

---

378. A client has received atropine sulfate preoperatively. The nurse monitors the client for which effect of the medication in the **immediate** postoperative period?

1 Diarrhea
2 Bradycardia
3 Urinary retention
4 Excessive salivation

Level of Cognitive Ability: Analyzing
Client Needs: Physiological Integrity
Clinical Judgment/Cognitive Skills: Take Action
Integrated Process: Nursing Process/Data Collection
Content Area: Pharmacology: Neurological: Anticholinergics
Health Problem: N/A

Answer: 3
Rationale: Atropine sulfate is an anticholinergic medication that causes tachycardia, drowsiness, blurred vision, dry mouth, constipation, and urinary retention. The nurse needs to monitor the client for any of these effects in the immediate postoperative period. None of the other options relate to this medication.
Priority Nursing Tip: Anticholinergic medications are contraindicated in the client with glaucoma.

Test-Taking Strategy: Note the strategic word *immediate,* and focus on the **subject**, effects of atropine sulfate. Recalling that atropine sulfate is an anticholinergic and recalling the effects of an anticholinergic will direct you to the correct option.

---

379. A client experiencing calcium oxalate renal calculi is told to limit dietary intake of oxalate. The nurse is confident that the teaching has been **effective** when the client includes which items on a list of foods high in oxalate? **Select all that apply.**

1 Beets
2 Spinach
3 Rhubarb
4 Black tea
5 Cantaloupe
6 Watermelon

Level of Cognitive Ability: Evaluating
Client Needs: Physiological Integrity
Clinical Judgment/Cognitive Skills: Evaluate Outcomes
Integrated Process: Teaching and Learning
Content Area: Adult Health: Renal and Urinary
Health Problem: Adult Health: Renal and Urinary: Obstructive Problems

Answer: 1, 2, 3, 4
Rationale: Food items that are high in oxalate include beets, spinach, rhubarb, black tea, Swiss chard, cocoa, wheat germ, cashews, almonds, pecans, peanuts, okra, chocolate, and lime peel.
Priority Nursing Tip: Encourage the client with renal calculi to increase fluid intake up to 3000 mL a day, unless contraindicated, to facilitate the passage of the stone and prevent infection.

Test-Taking Strategy: Focus on the **subject,** foods high in oxalate. Note the **strategic word,** *effective.* Knowledge regarding food items high in oxalate is needed to answer this question. Remembering that fruits are generally not sources of dietary oxalate will assist in answering questions similar to this one.

---

380. The nurse is gathering data from a client diagnosed with hyperparathyroidism. Which question asked to the client would elicit information about this condition?

1 "Do you have tremors in your hands?"
2 "Are you experiencing pain in your joints?"
3 "Have you had problems with diarrhea lately?"
4 "Do you notice any swelling in your legs at night?"

Answer: 2
Rationale: Hyperparathyroidism causes an oversecretion of parathyroid hormone (PTH), which causes excessive osteoblast growth and activity within the bones. When bone reabsorption is increased, calcium is released from the bones into the blood, causing hypercalcemia. The bones suffer demineralization as a result of calcium loss, leading to bone and joint pain and pathological fractures. Options 1 and 3 relate to assessment of hypoparathyroidism. Option 4 is unrelated to hyperparathyroidism.
Priority Nursing Tip: Safety is a priority in the care of the client with hyperparathyroidism. Move the client slowly and carefully because the client is at risk for pathological fractures.

Level of Cognitive Ability: Analyzing
Client Needs: Physiological Integrity
Clinical Judgment/Cognitive Skills: Recognize Cues
Integrated Process: Nursing Process/Data Collection
Content Area: Adult Health: Endocrine
Health Problem: Adult Health: Endocrine: Parathyroid Disorders

Test-Taking Strategy: Focus on the **subject**, hyperparathyroidism. Knowledge regarding the pathophysiology associated with hyperparathyroidism is required to answer the question. Eliminate options 1 and 3 first because these options provide information about hypoparathyroidism. From the remaining options, it is necessary to know the relationship among hyperparathyroidism, PTH, and joint pain to direct you to the correct option.

---

381. A client seeks medical attention for intermittent signs and symptoms that suggest a diagnosis of Raynaud's disease. The nurse needs to check the trigger of these signs/symptoms by asking which question?

1 "Does being exposed to heat seem to cause the episodes?"
2 "Do the signs and symptoms occur while you are asleep?"
3 "Does drinking coffee or ingesting chocolate seem related to the episodes?"
4 "Have you experienced any injuries that have limited your activity levels lately?"

Level of Cognitive Ability: Analyzing
Client Needs: Physiological Integrity
Clinical Judgment/Cognitive Skills: Recognize Cues
Integrated Process: Nursing Process/Data Collection
Content Area: Adult Health: Cardiovascular
Health Problem: Adult Health: Cardiovascular: Vascular Disorders

Answer: 3
Rationale: Raynaud's disease is vasospasm of the arterioles and arteries of the upper and lower extremities. It produces closure of the small arteries in the distal extremities in response to cold, vibration, or external stimuli. Episodes are characterized by pallor, cold, numbness, and possible cyanosis of the fingers, followed by erythema, tingling, and aching pain. Attacks are triggered by exposure to cold, nicotine, caffeine, trauma to the fingertips, and stress. Prolonged episodes of inactivity are unrelated to these episodes.
Priority Nursing Tip: Because stress can trigger vasospasm, the nurse would teach the client with Raynaud's disease stress management techniques.

Test-Taking Strategy: Focus on the **subject,** precipitating factors for Raynaud's disease. Recalling that symptoms occur with vasoconstriction will assist in eliminating options 1, 2, and 4 because these events are unlikely to cause vasoconstriction.

---

382. The nurse provides information to a client diagnosed with insulin-dependent diabetes mellitus. Which manifestations resulting from a blood glucose level less than 70 mg/dL would the nurse include in the information? **Select all that apply.**

1 Hunger
2 Sweating
3 Weakness
4 Nervousness
5 Cool, clammy skin
6 Increased urinary output

Level of Cognitive Ability: Analyzing
Client Needs: Physiological Integrity
Clinical Judgment/Cognitive Skills: Take Action
Integrated Process: Teaching and Learning
Content Area: Pharmacology: Endocrine: Insulin
Health Problem: Adult Health: Endocrine: Diabetes Mellitus

Answer: 1, 2, 3, 4, 5
Rationale: Hypoglycemia is characterized by a blood glucose level of less than 70 mg/dL. Clinical manifestations of hypoglycemia include hunger, sweating, weakness, nervousness, tachycardia, palpitations, blurred vision or double vision, and cool, clammy skin. Increased urinary output is a manifestation of hyperglycemia.
Priority Nursing Tip: If the client exhibits signs of a hypoglycemic reaction, perform a finger stick and check the client's glucose level. If hypoglycemia is confirmed, give the client a 10- to 15-g carbohydrate item to eat or drink, such as ½ cup of fruit juice.

Test-Taking Strategy: Focus on the **subject,** the manifestations of hypoglycemia. Recall that hypoglycemia is characterized by a blood glucose level lower than 70 mg/dL. Next think about the manifestations that occur when the blood glucose level is low. Also recalling the "3 P's" associated with hyperglycemia—polyuria, polydipsia, and polyphagia—will assist in eliminating option 6.

---

383. The nurse is checking a client with chronic sinusitis. The nurse determines that which manifestations reported by the client are related to this problem? **Select all that apply.**

1 Anosmia
2 Chronic cough
3 Blurry vision
4 Nasal stuffiness
5 Purulent nasal discharge
6 Headache that worsens in the evening

Level of Cognitive Ability: Analyzing
Client Needs: Physiological Integrity
Clinical Judgment/Cognitive Skills: Recognize Cues
Integrated Process: Nursing Process/Data Collection
Content Area: Adult Health: Respiratory
Health Problem: Adult Health: Respiratory: Upper Airway

Answer: 1, 2, 4, 5

Rationale: Chronic sinusitis is characterized by anosmia (loss of smell), a chronic cough resulting from nasal discharge, nasal stuffiness, persistent purulent nasal discharge, and headache that is worse upon arising after sleep. Blurred vision is not associated directly with this condition.

Priority Nursing Tip: Use a steam inhaler (15-minute vaporization of boiled water), bedside humidifier, or nasal saline spray to promote secretion drainage.

Test-Taking Strategy: Focus on the **subject,** chronic sinusitis. Think about the pathophysiology associated with this disorder. This will assist in determining the signs and symptoms and will direct you to the correct option. Remember that headache is worse upon arising after sleep.

---

384. A client is diagnosed with hypothyroidism. The nurse gathers data from the client, expecting to note which findings? **Select all that apply.**

1 Weight loss
2 Bradycardia
3 Hypotension
4 Dry, scaly skin
5 Heat intolerance
6 Decreased body temperature

Level of Cognitive Ability: Analyzing
Client Needs: Physiological Integrity
Clinical Judgment/Cognitive Skills: Recognize Cues
Integrated Process: Nursing Process/Data Collection
Content Area: Adult Health: Endocrine
Health Problem: Adult Health: Endocrine: Thyroid Disorders

Answer: 2, 3, 4, 6

Rationale: The manifestations of hypothyroidism are the result of decreased metabolism from low levels of thyroid hormones. Some of these manifestations are bradycardia; hypotension; cool, dry, scaly skin; decreased body temperature; dry, coarse, brittle hair; decreased hair growth; cold intolerance; slowing of intellectual functioning; lethargy; weight gain; and constipation.

Priority Nursing Tip: A severe complication of hypothyroidism is myxedema coma, a rare but serious disorder that results from persistently low thyroid production. It can be caused by acute illness, anesthesia and surgery, hypothermia, and the use of sedatives and opioids.

Test-Taking Strategy: Focus on the **subject,** hypothyroidism. Recall that it occurs as the result of decreased metabolism from low levels of thyroid hormones. Correlate *hypo*thyroidism with *decreased* body functioning to assist in answering the question. Weight loss and heat intolerance occur in hyperthyroidism.

---

385. A client is diagnosed with diabetes insipidus. The nurse would plan interventions to address which manifestations of this disorder? **Select all that apply.**

1 Bradycardia
2 Hypertension
3 Poor skin turgor
4 Increased urinary output
5 Dry mucous membranes
6 Decreased pulse pressure

Level of Cognitive Ability: Applying
Client Needs: Physiological Integrity
Clinical Judgment/Cognitive Skills: Generate Solutions
Integrated Process: Nursing Process/Planning
Content Area: Adult Health: Endocrine
Health Problem: Adult Health: Endocrine: Pituitary Disorders

Answer: 3, 4, 5, 6
Rationale: Diabetes insipidus is a water metabolism problem caused by an antidiuretic hormone (ADH) deficiency (either a decrease in ADH synthesis or an inability of the kidneys to respond to ADH). Clinical manifestations include poor skin turgor, increased urinary output, dry mucous membranes, decreased pulse pressure, tachycardia, hypotension, weak peripheral pulses, and increased thirst.
Priority Nursing Tip: Monitor for an electrolyte imbalance and signs of dehydration in the client with diabetes insipidus. If the condition is untreated, the client experiences a urine output of 4 to 24 L a day.

Test-Taking Strategy: Focus on the **subject,** diabetes insipidus. Think about the pathophysiology of this disorder, and recall that diabetes insipidus is caused by an ADH deficiency. This will assist in eliminating options 1 and 2.

---

386. A client diagnosed with pneumonia reports a decreased sense of taste that has greatly affected the motivation to eat and drink. Which intervention would the nurse implement to help increase the client's appetite?

1 Offer between-meal snacks.
2 Provide three large meals daily.
3 Provide mouth care before meals.
4 Offer to sit with the client during meals.

Level of Cognitive Ability: Applying
Client Needs: Physiological Integrity
Clinical Judgment/Cognitive Skills: Take Action
Integrated Process: Nursing Process/Implementation
Content Area: Adult Health: Respiratory
Health Problem: Adult Health: Respiratory: Viral, Bacterial, Fungal Infections

Answer: 3
Rationale: The client with pneumonia may experience decreased taste sensation as a result of sputum expectoration. To minimize this adverse effect, the nurse would provide oral hygiene before meals. The client would also have small, frequent meals because of dyspnea. The remaining options will not address the issue of impaired sense of taste.
Priority Nursing Tip: Unless contraindicated, encourage the client with pneumonia to consume fluids, up to 3 L per day, to thin secretions.

Test-Taking Strategy: Focus on the **subject,** anorexia and increasing the client's appetite. Eliminate options 1, 2, and 4 because they are **comparable or alike** and will not increase the client's appetite. Additionally, as a general measure, small frequent meals are better tolerated than large meals.

---

387. The nurse notes that a large number of clients reporting the presence of flulike symptoms are being seen in the clinic. Which recommendations would the nurse provide to these clients to minimize their risk for further illness? **Select all that apply.**

1 Get plenty of rest.
2 Increase intake of liquids.
3 Get a flu shot immediately.
4 Take antipyretics for fever.
5 Consume a well-balanced diet.

Answer: 1, 2, 4, 5
Rationale: Treatment for the flu includes getting rest, drinking fluids, and taking in nutritious foods and beverages. Medications such as antipyretics and analgesics may also be used for symptom management. Immunizations against influenza are a prophylactic measure and are not used to treat flu symptoms.
Priority Nursing Tip: Because the strain of influenza virus is different every year, annual vaccination is recommended.

Level of Cognitive Ability: Applying
Client Needs: Physiological Integrity
Clinical Judgment/Cognitive Skills: Take Action
Integrated Process: Teaching and Learning
Content Area: Adult Health: Respiratory
Health Problem: Adult Health: Viral, Bacterial, Fungal Infections

Test-Taking Strategy: Focus on the **subject,** interventions for influenza. Recalling that a flu shot is a prophylactic measure will assist in directing you to the correct options.

---

388. The nurse reinforcing instructions to a client with chronic pancreatitis about measures to prevent its exacerbation needs to provide which information? **Select all that apply.**

1 Eat bland foods.
2 Avoid alcohol ingestion.
3 Avoid cigarette smoking.
4 Avoid caffeinated beverages.
5 Eat small meals and snacks high in calories.
6 Eat high-fat, low-protein, high-carbohydrate meals.

Level of Cognitive Ability: Applying
Client Needs: Physiological Integrity
Clinical Judgment/Cognitive Skills: Take Action
Integrated Process: Teaching and Learning
Content Area: Adult Health: Gastrointestinal
Health Problem: Adult Health: Gastrointestinal: GI Accessory Organs

Answer: 1, 2, 3, 4, 5
Rationale: Chronic pancreatitis is a progressive, destructive disease of the pancreas, characterized by remissions and exacerbations (recurrence). Measures to prevent an exacerbation include eating bland, low-fat, high-protein, moderate-carbohydrate meals; avoiding alcohol ingestion, nicotine, and caffeinated beverages; eating small meals and snacks high in calories; and avoiding gastric stimulants such as spices.
Priority Nursing Tip: The pain that is associated with acute pancreatitis is aggravated if the client lies in a recumbent position.

Test-Taking Strategy: Focus on the **subject,** measures to prevent an exacerbation of chronic pancreatitis. Thinking about the pathophysiology associated with pancreatitis and noting the term *high-fat* in option 6 will direct you to eliminate this option.

---

389. The nurse notes this cardiac rhythm on the cardiac monitor. What would the nurse interpret that the client is experiencing? **Refer to the figure.**

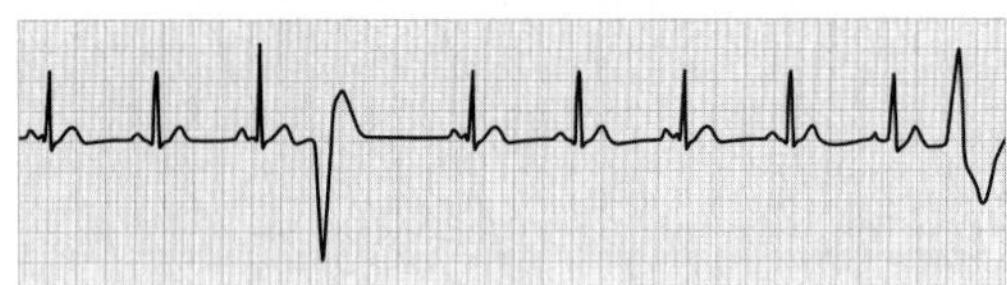

1 Atrial fibrillation
2 Sinus bradycardia
3 Ventricular fibrillation (VF)
4 Premature ventricular contractions (PVCs)

Level of Cognitive Ability: Analyzing
Client Needs: Physiological Integrity
Clinical Judgment/Cognitive Skills: Analyze Cues
Integrated Process: Nursing Process/Data Collection
Content Area: Adult Health: Cardiovascular
Health Problem: Adult Health: Cardiovascular: Dysrhythmias

Answer: 4
Rationale: PVCs are abnormal ectopic beats occurring in otherwise normal sinus rhythm, originating in the ventricles. They are characterized by an absence of P waves, wide and bizarre QRS complexes, and a compensatory pause that follows the ectopy. In atrial fibrillation, no definitive P wave usually can be observed; only fibrillatory waves before each QRS complex are observed. In sinus bradycardia, atrial and ventricular rhythms are regular, and the rates are less than 60 beats per minute. In ventricular fibrillation, impulses from many irritable foci in the ventricles fire in a totally disorganized manner, which appears as a chaotic rapid rhythm in which the ventricles quiver.
Priority Nursing Tip: The cardiologist is notified if the client experiences premature ventricular contractions so that their cause can be identified and they can be treated.

Test-Taking Strategy: Focus on the **subject,** the cardiac rhythm on the cardiac monitor. Remember that PVCs are characterized by wide and bizarre QRS complexes.

---

390. A client is diagnosed with cholecystitis. The nurse reviews the client's medical record, expecting to note documentation of which manifestations of this disorder? **Select all that apply.**

1 Dyspepsia
2 Dark stools
3 Light-colored and clear urine
4 Feelings of abdominal fullness
5 Rebound tenderness in the abdomen
6 Upper abdominal pain that radiates to the right shoulder

Level of Cognitive Ability: Analyzing
Client Needs: Physiological Integrity
Clinical Judgment/Cognitive Skills: Recognize Cues
Integrated Process: Nursing Process/Data Collection
Content Area: Adult Health: Gastrointestinal
Health Problem: Adult Health: Gastrointestinal: GI Accessory Organs

Answer: 1, 4, 5, 6
Rationale: Cholecystitis is an inflammation of the gallbladder. Manifestations include dyspepsia; feelings of abdominal fullness; rebound tenderness (Blumberg's sign); upper abdominal pain or discomfort that can radiate to the right shoulder; pain triggered by a high-fat meal; clay-colored stools, dark urine, and possible steatorrhea; anorexia, nausea, and vomiting; eructation; flatulence; fever; and jaundice.
Priority Nursing Tip: Instruct the client with cholecystitis to consume a diet that is low in fat.

Test-Taking Strategy: Focus on the **subject,** cholecystitis. Think about the function of the gallbladder and the pathophysiology associated with this disorder. This will assist in eliminating options 2 and 3. Remember that clay-colored stools and dark urine occur in this disorder.

---

391. A client is experiencing pulmonary edema as an exacerbation of chronic left-sided heart failure. The nurse assisting in the care of the client would check the client for what manifestation?

1 Weight loss
2 Bilateral crackles
3 Distended neck veins
4 Peripheral pitting edema

Level of Cognitive Ability: Analyzing
Client Needs: Physiological Integrity
Clinical Judgment/Cognitive Skills: Recognize Cues
Integrated Process: Nursing Process/Data Collection
Content Area: Adult Health: Cardiovascular
Health Problem: Adult Health: Cardiovascular: Pulmonary Edema

Answer: 2
Rationale: The client with pulmonary edema presents primarily with symptoms that are respiratory in nature because the blood flow is stagnant in the lungs, which lie behind the left side of the heart from a circulatory standpoint. The client would experience weight gain from fluid retention, not weight loss. Distended neck veins and peripheral pitting edema are classic signs of right-sided heart failure.
Priority Nursing Tip: If the client develops pulmonary edema, immediately place the client in a high-Fowler's position and contact the primary health care provider. Do not leave the client.

Test-Taking Strategy: Focus on the **subject,** pulmonary edema, and note the words *left-sided heart failure.* Knowing that blood flow is stagnant behind the area of failure allows you to eliminate each of the incorrect options. To remember the signs and symptoms of heart failure, remember "left, lungs" and "right, systemic." Option 2 relates to the lungs.

---

392. A client begins to experience a tonic-clonic seizure. Which actions would the nurse take to ensure client safety? **Select all that apply.**

1 Restrict the client's movements.
2 Turn the supine client to the side.
3 Open the unconscious client's airway.
4 Gently guide the standing client to the floor.
5 Place a padded tongue blade into the client's mouth.
6 Loosen any restrictive clothing that the client is wearing.

Level of Cognitive Ability: Applying
Client Needs: Physiological Integrity
Clinical Judgment/Cognitive Skills: Take Action
Integrated Process: Nursing Process/Implementation
Content Area: Adult Health: Neurological
Health Problem: Adult Health: Neurological: Seizure Disorder/Epilepsy

Answer: 2, 3, 4, 6
Rationale: Precautions are taken to prevent a client from sustaining injury during a seizure. The nurse would maintain the client's airway and turn the client to the side. The nurse would also protect the client from injury, guide the client's movements, and loosen any restrictive clothing. Restraints are never used because they could injure the client during the seizure. A padded tongue blade or any other object is never placed into the client's mouth after a seizure begins because the jaw may clench down.
Priority Nursing Tip: If a client experiences a seizure while standing or sitting, gently ease the client to the floor and protect the client's head and body.

Test-Taking Strategy: Focus on the **subject,** a client experiencing seizure activity. Focus on the **ABCs—airway, breathing, and circulation.** Visualize each of the actions to assist in answering correctly. Remember that restraints are never used because they could injure the client and that a padded tongue blade or any other object is never placed into the client's mouth.

---

393. The nurse is monitoring a client diagnosed with a ruptured appendix for signs of peritonitis. The nurse would check for which manifestations of this complication? **Select all that apply.**

1 Bradycardia
2 Distended abdomen
3 Subnormal temperature
4 Rigid, boardlike abdomen
5 Diminished bowel sounds
6 Inability to pass flatus or feces

Level of Cognitive Ability: Analyzing
Client Needs: Physiological Integrity
Clinical Judgment/Cognitive Skills: Recognize Cues
Integrated Process: Nursing Process/Data Collection
Content Area: Adult Health: Gastrointestinal
Health Problem: Adult Health: Gastrointestinal: Lower GI Disorders

Answer: 2, 4, 5, 6
Rationale: Peritonitis is an acute inflammation of the visceral and parietal peritoneum, the endothelial lining of the abdominal cavity. Clinical manifestations include distended abdomen; a rigid, boardlike abdomen; diminished bowel sounds; inability to pass flatus or feces; abdominal pain (localized, poorly localized, or referred to the shoulder or thorax); anorexia, nausea, and vomiting; rebound tenderness in the abdomen; high fever; tachycardia; dehydration from the high fever; decreased urinary output; hiccups; and possible compromise in respiratory status.
Priority Nursing Tip: Avoid the application of heat to the abdomen of a client with appendicitis because heat can cause rupture of the appendix, leading to peritonitis.

Test-Taking Strategy: Focus on the **subject,** signs of peritonitis. Remember that the suffix *-itis* indicates inflammation or infection. This will assist in determining that options 1 and 3 are incorrect. In inflammation, the client would experience an elevated temperature, and tachycardia is a physiological bodily response to fever.

---

394. While preparing to administer an intravenous (IV) piggyback medication, the nurse notes that the medication is incompatible with the IV solution. Which intervention would the nurse implement to ensure the client's safety?

1 Ask the registered nurse about using a different IV solution.
2 Collaborate with the registered nurse about a different administration route.
3 Flush the tubing before and after administering the medication with normal saline.
4 Ask the registered nurse to start a new IV catheter for the incompatible medication.

Level of Cognitive Ability: Applying
Client Needs: Physiological Integrity
Clinical Judgment/Cognitive Skills: Take Action
Integrated Process: Nursing Process/ Implementation
Content Area: Skills: Medication Administration
Health Problem: N/A

Answer: 3
Rationale: When giving a medication intravenously, if the medication is incompatible with the IV solution, the tubing is flushed before and after the medication with infusions of normal saline to prevent inline precipitation of the incompatible agents. Starting a new IV, changing the solution, or changing the administration route is unnecessary because a simpler, less risky, viable option exists.
Priority Nursing Tip: Normal saline is physiologically similar to body fluid and is generally the solution of choice to flush an intravenous line.

Test-Taking Strategy: Focus on the **subject**, intravenous medication administration. You can eliminate options 1, 2, and 4 because they are unnecessary; in addition, option 4 increases the risk of infection and is likely to cause the client discomfort.

---

395. The nurse is preparing to administer ear drops to an infant. The nurse would plan to proceed by taking which step to ensure the appropriate instillation of the medication?

1 Pull down and back on the auricle, and direct the solution onto the eardrum.
2 Pull up and back on the earlobe, and direct the solution toward the wall of the ear canal.
3 Pull up and back on the auricle, and direct the solution toward the wall of the ear canal.
4 Pull down and back on the auricle, and direct the solution toward the wall of the ear canal.

Level of Cognitive Ability: Applying
Client Needs: Physiological Integrity
Clinical Judgment/Cognitive Skills: Take Action
Integrated Process: Nursing Process/ Implementation
Content Area: Skills: Medication Administration
Health Problem: N/A

Answer: 4
Rationale: The infant would be turned on the side with the affected ear uppermost. With the nondominant hand, the nurse pulls down and back on the auricle. The wrist of the dominant hand is rested on the infant's head. The medication is administered by aiming it at the wall of the ear canal rather than directly onto the eardrum. The infant would be held or positioned with the affected ear uppermost for 10 to 15 minutes to retain the solution. In the adult, the auricle is pulled up and back to straighten the auditory canal.
Priority Nursing Tip: For an infant or child younger than 3 years, pull the auricle down and back to administer ear medications. For a child older than 3 years, pull the auricle up and back.

Test-Taking Strategy: Focus on the **subject**, administering ear medications. Basic safety principles related to the administration of ear medications would assist in eliminating option 1. Option 3 is eliminated because it is the adult procedure. It would be difficult to pull up and back on an earlobe; therefore, eliminate option 2.

---

396. A client seeks treatment in an ambulatory clinic for hoarseness that has persisted for 8 weeks. Based on the symptom, the nurse interprets that the client is at risk for which disorder?

1 Thyroid cancer
2 Acute laryngitis
3 Laryngeal cancer
4 Bronchogenic cancer

Level of Cognitive Ability: Analyzing
Client Needs: Physiological Integrity
Clinical Judgment/Cognitive Skills: Analyze Cues
Integrated Process: Nursing Process/Data Collection
Content Area: Adult Health: Respiratory
Health Problem: Adult Health: Respiratory: Upper Airway

Answer: 3

Rationale: Hoarseness is a common early sign of laryngeal cancer, but not of thyroid or bronchogenic cancer. Hoarseness that persists for 8 weeks is not associated with an acute problem, such as laryngitis.

Priority Nursing Tip: Risk factors for laryngeal cancer include smoking, heavy alcohol use, exposure to environmental pollutants such as asbestos or wood dust, and exposure to radiation.

Test-Taking Strategy: Focus on the **subject,** persistent hoarseness. Begin to answer this question by eliminating option 2, because an acute problem would not generally last for 8 weeks. From the remaining options, recall that the vocal cords are in the larynx when selecting the correct option.

---

397. A client is admitted to the cardiac intensive care unit after coronary artery bypass graft (CABG) surgery. The nurse assisting in caring for the client notes that in the first hour after admission, the mediastinal chest tube drainage was 75 mL. During the second hour, the drainage has dropped to 5 mL. The nurse interprets this data and implements which intervention?

1 Identifies that the tube is draining normally
2 Checks the tube to locate a possible occlusion
3 Auscultates the lungs for appropriate bilateral expansion
4 Assists the client with frequent coughing and deep breathing

Level of Cognitive Ability: Synthesizing
Client Needs: Physiological Integrity
Clinical Judgment/Cognitive Skills: Take Action
Integrated Process: Nursing Process/Implementation
Content Area: Complex Care: Emergency Situations/Management
Health Problem: Adult Health: Cardiovascular: Coronary Artery Disease

Answer: 2

Rationale: After CABG surgery, chest tube drainage would not exceed 100 to 150 mL/hr during the first 2 hours postoperatively, and approximately 500 mL of drainage is expected in the first 24 hours after CABG surgery. The sudden drop in drainage between the first and second hour indicates that the tube is possibly occluded and requires further assessment by the nurse. Options 1, 3, and 4 are incorrect interventions.

Priority Nursing Tip: After CABG surgery, monitor the client for hypotension and hypertension. Hypotension can cause collapse of a vein graft. Hypertension causes increased pressure and can promote leakage from the suture line and bleeding.

Test-Taking Strategy: Focus on the **subject,** chest tube drainage. Eliminate option 3 first because the mediastinal chest tubes remove fluid from the mediastinum and are unrelated to restoration of negative pleural pressure or bilateral expansion. Needing to cough and deep-breathe is a response that is unrelated to the client's problem, so option 4 is eliminated next. From the remaining options, knowing that the drainage would not drop so radically in 1 hour in the immediate postoperative period directs you to the correct option.

---

398. The nurse is checking a client diagnosed with pleurisy 48 hours ago. When auscultating the chest, the nurse is unable to detect the pleural friction rub, which was auscultated on admission. This change in the client's condition confirms which event has occurred?

1 The prescribed medication therapy has been effective.
2 The client has been taking deep breaths as instructed.
3 The effects of the inflammatory reaction at the site decreased.
4 There is now an accumulation of pleural fluid in the inflamed area.

Level of Cognitive Ability: Analyzing
Client Needs: Physiological Integrity
Clinical Judgment/Cognitive Skills: Analyze Cues
Integrated Process: Nursing Process/Data Collection
Content Area: Adult Health: Respiratory
Health Problem: Adult Health: Respiratory: Pleurisy

Answer: 4
Rationale: Pleurisy is the inflammation of the visceral and parietal membranes. These membranes rub together during respiration and cause pain. Pleural friction rub is auscultated early in the course of pleurisy, before pleural fluid accumulates. Once fluid accumulates in the inflamed area, there is less friction between the visceral and parietal lung surfaces, and the pleural friction rub disappears. Options 1, 2, and 3 are incorrect interpretations.
Priority Nursing Tip: Instruct the client with pleurisy to lie on the affected side to splint the chest. This will ease the pain when coughing and deep-breathing.

Test-Taking Strategy: Focus on the **subject,** pleurisy and pleural friction rub. Options 1 and 3 are **comparable or alike,** and because the question states that the problem was diagnosed 48 hours ago, these options would be eliminated. Eliminate option 2 because deep breaths would intensify the pain. Remember that fluid accumulation in the area provides a buffer between the lung and chest wall surfaces, which resolves the friction rub.

---

399. The nurse reinforces information to a client with a colostomy. When discussing measures to help manage colostomy odors, the nurse will encourage the client to regularly consume which foods? **Select all that apply.**

1 Parsley
2 Yogurt
3 Buttermilk
4 Cucumbers
5 Cauliflower
6 Cranberry juice

Level of Cognitive Ability: Applying
Client Needs: Physiological Integrity
Clinical Judgment/Cognitive Skills: Take Action
Integrated Process: Teaching and Learning
Content Area: Foundations of Care: Therapeutic Diets
Health Problem: Adult Health: Gastrointestinal: Lower GI Disorders

Answer: 1, 2, 3, 6
Rationale: The nurse would provide information about foods and measures that will prevent odor from a colostomy. Parsley, yogurt, buttermilk, and cranberry juice will prevent odor. Charcoal filters, pouch deodorizers, or placement of a breath mint in the pouch will also eliminate odors. Foods that cause flatus and thus odor, including broccoli, brussels sprouts, cabbage, cauliflower, cucumbers, mushrooms, and peas, need to be avoided.
Priority Nursing Tip: Body image is a concern for a client with a colostomy, and the nurse needs to be sensitive to the client when discussing this concern.

Test-Taking Strategy: Focus on the **subject,** foods to control odor. Eliminate options 4 and 5 using basic knowledge regarding nutrition because these foods cause flatus.

---

400. When a client experiences frequent runs of ventricular tachycardia, the cardiologist prescribes flecainide. Because of the effects of the medication, the nurse assisting in caring for the client plans for which intervention that is specific to this client's safety?

1 Monitor the client's urinary output.
2 Check the client for neurological problems.
3 Ensure that the bed rails remain in the up position.
4 Monitor the client's vital signs and electrocardiogram (ECG) frequently.

Level of Cognitive Ability: Analyzing
Client Needs: Physiological Integrity
Clinical Judgment/Cognitive Skills: Take Action
Integrated Process: Nursing Process/Implementation
Content Area: Pharmacology: Cardiovascular: Antidysrhythmics
Health Problem: Adult Health: Cardiovascular: Dysrhythmias

Answer: 4
Rationale: Flecainide is an antidysrhythmic medication that slows conduction and decreases excitability, conduction velocity, and automaticity. However, the nurse must monitor for the development of a new or worsening dysrhythmia. Options 1, 2, and 3 are components of standard care but are not specific to this medication.
Priority Nursing Tip: Monitor the client receiving flecainide for an increase in the number or severity of dysrhythmias. This adverse effect may warrant a decrease in dosage or discontinuation of the medication.

Test-Taking Strategy: Focus on the **subject,** flecainide. Note the relationship between the information in the question (the client has a dysrhythmia) and the nursing action in the correct option. Select the option that relates to cardiac status monitoring.

---

401. The nurse provides information to a client diagnosed with gastroesophageal reflux disease (GERD). What information would the nurse include when discussing foods that contribute to decreased lower esophageal sphincter (LES) pressure and thus worsen the condition? **Select all that apply.**

1 Alcohol
2 Fatty foods
3 Citrus fruits
4 Baked potatoes
5 Caffeinated beverages
6 Tomatoes and tomato products

Level of Cognitive Ability: Applying
Client Needs: Physiological Integrity
Clinical Judgment/Cognitive Skills: Take Action
Integrated Process: Nursing Process/Implementation
Content Area: Adult Health: Gastrointestinal
Health Problem: Adult Health: Gastrointestinal: Upper GI Disorders

Answer: 1, 2, 3, 5, 6
Rationale: GERD occurs as a result of the backward flow (reflux) of gastrointestinal contents into the esophagus. The most common cause of GERD is inappropriate relaxation of the LES, which allows the reflux of gastric contents into the esophagus and exposes the esophageal mucosa to gastric contents. Factors that influence the tone and contractility of the LES and lower LES pressure include alcohol; fatty foods; citrus fruits; caffeinated beverages such as coffee, tea, and cola; tomatoes and tomato products; chocolate; nicotine in cigarette smoke; calcium channel blockers; nitrates; anticholinergics; high levels of estrogen and progesterone; peppermint and spearmint; and nasogastric tube placement. Baked potatoes would not contribute to worsening the problem.
Priority Nursing Tip: Teach the client with GERD to avoid lying down with a full stomach; to avoid eating within 2 to 3 hours of bedtime; to avoid wearing tight-fitting clothing, particularly around the waist; and to sleep with the head of the bed raised at least 6 to 8 inches.

Test-Taking Strategy: Note the client's diagnosis of GERD and focus on the **subject,** factors that contribute to decreased LES pressure. Read each option and consider whether the item will aggravate the client's condition. The only item that will not is option 4, baked potatoes.

UNIT
III

Integrated Processes

CHAPTER

10

Integrated Processes and the NCLEX-PN® Test Plan

INTEGRATED PROCESSES

In the new test plan implemented in April 2020, the National Council of State Boards of Nursing (NCSBN) identified a test plan framework based on Client Needs. This framework was selected on the basis of the analysis of the findings in a practice analysis study of newly licensed practical nurses in the United States. This study identified the nursing activities performed by entry-level nurses across all settings for all clients. The NCSBN identified four major categories of Client Needs. These categories—Physiological Integrity, Safe and Effective Care Environment, Health Promotion and Maintenance, and Psychosocial Integrity—are described in Chapter 5.

The 2020 NCLEX-PN test plan also identifies five processes, titled Integrated Processes, that are fundamental to the practice of nursing. These processes are integrated throughout the four major categories of Client Needs and include Caring, Clinical Problem-Solving Process (Nursing Process), Communication and Documentation, Culture and Spirituality, and Teaching and Learning (Box 10.1).

CARING

Caring is the essence of nursing, and it is basic to any helping relationship; it is central to every encounter that the nurse has with a client. Through caring, the nurse humanizes the client. Treating the client with respect and dignity is a true expression of caring. In the technological environment of health care, emphasizing the client's individuality counteracts any potential process of depersonalization. Caring is an Integrated Process of the test plan of the NCLEX-PN, so this concept is central to all Client Needs categories of the plan. The NCSBN describes caring as the interaction of the nurse and client in an atmosphere of mutual respect and trust; in this collaborative environment, the nurse provides support and compassion to help achieve the desired outcomes.

In the NCLEX-PN, the concept of caring is primary. It is easy to become involved with looking at a question from a technological viewpoint. However, the concept of caring should be addressed when reading a test question and when selecting an option. Always address the client and the client's feelings and provide support. Remember that this examination is all about nursing and that nursing is caring (Box 10.2).

Box 10.1 ▲ INTEGRATED PROCESSES

Caring
Clinical Problem-Solving Process (Nursing Process)
Communication and Documentation
Culture and Spirituality
Teaching and Learning

Box 10.2 ▲ CARING

QUESTION

A client and her infant have undergone testing for human immunodeficiency virus (HIV), and both clients were found to be positive. The news is devastating, and the client is crying. Which is the appropriate intervention at this time?

1. Discuss with the client how she got HIV.
2. Listen quietly while the client talks and cries.
3. Describe the progressive stages and treatments of HIV.
4. Call an HIV counselor and make an appointment for the client.

ANSWER: 2

HIV is a retrovirus that causes acquired immunodeficiency syndrome. The client has just received devastating news and should have someone present with her as she begins to cope with this issue. The nurse should sit and actively listen while the client talks and cries. Calling an HIV counselor may be helpful, but it is not what the client needs at this time. The other options are inappropriate for this stage of coping with the news that both the client and the infant are HIV-positive. Remember to address the client's feelings and to support the client. The nurse should sit, listen, and provide support because this is the most caring response.

CLINICAL PROBLEM-SOLVING PROCESS (NURSING PROCESS)

The Clinical Problem-Solving Process (Nursing Process) provides a systematic and organized approach for delivering care to clients. The steps of this process are data collection, planning, implementation, and evaluation (Box 10.3).

Data Collection

Data collection is the first step of the nursing process, when the nurse participates in a systematic method of establishing a database about the client. This step of the nursing process includes gathering information about the client, recognizing cues, communicating the information gained during the data collection, analyzing cues and prioritizing hypotheses by collaborating with the registered nurse, and contributing to the formation of a plan of care.

Data collection begins with the first contact with the client. The database provides the foundation for the remaining steps of the nursing process. During all successive contacts, the nurse continues to collect information that is significant and relevant to the needs of the client. With each contact, the nurse uses all of the senses to gather data about the client and recognize cues.

The nurse collects data about the client from a variety of sources during this process. The client is the primary source of data. Family members or significant others are secondary sources of data, and these sources may supplement or verify the information provided by the client. Data may also be obtained from other health care team members and from the client's current and prior health records.

The information collected by the nurse includes both subjective and objective data. Subjective data include the information that the client states and that is based on the client's opinion. Objective data are the observable, measurable pieces of information about the client. Objective data include measurements (e.g., vital signs, laboratory findings) and information obtained from the observation of the client. Objective data also include clinical manifestations (e.g., the signs and symptoms of an illness or disease).

As part of the process of data collection, the nurse is responsible for recognizing significant cues in the client, determining the need for additional information, reporting findings to the registered nurse (RN) or other relevant health care team members (e.g., the health care provider), and documenting findings thoroughly and accurately.

The nurse contributes to the formation of a nursing care plan by assisting the registered nurse with analyzing cues and prioritizing hypotheses, organizing relevant health care data, and determining significant relationships between the data and client needs, problems, or both.

On the NCLEX-PN, remember that data collection is the first step of the nursing process. When answering these types of questions, focus on the data in the question, and select the option that addresses a data collection action. The exception to this guideline is if the question identifies an emergency situation; in an emergency situation, a nursing action may be the priority. In addition, use the skills of prioritizing (e.g., the ABCs—airway, breathing, and circulation; Maslow's Hierarchy of Needs theory) to answer the question. Additionally, if the question asks about the procedure for administering cardiopulmonary resuscitation, then follow the CAB (circulation, airway, breathing) guidelines (Box 10.4).

Box 10.3 ▲ CLINICAL PROBLEM-SOLVING PROCESS (NURSING PROCESS)

Data Collection
Planning
Implementation
Evaluation

PLANNING

Planning is the second step of the nursing process. In this step, the nurse provides input into plan development, participates in setting goals for meeting the client's needs, and helps generate solutions to achieve these goals.

Box 10.4 ▲ CLINICAL PROBLEM-SOLVING PROCESS: DATA COLLECTION

QUESTION

The nurse assigned to care for a client with a tracheostomy tube is asked to check the client for subcutaneous emphysema. The nurse checks the client for which data associated with subcutaneous emphysema?

1. Signs of respiratory distress
2. Crackling sounds heard in the lungs
3. Abnormal skin and mucous membrane color
4. A crackling sensation on palpation of the tissues surrounding the tracheostomy site

ANSWER: 4

Subcutaneous emphysema, which is also known as *crepitus*, is a complication of a tracheostomy. It occurs when air escapes from the tracheostomy incision into the tissues; dissects fascial planes under the skin; and accumulates around the face, neck, and upper chest. These areas appear puffy, and slight finger pressure will produce a crackling sound and sensation. This is not generally a serious condition because the air will eventually be absorbed. Options 1, 2, and 3 are not characteristics of subcutaneous emphysema.

During the planning phase, the nurse assists with the formation of the goals of care by participating in the identification of nursing interventions to achieve goals and by communicating client needs that may require the alteration of the goals of care. The nurse reviews the data collected with the RN and then assists to set goals, generate solutions, and list interventions. When evidence of a new client problem emerges, the nurse again collects data about the problem and collaborates with the RN; then the plan of care is revised accordingly. Prioritizing hypotheses and setting priorities assist the nurse with organizing and planning care that solves the most urgent problems. The client should be included in discussions when identifying the priorities of care. Priorities may change as the client's level of wellness changes. The most important problems—those that are potentially life threatening—must be taken care of immediately.

After priorities are established, the client and the nurse mutually decide on the expected goals. A goal must be set for each priority or client need. The selected goals serve as a guide for individualizing the care of the client. The goals must be client-centered, measurable, realistic, time-referenced, and determined by the client and nurse together. Unless criteria for the goals have been predetermined, it is difficult to know whether the goal is achieved and if the problem has been resolved.

The nurse assists with the development of the plan of care by collaborating with the client, the RN, and other health care team members to generate solutions and select nursing interventions that will achieve the goals and by planning for client safety, comfort, and the maintenance of optimal functioning. The nurse participates in the identification of health and social resources available to the client and family and collaborates with other health care team members when planning the delivery of care. The nurse should communicate client needs, review the plan of care with the RN, and document the plan of care thoroughly and accurately.

When answering questions on the NCLEX-PN, remember that this is a nursing examination. The answer to the question most likely will involve something that is included in the nursing care plan rather than the medical plan, unless the question asks what the nurse anticipates that the primary health care provider will prescribe. In addition, remember that actual problems are usually more important than potential or at-risk problems and that physiological needs are usually the priority (Box 10.5).

Box 10.5 ▲ CLINICAL PROBLEM-SOLVING PROCESS: PLANNING

QUESTION

The nurse is planning care for a child admitted to the hospital with an infectious and communicable disease. The nurse would identify which as a **priority** goal?

1. The public health department will be notified.
2. The child will not spread the infection to others.
3. The child will experience only minor complications.
4. The nursing supervisor will be notified about the child's diagnosis.

ANSWER: 2

Note the **strategic word,** *priority.* From the options provided, the priority goal for a child with an infectious and communicable disease is to prevent the spread of infection to others. Although the nursing supervisor would be notified of the child's diagnosis and the health department may need to be notified at some point, these are not priority goals. The child should experience no complications.

Implementation

Implementation is the third step of the nursing process, and it includes initiating and completing the nursing actions that are required to accomplish the defined goals. This step is the take action phase, and it involves assisting with organizing and managing client care, providing care to achieve established goals of care, and communicating nursing interventions.

The nurse assists with organizing and managing the client's care by implementing the established plan of care and by participating in client care conferences. The nurse is responsible for using safe and appropriate techniques and precautionary and preventive interventions when providing care to a client. The nurse is also responsible for taking action if adverse responses occur, initiating lifesaving interventions for emergency situations, and providing an environment that is conducive to the attainment of the goals of care.

This step of the nursing process also includes providing care based on the client's needs, preferences, or both; encouraging the client to follow the prescribed treatment plan; and assisting the client with maintaining optimal functioning. In addition, the process of implementation includes monitoring the client care administered by other health care providers such as other licensed practical nurses and assistive personnel and reinforcing teaching about the principles, procedures, and techniques required for the maintenance and promotion of health.

The implementation step concludes when the nurse's actions are completed and when these actions, including their effects and the client's response, are communicated to the relevant members of the health care team and documented.

The NCLEX-PN is an examination about nursing, so focus on the nursing action rather than the medical action unless the question is asking what prescribed medical action is anticipated (Box 10.6).

Box 10.6 ▲ CLINICAL PROBLEM-SOLVING PROCESS: IMPLEMENTATION

QUESTION

The nurse is changing a dressing on a hospitalized client who had abdominal surgery. When the nurse removes the abdominal dressing, the nurse notes a protrusion of the bowel through the incision. Which action would the nurse take **first**?

1. Notify the registered nurse.
2. Check the client's vital signs.
3. Prepare the client for surgery.
4. Document the findings, actions taken, and client response.

ANSWER: 1

Evisceration is the protrusion of an internal organ (e.g., a bowel loop) through an incision. Wound eviscerations are emergencies, and if an evisceration occurs, the registered nurse is immediately notified and will then contact the surgeon. The client is then immediately placed in a supine (on the back) and semi-Fowler's position, with the knees slightly flexed. This position eases pressure on the wound, prevents further tearing of the wound edges, and reduces the risk of further evisceration. The nurse next covers the protruding bowel with a sterile dressing that has been moistened with sterile normal saline solution to help prevent wound contamination and to keep the abdominal contents moist. After these immediate interventions have been performed, the nurse checks the client's vital signs and pulse oximetry for abnormalities and signs of shock. An intravenous device will be inserted if one is not in place, and the client will be placed on NPO (nothing by mouth) status because surgery will most likely be needed to repair the wound. Finally, the nurse documents the findings, the actions taken, and the client's response.

Evaluation

Evaluation is the fourth step of the nursing process, and it is a way of evaluating outcomes and measuring client progress toward the meeting of established goals. Although evaluation is the final step of the nursing process, it is an ongoing and integral component of each step. The process of data collection is reviewed to determine whether sufficient information was obtained and whether the information obtained was specific and appropriate. The plan and expected outcomes are examined to determine whether they are realistic, achievable, time-referenced, measurable, and effective. Interventions are examined to determine their effectiveness in achieving the expected outcomes.

Because evaluation is ongoing, it is vital to all steps of the nursing process. Evaluation is the continuous process of comparing actual outcomes with the expected outcomes of care, and it provides the means for determining the need to modify the plan of care. Inherent in this step of the nursing process are the communication of evaluation findings, the process of documenting and reporting the client's response to treatment and care, and the determination of the effectiveness of teaching to relevant members of the health care team.

Evaluation questions on the NCLEX-PN may be written to address a client's response to treatment measures or to determine a client's understanding of the prescribed treatment measures (Box 10.7).

Box 10.7 ▲ CLINICAL PROBLEM-SOLVING PROCESS: EVALUATION

QUESTION

The nurse administers hydralazine hydrochloride to a client with autonomic dysreflexia. Which finding indicates that the medication is **effective**?

1. Muscle spasms subside.
2. The blood pressure declines.
3. The client says, "I feel better."
4. The intensity of seizure activity declines.

ANSWER: 2

Hydralazine hydrochloride is an antihypertensive agent that decreases the blood pressure by providing vasodilation. Options 1, 3, and 4 either do not indicate a specific response or are unrelated to the action of the medication.

COMMUNICATION AND DOCUMENTATION

The process of communication occurs as the nurse interacts either verbally or nonverbally with a client. Therapeutic communication techniques are essential to an effective nurse–client relationship. Communication questions are integrated throughout the NCLEX-PN test plan, and they may address a client situation in any health care setting. The NCSBN describes communication and documentation as both the verbal and nonverbal interactions between the client, the significant others, and the members of the health care team, as well as the events and activities associated with client care as validated through a written or electronic record that reflects standards of practice and accountability into the provision of care.

When answering a question on the NCLEX-PN, the use of an effective communication technique indicates a correct option, and the use of an ineffective communication technique indicates an incorrect option. In addition, some communication questions may focus on psychosocial issues or issues related to client anxiety, fears, and concerns. With these types of questions, always focus on the client's feelings, concerns, and anxieties first, and select the option that reflects these.

Documentation is a critical component of a nurse's responsibilities. The process of documentation serves many purposes and provides a comprehensive representation of the client's health status and of the care provided by all members of the health care team. There are many methods of documentation, but the responsibilities surrounding this practice remain the same.

When answering a question on the NCLEX-PN that is related to documentation, consider the associated ethical and legal responsibilities and the specific guidelines that are related to both narrative and computerized documentation systems (Box 10.8).

CULTURE AND SPIRITUALITY

Culture can be described as the knowledge, beliefs, and patterns of behavior; ideas; attitudes; values; and norms that are unique to a particular group of people. Spirituality is a broad concept that carries different meanings for different individuals. It can relate to religious beliefs and values and to the soul or human spirit, rather than to material and physical things. Spirituality is reflected in how a person lives their life, and is shown in their values and beliefs. These values and beliefs can directly affect a person's health choices.

Nurses often care for clients who come from ethnic, cultural, religious, and spiritual backgrounds that are different from their own. The nurse is responsible for providing quality care, including culturally competent care, to all members of society. Awareness of and sensitivity to the unique health and illness beliefs and practices of people of different backgrounds are essential for the delivery of safe and effective care.

The NCLEX-PN test plan describes culture and spirituality as an interaction between the nurse and client that recognizes and considers unique and individual preferences to client care.

Providing individualized and holistic client care that addresses individual beliefs, customs, and practices is a role of the nurse. Cultural awareness is learning about the cultures of clients being cared for; this includes a self-examination of one's own background and a recognition of biases, prejudices, and assumptions about other people. The nurse needs to ask the client about their cultural and spiritual health care practices and preferences so that the nurse can create plans of care that address individualized cultural and spiritual needs and goals. This is an essential nursing responsibility to provide culturally competent health care.

When taking the NCLEX examination, remember that cultural sensitivity is a nursing responsibility and that it is important to ask clients about their cultural and spiritual preferences so that culturally congruent plans of care can be developed (Box 10.9).

TEACHING AND LEARNING

Client and family education are primary nursing responsibilities. The NCSBN describes teaching and learning as facilitating the acquisition of knowledge, skills, and attitudes that lead to a change in behavior. The principles related to the teaching and learning process are used when the nurse functions in the role of a teacher. The nurse should remember that determining the client's readiness and motivation to learn is the initial step of the teaching and learning process.

When answering a question on the NCLEX-PN that is related to the teaching and learning process, use the principles related to Teaching and Learning theory. If a test question addresses client education, remember that a client's motivation and readiness to learn are the first priorities (Box 10.10).

Box 10.8 ▲ COMMUNICATION AND DOCUMENTATION

COMMUNICATION QUESTION

A client with depression states to the nurse that he is going to "put an end to my misery." The nurse would provide which response to the client?

1. "We all feel like that at times."
2. "Why do you feel as if you need to say that?"
3. "Can you tell me more about what you plan to do?"
4. "You feel like that now, but soon you'll regain your will to live."

ANSWER: 3

All suicidal threats must be taken seriously, and their meaning must be thoroughly explored. Options 1 and 4 devalue and ignore the client's feelings. Option 2 is incorrect because "why" questions are demeaning and belittling, and they will make the client feel guilty. Also, the client may not know the reason for his thoughts or intended actions.

DOCUMENTATION QUESTION

The nurse hears a client calling out for help. The nurse hurries down the hallway to the client's room and finds the client lying on the floor. The nurse checks the client thoroughly and assists the client back to bed. The nurse notifies the registered nurse of the incident and completes an incident report. Which would the nurse document in the incident report?

1. The client fell out of bed.
2. The client climbed over the side rails.
3. The client was found lying on the floor.
4. The client became restless and tried to get out of bed.

ANSWER: 3

Rationale: The incident report should contain the client's name, age, and diagnosis. It should contain a factual description of the incident, any injuries experienced by those involved, and the outcome of the situation. Option 3 is the only option that describes the facts as observed by the nurse. Options 1, 2, and 4 are interpretations of the situation and are not factual data as observed by the nurse. Remember to focus on factual information when documenting and to avoid including interpretations.

Box 10.9 ▲ CULTURE AND SPIRITUALITY

CULTURE QUESTION

The nurse is caring for a client who does not speak English. An interpreter is currently unavailable. The nurse needs to perform a dressing change. What would the nurse do to enhance communication with this client before changing the dressing?

1. Ask relatives to interpret because an interpreter is unavailable.
2. Speak slowly and allow the client time to interpret what is being said.
3. Use many nonverbal cues and repetition to reinforce what is being said.
4. Use common words in the nurse's language, because the client is likely to be familiar with them.

ANSWER: 2

When caring for a client who speaks a language that is different from the nurse's, it is ideal for the nurse to call on a dialect-specific interpreter designated by the health care agency. If an interpreter is unavailable, the nurse would speak slowly and allow the client time to interpret what is being said. The nurse would avoid asking relatives to be interpreters to minimize bias and misinterpretation. The nurse would avoid using nonverbal cues, because they could be misinterpreted by the client. The nurse would use common words in the client's language if known.

SPIRITUALITY QUESTION

The nurse is attending an educational session on incorporating spiritual assessment in client care. Which statement, if made by one of the participants attending the session, indicates a **need for further education** regarding spirituality in health care?

1. "Spirituality has different meanings for different people."
2. "Spirituality can positively influence health and quality of life."
3. "Nurses need to be aware of their own spirituality to address this topic with others."
4. "Spirituality can be a comforting influence; however, there is no scientific evidence of the benefits."

ANSWER: 4

Note the **strategic words,** *need for further education.* These words indicate a **negative event query** and the need to select the incorrect statement. Spirituality is a broad concept that is central to a person's life and their "spirit." The spirit is what defines a person and is at the center of all aspects of a person's life. Spirituality has different meanings for different people. It can positively influence health, quality of life, health promotion behaviors, and disease prevention behaviors. Nurses need to be aware of their own spirituality to accurately assess and address spirituality needs for others. Spirituality can have a comforting influence, and there is research that shows the positive influence it can have on a person's overall well-being.

Box 10.10 ▲ TEACHING AND LEARNING

QUESTION

Digoxin and furosemide are prescribed for a client with heart failure, and the nurse provides instructions to the client about the medications. Which client statement indicates the **need for further instruction**?

1. "These medications cause an increase in urine output."
2. "I should take my radial pulse before taking these medications."
3. "I should decrease my intake of foods high in potassium, such as bananas."
4. "These medications should be taken in the morning rather than in the evening."

ANSWER: 3

Note the **strategic words,** *need for further education.* These words indicate a **negative event query** and the need to select the incorrect statement. Digoxin is a cardiac glycoside, and furosemide is a diuretic. Clients who are taking digoxin have an increased risk of toxicity from the potassium-depleting effect of the furosemide. Therefore, the diet should be high in potassium. The client needs to take their pulse before taking cardiac glycosides. For the best therapeutic effects, these medications should be taken at the same time in the morning. A combined therapeutic effect of these medications is to increase urine output. The increased blood flow to the kidneys as a result of enhanced cardiac contractility caused by the digoxin promotes urinary output. Furosemide is a loop diuretic that works by acting on the kidneys to increase the flow of urine and urine output.

CHAPTER

11

Integrated Processes Practice Questions

CARING

1. A client diagnosed with diabetes mellitus requires the immediate amputation of a leg. The client is very upset and states, "This is the doctor's fault! I did everything that I was told to do!" When considering the grieving process, how would the nurse respond to the client's statement?
   1 Notify the agency's risk management department.
   2 Help the client consider alternatives to treatment.
   3 Allow the client to use anger as a coping mechanism.
   4 Ask the client to list all previous health care providers.

Level of Cognitive Ability: Applying
Client Needs: Psychosocial Integrity
Clinical Judgment/Cognitive Skills: Generate Solutions
Integrated Process: Caring
Content Area: Adult Health: Endocrine
Health Problem: Adult Health: Musculoskeletal: Amputation

Answer: 3
Rationale: Anger is a stage in the grieving process and an expected response to impending loss. Usually a client directs the anger toward himself or herself, God or another spiritual being, or the caregivers; thus far, the client's behavior demonstrates effective coping. Notifying the risk management department is premature, especially because the client has said nothing about legal action. Analyzing alternative treatment options and previous health care providers is likely to interfere with effective coping, and it can delay lifesaving treatment.
Priority Nursing Tip: A coping mechanism is a method used to decrease anxiety.

Test-Taking Strategy: Focus on the **subject,** a very upset client. Noting that the client is blaming the doctor and knowledge of the stages of grief associated with loss will direct you to the correct option.

---

2. The nurse has an established relationship with the family of a client whose death is imminent. Which intervention would the nurse focus on in order to help the family **most effectively** cope with this experience?
   1 Limiting time in the client's room to promote privacy
   2 Providing education regarding coping mechanisms
   3 Identifying spiritual measures that work best for dying clients
   4 Answering questions clearly and providing resources as requested

Answer: 4
Rationale: Maintaining effective and open communication among family members affected by death and grief is important to facilitate decision making and effective coping. The nurse maintains and enhances communication and preserves the family's sense of self-direction and control effectively by answering questions clearly and providing information and resources for decision making as requested by the family. Isolating the family from the client by limiting time in the client's room is inappropriate. The nurse would not provide education about coping mechanisms for family members because coping mechanisms directed by the nurse are unlikely to be as effective as the methods that the individuals choose for themselves. Identifying spiritual measures that work best for the dying client generalizes and does not reflect individualized care.

Level of Cognitive Ability: Applying
Client Needs: Psychosocial Integrity
Clinical Judgment/Cognitive Skills: Generate Solutions
Integrated Process: Caring
Content Area: Developmental Stages: End-of-Life Care
Health Problem: Mental Health: Coping

Priority Nursing Tip: People dealing with crisis usually feel helpless and are unable to control the circumstances; therefore, the nurse must facilitate open communication to determine and then meet each person's needs.

Test-Taking Strategy: Note the **strategic words,** *most effectively.* Focus on **therapeutic communication techniques** and the role of the nurse in grieving, loss, and crisis; then choose the most effective intervention. Also note that the correct option uses the words *as requested.*

---

3. A client comes into the emergency department demonstrating manifestations indicative of a severe state of anxiety. What is the **priority** nursing intervention at this time?

1 Remaining with the client
2 Placing the client in a quiet room
3 Teaching the client deep-breathing exercises
4 Encouraging the expression of feelings and concerns

Answer: 1
Rationale: If the client is left alone with severe anxiety, the client may feel abandoned and become overwhelmed. Placing the client in a quiet room is also indicated, but the nurse must stay with the client. It is not possible to teach the client deep-breathing or relaxation exercises until the anxiety decreases. Encouraging the client to discuss concerns and feelings would not take place until the anxiety has decreased.
Priority Nursing Tip: Anxiety occurs as the result of a threat that may be misperceived or misinterpreted or of a threat to identity or self-esteem.

Level of Cognitive Ability: Applying
Client Needs: Psychosocial Integrity
Clinical Judgment/Cognitive Skills: Take Action
Integrated Process: Caring
Content Area: Mental Health
Health Problem: Mental Health: Anxiety disorder

Test-Taking Strategy: Because the anxiety state is severe, eliminate options 3 and 4. From the remaining choices, consider the **strategic word,** *priority,* in the question. Focus on the **subject,** a client in a severe state of anxiety. This will direct you to the correct option.

---

4. When a client is dead on arrival (DOA) to the emergency department, the family members state that they do not want an autopsy performed. Which statement would the nurse make in response to the family?

1 "Autopsies are mandatory for clients who are DOA."
2 "Federal law requires autopsies for clients who are DOA."
3 "The medical examiner makes the decision about autopsies."
4 "I will make sure the medical examiner is aware of your request."

Answer: 4
Rationale: The nurse would notify the medical examiner or the coroner when a family wishes to avoid having an autopsy on a deceased family member. Normally, the medical examiner will honor the family's request unless there is a state law requiring the autopsy. Depending on the state, it is not mandatory for every client who is DOA to have an autopsy. However, many states require an autopsy in specific circumstances, including sudden death, a suspicious death, and death within 24 hours of admission to the hospital. Autopsy is not a requirement under federal law.
Priority Nursing Tip: Special consents are required for performing an autopsy, using restraints, receiving blood transfusions, photographing the client, disposing of body parts during surgery, and donating organs after death. It is often within the client's or family's right to deny such requests.

Level of Cognitive Ability: Applying
Client Needs: Safe and Effective Care Environment

Clinical Judgment/Cognitive Skills: Take Action
Integrated Process: Caring
Content Area: Developmental Stages: End-of-Life Care
Health Problem: Mental Health: Grief/Loss

Test-Taking Strategy: Focus on the **subject,** the laws and issues surrounding autopsy, and use **therapeutic communication techniques** to answer the question. Eliminate options 1 and 2 because these statements are inaccurate. From the remaining choices, option 4 is the most therapeutic and caring response to the family.

---

5. The nurse is interacting with the family of a client who is unconscious as a result of a head injury. Which approach would the nurse use to help the family cope with their concerns?

1 Explain equipment and procedures on an ongoing basis.
2 Discuss that the family should display their grief only when not in the room with the client.
3 Discourage them from touching the client in order to minimize stimulation.
4 Explain that they need their rest, so they should adhere to regular visiting hours.

Level of Cognitive Ability: Applying
Client Needs: Psychosocial Integrity
Clinical Judgment/Cognitive Skills: Take Action
Integrated Process: Caring
Content Area: Adult Health: Neurological
Health Problem: Adult Health: Neurological: Head Injury/Trauma

Answer: 1
Rationale: Families often need assistance to cope with the sudden severe illness of a loved one. The nurse needs to explain all equipment, treatments, and procedures, and he or she would supplement or reinforce the information given by the health care providers. Displaying grief is a normal process and would not be discouraged. The family would be encouraged to touch and speak to the client and become involved in the client's care in some way if they are comfortable with doing so. The nurse would allow the family to stay with the client whenever possible. This is important for both the client and the family.
Priority Nursing Tip: Families of clients who are acutely ill may experience anticipatory grief. Anticipatory grief occurs before the loss and is associated with an acute, chronic, or terminal illness.

Test-Taking Strategy: Use **therapeutic communication techniques** to answer this question. The correct option provides the family with information that will help them cope with the situation. Each of the incorrect options puts distance between the family and the client.

---

6. The nurse assists in admitting a client who is demonstrating right-sided weakness, aphasia, and urinary incontinence. The woman's daughter states, "If this is a stroke, it's the kiss of death." What **initial** response would the nurse make?

1 "Why would you think like that?"
2 "You feel your mother is dying?"
3 "These symptoms are reversible."
4 "A stroke is not the kiss of death."

Level of Cognitive Ability: Applying
Client Needs: Psychosocial Integrity
Clinical Judgment/Cognitive Skills: Take Action
Integrated Process: Caring
Content Area: Foundations of Care: Communication
Health Problem: Adult Health: Neurological: Stroke

Answer: 2
Rationale: Option 2 allows the daughter to verbalize her feelings, begin coping, and adapt to what is happening. By restating, the nurse seeks clarification of the daughter's feelings and offers information that potentially helps ease some of the fears and concerns related to the client's condition and prognosis. Option 1 is a disapproving comment that is likely to interfere with communication. Option 3 is potentially misleading and offers false hope. The nurse could reflect back the statement in option 4 to the daughter to promote communication. However, as it stands, option 4 is a barrier to communication that contradicts the daughter's feelings.
Priority Nursing Tip: Critical factors in the early intervention and treatment of stroke include accurately identifying stroke manifestations and establishing the onset of manifestations.

Test-Taking Strategy: Note the **strategic word,** *initial.* Use the principles of **therapeutic communication** to arrive at the option that allows for clarification of the daughter's feelings.

---

7. A client and her infant have been diagnosed as being positive for human immunodeficiency virus (HIV). When the client is observed crying, the nurse determines that which intervention will meet the client's **initial** needs?
   1 Discussing how the client was exposed to HIV
   2 Sitting quietly with the client as she talks and cries
   3 Describing the progressive stages and treatments of HIV
   4 Calling an HIV counselor to make an appointment for the client and infant

Level of Cognitive Ability: Analyzing
Client Needs: Psychosocial Integrity
Clinical Judgment/Cognitive Skills: Generate Solutions
Integrated Process: Caring
Content Area: Pediatrics: Immune
Health Problem: Pediatric-Specific: Immunodeficiency Disease

Answer: 2
Rationale: This client has just received devastating news and needs to have someone present with her as she begins to cope with this issue. The nurse needs to sit and actively listen while the client talks and cries. Discussing how the client was exposed to HIV and describing the progression and treatment of HIV are inappropriate for this stage of coping. Calling an HIV counselor may be helpful, but it is not what the client needs initially.
Priority Nursing Tip: The nurse must maintain issues of confidentiality surrounding HIV and acquired immunodeficiency syndrome testing while addressing the client's feelings.

Test-Taking Strategy: Note the **strategic word,** *initial.* Use **therapeutic communication techniques,** and remember to focus on the client's feelings. This will direct you to the correct option.

---

8. The nurse cared for a client who died a few minutes ago. Which event supports the nurse's belief that the client died with dignity?
   1 The family thanks the nurse for facilitating such a peaceful death.
   2 The nurse states that it is difficult to give that kind of care to a dying client.
   3 The primary health care provider acknowledges that all of the prescriptions were carried out.
   4 The nurse kept the client's last hours comfortable with increasing doses of pain medication.

Level of Cognitive Ability: Evaluating
Client Needs: Psychosocial Integrity
Clinical Judgment/Cognitive Skills: Evaluate Outcomes
Integrated Process: Caring
Content Area: Developmental Stages: End-of-Life Care
Health Problem: Mental Health: Grief/Loss

Answer: 1
Rationale: The family response is an external perception, and it is extremely important. Families derive a great deal of comfort from knowing that their loved one received the best care possible. The correct option provides external validation that the client received comprehensive, quality care. Option 2 focuses on the feelings of the nurse, who may be expressing his or her own anxiety. Option 3 focuses on the provider's prescriptions rather than client care. Option 4 reflects on only one aspect of the care of a dying client.
Priority Nursing Tip: Outcomes related to care during illness and the dying experience would be based on the client's wishes. Pain must be controlled; the dying client needs to be as pain-free and comfortable as possible.

Test-Taking Strategy: Focus on the **subject,** whether the client died with dignity. The only choice that addresses this subject is the correct option.

---

9. A client diagnosed with Parkinson's disease is having difficulty adjusting to the disorder. The nurse provides education to the family that focuses on addressing the client's activities of daily living. Which statement indicates that the teaching has been **effective?**

1 "We need to plan for only a few activities during the day."
2 "We need to assist with activities of daily living as much as possible."
3 "We need to cluster activities at the end of the day to help conserve energy."
4 "We need to encourage and praise efforts to exercise and perform activities of daily living."

Level of Cognitive Ability: Evaluating
Client Needs: Psychosocial Integrity
Clinical Judgment/Cognitive Skills: Evaluate Outcomes
Integrated Process: Caring
Content Area: Adult Health: Neurological
Health Problem: Adult Health: Neurological: Parkinson's Disease

Answer: 4
Rationale: The client with Parkinson's disease has a tendency to become withdrawn and depressed, which can be limited by encouraging the client to be an active participant in his or her own care. The family would plan activities intermittently throughout the day to inhibit daytime sleeping and boredom. Family members need to give the client encouragement and praise for his or her perseverance in these efforts and help only when necessary.
Priority Nursing Tip: The client with Parkinson's disease needs to exercise in the morning, when energy levels are highest.

Test-Taking Strategy: Focus on the **strategic word,** *effective,* and the **subject,** supporting the client in coping with the effects of Parkinson's disease. Recalling that the client would be an active participant in his or her own care will direct you to the correct option.

---

10. A licensed practical nurse is helping a community health nurse in caring for a group of homeless people. What is the **most immediate** concern when planning for the potential needs of this group?

1 Finding affordable housing for the group
2 Setting up a 24-hour crisis center and hotline
3 Providing peer support through structured support groups
4 Ensuring that adequate food, shelter, and clothing are available

Level of Cognitive Ability: Analyzing
Client Needs: Physiological Integrity
Clinical Judgment/Cognitive Skills: Prioritize Hypotheses
Integrated Process: Caring
Content Area: Foundations of Care: Community Health
Health Problem: Mental Health: Crisis

Answer: 4
Rationale: The question asks about the situation's most immediate concern. The initial community health concern is always attending to people's basic physiological needs of food, shelter, and clothing. Finding affordable housing and providing crisis intervention and peer support are meaningful interventions that may be completed at a later time.
Priority Nursing Tip: Nursing's primary concern is always initially focused on meeting a client's physiological needs.

Test-Taking Strategy: Note the **strategic words,** *most immediate.* Use **Maslow's Hierarchy of Needs theory** to answer the question. The correct option addresses basic physiological needs. Although the remaining options are also appropriate actions, the correct option is the most immediate concern.

---

11. A stillborn baby was delivered a few hours ago. After the birth, the family has remained together, holding and touching the baby. Which statement by the nurse is **most appropriate**?

1 "How can I assist you with ways to remember your baby?"
2 "You seem upset. Do you think a tranquilizer would help?"
3 "I feel so bad. I don't understand why this happened either."
4 "I can allow another 15 minutes together for you to grieve."

Level of Cognitive Ability: Evaluating
Client Needs: Psychosocial Integrity
Clinical Judgment/Cognitive Skills: Evaluate Outcomes
Integrated Process: Caring
Content Area: Developmental Stages: End-of-Life Care
Health Problem: Maternity: Fetal Distress/Demise

Answer: 1

Rationale: Nurses would be able to explore measures that assist the family with creating memories of the infant so that the existence of the child is confirmed and the parents can complete the grieving process. The correct option identifies this measure and also demonstrates a caring and empathetic client-focused response while providing the family with the option to express their needs. Option 2 devalues the parents' feelings and is inappropriate. Option 3 is inappropriate and reflects a lack of knowledge on the nurse's part. Option 4 makes the nurse seem uncaring.

Priority Nursing Tip: Loss and grief may occur with the birth of a preterm infant, an infant with complications of birth, or an infant with congenital anomalies; it may also occur in a client who is giving up a child for adoption. Beliefs and needs vary widely across individuals, cultures, and religions.

Test-Taking Strategy: Focus on the **strategic words,** *most appropriate.* Use **therapeutic communication techniques** to choose the option that demonstrates a caring and empathetic response by the nurse and that meets the psychosocial needs of the grieving client and family.

---

12. The nurse is caring for a depressed, withdrawn client who was responsible for an automobile accident that recently resulted in the death of a child. What is the nurse's **initial** action?

1 Allow the client to have some time alone to grieve over the loss.
2 Reinforce to the client that the child's death was the result of an accident.
3 Communicate in a manner that acknowledges and respects the client's depressed state.
4 Inform the primary health care provider of the client's possible need for medication to cope.

Level of Cognitive Ability: Applying
Client Needs: Psychosocial Integrity
Clinical Judgment/Cognitive Skills: Take Action
Integrated Process: Caring
Content Area: Mental Health
Health Problem: Mental Health: Mood Disorders

Answer: 3

Rationale: The nurse's initial intervention is to encourage the client to express feelings, which is facilitated by establishing a nurse–client relationship that is based on respect. The correct option validates the perception that the client is depressed. This action also allows the nurse to collect data about the situation. Options 1, 2, and 4 address interventions before collecting data about the situation and identifying the client's actual needs.

Priority Nursing Tip: For any client experiencing depression after a traumatic event, the nurse would be nonjudgmental and supportive. Encourage the client to express her or his feelings.

Test-Taking Strategy: Note the **strategic word,** *initial,* while using **therapeutic communication techniques.** Select the option that encourages the client to express feelings and that maintains communication. Remember to always address the client's feelings.

---

13. The nurse is bathing a client when the client begins to cry. Which action by the nurse is therapeutic at this time?
  1 Continue bathing the client and say nothing.
  2 Stop the bath, cover the client, and sit with the client.
  3 Stop the bath, cover the client, and allow the client private time.
  4 Call the primary health care provider to report the signs of depression.

Level of Cognitive Ability: Applying
Client Needs: Psychosocial Integrity
Clinical Judgment/Cognitive Skills: Take Action
Integrated Process: Caring
Content Area: Mental Health
Health Problem: Mental Health: Coping

Answer: 2
Rationale: If a client begins to cry, the nurse needs to stay with the client and let the client know that it is all right to cry. The nurse would ask the client what the client is thinking or feeling at the time. By continuing the bath or by leaving the client, the nurse appears to be ignoring the client's feelings. Crying alone is not necessarily an indication of depression, and calling the primary health care provider is a premature action.
Priority Nursing Tip: Used appropriately, silence and listening are therapeutic communication techniques.

Test-Taking Strategy: Focus on the **subject,** a client who begins to cry. The nurse needs to acknowledge the client's crying and provide emotional support. The correct option is the only one that provides the appropriate care for an emotional client.

---

14. An older couple was emotionally despondent when their home was severely damaged by flooding. When planning for the couple's **initial** needs, what intervention would the nurse plan to implement?
  1 Contacting their families
  2 Attending to their emotional needs
  3 Arranging for the repair of their home
  4 Attending to their basic physiological needs

Level of Cognitive Ability: Analyzing
Client Needs: Physiological Integrity
Clinical Judgment/Cognitive Skills: Prioritize Hypotheses
Integrated Process: Caring
Content Area: Foundations of Care: Community Health
Health Problem: Mental Health: Crisis

Answer: 4
Rationale: The question asks about the first thing that the nurse needs to consider when planning for the rescue and relocation of these older residents. The initial concerns of community health are always attending to people's basic needs of food, shelter, and clothing. Contacting family, addressing emotional needs, and arranging for home repairs are needs that may be addressed as needed after physiological needs are met.
Priority Nursing Tip: For any client, the nurse would address physiological needs first; then the nurse would determine safety and psychosocial needs.

Test-Taking Strategy: Note the **strategic word,** *initial.* Use **Maslow's Hierarchy of Needs theory** to answer the question. The correct option addresses basic physiological needs. Although the remaining options may be appropriate actions at a later time, the correct option is the immediate concern.

---

15. The nurse is assisting in planning the care of a client newly admitted to the mental health unit for suicidal ideations. To provide a caring, therapeutic environment, which intervention would be included in the nursing care plan?
  1 Placing the client in a private room to ensure privacy and confidentiality
  2 Interacting with the client and demonstrating examples of unconditional positive regard

Answer: 2
Rationale: The establishment of a therapeutic relationship with the suicidal client increases feelings of acceptance. Although the suicidal behavior and the client's thinking are unacceptable, the use of unconditional positive regard acknowledges the client in a human-to-human context and increases the client's sense of self-worth. The client would not be placed in a private room because this is an unsafe action that may intensify the client's feelings of worthlessness. A distance of 18 inches or less between two individuals constitutes intimate space. The invasion of this space may be misinterpreted by the client and increase the client's tension

3 Maintaining a distance of 10 inches in order to ensure the client that personal control will be provided
4 Placing the client in charge of a meaningful unit activity, such as the morning chess tournament

Level of Cognitive Ability: Applying
Client Needs: Psychosocial Integrity
Clinical Judgment/Cognitive Skills: Generate Solutions
Integrated Process: Caring
Content Area: Mental Health
Health Problem: Mental Health: Suicide

and feelings of helplessness. Placing the client in charge of the morning chess tournament is a premature intervention that can overwhelm the client and cause the client to fail; this can reinforce the client's feelings of worthlessness.
Priority Nursing Tip: Monitor a depressed client closely for signs of suicidal ideation. If the client presents with increased energy, monitor the client closely because it could mean that the client now has the energy to perform the act of suicide.

Test-Taking Strategy: Focus on the **subject,** providing a therapeutic environment for a client who is suicidal. The correct option is the only choice that addresses a caring and therapeutic environment.

---

16. Shortly after a client dies, the nurse asks the family about funeral arrangements. When the family refuses to discuss the issue, which intervention by the nurse is appropriate for their stage of grief at this time?
1 Displaying acceptance of the family's issues
2 Providing information about funerals in general
3 Probing for information about funeral arrangements
4 Asking the family if they would like time alone with the client

Level of Cognitive Ability: Applying
Client Needs: Psychosocial Integrity
Clinical Judgment/Cognitive Skills: Generate Solutions
Integrated Process: Caring
Content Area: Developmental Stages: End-of-Life
Health Problem: Mental Health: Grief/Loss

Answer: 4
Rationale: The family is exhibiting the first stage of grief: denial. By asking the family if they would like time alone with the client, the nurse supports the family's feelings and allows the family to process the death. Option 1 is a suitable intervention for the acceptance or reorganization and restitution stage of grief. Eliminate options 2 and 3 because they are inappropriate at this time, since the family has indicated their desire not to discuss funeral arrangements.
Priority Nursing Tip: Grief usually involves moving through a series of stages or tasks to help resolve the grief. Feelings associated with grief include anger, frustration, loneliness, sadness, guilt, regret, and peace.

Test-Taking Strategy: Focus on the **subject,** a grieving family. Note the words *at this time* and the stage of grief that the family is demonstrating. This will help you recognize that the family is in denial and will direct you to choose the correct option.

---

17. A client diagnosed with incurable cancer has a life expectancy of a few weeks. Which response indicates that the client's partner is reacting with an expected coping response?
1 Refusing to visit the client
2 Expressing anger with her or his God
3 Not allowing the death to occur at home
4 Sending the children to live with relatives

Level of Cognitive Ability: Applying
Client Needs: Psychosocial Integrity

Answer: 2
Rationale: The expression of anger is a normal response to impending loss, and often the anger is directed internally or at the dying person, God or another spiritual being, or the caregivers. In option 1, the partner is avoiding the client's situation and needs by refusing to visit. Options 3 and 4 are unilateral decisions made by the partner without considering anyone else's feelings.
Priority Nursing Tip: A coping mechanism is a method used to decrease anxiety. The use of a coping mechanism can be conscious, unconscious, constructive, destructive, task-oriented in relation to direct problem-solving, or defense-oriented and regulating in response to self-protection.

Clinical Judgment/Cognitive Skills: Analyze Cues
Integrated Process: Caring
Content Area: Developmental Stages: End-of-Life
Health Problem: Mental Health: Coping

Test-Taking Strategy: Focus on the **subject,** *an expected coping response.* Recalling the stages of grief associated with loss will direct you to the correct option.

COMMUNICATION AND DOCUMENTATION

18. The nurse working on the mental health unit is in the orientation (introductory) phase of the therapeutic nurse–client relationship. Which intervention is representative of this phase of the relationship?

1 The nurse and client determine the contract plan for meetings.
2 The client is encouraged to make use of all services, depending on need.
3 The client begins to identify with the nurse, and trust and rapport are maintained.
4 The nurse focuses on facilitating the therapeutic expression of the client's feelings.

Level of Cognitive Ability: Applying
Client Needs: Psychosocial Integrity
Clinical Judgment/Cognitive Skills: Generate Solutions
Integrated Process: Communication and Documentation
Content Area: Mental Health
Health Problem: N/A

Answer: 1
Rationale: In the orientation (introductory) phase of the therapeutic nurse–client relationship, the client and nurse meet and determine the plan for time, such as how often to meet, the length of the meetings, and when termination is anticipated to occur. Utilizing services, identification with the nurse, and expression of feelings are appropriate for the working phase of the therapeutic nurse–client relationship.
Priority Nursing Tip: Acceptance, trust, and boundaries are established in the orientation (introductory) phase of the therapeutic nurse–client relationship.

Test-Taking Strategy: Focus on the **subject,** the orientation (introductory) phase of the therapeutic nurse–client relationship. Recognizing that the correct option contains the only "orienting" actions will assist you in selecting it as the correct option.

---

19. The partner of a client who has an esophageal tube introduced for a second time tells the nurse, "I thought having this tube down the nose the first time would convince anyone to quit drinking." Which response to the statement would the nurse make?

1 "I think you are a good person to stay with him."
2 "Alcoholism is a disease that affects the whole family."
3 "Have you discussed this subject at the Al-Anon meetings?"
4 "You sound frustrated dealing with such a drinking problem."

Answer: 4
Rationale: In option 4, the nurse uses the therapeutic communication techniques of clarifying and focusing to assist the client's partner with expressing feelings about the client's chronic illness. Showing approval, stereotyping, and changing the subject are nontherapeutic techniques that block communication.
Priority Nursing Tip: Alcohol abuse is an addiction, and a relapse in behavior can occur. This can be very frustrating for families to understand and accept.

Level of Cognitive Ability: Applying
Client Needs: Psychosocial Integrity
Clinical Judgment/Cognitive Skills: Take Action
Integrated Process: Communication and Documentation
Content Area: Foundations of Care: Communication
Health Problem: Mental Health: Addictions

Test-Taking Strategy: Note the client of the question, the client's partner. Use **therapeutic communication techniques.** Remembering to always address the client's feelings will direct you to the correct option.

---

20. The nurse is caring for a client diagnosed with type 2 diabetes mellitus, who was recently hospitalized for hyperglycemic hyperosmolar syndrome (HHS). When preparing for discharge from the hospital, the client expresses anxiety and concerns about the recurrence of HHS. Which response is **best**?

1 "Do you have concerns about managing your condition?"
2 "Do you think you might need to go to the nursing home?"
3 "If you take the correct medications, I doubt this will happen again."
4 "Don't worry. I'm sure your family will provide all the help you need."

Level of Cognitive Ability: Applying
Client Needs: Psychosocial Integrity
Clinical Judgment/Cognitive Skills: Take Action
Integrated Process: Communication and Documentation
Content Area: Foundations of Care: Communication
Health Problem: Adult Health: Endocrine: Diabetes Mellitus

Answer: 1
Rationale: The nurse would provide time and listen to the client's concerns while attempting to clarify the client's feelings, as in the correct option. Option 2 is an inappropriate nursing response because it is making suggestions regarding care options without appropriately identifying the client's true concerns. Options 3 and 4 provide inappropriate false hope and disregard the client's concerns.
Priority Nursing Tip: It is inappropriate to tell a client to "not worry" because it is a barrier to effective communication between the client and the nurse.

Test-Taking Strategy: Focus on the **strategic word,** *best,* and use **therapeutic communication techniques** to always address the client's feelings, especially anxiety, to direct you to the correct option.

---

21. The nurse checks the client's peripheral intravenous (IV) site and notes that it is cool, pale, and swollen, and that the fluid is not infusing. Which condition would the nurse report and document?

1 Phlebitis
2 Infection
3 Infiltration
4 Thrombosis

Level of Cognitive Ability: Analyzing
Client Needs: Physiological Integrity
Clinical Judgment/Cognitive Skills: Analyze Cues

Answer: 3
Rationale: The infusion stops when the pressure in the tissue exceeds the pressure in the tubing. The pallor, coolness, and swelling of the IV site are the result of IV fluid infusing into the subcutaneous tissue. An IV site is infiltrated when it becomes dislodged from the vein and is lying in subcutaneous tissue, so the nurse concludes that the IV is infiltrated. The nurse needs to remove the infiltrated catheter and plan for insertion of a new IV. All the remaining options are likely to be accompanied by warmth at the site. Eliminate options 1, 2, and 4, which suggest that the site appearance would be reddened.
Priority Nursing Tip: An infusion catheter would be inserted at a distal site to provide the option of proceeding up the

Integrated Process: Communication and Documentation
Content Area: Complex Care: Intravenous Therapy
Health Problem: Adult Health: Integumentary: Inflammations/Infections

extremity if the vein is ruptured or infiltration occurs; for example, if infiltration occurs from the antecubital vein, the lower veins in the same arm usually cannot be used for further puncture sites.

Test-Taking Strategy: Focus on the **subject,** an IV site that is cool, pale, swollen, and not infusing. Use your knowledge regarding the clinical indicators of the complications associated with IV therapy to direct you to the correct option. Eliminate options 1, 2, and 4, which are **comparable or alike** and are characteristic of warmth at the site.

---

22. The nurse has provided education to the assistive personnel (AP) in preparation for communicating with a hearing-impaired client. Which statements by the AP indicate that teaching has been **effective? Select all that apply.**

❒ 1 "Speak using a normal tone of voice."
❒ 2 "Speak clearly when communicating with the client."
❒ 3 "Speak slowly and directly into the client's impaired ear."
❒ 4 "Face the client directly when carrying on a conversation."
❒ 5 "Be aware of signs that the client does not understand the conversation."

Level of Cognitive Ability: Evaluating
Client Needs: Safe and Effective Care Environment
Clinical Judgment/Cognitive Skills: Evaluate Outcomes
Integrated Process: Communication and Documentation
Content Area: Foundations of Care: Communication
Health Problem: Adult Health: Ear: Hearing Loss

Answer: 1, 2, 4, 5
Rationale: When communicating with a hearing-impaired client, the caregiver would speak in a normal tone to the client and would not shout. One needs to talk directly to the client while facing the client and speak clearly. If the client does not seem to understand what is being said, the caregiver would express the statement differently. Moving closer to the client and toward the better ear may facilitate communication, but one must avoid talking directly into the impaired ear.
Priority Nursing Tip: Hearing impairment occurs with aging; usually high-frequency tones are less perceptible.

Test-Taking Strategy: Focus on the **strategic word,** *effective,* and the **subject,** communication techniques for a hearing-impaired client. Knowledge regarding effective **therapeutic communication techniques** will direct you to the correct options.

---

23. The nurse assists to create a plan of care to facilitate effective communication for a client who requests assistance in order to live independently. Which intervention has **highest priority**?

1 Directing the discussions so that teaching needs are met
2 Focusing directly on the client's message regarding needs
3 Reflecting only facts related to the client's expressed concerns
4 Reacting to the client's responses in a matter-of-fact, professional manner

Level of Cognitive Ability: Creating
Client Needs: Psychosocial Integrity
Clinical Judgment/Cognitive Skills: Prioritize Hypotheses
Integrated Process: Communication and Documentation
Content Area: Foundations of Care: Communication
Health Problem: Mental Health: Coping

Answer: 2
Rationale: For effective communication, the nurse uses active listening and checks for verbal and nonverbal communication to receive the client's intended message, thus creating an environment in which the client feels comfortable expressing feelings. An authoritarian approach is directive and not permissive, and it is unlikely to create an environment for the free exchange of thoughts and ideas. Reflecting facts only is a barrier to effective communication because subjective information can also provide a stimulus for effective communication. Reacting in a matter-of-fact manner can be an ineffective strategy for facilitating communication.
Priority Nursing Tip: The nurse would use both verbal and nonverbal communication cues to interpret what the client is trying to express.

Test-Taking Strategy: Note the **strategic words,** *highest priority.* Eliminate option 3 because of the **closed-ended word** *"only."* Next, use **therapeutic communication techniques.** This will direct you to the correct option.

---

24. The nursing student is listening to a lecture on correcting errors in a written narrative in a medical record. Which statement by the nursing student indicates that the teaching has been **effective?**

1 "The correct procedure is to document the correction as a late entry."
2 "The correct procedure is to delete the error so that it cannot be read."
3 "The correct procedure is to draw a line through the error and initial and date it."
4 "The correct procedure is to cover the error completely using a black permanent marker."

Level of Cognitive Ability: Evaluating
Client Needs: Safe and Effective Care Environment
Clinical Judgment/Cognitive Skills: Evaluate Outcomes
Integrated Process: Communication and Documentation
Content Area: Leadership/Management: Ethical/Legal
Health Problem: N/A

Answer: 3
Rationale: If the nurse makes a narrative documentation error in the client's record, the agency's policy would be followed to correct the error. Agency policy usually includes drawing one line through the error, initialing and dating the line, and then providing the correct information. The nurse uses a late entry to document additional information that was not documented at the time that it occurred. The nurse avoids attempting to remove the error by any means because these actions raise the suspicion of wrongdoing.
Priority Nursing Tip: Principles of documentation must be followed and data recorded accurately, concisely, completely, legibly, and objectively without bias or opinions. Always follow agency protocol for documentation.

Test-Taking Strategy: Focus on the **strategic word,** *effective,* and the **subject,** the principles related to a documentation error. The correct option is the only option that represents application of documentation principles because the remaining options either alter the record in some fashion or incorrectly identify the documentation.

---

25. When responding to the call bell, the nurse finds the client lying on the floor beside the bed. After thoroughly collecting data and providing appropriate care, the nurse completes an incident report. How would the incident be described in the report?

1 The client fell out of bed and was found on the floor.
2 The client fell while climbing over the bed's side rails.
3 The client was found lying on the floor beside the bed.
4 The client was restless and fell while getting out of bed.

Level of Cognitive Ability: Applying
Client Needs: Safe and Effective Care Environment
Clinical Judgment/Cognitive Skills: Take Action
Integrated Process: Communication and Documentation
Content Area: Leadership/Management: Ethical/Legal
Health Problem: N/A

Answer: 3
Rationale: The incident report would contain the client's name, age, and diagnosis. It would contain a factual description of the incident, any injuries experienced by those involved, and the outcome of the situation. The correct option is the only option that describes the facts as observed by the nurse. All the remaining options are interpretations of the situation and are not factual data as observed by the nurse.
Priority Nursing Tip: The incident report is used as a means of identifying risk situations and improving client care. The report form would not be copied or placed in the client's record.

Test-Taking Strategy: Focus on the **subject,** an incident report, and use general documentation guidelines and principles to answer the question. Remembering to focus on factual information when documenting and to avoid the inclusion of interpretations will direct you to option 3.

---

26. A client diagnosed with angina pectoris appears to be very anxious and states, "So, I had a heart attack, right?" Which response would the nurse make to the client?

1 "No. That is not why you are hospitalized."
2 "No, but there could be some minimal damage to your heart."
3 "No, not this time, and we will do our best to prevent a future heart attack."
4 "No, but it's necessary to monitor you and control or eliminate your pain."

Level of Cognitive Ability: Applying
Client Needs: Psychosocial Integrity
Clinical Judgment/Cognitive Skills: Take Action
Integrated Process: Communication and Documentation
Content Area: Foundations of Care: Communication
Health Problem: Adult Health: Cardiovascular: Coronary Artery Disease

Answer: 4
Rationale: Angina pectoris occurs as a result of an inadequate blood supply to the myocardium, causing pain; managing the condition will help address the client's pain. The nurse will want to correct the client's misconception regarding a heart attack while addressing the client's concerns. Option 1 does not address the client's concerns. Option 2 is incorrect because angina involves interrupted blood supply but does not result in cardiac tissue damage. Neither the nurse nor the primary health care provider can guarantee that a heart attack will not occur, whereas option 3 seems to indicate otherwise.
Priority Nursing Tip: By clarifying the client's condition with the client, the nurse will help minimize stress, which is a contributing factor of angina attacks.

Test-Taking Strategy: Use **therapeutic communication techniques** and focus on the **subject,** the difference between the pathology of a heart attack and angina. The correct option is the only option that demonstrates correct communication techniques and provides accurate information on the client's condition.

---

27. A client diagnosed with delirium anxiously states, "Look at the spiders on the wall." Which response by the nurse addresses the client's concerns therapeutically?

1 "Would you like me to kill the spiders for you?"
2 "While there may be spiders on the wall, they are not going to hurt you."
3 "I know that you are frightened, but I do not see any spiders on the wall."
4 "You are having a hallucination; I'm sure there are no spiders in this room."

Level of Cognitive Ability: Applying
Client Needs: Psychosocial Integrity
Clinical Judgment/Cognitive Skills: Take Action
Integrated Process: Communication and Documentation
Content Area: Mental Health
Health Problem: Mental Health: Neurocognitive Impairment

Answer: 3
Rationale: When hallucinations are present, the nurse would reinforce reality with the client while acknowledging the client's feelings as the correct option does. Eliminate options 1, 2, and 4 because they do not reinforce reality but rather support the legitimacy of the hallucination, or reinforce reality but do not address the client's feelings.
Priority Nursing Tip: If the client is hallucinating, ask the client to describe the hallucinations. Avoid reacting to the hallucination as if it were real.

Test-Taking Strategy: Use **therapeutic communication techniques** and focus on the **subject,** therapeutically responding to a client who is hallucinating. The correct option is the only option that both supports reality and addresses the client's feelings.

---

28. While in the hospital, a client was diagnosed with coronary artery disease (CAD). Which question by the nurse is likely to elicit the **most** useful response for determining the client's degree of adjustment to the new diagnosis?

1 "Is there anyone to help with housework and shopping?"
2 "How do you feel about making changes to your lifestyle?"
3 "Do you understand the schedule for your new medications?"
4 "Did you make a follow-up appointment with your provider?"

Level of Cognitive Ability: Applying
Client Needs: Health Promotion and Maintenance
Clinical Judgment/Cognitive Skills: Generate Solutions
Integrated Process: Communication and Documentation
Content Area: Foundations of Care: Communication
Health Problem: Adult Health: Cardiovascular: Coronary Artery Disease

Answer: 2
Rationale: Exploring feelings assists the nurse with determining the individualized plan of care for the client who is adjusting to a new diagnosis. The correct option is the best question to ask the client because it is likely to elicit the most revealing information about the client's feelings about CAD and the requisite lifestyle changes that can help maintain health and wellness. The remaining choices are aspects of post-hospital care, but they are unlikely to uncover as much information about the client's adjustment to CAD because they are closed-ended questions.
Priority Nursing Tip: Increased cholesterol levels, low-density lipoprotein (LDL) levels, and triglyceride levels place the client at risk for CAD.

Test-Taking Strategy: Note the **strategic word,** *most.* Use **therapeutic communication techniques.** Open-ended questions are needed to explore the client's reactions to or feelings about an identified situation. Closed-ended responses generally elicit a "yes" or "no" response exclusively. All of the incorrect options are closed-ended responses.

---

29. A client has been using crutches to ambulate for 1 week and now reports pain, fatigue, and frustration with crutch walking. How would the nurse respond when the client states, "I feel as if I will always be crippled"?
1 "Tell me what makes this so bothersome for you."
2 "I know how you feel. I had to use crutches before too."
3 "Why don't you take a couple of days off of work and rest?"
4 "Just remember, you'll be done with the crutches in another month."

Level of Cognitive Ability: Applying
Client Needs: Psychosocial Integrity
Clinical Judgment/Cognitive Skills: Take Action
Integrated Process: Communication and Documentation
Content Area: Foundations of Care: Communication
Health Problem: Adult Health: Musculoskeletal: Skeletal Injury

Answer: 1
Rationale: The correct option demonstrates the therapeutic communication technique of clarification and validation and indicates that the nurse is dealing with the client's problem from the client's perspective. Option 2 devalues the client's feelings and thus blocks communication. Option 3 gives advice and is a communication block. Option 4 provides false reassurances because the client may not be done with the crutches in another month. Additionally, it does not focus on the present problem.
Priority Nursing Tip: The nurse would monitor for compartment syndrome in a client who has a cast. This is a condition in which pressure increases in a confined anatomical space, leading to decreased blood flow, ischemia, and dysfunction of the tissues.

Test-Taking Strategy: Use **therapeutic communication techniques.** The correct option is the only response that encourages communication. The remaining options are **comparable or alike** because they are blocks to communication.

---

30. A teenaged client is discharged from the hospital after surgery with instructions to use a cane for the next 6 months. What question **best** demonstrates the nurse's ability to use therapeutic communication techniques to **effectively** interpret the teenager's feelings about using a cane?
1 "How do you feel about needing a cane to walk?"
2 "Do you have questions about ambulating with a cane?"
3 "Are you worried about what your friends will think about your cane?"
4 "What types of problems do you think you'll have ambulating with a cane?"

Level of Cognitive Ability: Applying
Client Needs: Psychosocial Integrity
Clinical Judgment/Cognitive Skills: Take Action
Integrated Process: Communication and Documentation
Content Area: Developmental Stages: Adolescent
Health Problem: Adult Health: Musculoskeletal: Skeletal Injury

Answer: 1
Rationale: The nurse effectively uses therapeutic communication techniques when posing an open-ended question to elicit data about how the teenager feels about using a cane. The remaining options are closed-ended questions. Option 3 makes assumptions about how the teenager feels, and options 2 and 4 focus on the physical aspects of using the cane.
Priority Nursing Tip: The nurse would instruct the client using a cane to inspect the rubber tip on the cane regularly for worn places. A worn tip will need to be replaced.

Test-Taking Strategy: Note the **strategic words,** *best* and *effectively,* in the question. Focus on the **subject,** the teenager's feelings about the use of the cane. Note the relationship between the subject and the correct option. Also use **therapeutic communication techniques,** and avoid responses that include communication blocks.

31. After the surgical repair of a fractured hip, a client has consistently refused to engage in ambulation as prescribed. Which statement by the nurse will **best** encourage the client's need to ambulate?

1 "What is it about getting out of bed that concerns you?"
2 "If you are afraid of the pain, I can give you medication to help."
3 "If you don't get up and start walking, your recovery will take much longer."
4 "Being dependent on others must be depressing for an active person like yourself."

Level of Cognitive Ability: Applying
Client Needs: Psychological Integrity
Clinical Judgment/Cognitive Skills: Take Action
Integrated Process: Communication and Documentation
Content Area: Foundations of Care: Communication
Health Problem: Adult Health: Musculoskeletal: Skeletal Injury

Answer: 1

Rationale: Early ambulation during the postoperative period is very important to a client's health and recovery, but many different factors may be contributing to the client's refusal to ambulate as prescribed. Asking an open-ended question that encourages a discussion about getting out of bed is the best option available to allow the nurse to facilitate the client's plan of care. Pain may be a concern for the client, but again, the nurse is making an unfounded assumption. Although it is true that the recovery might be prolonged by not ambulating and that the client may be depressed, these statements make assumptions about the reason the client is refusing to comply with the plan of care.

Priority Nursing Tip: Effective communication with the client is a necessary factor in determining the underlying reasons for nonadherence with the plan of care.

Test-Taking Strategy: Note the **strategic word,** *best.* Use the principles of **therapeutic communication techniques** and your understanding that nonadherence may have many and varied reasons to help direct you to the correct option.

---

32. The student nurse is listening to a lecture on caring for clients with thrombophlebitis. Which statement by the student nurse indicates that the teaching has been **effective?**

1 "Elevating the affected leg is indicated."
2 "Keeping the affected leg flat encourages healing."
3 "Engaging in activity as tolerated would be encouraged."
4 "Maintaining bathroom privileges is the most important action."

Level of Cognitive Ability: Evaluating
Client Needs: Physiological Integrity
Clinical Judgment/Cognitive Skills: Evaluate Outcomes
Integrated Process: Communication and Documentation
Content Area: Adult Health: Cardiovascular
Health Problem: Adult Health: Cardiovascular: Vascular Disorders

Answer: 1

Rationale: The nurse plans to elevate the affected extremity because this facilitates venous return by using gravity to improve blood return to the heart, decreases venous pressure, and helps relieve edema and pain. Option 2 does not facilitate venous return and thus is not indicated for a client with thrombophlebitis. Options 3 and 4 are unsuitable activities for a client on bed rest.

Priority Nursing Tip: Thrombophlebitis is an inflammation of a vein, often accompanied by clot formation. It can present serious circulatory problems.

Test-Taking Strategy: Note the **strategic word,** *effective,* and focus on the **subject,** thrombophlebitis. Think about what pathophysiology is associated with this condition and how gravity affects venous blood flow and edema. This will direct you to the correct option.

---

33. A client who is experiencing paranoid thinking involving food being poisoned is admitted to the mental health unit. Which communication technique would the nurse use to encourage the client to communicate her fears?
   1 Open-ended questions and silence
   2 Offering personal opinions about the need to eat
   3 Verbalizing reasons why the client may choose not to eat
   4 Focusing on self-disclosure of the nurse's own food preferences

Level of Cognitive Ability: Applying
Client Needs: Physiological Integrity
Clinical Judgment/Cognitive Skills: Take Action
Integrated Process: Communication and Documentation
Content Area: Foundations of Care: Communication
Health Problem: Mental Health: Personality Disorders

Answer: 1
Rationale: Open-ended questions and silence are strategies that are used to encourage clients to discuss their feelings in a descriptive manner. Options 2 and 3 are not helpful to the client because they do not encourage the expression of personal feelings. Option 4 is not a client-centered intervention.
Priority Nursing Tip: Avoid whispering in the presence of a client who is paranoid because this will intensify feelings of paranoia.

Test-Taking Strategy: Use your knowledge of **therapeutic communication techniques** to identify the usefulness of the techniques suggested in the correct option. The communication techniques identified in the remaining options are nontherapeutic and are blocks to communication.

---

34. The nurse is preparing a client for electroconvulsive therapy (ECT). After the client signs the informed consent form for the procedure, a family member states, "I don't think that this ECT will be helpful, especially since it makes people's memory worse." What communication technique would the nurse implement to address the family member's concern?
   1 Ask other family members and the client whether they think that ECT makes memory worse.
   2 Immediately reassure the client and family that ECT will help and that the memory loss is only temporary.
   3 Involve the family member in a dialogue to ascertain how the family member arrived at this conclusion.
   4 Reinforce with the client and the family member that depression causes more memory impairment than ECT.

Answer: 3
Rationale: In option 3, the nurse is looking for data to assist with clarifying information about the procedure with the family, which is necessary in order to deal effectively with their concerns. Option 1 may place family members on the defensive and promote conflict among them. Option 2 does not acknowledge the family member's statement and concerns. Option 4 addresses content clarification but not the data collection process, and it is not the most therapeutic action.
Priority Nursing Tip: ECT may be prescribed to treat depression. It consists of inducing a seizure by passing an electrical current through the brain via electrodes attached to the temples. ECT is not a permanent cure. It is true that some clients experience temporary memory loss, but it usually centers on the time period around the treatment itself.

Level of Cognitive Ability: Applying
Client Needs: Psychosocial Integrity
Clinical Judgment/Cognitive Skills: Generate Solutions
Integrated Process: Communication and Documentation
Content Area: Foundations of Care: Communication
Health Problem: Mental Health: Therapeutic Communication

Test-Taking Strategy: Use **therapeutic communication techniques** and the **steps of the nursing process.** Remember that data collection is the first step in the nursing process. In the correct option, the nurse gathers more data via the data collection process and addresses the family member's thoughts and feelings.

CULTURE AND SPIRITUALITY

35. The nurse is caring for a postoperative client with spiritually and culturally based eating and food requirements. Which interventions demonstrate the nurse's spiritual and cultural consideration of the client? **Select all that apply.**

- ❒ 1 Encouraging the client to try new foods only until healing is complete
- ❒ 2 Suggesting the substitution of similar foods for the culturally appropriate ones
- ❒ 3 Asking the client to explain the factors that are important to his meal practices
- ❒ 4 Including the family in discussions regarding the preparation of accepted foods
- ❒ 5 Discussing the nutritional requirements the client currently has postoperatively

Level of Cognitive Ability: Applying
Client Needs: Safe and Effective Care Environment
Clinical Judgment/Cognitive Skills: Take Action
Integrated Process: Culture/Spirituality
Content Area: Foundations of Care: Spirituality, Culture, and Ethnicity
Health Problem: N/A

Answer: 3, 4, 5

Rationale: Spiritual and cultural consideration reflects attempts to maintain familiar customs to achieve healthy responses. Gaining knowledge of the customs and their importance to the client will be the basis for an understanding that allows for flexibility and compromise when necessary. Including the family in the discussion will assist with the process, as will discussing the needs the client has at this particular time in order to formulate a plan that meets the needs while maintaining cultural customs. Encouraging new foods in place of the usual foods may be viewed as being insensitive and showing a lack of concern. Substitution is not always necessary.

Priority Nursing Tip: Spiritual and cultural consideration is a critical factor in providing quality nursing care and has a direct effect on client recovery and ultimate wellness.

Test-Taking Strategy: Focus on the **subject,** spiritual and cultural considerations. Eliminate option 1 because of the **closed-ended word** "only." Recall that encouraging clients to move away from their usual customs is considered to show a lack of sensitivity and does not indicate cultural competency. Understanding the goals of spiritually and culturally considerate care will direct you to the correct options.

---

36. The nurse is caring for a client of an unfamiliar ethnic culture. The nurse shows an understanding of the general principles of culturally sensitive interaction when implementing which interventions? **Select all that apply.**

- ☐ 1 Addressing the client using the client's full surname to display respect
- ☐ 2 Maintaining eye contact with the client so as to show respect for the client
- ☐ 3 Utilizing the position of authority nurses hold to provide an explanation of facility rules
- ☐ 4 Touching the client is not readily accepted in many cultures
- ☐ 5 Avoiding any frequent engagement with the client in conversation of a personal nature

Level of Cognitive Ability: Applying
Client Needs: Safe and Effective Care Environment
Clinical Judgment/Cognitive Skills: Take Action
Integrated Process: Culture and Spirituality
Content Area: Foundations of Care: Spirituality, Culture, and Ethnicity
Health Problem: N/A

Answer: 1, 4, 5
Rationale: Although cultural sensitivities vary, it is generally prudent to show respect for any client of any ethnic background by using a formal name. Personal conversations not required as part of the data collection process would be avoided, as would a show of authority. Maintaining eye contact is not universally taken to be a positive behavior and so may be limited until it is determined to be acceptable by the client. Physical touching by strangers is not readily accepted in many cultures and would be engaged in cautiously and only when necessary and with permission from the client.
Priority Nursing Tip: Cultural and spiritual practices vary greatly, and the nurse is responsible for acquiring such knowledge in order to provide culturally sensitive care.

Test-Taking Strategy: Focus on the **subject,** general principles of cultural sensitivity. Remember that close and intimate contact generally is avoided in order to show respect. Understanding the basic principles of culturally sensitive care will direct you to the correct options.

---

37. The nurse is participating in end-of-life care for a client who has recently immigrated. Which interventions would the nurse consider in the plan of care for this client? **Select all that apply.**

- ☐ 1 Respect family requests for the use of herbal medicines.
- ☐ 2 Have direct conversations with the matriarch of the family only.
- ☐ 3 Acknowledge that lack of eye contact does not mean disinterest.
- ☐ 4 Allow someone from the family to stay with the client after death if requested.
- ☐ 5 Recognize that the use of healers is a common practice in all non-Western cultures.

Level of Cognitive Ability: Applying
Client Needs: Psychosocial Integrity

Answer: 1, 3, 4
Rationale: Herbal medicine plays an important role in many cultures in the care of the dying client, and family requests to incorporate its use in care would be acknowledged and discussed with the primary health care provider. The nurse must realize that lack of direct eye contact would not be interpreted as a sign of disinterest. If requested, someone from the family would be allowed to stay with the client after death. The use of healers is not a practice of every culture. The nurse needs to assess and determine whom the family wishes to be the person of direct contact for conversations.
Priority Nursing Tip: An initial step in ensuring culturally competent care is to assess the needs of the client and what the client wishes to be part of the plan of care.

Clinical Judgment/Cognitive Skills: Generate Solutions
Integrated Process: Culture and Spirituality
Content Area: Foundations of Care: Spirituality, Culture, and Ethnicity
Health Problem: N/A

Test-Taking Strategy: Focus on the **subject**, specific knowledge of different cultural groups and religious and spiritual practices. Read each option carefully, and eliminate option 5 because of the **closed-ended word** *all* and option 2 because of the **closed-ended word** *only*.

---

38. The nurse is caring for a client who does not speak English. An interpreter is currently unavailable. The nurse must perform a dressing change. What would the nurse do to enhance communication with this client before changing the dressing?

1 Ask relatives to interpret because an interpreter is unavailable.
2 Speak slowly and allow the client time to interpret what is being said.
3 Use many nonverbal cues and repetition to reinforce what is being said.
4 Use common words in the nurse's language, because the client is likely to be familiar with them.

Level of Cognitive Ability: Applying
Client Needs: Psychosocial Integrity
Clinical Judgment/Cognitive Skills: Take Action
Integrated Process: Culture and Spirituality
Content Area: Foundations of Care: Spirituality, Culture, and Ethnicity
Health Problem: Adult Health: Integumentary: Wounds

Answer: 2
Rationale: When caring for a client who speaks a language that is different from the nurse's, it is ideal for the nurse to call on a dialect-specific interpreter designated by the health care agency that is the same age and same gender as the client. If an interpreter is unavailable, the nurse would speak slowly and allow the client time to interpret what is being said. The nurse would avoid asking relatives to be interpreters to minimize bias and misinterpretation. The nurse would avoid using nonverbal facial expressions and body language, because they could be misinterpreted by the client. The nurse would use common words in the client's language if known.
Priority Nursing Tip: Client confidentiality, as well as the delivery of accurate information, may be compromised when a family member or a non–health care provider acts as interpreter.

Test-Taking Strategy: Focus on the **subject**, communication and language barrier. Recalling that family members would not be used as interpreters because of the risk of bias or misinterpretation will assist you in eliminating option 1. Also recalling that nonverbal cues and body language mean different things in different cultures will assist you in eliminating option 3. From the remaining options, read carefully; it is necessary to know that speaking slowly enhances interpretation on the part of the client.

---

39. The nurse is collecting cultural and spiritual data on a newly admitted client. Which factors specifically related to culture and spirituality would the nurse address? **Select all that apply.**

❒ 1 Nutrition
❒ 2 Communication
❒ 3 Insurance coverage
❒ 4 High-risk behaviors
❒ 5 Health care practices
❒ 6 Family roles and organization

Level of Cognitive Ability: Applying
Client Needs: Psychosocial Integrity
Clinical Judgment/Cognitive Skills:
Integrated Process: Culture and Spirituality
Content Area: Foundations of Care: Spirituality, Culture, and Ethnicity
Health Problem: N/A

Answer: 1, 2, 4, 5, 6
Rationale: When collecting cultural and spiritual data, the nurse would focus on the following factors: nutrition, communication, high-risk behaviors, health care practices, family roles and organization, workforce issues, biocultural ecology, overview (e.g., heritage), pregnancy and childbirth practices, death rituals, spirituality preferences, and health care practitioners. Asking the client about insurance coverage is not specifically related to cultural or spiritual practices.
Priority Nursing Tip: Nurses often care for clients who come from ethnic, cultural, or religious backgrounds that are different from their own. Awareness of and sensitivity to the unique health and illness beliefs and practices of people of different backgrounds are essential for the delivery of safe and effective care.

Test-Taking Strategy: Focus on the **subject**, collecting cultural and spiritual data. Recognizing that option 3 is the only option that does not specifically relate to values, beliefs, and customs will assist you in eliminating this option.

---

40. The nurse is caring for an Orthodox Jewish client of the opposite sex whose condition is terminal. The nurse is implementing a plan of care and wishes to communicate this plan with the client and family. The nurse would be aware of the possibility of which end-of-life spiritual and religious practices when planning and communicating with the client and family? **Select all that apply.**

❒ 1 Religious laws are suspended during times of severe illness.
❒ 2 Family members may not shake hands with members of the opposite sex.
❒ 3 Clients are usually very quiet and do not express what they are thinking or feeling.
❒ 4 During the process of dying, visitors and conversation would be kept to a minimum.
❒ 5 Family members may not make direct eye contact with members of the opposite sex.

Level of Cognitive Ability: Analyzing
Client Needs: Psychosocial Integrity
Clinical Judgment/Cognitive Skills: Generate Solutions
Integrated Process: Culture and Spirituality
Content Area: Foundations of Care: Spirituality, Culture, and Ethnicity
Health Problem: N/A

Answer: 1, 2, 5
Rationale: The Orthodox Jew strictly follows the laws of Judaism; however, during times of severe illness, Jewish laws are not observed if doing so will endanger the client's health. In the Orthodox Jewish faith, members generally will not shake hands or make direct eye contact with members of the opposite sex. During times of illness or death, the Orthodox Jewish community, including family and friends, will frequently visit and are considered the nucleus of the Jewish culture. Clients of the Orthodox Jewish faith are generally very verbal about what they are feeling.
Priority Nursing Tip: According to Jewish law and custom, it is very important for the client not to be left alone to die.

Test-Taking Strategy: Note the **subject,** end-of-life spiritual and religious beliefs of Orthodox Judaism. Think about these religious beliefs to answer correctly. Also, eliminate options 3 and 4 because they are **comparable or alike** options.

---

41. The nurse is caring for a client who reports being a practicing Roman Catholic. Which action by the nurse demonstrates spiritual and cultural sensitivity?

1 Observe fasting rules on Sundays.
2 Inform dietary staff that meat cannot be served on Fridays.
3 Allow the client to observe communion daily if requested.
4 Discourage anointing by the priest unless the condition becomes terminal.

Level of Cognitive Ability: Applying
Client Needs: Psychosocial Integrity
Clinical Judgment/Cognitive Skills:
Integrated Process: Culture and Spirituality
Content Area: Foundations of Care: Spirituality, Culture, and Ethnicity
Health Problem: N/A

Answer: 3
Rationale: During response to illness, practicing Roman Catholics may request to be anointed while sick. They may also practice daily Holy Communion. Fasting on Sundays and avoidance of meat on Fridays are not current practices of the Roman Catholic.
Priority Nursing Tip: It is important to understand the client's religious and spiritual beliefs and how they affect a client's health status. It is also important to have background information regarding holy days and practices for various religions.

Test-Taking Strategy: Focus on the subject, practices of a Roman Catholic client and spiritual and cultural sensitivity. Use knowledge regarding the spiritual practices of the Roman Catholic to answer correctly. Remember that Roman Catholics often practice daily communion and may request to be anointed while sick.

---

42. The nurse is caring for a client who follows a kosher diet. Which foods would the nurse use in meal planning for the client? **Select all that apply.**

❒ 1 Pork
❒ 2 Tuna
❒ 3 Apples
❒ 4 Chicken
❒ 5 Potatoes

Level of Cognitive Ability: Applying
Client Needs: Psychosocial Integrity
Clinical Judgment/Cognitive Skills: Generate Solutions
Integrated Process: Culture and Spirituality
Content Area: Foundations of Care: Spirituality, Culture, and Ethnicity
Health Problem: N/A

Answer: 2, 3, 4, 5

Rationale: Clients who follow a kosher diet avoid meat from carnivores, pork products, and fish without scales or fins. Fruits and vegetables are considered kosher. Tuna, chicken, potatoes, and apples are also considered kosher and appropriate.

Priority Nursing Tip: A kosher diet is a healthy diet because of the strict rules under which the foods allowed on the diet are prepared. Foods are prepared so that harmful hormones that transfer from meat and dairy products into the body are eliminated.

Test-Taking Strategy: Focus on the **subject**, a kosher diet. Most cultures do not abstain from fruits and vegetables, so select option 3. Think about what you know about a kosher diet. Clients who follow a kosher diet avoid meat from carnivores, pork products, and fish without scales or fins. This will assist in directing you to the remaining correct options.

---

43. The nurse is caring for a client who has been admitted for asthma. The nurse is unfamiliar with the cultural and spiritual practices and beliefs of the client's homeland. Which questions are **most appropriate** for the nurse to ask during the admission process? **Select all that apply.**

❒ 1 "What do you believe is causing your illness?"
❒ 2 "Why don't you take some asthma medication?"
❒ 3 "Why do you wear that amulet around your neck?"
❒ 4 "Are there any remedies you have used in the past?"
❒ 5 "Who do you usually see for help when you are sick?"

Level of Cognitive Ability: Applying
Client Needs: Safe and Effective Care Environment
Clinical Judgment/Cognitive Skills: Generate Solutions
Integrated Process: Culture and Spirituality
Content Area: Foundations of Care: Spirituality, Culture, and Ethnicity
Health Problem: Adult Health: Respiratory/ Asthma

Answer: 1, 4, 5

Rationale: Data collection includes cultural and spiritual information. It includes questions regarding clients' health beliefs and practices, their health care providers, and their beliefs regarding the origin of illness. Option 2 may have an accusatory undertone. This type of question will not assist the nurse in developing a rapport. A person's reason for wearing an amulet is not relevant to this situation; this question may be perceived as intrusive.

Priority Nursing Tip: It is important to ask questions that will assist in gaining information about a client's health care practices. The nurse would avoid gesturing because certain hand or body movements may have adverse connotations in other cultures. The nurse would also evaluate whether questions or instructions have been understood because some clients will nod "yes" but not really comprehend.

Test-Taking Strategy: Note the **strategic words,** *most appropriate.* Focus on the **subject,** therapeutic communication with a client whose cultural practices are unfamiliar to the nurse. It is also important to keep in mind that the nurse needs to be sensitive to ways in which cultural beliefs and faith impact the client's health care experiences. Think about **therapeutic communication techniques,** review each option, and then sort the options into therapeutic or nontherapeutic responses to help you eliminate nontherapeutic responses.

---

44. The nurse is collecting data from a client who recently moved to America. The client presented to the emergency department with complaints of a headache and nausea. The client is accompanied by an adult son. On data collection, the nurse notes long, pale red welts on both arms. Which actions would the nurse take **next? Select all that apply.**

- ❒ 1 Report findings to social services.
- ❒ 2 Ask whether she has used any home remedies.
- ❒ 3 Determine cultural health beliefs and practices.
- ❒ 4 Remove the adult son from the room immediately.
- ❒ 5 Recognize the redness as a result of a traditional form of healing.

Level of Cognitive Ability: Analyzing
Client Needs: Physiological Integrity
Clinical Judgment/Cognitive Skills: Analyze Cues
Integrated Process: Culture and Spirituality
Content Area: Foundations of Care: Spirituality, Culture, and Ethnicity
Health Problem: N/A

Answer: 2, 3, 5
Rationale: The nurse would ask the client whether she has used any home remedies. The nurse would determine cultural health beliefs and practices and understand that "coining or coin rubbing" is a traditional form of healing. The nurse would recognize the redness as a result of coining. The nurse would not report the welts to social services because the practice is not abuse. The son would not be removed from the room unless the client requests it.
Priority Nursing Tip: Coining leaves distinct markings and is often misconstrued as a sign of abuse. Coining begins with the use of warm massage oil mixed with essential oils such as peppermint to irritate the skin slightly. The massage relaxes the client in preparation for the next stage, in which a coin is repeatedly rubbed against the skin in long, flowing movements away from the heart. Blood then rises to the top of the skin. The markings will subside in a few days.

Test-Taking Strategy: Note the **strategic word,** *next.* Focus on the **subject,** data collection from a client who presents with long, pale red welts on her arms. Think about the relationship between cultural health beliefs and health care practices. Specific knowledge that coining is a common practice in some cultures is necessary to answer correctly.

---

45. The hospice nurse is caring for a client of the Muslim faith. Which religious belief would the nurse expect to observe?

1 The client's bed is positioned toward Mecca.
2 The client is left alone except for bathing and feeding.
3 The religious leader is not allowed to visit until the client has died.
4 Fasting is implemented to promote healing.

Level of Cognitive Ability: Analyzing
Client Needs: Psychosocial Integrity
Clinical Judgment/Cognitive Skills: Recognize Cues
Integrated Process: Culture and Spirituality
Content Area: Foundations of Care: Spirituality, Culture, and Ethnicity
Health Problem: N/A

Answer: 1
Rationale: Mecca is Islam's holiest city. Those of the Muslim faith desire their body to be facing Mecca. It is not common practice to leave the client alone. If appropriate medically, a family member may wish to remain with the client at all times. A religious leader needs to be made available anytime the client or family makes that request. Fasting to promote healing is not a common practice.
Priority Nursing Tip: Clients and families of different faiths may deal with and face imminent death differently based on their spiritual beliefs. It is important for the nurse to be familiar with death and dying beliefs and cultural and spiritual practices in order to provide culturally congruent care.

Test-Taking Strategy: Focus on the **subject,** religious practices of a Muslim client. It is necessary to have knowledge of these religious practices and beliefs in order to answer correctly.

---

46. A Muslim female client has been stabilized after an assault in the parking lot of a local restaurant. The nurse understands that which intervention is the **most appropriate** to ensure the client's comfort if requested?

1 Assigning the best male nurse to the client.
2 Assigning the client a female nurse for every shift.
3 Allowing the client to pick which nurses she would like to care for her.
4 Removing all of the client's clothing each shift to perform a skin check.

Level of Cognitive Ability: Applying
Client Needs: Psychosocial Integrity
Clinical Judgment/Cognitive Skills: Take Action
Integrated Process: Culture and Spirituality
Content Area: Foundations of Care: Spirituality, Culture, and Ethnicity
Health Problem: Mental Health: Abuse/Neglect

Answer: 2
Rationale: Information about family and gender roles will greatly influence the nurse's plan of care. Muslim women can be cared for only by a female. Assigning a male nurse to care for this client would be inappropriate. It would also be inappropriate to place the client in a position to choose which nurse will care for her. Unless medically necessary, the client would not need to have a skin check every shift. If it is required, a female must be present to assist in the skin check.
Priority Nursing Tip: When assigned to a client, note the client's culture and review any specific beliefs and practices that would be taken into consideration when planning care.

Test-Taking Strategy: Focus on the **strategic words,** *most appropriate.* Note that the client in the question is a female. Next, think about the cultural beliefs of a Muslim and that the subject of the question is an intervention.

---

47. The unit manager working on a medical-surgical unit is conducting an in-service session on the provision of spiritually and culturally competent care and factors that contribute to health disparities. Which factors does the manager incorporate into this teaching session? **Select all that apply.**

❒ 1 Age
❒ 2 Genetics
❒ 3 Ethnicity
❒ 4 Education
❒ 5 Past medical history
❒ 6 Health care provider attitudes

Level of Cognitive Ability: Applying
Client Needs: Psychosocial Integrity
Clinical Judgment/Cognitive Skills: Generate Solutions
Integrated Process: Culture and Spirituality
Content Area: Foundations of Care: Spirituality, Culture, and Ethnicity
Health Problem: N/A

Answer: 1, 3, 4, 6
Rationale: Many factors contribute to health disparities, including age; ethnicity, race, and culture; education; health care provider attitudes; geographic location; income; occupation; health literacy; and gender. Genetics and past medical history are not factors that influence health disparities.
Priority Nursing Tip: In the provision of spiritually and culturally competent care, the nurse needs to avoid stereotyping and needs to be aware that there are several subcultures within cultures and that there are several dialects within languages.

Test-Taking Strategy: It is necessary to understand the subject of health disparities to answer this question. Recall that disparities relate to a person's position in society. Analyze each of the options, and determine whether they would contribute to health disparities.

---

48. The nurse is caring for a client of a different culture and is checking for client perceptions regarding nutrition. Which, in addition to the impact of food on disease and illness, would the nurse consider in order to provide culturally competent care?

1 Educational background and employment history
2 Familial support systems and financial well-being
3 Client perception of body weight and size relative to culture
4 Ability to purchase foods necessary for disease management

Level of Cognitive Ability: Applying
Client Needs: Psychosocial Integrity
Clinical Judgment/Cognitive Skills: Generate Solutions
Integrated Process: Culture and Spirituality
Content Area: Foundations of Care: Spirituality, Culture, and Ethnicity
Health Problem: Adult Health: Gastrointestinal: Nutrition/Malabsorption Problems

Answer: 3
Rationale: When addressing nutrition for clients with diverse cultural backgrounds, dietary preferences, the impact of food on disease and illness, and client perception of body weight and size relative to culture must be considered. For example, some cultures may not consider obesity to be a major health indicator; therefore, teaching regarding weight reduction may be difficult. The other options address social and financial status and are not directly related to cultural considerations with regard to nutrition.
Priority Nursing Tip: Learn about the cultures of clients with whom you will be working; also, ask clients about their health care practices and preferences.

Test-Taking Strategy: Focus on the **subject,** cultural considerations in relation to nutrition. Recognizing that options 1, 2, and 4 are **comparable or alike** and are in some way related to financial status will assist you in eliminating these options. In addition, note the similarity between the question and the correct option in that both contain the word *culture.*

---

49. The nurse is caring for a client in labor who is from the Philippines. The client is 4 cm dilated and 30% effaced. This is her first child. The client is grimacing; her pulse, respiratory rate, and blood pressure are elevated. The nurse offers to contact the obstetrician for an epidural prescription. The client declines. The nurse would hypothesize that the client declined the epidural for which reason?

1 Filipino clients tend to decrease their pain through a verbal release.
2 Filipino clients will only accept treatments for pain from their partners.
3 Filipino clients are often stoic and view childbirth pain as a normal part of life.
4 Filipino clients believe that pain is a form of spiritual atonement for one's past deeds.

Level of Cognitive Ability: Analyzing
Client Needs: Psychosocial Integrity
Clinical Judgment/Cognitive Skills: Prioritize Hypotheses
Integrated Process: Culture and Spirituality
Content Area: Foundations of Care: Spirituality, Culture, and Ethnicity
Health Problem: Maternity: Discomforts of Pregnancy

Answer: 4
Rationale: Childbirth experiences differ among different cultures. Filipinos may view pain as part of living an honorable life and view this as an opportunity to reach a fuller spiritual life or to atone for past wrongdoings. The client will not complain of pain despite physiological indicators. The remaining options give incorrect information.
Priority Nursing Tip: When planning any intervention, the nurse must take a client's culture into consideration.

Test-Taking Strategy: Focus on the **subject,** the Filipino culture. To plan effective care for clients, the nurse must collect cultural data from each client. To answer correctly, it is necessary to know that Filipinos believe that pain is a form of spiritual atonement.

TEACHING AND LEARNING

50. The nurse is reinforcing discharge teaching to a client treated for tuberculosis (TB). Which statement by the client indicates that teaching has been **effective? Select all that apply.**

❒ 1 "All used dishes need to be sterilized."
❒ 2 "My close contacts need to be tested for TB."
❒ 3 "Soiled tissues need to be disposed of properly."
❒ 4 "House isolation is required for at least 8 months."
❒ 5 "The mouth needs to be covered when coughing."

Level of Cognitive Ability: Evaluating
Client Needs: Safe and Effective Care Environment
Clinical Judgment/Cognitive Skills: Evaluate Outcomes
Integrated Process: Teaching and Learning
Content Area: Foundations of Care: Infection Control
Health Problem: Adult Health: Respiratory: Tuberculosis

Answer: 2, 3, 5
Rationale: TB is a communicable disease, and the nurse must teach the client measures to prevent its spread. Any close contacts with the client must be tested and treated if the results of the screening test are positive. Because it is an airborne disease, the client must properly dispose of used tissues and needs to cover the mouth when coughing. There is no evidence to suggest that sterilizing dishes would break the chain of infection with pulmonary TB. It is not necessary for the client to isolate herself or himself to the house. Once the client is treated and the results of three sputum cultures are negative, the client will not spread the infection.
Priority Nursing Tip: Multidrug-resistant strains of TB can result from improper adherence, nonadherence with treatment programs, or development of mutations in tubercle bacillus; the nurse must include the importance of medication adherence when teaching the client with tuberculosis (TB).

Test-Taking Strategy: Focus on the **strategic word,** *effective,* and the **subject,** minimizing the spread of TB. Also focusing on the pathophysiology of TB and on the associated communicability factors and risks will assist you in answering correctly.

---

51. A client is receiving intravenous (IV) antibiotic therapy at home via an intermittent IV catheter. To facilitate the early detection of IV therapy complications, which intervention would be included in the client's education?

1 Protect the IV site continually.
2 Keep the IV site clean and dry.
3 Report local pain, drainage, or edema.
4 Apply pressure to the IV site if it dislodges.

Level of Cognitive Ability: Applying
Client Needs: Safe and Effective Care Environment
Clinical Judgment/Cognitive Skills: Take Action
Integrated Process: Teaching and Learning
Content Area: Foundations of Care: Client Teaching
Health Problem: N/A

Answer: 3
Rationale: The nurse instructs the client to report clinical indicators of an IV site infection, including pain, drainage, and edema, because the early detection of infection decreases the risk of septicemia, tissue loss, and devastating complications. The remaining options are reasonable aspects of client teaching for IV therapy at home, but they are not surveillance methods.
Priority Nursing Tip: Any solution administered by the IV route directly enters the client's circulatory system. Strict aseptic technique is necessary to prevent infection.

Test-Taking Strategy: Focus on the **subject,** early detection of IV therapy complications. Eliminate options 1, 2, and 4 because these choices describe aspects of IV care to help prevent complications, but they do not contribute to early detection.

---

52. The nurse reinforces instructions about the management of pruritus to a client diagnosed with hepatitis who developed jaundice. Which statement made by the client suggests to the nurse that the client **needs further teaching?**

1 "I need to wear loose cotton clothing."
2 "A tepid water bath would help stop the itching."
3 "Keeping the house warmer is likely to lessen the itching."
4 "I need to take the prescribed antihistamines as I'm supposed to."

Level of Cognitive Ability: Evaluating
Client Needs: Physiological Integrity
Clinical Judgment/Cognitive Skills: Evaluate Outcomes
Integrated Process: Teaching and Learning
Content Area: Adult Health: Gastrointestinal
Health Problem: Adult Health: Gastrointestinal: Hepatitis

Answer: 3
Rationale: Pruritus is caused by the accumulation of bile salts in the skin and results from obstructed biliary excretion. The client would be instructed to keep the house temperature cool in order to minimize the itching. The client would avoid the use of alkaline soap, and he or she would wear loose, soft cotton clothing. Antihistamines may relieve the itching, as will tepid water and emollient baths.
Priority Nursing Tip: Jaundice results when the liver is unable to metabolize bilirubin or when edema, fibrosis, and scarring of the hepatic bile ducts interfere with normal bile and bilirubin secretion.

Test-Taking Strategy: Note the **strategic words,** *needs further teaching*. These words indicate a **negative event query** and ask you to select an option that is an incorrect statement. Recalling that heat causes vasodilation will assist with directing you to the correct option.

---

53. The nurse has reinforced home care instructions to a client with prostate cancer who has been hospitalized for a transurethral resection of the prostate (TURP). Which statement by the client indicates the **need for further teaching?**

1 "Prune juice needs to be included in my diet."
2 "I need to avoid strenuous activity for 4 to 6 weeks."
3 "I can't lift or push objects that weigh more than 30 pounds."
4 "My intake of water needs to be at least six to eight glasses daily."

Level of Cognitive Ability: Evaluating
Client Needs: Physiological Integrity
Clinical Judgment/Cognitive Skills: Evaluate Outcomes
Integrated Process: Teaching and Learning
Content Area: Adult Health: Renal and Urinary
Health Problem: Adult Health: Cancer: Prostate

Answer: 3
Rationale: The client needs to be advised to avoid strenuous activity for 4 to 6 weeks and to avoid lifting items that weigh more than 20 pounds. Straining during defecation is avoided to prevent bleeding. Prune juice is a satisfactory bowel stimulant. The client needs to consume a daily intake of at least six to eight glasses of nonalcoholic fluids to minimize clot formation.
Priority Nursing Tip: After TURP, monitor for hemorrhage. Postoperative continuous bladder irrigation may be prescribed, which prevents catheter obstruction from clots.

Test-Taking Strategy: Note the **strategic words,** *need for further teaching*. These words indicate a **negative event query** and ask you to select an option that is an incorrect statement. Eliminate options that suggest general postoperative teaching points. Considering the anatomical location of the surgical procedure, it is reasonable to think that constipation needs to be avoided. Also note that lifting items that weigh 30 pounds is excessive.

---

54. A client is being treated for an atrial dysrhythmia with quinidine gluconate. Which statement by the client indicates to the nurse that the medication instructions about what to do if a dose is missed have been understood?

1 "I need to call my cardiologist."
2 "I would take the next prescribed dose as usual."
3 "I would take the dose as soon as I realize I've missed it."
4 "I take two doses of the medication at the next scheduled time."

Level of Cognitive Ability: Evaluating
Client Needs: Physiological Integrity
Clinical Judgment/Cognitive Skills: Evaluating Outcomes
Integrated Process: Teaching and Learning
Content Area: Pharmacology: Cardiovascular: Antidysrhythmic
Health Problem: Adult Health: Cardiovascular: Dysrhythmias

Answer: 2
Rationale: Quinidine gluconate needs to be taken exactly as prescribed. Because of the action and effects of this medication, the client would be instructed to take the medication if remembered within 2 hours of the missed dose, or to omit the dose and then resume the normal schedule. There is no need to call the doctor. It is not safe to take the dose whenever it is remembered or to take an extra dose.
Priority Nursing Tip: Quinidine gluconate is an antidysrhythmic medication. The client must be instructed to take the medication exactly as prescribed.

Test-Taking Strategy: Focus on the **subject**, the principles related to quinidine gluconate administration. Think about the action and effect of the medication. Only the correct option expresses the appropriate measures to take when this medication dose is forgotten.

---

55. The nurse is educating the client on how to save lives and prevent burn injuries in the event of a fire in the home. Which statement by the client indicates that the teaching has been **effective?**

1 "I should put escape ladders in the bedrooms."
2 "I should install a whole-house sprinkler system."
3 "I should keep fresh batteries in smoke detectors."
4 "I should mount fire extinguishers in several areas."

Level of Cognitive Ability: Evaluating
Client Needs: Safe and Effective Care Environment
Clinical Judgment/Cognitive Skills: Evaluate Outcomes
Integrated Process: Teaching and Learning
Content Area: Foundations of Care: Safety
Health Problem: N/A

Answer: 3
Rationale: The early detection of smoke using a smoke detector and immediate evacuation from the house have significant and positive effects on mortality rates. This is because the smoke alarm activates before the appearance of open flames, which gives people in the house a chance to evacuate without burn injuries. Option 1 helps people in the house escape from second-story rooms safely, but it does not alert the people to the fire before flames are evident, thus exposing them to the risk of burn injury. Installing a sprinkler system is very expensive, and this is usually not done in private residences. Fire extinguishers are a good idea to have in the kitchen and other areas for small fires, but they are not designed to extinguish large fires.
Priority Nursing Tip: In the hospital, remember the mnemonic RACE (Rescue the client, Activate the fire alarm, Confine the fire, and Extinguish the fire) to set priorities in the event of a fire.

Test-Taking Strategy: Note the **strategic word,** *effective*. Focus on the **subject,** measures to save lives and prevent burn injuries in the event of a fire in the home. This will direct you to the correct option.

---

56. A client has had same-day surgery to insert a ventilating tube into the tympanic membrane. Which statement assures the nurse that the client understands the discharge instructions?

1 "I will use a shower cap when taking a shower."
2 "I was told to try to avoid taking medications for pain."
3 "I need to wash my hair quickly, taking 2 minutes or less."
4 "Swimming is allowed only if I keep my head above water."

Answer: 1

Rationale: After the insertion of tubes into the tympanic membrane, it is important to avoid getting water in the ears. A shower cap or earplug may be used when showering if allowed by the primary health care provider. Swimming, showering without a shower cap or earplugs, and washing the hair are avoided after surgery until the time frame designated for each is identified by the surgeon. The client would take medication as advised for postoperative discomfort.

Priority Nursing Tip: Ventilating tubes inserted into the tympanic membranes are tiny white spool-shaped tubes. If the tubes fall out, it is not an emergency, but the primary health care provider would be notified.

Test-Taking Strategy: Note the words *understands the discharge instructions*. Eliminate options 3 and 4 because of the word *quickly* and the closed-ended word "only." From the remaining choices, focusing on the anatomical location of the surgery will direct you to the correct option.

Level of Cognitive Ability: Evaluating
Client Needs: Physiological Integrity
Clinical Judgment/Cognitive Skills: Evaluate Outcomes
Integrated Process: Teaching and Learning
Content Area: Adult Health: Ear
Health Problem: Adult Health: Ear: Inflammatory/Infections/Structural Problems

---

57. The nurse has completed diet teaching for a client on a low-sodium diet for the treatment of hypertension. Which statement by the client would indicate to the nurse that there is a **need for further teaching?**

1 "Frozen foods are usually lowest in sodium."
2 "This diet will help lower my blood pressure."
3 "This diet is not a replacement for my antihypertensive medications."
4 "The reason I need to lower my salt intake is to reduce fluid retention."

Answer: 1

Rationale: A low-sodium diet is used as an adjunct to antihypertensive medications for the treatment of hypertension. Sodium retains fluid, which leads to hypertension as a result of increased fluid volume. Frozen foods use salt as a preservative, which increases their sodium content. Canned foods are extremely high in sodium. Fresh foods are best.

Priority Nursing Tip: Emphasize to the client with hypertension that dietary changes are not temporary and must be maintained for life.

Test-Taking Strategy: Note the **strategic words,** *need for further teaching*. These words indicate a **negative event query** and ask you to select an option that is an incorrect statement. Eliminate options that are accurate statements related to hypertension. Also, recall that "fresh is best"; fresh foods are lowest in sodium.

Level of Cognitive Ability: Evaluating
Client Needs: Physiological Integrity
Clinical Judgment/Cognitive Skills: Evaluate Outcomes
Integrated Process: Teaching and Learning
Content Area: Foundations of Care: Therapeutic Diets
Health Problem: Adult Health: Cardiovascular: Hypertension

---

58. The nurse is reinforcing dietary instructions to a client who had a kidney transplant and has been prescribed cyclosporine. Which statement by the client indicates the **need for further teaching?**

1 "Red meats are all right to eat."
2 "Orange juice is a great choice for breakfast."
3 "Grapefruit juice will not interfere with the medication."
4 "Green leafy vegetables should be eaten as often as possible."

Level of Cognitive Ability: Evaluating
Client Needs: Physiological Integrity
Clinical Judgment/Cognitive Skills: Evaluate Outcomes
Integrated Process: Teaching and Learning
Content Area: Pharmacology: Immune: Immunosuppressants
Health Problem: Adult Health: Immune: Transplantation

Answer: 3
Rationale: A compound in grapefruit juice inhibits the metabolism of cyclosporine. Thus, drinking grapefruit juice can raise cyclosporine levels by 50% to 100%, greatly increasing the risk of toxicity. The foods in options 1, 2, and 4 are acceptable to consume.
Priority Nursing Tip: Cyclosporine is an immunosuppressant medication that can be toxic and cause kidney damage.

Test-Taking Strategy: Focus on the **strategic words,** *need for further teaching,* and the **subject,** dietary instructions. This creates a **negative event query** and requires you to select something the client would avoid ingesting. Use general medication guidelines to assist in answering the question, and remember that grapefruit juice would not be administered with medications.

---

59. The nurse notes that the initial assessment on a pregnant client determined that the client is at risk for toxoplasmosis. The nurse reinforces education to the client on how to prevent the disease. Which statement by the client indicates that teaching has been **effective?**

1 "It's all right to eat raw meats."
2 "I need to wash hands only before meals."
3 "I need to avoid exposure to litter boxes used by my cat."
4 "I need to use topical corticosteroid treatments prophylactically."

Level of Cognitive Ability: Evaluating
Client Needs: Safe and Effective Care Environment
Clinical Judgment/Cognitive Skills: Evaluate Outcomes
Integrated Process: Teaching and Learning
Content Area: Foundations of Care: Infection Control
Health Problem: Maternity: Infections/ Inflammations

Answer: 3
Rationale: Infected house cats transmit toxoplasmosis through the feces. Handling litter boxes can transmit the disease to the pregnant client. Meats that are undercooked can harbor microorganisms that can cause infection. Hands need to be washed frequently throughout the day. The use of topical corticosteroids will not prevent exposure to the disease.
Priority Nursing Tip: Toxoplasmosis is an infection that can be transmitted to the fetus across the placenta. This infection can cause spontaneous abortion in the first trimester.

Test-Taking Strategy: Focus on the **strategic word,** *effective.* Eliminate option 2 because of the **closed-ended word** "only." Eliminate option 1 because of the word *raw.* From the remaining choices, focusing on the words *prevent the disease* in the question will direct you to the correct option.

---

60. The nurse is reinforcing instructions to a parent of a child diagnosed with cystic fibrosis (CF) about the appropriate dietary measures. Which diet would the nurse tell the parent that the child needs to consume?

1 Low-calorie, low-fat diet
2 High-calorie, restricted fat
3 Low-calorie, low-protein diet
4 High-calorie, high-protein diet

Level of Cognitive Ability: Applying
Client Needs: Physiological Integrity
Clinical Judgment/Cognitive Skills: Generate Solutions
Integrated Process: Teaching and Learning
Content Area: Foundations of Care: Therapeutic Diets
Health Problem: Pediatric–Specific: Cystic Fibrosis

Answer: 4
Rationale: Children with CF are managed with a high-calorie, high-protein diet. Pancreatic enzyme replacement therapy and fat-soluble vitamin supplements are administered. Fat restriction is unnecessary.
Priority Nursing Tip: CF is a progressive and incurable disorder, and respiratory failure is a common cause of death; organ transplantations may be an option to increase survival rates.

Test-Taking Strategy: Eliminate options 1 and 2 first because they are **comparable or alike,** and both restrict fat. From the remaining choices, focus on the **subject,** nutritional needs of a child with CF and the pathophysiology related to CF; this will direct you to the correct option.

---

61. The student nurse is listening to an orthopedic lecture on preoperative education and knee surgeries. Which statement by the student nurse indicates that the teaching has been **effective?**

1 "Crutch-walking instructions would be scheduled before surgery."
2 "Crutch-walking instructions would be given on the first postoperative day."
3 "Crutch-walking instructions would be scheduled on the second postoperative day."
4 "Crutch-walking instructions would be scheduled at the time of discharge after surgery."

Level of Cognitive Ability: Evaluating
Client Needs: Physiological Integrity
Clinical Judgment/Cognitive Skills: Evaluate Outcomes
Integrated Process: Teaching and Learning
Content Area: Skills: Activity/Mobility
Health Problem: Adult Health: Musculoskeletal: Skeletal Injury

Answer: 1
Rationale: It is best to check crutch-walking ability and instruct the client with regard to the use of the crutches before surgery because this task can be difficult to learn when the client is in pain and not used to the imbalance that may occur after surgery. None of the remaining options are appropriate times to teach a client about crutch walking.
Priority Nursing Tip: For the client undergoing knee replacement surgery, the nurse would plan to begin continuous passive motion 24 to 48 hours postoperatively as prescribed to exercise the knee and provide moderate flexion and extension.

Test-Taking Strategy: Focus on the **strategic word,** *effective,* and the **subject,** the time to schedule crutch-walking instructions. Eliminate options 2, 3, and 4, which are **comparable or alike** in that they address the postoperative period.

---

62. A client with a short leg plaster cast reports intense itching under the cast. The nurse reinforces instructions to the client regarding relief measures for the itching. Which statement by the client indicates an understanding of the measures used to relieve the itching?

1 "I can use the blunt part of a ruler to scratch the area."
2 "I can trickle small amounts of water down inside the cast."
3 "I need to obtain assistance when placing an object into the cast for the itching."
4 "I can use a hair dryer on the low setting and allow the air to blow into the cast."

Level of Cognitive Ability: Evaluating
Client Needs: Physiological Integrity
Clinical Judgment/Cognitive Skills: Evaluate Outcomes
Integrated Process: Teaching and Learning
Content Area: Foundations of Care: Safety
Health Problem: Adult Health: Musculoskeletal: Skeletal Injury

Answer: 4
Rationale: Itching is a common complaint of clients with casts. Objects would not be put inside a cast because of the risk of scratching the skin and providing a point of entry for bacteria. A plaster cast can break down when wet. Therefore, the best way to relieve itching is with the forceful injection of air inside the cast.
Priority Nursing Tip: The orthopedic specialist is notified immediately if circulatory impairment occurs in the extremity with a cast.

Test-Taking Strategy: Eliminate options that are **comparable or alike** and indicate putting objects inside the cast. Next, focus on the **subject,** proper cast care, to direct you to the correct option.

---

63. Disulfiram has been prescribed for a client, and the nurse reinforces instructions to the client about the medication. Which statement by the client indicates the **need for further teaching?**

1 "I must be careful taking cold medicines."
2 "I will have to check my aftershave lotion."
3 "I'll be fine as long as I don't drink alcohol."
4 "I need to be careful with ingredients when I cook."

Level of Cognitive Ability: Evaluating
Client Needs: Physiological Integrity
Clinical Judgment/Cognitive Skills:
Integrated Process: Teaching and Learning
Content Area: Pharmacology: Psychotherapeutics: Alcohol Deterrents
Health Problem: Mental Health: Addictions

Answer: 3
Rationale: Clients who are taking disulfiram must be taught that substances that contain alcohol can trigger an adverse reaction. Sources of hidden alcohol include foods (soups, sauces, and vinegars), medicine (cold medicine), mouthwashes, and skin preparations (alcohol rubs and aftershave lotions).
Priority Nursing Tip: Disulfiram is an alcohol deterrent that may be prescribed for alcoholic dependence. The medication sensitizes the client to alcohol, so a disulfiram–alcohol reaction occurs if alcohol is ingested.

Test-Taking Strategy: Note the **strategic words,** *need for further teaching.* These words indicate a **negative event query** and ask you to select an option that is an incorrect statement. Remember that disulfiram is used for clients who have alcoholism, and any form of alcohol must be avoided with this medication.

---

64. The nurse has reinforced instructions to a client who is receiving external radiation therapy for breast cancer. Which statement by the client indicates a **need for further teaching** regarding self-care related to the radiation therapy?

1 "I need to eat a high-protein diet."
2 "I need to avoid exposure to sunlight."
3 "I need to wash my skin with a mild soap and pat it dry."
4 "I need to apply pressure on the irritated area to prevent bleeding."

Level of Cognitive Ability: Evaluating
Client Needs: Physiological Integrity
Clinical Judgment/Cognitive Skills:
Integrated Process: Teaching and Learning
Content Area: Adult Health: Oncology
Health Problem: Adult Health: Cancer: Breast

Answer: 4
Rationale: The client receiving external radiation therapy needs to avoid pressure on the irritated area and wear loose-fitting clothing. Specific health care provider instructions would be necessary to obtain if an alteration in skin integrity occurs as a result of the radiation therapy. The remaining options are accurate measures regarding radiation therapy.
Priority Nursing Tip: The client undergoing external radiation therapy does not emit radiation and does not pose a hazard to anyone else.

Test-Taking Strategy: Note the **strategic words,** *need for further teaching*. These words indicate a **negative event query** and ask you to select an option that is an incorrect statement. The word *pressure* in the correct option is an indication that this is an inappropriate measure.

---

65. The nurse reinforces instructions to a client regarding the testicular self-examination (TSE). Which statement by the client indicates that the client **needs further teaching** regarding TSE?

1 "I know to report any small lumps."
2 "I need to examine myself every 2 months."
3 "I need to examine myself after I take a warm shower."
4 "I know it's normal to feel something that is cordlike in the back."

Level of Cognitive Ability: Evaluating
Client Needs: Health Promotion and Maintenance
Clinical Judgment/Cognitive Skills: Evaluate Outcomes
Integrated Process: Teaching and Learning
Content Area: Health Assessment/Physical Exam: Client Teaching
Health Problem: Adult Health: Cancer: Testicular

Answer: 2
Rationale: TSE would be performed every month. Small lumps or abnormalities would be reported. The spermatic cord finding is normal. After a warm bath or shower, the scrotum is relaxed, which makes it easier to perform TSE.
Priority Nursing Tip: Teach the client how to perform TSE; a day of the month is selected, and the examination is performed on the same day each month after a shower or bath, when the hands are warm and soapy and the scrotum is warm.

Test-Taking Strategy: Note the **strategic words,** *needs further teaching*. These words indicate a **negative event query** and the need to select the incorrect client statement. Remembering that breast self-examination needs to be performed monthly may assist you with recalling that TSE is also performed monthly.

---

66. A client diagnosed with acquired immunodeficiency syndrome (AIDS) is reporting fatigue. The nurse provides the client information on ways to conserve energy. Which statement indicates that the teaching was **effective?**

1 "Bathe before eating breakfast."
2 "Sit for as many activities as possible."
3 "Stand in the shower instead of taking a bath."
4 "Group all tasks to be performed early in the morning."

Level of Cognitive Ability: Evaluating
Client Needs: Physiological Integrity
Clinical Judgment/Cognitive Skills: Evaluate Outcomes
Integrated Process: Teaching and Learning
Content Area: Adult Health: Immune
Health Problem: Adult Health: Immune: Immunodeficiency Syndrome

Answer: 2

Rationale: The client is taught to conserve energy by sitting for as many activities as possible, including dressing, shaving, preparing food, and ironing. The client would also sit in a shower chair instead of standing while showering. The client needs to prioritize activities such as eating breakfast before bathing, and the client would intersperse each major activity with a period of rest.

Priority Nursing Tip: AIDS is a disorder caused by the human immunodeficiency virus (HIV) and is characterized by generalized dysfunction of the immune system.

Test-Taking Strategy: Focus on the **strategic word,** *effective,* and the **subject,** conserving energy. Think about the amount of exertion required by the client to perform each of the activities described in the options. Eliminate options that are obviously taxing for the client. From the remaining choices, recall that bathing may take away energy that could be used for eating and so is not helpful.

---

67. A 10-year-old child has been diagnosed with type 1 diabetes mellitus. What instruction would the nurse reinforce concerning the monitoring of the child's insulin needs?

1 The child would be taught to self-monitor insulin needs.
2 The parents will need to be available to monitor the child's insulin needs.
3 The child's teacher will assume responsibility for monitoring the child's insulin needs.
4 Friends and family will need to be involved with monitoring the child's insulin needs.

Level of Cognitive Ability: Applying
Client Needs: Physiological Integrity
Clinical Judgment/Cognitive Skills: Generate Solutions
Integrated Process: Teaching and Learning
Content Area: Pediatrics: Metabolic/Endocrine
Health Problem: Pediatric-Specific: Diabetes Mellitus

Answer: 1

Rationale: Most children age 9 years or older can understand the principles of monitoring their own insulin requirements. They are usually responsible enough to determine the appropriate intervention needed to maintain their health. Parents, friends, and family cannot always be available. The teacher would not be expected to take responsibility for health care interventions.

Priority Nursing Tip: The abdomen is the preferred site for infusion set sites and injections. It is easy to see and reach, and offers the quickest absorption.

Test-Taking Strategy: Focus on the **subject,** a 10-year-old child with type 1 diabetes mellitus. Noting the age of the child will indicate that the child is able to take control and responsibility regarding her or his health care situation. Eliminate options 2, 3, and 4, which are **comparable or alike** in that they rely on other individuals to care for the child.

---

68. The nurse reinforces instructions for a client diagnosed with oral candidiasis (thrush) about caring for the disorder. Which statement by the client indicates a **need for additional teaching?**

1 "I can eat foods that are liquid or pureed."
2 "I need to eliminate spicy foods from my diet."
3 "It's best if I don't drink citrus juices or hot liquids."
4 "I need to rinse my mouth 4 times daily with commercial mouthwash."

Level of Cognitive Ability: Evaluating
Client Needs: Physiological Integrity
Clinical Judgment/Cognitive Skills: Evaluate Outcomes
Integrated Process: Teaching and Learning
Content Area: Adult Health: Immune
Health Problem: Adult Health: Integumentary: Inflammations/Infections

Answer: 4
Rationale: Clients with thrush cannot tolerate commercial mouthwashes because the high alcohol concentration in these products can cause pain and discomfort of the lesions. A solution of warm water or mouthwash formulas without alcohol are better tolerated and may promote healing. A change in diet to liquid or pureed food often eases the discomfort of eating. The client would avoid spicy foods, citrus juices, and hot liquids.
Priority Nursing Tip: Candidiasis can be oral or vaginal. Antifungal medications are used to treat this infection. The nurse would encourage increased fluid intake and monitor the client's temperature when the client has an infection and is taking antifungal medication.

Test-Taking Strategy: Note the **strategic words,** *need for further teaching*. These words indicate a **negative event query** and ask you to select an option that is an incorrect statement. In addition, noting the words *commercial mouthwash* in the correct option will direct you to this option.

---

69. The nurse has reinforced instructions about site care to a hemodialysis client who had an implantation of an arteriovenous (AV) fistula in the right arm. Which statement by the client indicates a **need for further teaching?**

1 "I will need to sleep on my right side."
2 "It's important that I don't carry heavy objects with the right arm."
3 "I will perform range-of-motion exercises routinely on my right arm."
4 "It's important that I report any right arm redness or drainage at the site."

Level of Cognitive Ability: Evaluating
Client Needs: Physiological Integrity
Clinical Judgment/Cognitive Skills: Evaluate Outcomes
Integrated Process: Teaching and Learning
Content Area: Adult Health: Renal and Urinary
Health Problem: Adult Health: Renal and Urinary: Acute Kidney Injury and Chronic Kidney Disease

Answer: 1
Rationale: Routine instructions to the client with an AV fistula, graft, or shunt include avoiding sleeping with the body weight on the extremity with the access site, avoiding carrying heavy objects with or compressing the extremity that has the access site, performing routine range-of-motion exercises of the affected extremity, and reporting signs and symptoms of infection.
Priority Nursing Tip: Arterial steal syndrome can occur as a result of the presence of an AV fistula. This is a syndrome that can develop after the insertion of an AV fistula when too much blood is diverted to the vein and arterial perfusion to the hand is compromised.

Test-Taking Strategy: Note the **strategic words,** *need for further teaching*. These words indicate a **negative event query** and ask you to select an option that is an incorrect statement. Recalling the importance of maintaining the patency of the AV fistula will direct you to the correct option.

---

70. The nurse reinforces instructions about applying a nitroglycerin patch. What statement indicates that the client is using correct technique?

1 "A second patch will be applied if chest pain occurs."
2 "I will apply the patch to a nonhairy area of the body."
3 "I will remove the patch when bathing and reapply it after the bath."
4 "I will remove the patch after gently rubbing the area to activate the medication."

Level of Cognitive Ability: Evaluating
Client Needs: Physiological Integrity
Clinical Judgment/Cognitive Skills: Evaluate Outcomes
Integrated Process: Teaching and Learning
Content Area: Pharmacology: Cardiovascular: Vasodilators
Health Problem: Adult Health: Cardiovascular: Coronary Artery Disease

Answer: 2

Rationale: Topical nitroglycerin is applied to a nonhairy part of the body. It is used on a scheduled basis and is not prescribed specifically for the occurrence of chest pain. The ointment is not rubbed into the skin; it is reapplied only as directed.

Priority Nursing Tip: Nitroglycerin is a vasodilator and will lower the blood pressure. The nurse needs to wear gloves when applying the topical preparation to a client.

Test-Taking Strategy: Focus on the **subject,** understanding the instructions for applying a nitroglycerin patch. Noting the word *nonhairy* in the correct option will direct you to this choice.

---

71. The nurse is reinforcing medication instructions to a client who is receiving furosemide. Which client statement indicates a **need for further teaching?**

1 "I need to change positions slowly."
2 "I need to talk to my doctor about the use of alcohol."
3 "I need to be careful not to get overheated in warm weather."
4 "I need to avoid the use of salt substitutes because they contain potassium."

Level of Cognitive Ability: Evaluating
Client Needs: Physiological Integrity
Clinical Judgment/Cognitive Skills: Evaluate Outcomes
Integrated Process: Teaching and Learning
Content Area: Pharmacology: Cardiovascular: Diuretics
Health Problem: Adult Health: Cardiovascular: Heart Failure

Answer: 4

Rationale: Furosemide is a potassium-losing diuretic, so there is no need to avoid high-potassium products, such as a salt substitute. Orthostatic hypotension is a risk, and the client must use caution when changing positions and with exposure to warm weather. The client needs to discuss the use of alcohol with the primary health care provider.

Priority Nursing Tip: The nurse would monitor the electrolyte values, specifically the potassium value, when the client is receiving a potassium-losing diuretic.

Test-Taking Strategy: Note the **strategic words,** *need for further teaching.* These words indicate a **negative event query** and ask you to select an option that is an incorrect statement. Focus on the **subject,** a client who is receiving furosemide. Recalling that furosemide is a potassium-losing diuretic and that diuretic therapy can induce orthostatic hypotension will direct you to the correct option.

---

72. A client with hypertension has been prescribed a clonidine patch. The nurse has reinforced instructions to the client regarding the use of the patch. Which client statement indicates a **need for further teaching?**

1 "I intend to change the patch every 7 days."
2 "I need to trim the patch if an edge becomes loose."
3 "It's important to put the patch on a hairless site on my torso."
4 "It's all right to leave the patch in place during bathing or showering."

Level of Cognitive Ability: Evaluating
Client Needs: Physiological Integrity
Clinical Judgment/Cognitive Skills: Evaluate Outcomes
Integrated Process: Teaching and Learning
Content Area: Pharmacology: Cardiovascular: Antihypertensives
Health Problem: Adult Health: Cardiovascular Hypertension

Answer: 2
Rationale: The clonidine patch would not be trimmed because it will alter the medication dose. If it becomes slightly loose, it would be covered with an adhesive overlay from the medication package. If it becomes very loose or falls off, it would be replaced. It is changed every 7 days, and it is left in place when bathing or showering. The clonidine patch would be applied to a hairless site on the torso or the upper arm. The patch is discarded by folding it in half with the adhesive sides together.
Priority Nursing Tip: Clonidine is a centrally acting sympatholytic that is used to treat hypertension. The client is instructed not to discontinue the medication because abrupt withdrawal can cause severe rebound hypertension.

Test-Taking Strategy: Note the **strategic words,** *need for further teaching*. These words indicate a **negative event query** and ask you to select an option that is an incorrect statement. Noting the words *trim the patch* will direct you to the correct option because this client's action would alter the medication dose.

---

73. The nurse reinforces instructions to the client about the use of cholestyramine. Which client statement indicates a **need for further teaching?**

1 "I need to take this medication with meals."
2 "I need to mix the medication with juice or applesauce."
3 "I need to call my doctor immediately if it causes constipation."
4 "I need to increase my fluid intake while taking this medication."

Level of Cognitive Ability: Evaluating
Client Needs: Physiological Integrity
Clinical Judgment/Cognitive Skills: Evaluate Outcomes
Integrated Process: Teaching and Learning
Content Area: Pharmacology: Cardiovascular: Antilipemics
Health Problem: Adult Health: Cardiovascular: Coronary Artery Disease

Answer: 3
Rationale: Common side effects of cholestyramine include constipation, nausea, indigestion, and flatulence. Therefore, it is unnecessary to contact the primary health care provider immediately if constipation occurs. Cholestyramine must be administered with food to be effective. This medication would not be taken dry, and it can be mixed in water, juice, carbonated beverages, applesauce, or soup. Increasing fluids will minimize the constipating effects of the medication.
Priority Nursing Tip: Cholestyramine is a bile acid sequestrant used to lower the cholesterol level, and client adherence is a problem because of its taste and palatability. Mixing the medication with flavored products or fruit juices can improve the taste.

Test-Taking Strategy: Note the **strategic words,** *need for further teaching*. These words indicate a **negative event query** and ask you to select an option that is an incorrect statement. Select the correct option because of the word *immediately* and because normally measures can be taken to prevent constipation.

---

74. The nurse is reviewing written medication instructions with a client who is prescribed colestipol hydrochloride as part of the treatment plan for coronary artery disease. Which statement by the client indicates that the teaching has been **effective?**

1 "Vitamin C will help control unintended side effects."
2 "Vitamin B_{12} will help control unintended side effects."
3 "B-complex vitamins will help control unintended side effects."
4 "Fat-soluble vitamins will help control unintended side effects."

Level of Cognitive Ability: Evaluating
Client Needs: Physiological Integrity
Clinical Judgment/Cognitive Skills: Evaluate Outcomes
Integrated Process: Teaching and Learning
Content Area: Pharmacology: Cardiovascular: Antilipemics
Health Problem: Adult Health: Cardiovascular: Coronary Artery Disease

Answer: 4
Rationale: Colestipol hydrochloride, which is a bile-sequestering agent, is used to lower blood cholesterol levels. However, the bile salts (which are rich in cholesterol) interfere with the absorption of the fat-soluble vitamins A, D, E, and K, as well as folic acid. With ongoing therapy, the client is at risk for the deficiency of these vitamins and is counseled to take them as supplements.
Priority Nursing Tip: Bile acid sequestrants bind with acids in the intestines, which prevents reabsorption of cholesterol.

Test-Taking Strategy: Focus on the **strategic word,** *effective,* and the **subject,** considerations for administration of colestipol hydrochloride and counteracting unintended medication effects. This will help you recall that bile-sequestering agents interfere with the absorption of fat-soluble vitamins and will assist you with eliminating the remaining options. Also, option 4 is the correct option because it is the **umbrella option.**

NURSING PROCESS: DATA COLLECTION

75. Which data would the nurse expect to obtain to support the diagnosis of irritable bowel syndrome in a child?

1 Frequent incidents of frothy diarrhea
2 Frequent foul-smelling ribbon stools
3 Profuse, watery diarrhea and vomiting daily
4 Diffuse abdominal pain unrelated to meals or activity

Level of Cognitive Ability: Analyzing
Client Needs: Physiological Integrity
Clinical Judgment/Cognitive Skills: Analyze Cues
Integrated Process: Nursing Process/Data Collection
Content Area: Pediatrics: Gastrointestinal
Health Problem: Pediatric-Specific: GI and Rectal Problems

Answer: 4
Rationale: Irritable bowel syndrome causes diffuse abdominal pain unrelated to meals or activity. Alternating constipation and diarrhea with the presence of undigested food and mucus in the stools may also be noted. Option 1 is a clinical manifestation of lactose intolerance. Option 2 is a clinical manifestation of Hirschsprung's disease. Option 3 is a clinical manifestation of celiac disease.
Priority Nursing Tip: Stress and emotional factors may contribute to the occurrence of irritable bowel syndrome.

Test-Taking Strategy: Focus on the **subject,** manifestations of irritable bowel syndrome. Noting the name of the syndrome will direct you to the correct option because you would expect abdominal pain to occur in clients with this disorder.

---

76. The nurse caring for a child diagnosed with rubeola (measles) notes that the pediatrician has documented the presence of Koplik's spots. On the basis of this documentation, which observation is expected?

1 Pinpoint petechiae noted on both legs
2 Whitish vesicles located across the chest
3 Petechiae spots that are reddish and pinpoint on the soft palate
4 Small blue-white spots with a red base found on the buccal mucosa

Level of Cognitive Ability: Analyzing
Client Needs: Physiological Integrity
Clinical Judgment/Cognitive Skills: Recognize Cues
Integrated Process: Nursing Process/Data Collection
Content Area: Pediatrics: Infectious and Communicable Diseases
Health Problem: Pediatric-Specific: Communicable Diseases

Answer: 4

Rationale: In rubeola (measles), Koplik's spots appear approximately 2 days before the appearance of the rash. These are small blue-white spots with a red base that are found on the buccal mucosa. The spots last approximately 3 days, after which time they slough off. Based on this information, the remaining options are all incorrect.

Priority Nursing Tip: Rubeola (measles) is transmitted via airborne particles, direct contact with infectious droplets, or transplacental contact. The nurse must implement airborne precautions when caring for the hospitalized client with rubeola.

Test-Taking Strategy: Eliminate options 1 and 3, which are **comparable or alike** and address petechiae spots. Focusing on the **subject,** Koplik's spots, will direct you to the correct option.

---

77. Which finding would the nurse expect to note in the child hospitalized with a diagnosis of nephrotic syndrome?

1 Weight loss
2 Constipation
3 Hypotension
4 Abdominal pain

Level of Cognitive Ability: Analyzing
Client Needs: Physiological Integrity
Clinical Judgment/Cognitive Skills: Recognize Cues
Integrated Process: Nursing Process/Data Collection
Content Area: Pediatrics: Renal and Urinary
Health Problem: Pediatric-Specific: Nephrotic Syndrome

Answer: 4

Rationale: Clinical manifestations associated with nephrotic syndrome include edema, anorexia, fatigue, and abdominal pain from the presence of extra fluid in the peritoneal cavity. Diarrhea caused by the edema of the bowel occurs and may cause decreased absorption of nutrients. Increased weight from fluid buildup and a normal blood pressure are noted.

Priority Nursing Tip: The primary objectives of therapeutic management for nephrotic syndrome are to reduce the excretion of urinary protein, maintain protein-free urine, reduce edema, prevent infection, and minimize complications.

Test-Taking Strategy: Focus on the **subject,** the physiology and manifestations associated with nephrotic syndrome. Recalling that edema is a clinical manifestation will direct you to the correct option.

---

78. A child is admitted to the hospital with a suspected diagnosis of von Willebrand's disease. On data collection of the child, which symptom would **most likely** be noted?

1 Hematuria
2 Presence of hematomas
3 Presence of hemarthrosis
4 Bleeding from the mucous membranes

Level of Cognitive Ability: Analyzing
Client Needs: Physiological Integrity
Clinical Judgment/Cognitive Skills: Recognize Cues
Integrated Process: Nursing Process/Data Collection
Content Area: Pediatrics: Hematological
Health Problem: Pediatric-Specific: Bleeding Disorders

Answer: 4
Rationale: The primary clinical manifestations of von Willebrand's disease are bruising and mucous membrane bleeding from the nose, mouth, and gastrointestinal tract. Prolonged bleeding after trauma and surgery, including tooth extraction, may be the first evidence of abnormal hemostasis in those with mild disease. In females, menorrhagia and profuse postpartum bleeding may occur. Bleeding associated with von Willebrand's disease may be severe and lead to anemia and shock, but unlike what is seen in clients with hemophilia, deep bleeding into joints and muscles is rare. Options 1, 2, and 3 are characteristic of those signs found in clients with hemophilia.
Priority Nursing Tip: Von Willebrand's disease is a disorder that causes platelets to adhere to damaged endothelium and is characterized by an increased tendency to bleed from mucous membranes.

Test-Taking Strategy: Note the **strategic words,** *most likely.* Think about the pathophysiology of this disorder and recall that the remaining options are characteristic of hemophilia to assist you with eliminating these options and to direct you to the correct option.

---

79. A client prescribed dextroamphetamine reports difficulty falling asleep at night. The nurse reinforces instructions to the client on how to minimize sleep disorders. Which statement by the client indicates that teaching has been **effective?**

1 "I'll take the medication with a bedtime snack."
2 "I'll take the medication 3 hours after eating dinner."
3 "I'll take the medication 2 hours before going to bed."
4 "I'll take the medication at least 6 hours before bedtime."

Level of Cognitive Ability: Evaluating
Client Needs: Physiological Integrity
Clinical Judgment/Cognitive Skills: Evaluate Outcomes
Integrated Process: Nursing Process/Evaluation
Content Area: Pharmacology: Neurological: Central Nervous System Stimulants
Health Problem: N/A

Answer: 4
Rationale: Dextroamphetamine is a central nervous system (CNS) stimulant that acts by releasing norepinephrine from the nerve endings. The client would take the medication at least 6 hours before going to bed at night to prevent disturbances with sleep. Therefore, the remaining options are incorrect.
Priority Nursing Tip: The client taking a CNS stimulant needs to be instructed to avoid foods containing caffeine to prevent additional stimulation.

Test-Taking Strategy: Focus on the **strategic word,** *effective,* and the **subject,** dextroamphetamine and difficulty sleeping. Think about the action and purpose of this medication. Evaluate each of the options in terms of how far removed the scheduled dose is from the client's bedtime. This will direct you to option 4.

---

80. The nurse checking the level of consciousness of a child with a head injury documents that the child is obtunded. On the basis of this documentation, which observation did the nurse note?

1 The child is unable to think clearly and rapidly.
2 The child is unable to recognize place or person.
3 The child always requires considerable stimulation for arousal.
4 The child has limited interaction with the environment unless aroused.

Level of Cognitive Ability: Analyzing
Client Needs: Physiological Integrity
Clinical Judgment/Cognitive Skills: Recognize Cues
Integrated Process: Nursing Process/Data Collection
Content Area: Pediatrics: Neurological
Health Problem: Pediatric-Specific: Head Injury

Answer: 4
Rationale: If the child is obtunded, the child sleeps unless aroused and, when aroused, has limited interaction with the environment. The remaining options describe confusion, disorientation, and stupor.
Priority Nursing Tip: Do not place a client with a head injury in a flat or Trendelenburg's position because of the risk of increased intracranial pressure.

Test-Taking Strategy: Focus on the **subject,** the child is obtunded. Knowledge regarding the standard terms used to identify level of consciousness will direct you to the correct option.

---

81. The nurse is caring for a client diagnosed with acquired immunodeficiency syndrome (AIDS). Which sign/symptom indicates the presence of an opportunistic respiratory infection?

1 Nausea and vomiting
2 Fever and exertional dyspnea
3 An arterial blood gas pH of 7.40
4 A respiratory rate of 20 breaths per minute

Level of Cognitive Ability: Analyzing
Client Needs: Physiological Integrity
Clinical Judgment/Cognitive Skills: Recognize Cues
Integrated Process: Nursing Process/Data Collection
Content Area: Adult Health: Immune
Health Problem: Adult Health: Immune: Immunodeficiency Syndrome

Answer: 2
Rationale: Fever and exertional dyspnea are signs of *Pneumocystis jiroveci* pneumonia, which is a common, life-threatening opportunistic infection that afflicts those with AIDS. Option 1 is not associated with respiratory infection. Options 3 and 4 are normal findings.
Priority Nursing Tip: A client with human immunodeficiency virus (HIV) or AIDS is at risk for developing a life-threatening opportunistic infection. Monitor the client closely for signs or symptoms of infection, and report these signs immediately if they occur.

Test-Taking Strategy: Focus on the **subject,** opportunistic respiratory infection in a client with AIDS. Eliminate options that are **comparable or alike** and are normal findings. For the remaining options, focusing on the **subject,** a respiratory infection, will direct you to the correct option.

---

82. An adult client seeks treatment in an ambulatory care clinic for reports of a left earache, nausea, and a full feeling in the left ear. The client has an elevated temperature. Which question would the nurse ask **first?**

1 "Do you have a history of a recent brain abscess?"
2 "Do you have a chronic hearing problem in the left ear?"
3 "Do you successfully obtain pain relief with acetaminophen?"
4 "Do you have a history of a recent upper respiratory infection?"

Level of Cognitive Ability: Analyzing
Client Needs: Physiological Integrity
Clinical Judgment/Cognitive Skills: Recognize Cues
Integrated Process: Nursing Process/Data Collection
Content Area: Adult Health: Ear
Health Problem: Adult Health: Ear: Inflammation/Infections/Structural Problems

Answer: 4

Rationale: Otitis media in the adult is typically one-sided and presents as an acute process with earache, nausea and possible vomiting, fever, and fullness in the ear. The client may report diminished hearing in that ear during the acute process. The nurse takes a client history first, checking whether the client has had a recent URI. It is unnecessary to question the client about a brain abscess. The nurse may ask the client whether anything relieves the pain, but ear infection pain is usually not relieved until antibiotic therapy is initiated.

Priority Nursing Tip: Infants and children have eustachian tubes that are shorter, wider, and straighter, which makes them more prone to otitis media.

Test-Taking Strategy: Note the **data in the question** and focus on the **subject,** the relationship between an upper respiratory infection and otitis media. Noting the **strategic word,** *first,* will direct you to the correct option.

---

83. The licensed practical nurse assists the registered nurse in preparing to administer a continuous intravenous (IV) infusion through a peripheral IV to a dehydrated client. Which **priority** item would be checked before initiating the IV infusion?

1 Daily body weight
2 Serum electrolytes
3 Intake and output records
4 Identifying the client's dominant side

Level of Cognitive Ability: Analyzing
Client Needs: Physiological Integrity
Clinical Judgment/Cognitive Skills: Prioritize Hypotheses
Integrated Process: Nursing Process/Data Collection
Content Area: Foundations of Care: Fluids & Electrolytes
Health Problem: Adult Health: Gastrointestinal: Dehydration

Answer: 1

Rationale: The nurse obtains the client's baseline body weight as a priority before beginning the IV infusion because body weight is a sensitive and specific indicator of fluid volume status when body weights are compared on a daily basis. This means that as a client receives or accumulates fluid, body weight quickly and proportionately increases, and vice versa. The remaining options may also be reasonable items to check before initiating an IV infusion. However, intake, output, and serum electrolytes are potentially affected by more confounding factors; thus, they are less specific and are sensitive to fluctuations in body fluid. Determining the client's dominant side assists in deciding a site for inserting the initial IV catheter, but it provides no information about fluid volume status.

Priority Nursing Tip: Clients with respiratory, cardiac, renal, or liver disease; older clients; and very young children are at risk for circulatory overload and may not be able to tolerate an excessive body fluid volume.

Test-Taking Strategy: Focus on the **subject,** continuous IV infusion through a peripheral IV to a dehydrated client. Note the **strategic word,** *priority.* Review the options to determine the best method for the nurse to use to evaluate fluid status. Body weight is the best option because it is the most sensitive and specific measurement listed.

---

84. A client with coronary artery disease is scheduled for an arteriogram using a radiopaque dye. What is the **most important** information the nurse would determine before the procedure to ensure the client's safety?

1 Vital signs
2 Intake and output
3 Height and weight
4 Allergy to iodine or shellfish

Level of Cognitive Ability: Analyzing
Client Needs: Physiological Integrity
Clinical Judgment/Cognitive Skills: Prioritize Hypotheses
Integrated Process: Nursing Process/Data Collection
Content Area: Foundations of Care: Diagnostic Tests
Health Problem: Adult Health: Cardiovascular: Coronary Artery Disease

Answer: 4
Rationale: Allergy to iodine or seafood is associated with allergy to the radiopaque dye that is used for medical imaging examinations. Informed consent is necessary because an arteriogram requires the injection of a radiopaque dye into the blood vessel. Although the remaining options are components of the preprocedure assessment, the risks of allergic reaction and possible anaphylaxis are the most critical to the client's safety.
Priority Nursing Tip: If anaphylaxis occurs after the injection of a radiopaque dye, the nurse immediately checks the client's respiratory status and provides respiratory support and asks another nursing staff member to contact the primary health care provider.

Test-Taking Strategy: Note the **strategic words,** *most important.* Focusing on the **subject,** arteriogram using a radiopaque dye, will help you recall the risk of anaphylaxis related to the dye; this will direct you to the correct option.

---

85. The nurse is collecting cardiovascular data on a client with heart failure. Which item would the nurse check to obtain the **best** information about the client's left-sided heart function?

1 The status of breath sounds
2 The presence of peripheral edema
3 The presence of hepatojugular reflux
4 The presence of jugular vein distention

Level of Cognitive Ability: Analyzing
Client Needs: Physiological Integrity
Clinical Judgment/Cognitive Skills: Recognize Cues
Integrated Process: Nursing Process/Data Collection
Content Area: Health Assessment/Physical Exam: Heart and Peripheral Vascular
Health Problem: Adult Health: Cardiovascular: Heart Failure

Answer: 1
Rationale: The client with heart failure may present different symptoms depending on whether the right or the left side of the heart is failing. Checking breath sounds provides information about left-sided heart function. Peripheral edema, hepatojugular reflux, and jugular vein distention are all signs of right-sided heart failure.
Priority Nursing Tip: Signs of left ventricular failure are evident in the pulmonary system. Signs of right ventricular failure are evident in the systemic circulation.

Test-Taking Strategy: Focus on the **subject,** the status of left-sided heart function and the **strategic word,** *best.* Remember "left" and "lungs." The remaining options reflect right-sided heart failure.

---

86. The nurse is collecting data from a client who was admitted to the hospital with a thrombotic brain attack (stroke). What are the **most likely** signs/symptoms the client experienced before the stroke occurred? **Select all that apply.**

❒ 1 Temporary aphasia
❒ 2 Throbbing headaches
❒ 3 Transient hemiplegia
❒ 4 Paresthesia on one side of the body
❒ 5 Unexplained loss of consciousness

Level of Cognitive Ability: Analyzing
Client Needs: Physiological Integrity
Clinical Judgment/Cognitive Skills: Recognize Cues
Integrated Process: Nursing Process/Data Collection
Content Area: Adult Health: Neurological
Health Problem: Adult Health: Neurological: Stroke

Answer: 1, 3, 4
Rationale: Cerebral thrombosis does not occur suddenly. During the few hours or days before a thrombotic stroke, the client may experience a transient loss of speech (aphasia), hemiplegia, or paresthesia on one side of the body. Other signs and symptoms of thrombotic stroke vary, but they may include dizziness, cognitive changes, or seizures. Headache is rare, and a loss of consciousness is unlikely to occur.
Priority Nursing Tip: A stroke is a syndrome in which the cerebral circulation is interrupted, causing neurological deficits. Cerebral anoxia lasting longer than 10 minutes causes cerebral infarction with irreversible change.

Test-Taking Strategy: Focus on the **subject,** symptoms of a thrombotic brain attack (stroke), and the **strategic words,** *most likely.* Use the knowledge about the manifestations of this type of stroke to answer correctly. The remaining options are not associated commonly with this type of stroke and so can be eliminated.

---

87. A client with gastritis in a long-term care facility has had a series of gastrointestinal (GI) diagnostic tests, including an upper and lower GI series and endoscopies. Upon return to the long-term care facility, which **priority** item would the nurse focus on during data collection?

1 The comfort level
2 Activity tolerance
3 The level of consciousness
4 The hydration and nutrition status

Level of Cognitive Ability: Analyzing
Client Needs: Physiological Integrity
Clinical Judgment/Cognitive Skills: Prioritize Hypotheses
Integrated Process: Nursing Process/Data Collection
Content Area: Foundations of Care: Diagnostic Tests
Health Problem: Adult Health: Gastrointestinal: Gastritis/Gastroenteritis

Answer: 4
Rationale: Many of the diagnostic studies to identify GI disorders require that the GI tract be cleaned (usually with laxatives and enemas) before testing. In addition, the client most often takes nothing by mouth before and during the testing period. Because the studies may be done over a period that exceeds 24 hours, the client may become dehydrated and/or malnourished. Although the remaining options may be components of data collection, the correct option is the priority.
Priority Nursing Tip: After endoscopic procedures that involve the use of a local throat anesthetic, monitor for the return of a gag reflex before giving the client any oral substance. If the gag reflex has not returned, the client could aspirate.

Test-Taking Strategy: Note the **strategic word,** *priority.* Use **Maslow's Hierarchy of Needs theory** to direct you to the correct option. Hydration and nutrition are the priorities.

---

88. Which aspect would the nurse focus on when checking a client for the vegetative signs of depression? **Select all that apply.**

- ❒ 1 Weight
- ❒ 2 Appetite
- ❒ 3 Sleep patterns
- ❒ 4 Suicidal ideations
- ❒ 5 Psychomotor activity
- ❒ 6 Rational decision making

Level of Cognitive Ability: Analyzing
Client Needs: Physiological Integrity
Clinical Judgment/Cognitive Skills: Recognize Cues
Integrated Process: Nursing Process/Data Collection
Content Area: Mental Health
Health Problem: Mental Health: Mood Disorders

Answer: 1, 2, 3, 5
Rationale: The vegetative signs of depression are changes in physiological functioning that occur during depression. These include changes in appetite, weight, sleep patterns, and psychomotor activity. The remaining options represent psychological data collection categories.
Priority Nursing Tip: An inappropriate appearance and indications of poor hygiene practices may be signs of depression, manic disorder, dementia, organic brain disease, or another disorder.

Test-Taking Strategy: Focus on the **subject,** the vegetative signs of depression. Recalling that these are physiological changes and using **Maslow's Hierarchy of Needs theory** will direct you to the correct options.

---

89. A client diagnosed with cirrhosis of the liver is receiving oral triamterene daily. Which sign/symptom would indicate to the nurse that the client is experiencing an adverse effect of the medication?

1 Dry skin
2 Excitability
3 Constipation
4 Hyperkalemia

Level of Cognitive Ability: Analyzing
Client Needs: Physiological Integrity
Clinical Judgment/Cognitive Skills: Recognize Cues
Integrated Process: Nursing Process/Data Collection
Content Area: Pharmacology: Cardiovascular: Diuretics
Health Problem: Adult Health: Gastrointestinal: Cirrhosis

Answer: 4
Rationale: Triamterene is a potassium-sparing diuretic. Adverse effects include hyperkalemia, dehydration, hyponatremia, and lethargy. Although the concern with most diuretics is hypokalemia, this is a potassium-sparing medication, which means that the concern with the administration of this medication is hyperkalemia. Other effects include nausea, vomiting, cramping, diarrhea, headache, ataxia, drowsiness, confusion, and fever.
Priority Nursing Tip: The client with cirrhosis needs to consume foods high in thiamine. Thiamine is present in a variety of foods of plant and animal origin. Pork products are especially rich in this vitamin.

Test-Taking Strategy: Focus on the **subject,** oral triamterene, and think about the classification of the medication. Recalling that this is a potassium-sparing medication will direct you to the correct option.

---

90. The nurse is preparing a woman in early labor who is experiencing a significant increase in blood pressure for an amniotomy. Which **priority** data would the nurse check before the procedure?

1 Fetal heart rate
2 Maternal heart rate
3 Fetal scalp sampling
4 Maternal blood pressure

Answer: 1
Rationale: Fetal well-being must be confirmed before and after amniotomy. Fetal heart rate needs to be checked by Doppler or with the application of the external fetal monitor. Although maternal vital signs may be checked, fetal heart rate is the priority. A fetal scalp sampling cannot be done when the membranes are intact.
Priority Nursing Tip: Amniotomy (artificial rupture of the membranes) can be used to induce labor when the condition of the

Level of Cognitive Ability: Analyzing
Client Needs: Physiological Integrity
Clinical Judgment/Cognitive Skills: Prioritize Hypotheses
Integrated Process: Nursing Process/Data Collection
Content Area: Maternity: Antepartum
Health Problem: Maternity: Gestational Hypertension/Preeclampsia and Eclampsia

cervix is favorable (ripe) or to augment labor if the progress begins to slow.

Test-Taking Strategy: Note the **strategic word,** *priority.* Eliminate option 3 first, knowing that a fetal scalp sampling cannot be done before an amniotomy. Then eliminate options 2 and 4, which are **comparable or alike** and address maternal vital signs. The correct option addresses fetal well-being.

---

91. The nurse is monitoring a client whose membranes ruptured and who is now receiving an oxytocin infusion for the induction of labor. The nurse would suspect water intoxication if which sign or symptom is noted?

1 Fatigue
2 Lethargy
3 Sleepiness
4 Tachycardia

Level of Cognitive Ability: Analyzing
Client Needs: Physiological Integrity
Clinical Judgment/Cognitive Skills: Recognize Cues
Integrated Process: Nursing Process/Data Collection
Content Area: Pharmacology: Maternity/Newborn: Uterine Stimulants
Health Problem: N/A

Answer: 4
Rationale: Oxytocin is a uterine stimulant. During an oxytocin infusion, the woman is monitored closely for signs of water intoxication, including tachycardia, cardiac dysrhythmias, shortness of breath, nausea, and vomiting. The remaining options are not associated with water intoxication.
Priority Nursing Tip: An oxytocin infusion is discontinued if uterine contraction frequency is less than 2 minutes, the duration is longer than 90 seconds, or fetal distress is noted.

Test-Taking Strategy: Focus on the **subject,** water intoxication. Think about the physiological response that occurs when fluid overload exists to direct you to the correct option. In addition, eliminate options 1, 2, and 3 because they are **comparable or alike** and are related to energy levels.

---

92. The nurse reviews the record of a client who is receiving external radiation therapy and notes documentation of a skin finding as moist desquamation. Which finding on data collection of the client would the nurse expect to observe?

1 A rash
2 Dermatitis
3 Reddened skin
4 Weeping of the skin

Level of Cognitive Ability: Analyzing
Client Needs: Physiological Integrity
Clinical Judgment/Cognitive Skills: Recognize Cues

Answer: 4
Rationale: Moist desquamation occurs when the basal cells of the skin are destroyed. The dermal level is exposed, which results in the leakage of serum. A rash, dermatitis, and reddened skin may occur with external radiation, but these conditions are not described as moist desquamation.
Priority Nursing Tip: The nurse would teach the client receiving radiation therapy to wash the irradiated area gently each day with warm water alone or mild soap and water. The client needs to use the hand rather than a washcloth to wash the area.

Integrated Process: Nursing Process/Data Collection
Content Area: Adult Health: Integumentary
Health Problem: Adult Health: Integumentary: Inflammations/Infections

Test-Taking Strategy: Options 1, 2, and 3 are eliminated because they are **comparable or alike,** and they describe a dry rather than a moist skin alteration. In addition, note the relationship between the word *moist* in the question and *weeping* in the correct option.

---

93. The nurse is collecting data on a pregnant client with a history of cardiac disease. Which body area will venous congestion **most** commonly be noted in?
1 Vulva
2 Around the eyes
3 Fingers of the hands
4 Around the abdomen

Level of Cognitive Ability: Analyzing
Client Needs: Physiological Integrity
Clinical Judgment/Cognitive Skills: Recognize Cues
Integrated Process: Nursing Process/Data Collection
Content Area: Health Assessment/Physical Exam: Heart and Peripheral Vascular
Health Problem: Maternity: Cardiac Disease

Answer: 1
Rationale: Collecting data about the cardiovascular system includes observation for venous congestion that can develop into varicosities. Venous congestion is most commonly noted in the legs, the vulva, or the rectum. Although edema may be noted in the fingers and around the eyes, edema in these areas would not be directly associated with venous congestion. It would be difficult to check for edema in the abdominal area of a client who is pregnant.
Priority Nursing Tip: Varicose veins can occur in the second and the third trimesters of pregnancy. They result from weakening walls of the veins or valves and venous congestion.

Test-Taking Strategy: Focus on the **strategic word,** *most,* and note the **subject,** venous congestion. From the options provided, the only body area in which venous congestion would be noted is the vulva.

---

94. A client who has been receiving long-term diuretic therapy is admitted to the hospital with a diagnosis of dehydration. The nurse would check for which sign that correlates with this fluid imbalance?
1 Decreased pulse
2 Bibasilar crackles
3 Increased blood pressure
4 Increased urinary specific gravity

Level of Cognitive Ability: Applying
Client Needs: Physiological Integrity
Clinical Judgment/Cognitive Skills: Recognize Cues
Integrated Process: Nursing Process/Data Collection
Content Area: Foundations of Care: Fluids & Electrolytes
Health Problem: Adult Health: Gastrointestinal: Dehydration

Answer: 4
Rationale: Findings with fluid volume deficit are increased pulse and respirations, weight loss, poor skin turgor, dry mucous membranes, decreased urine output, concentrated urine with increased specific gravity, increased hematocrit, and altered level of consciousness. The findings in the remaining options are not associated with dehydration.
Priority Nursing Tip: The nurse needs to monitor for signs of dehydration and electrolyte imbalances in a client receiving diuretic therapy.

Test-Taking Strategy: Focus on the **subject,** a client with dehydration. Think about the pathophysiology associated with dehydration to direct you to the correct option.

---

95. A client at 35 weeks of gestation reports a sudden discharge of fluid from the vagina. Based on the data provided, which condition would the nurse suspect?

1 Miscarriage
2 Preterm labor
3 Intrauterine fetal demise
4 Premature rupture of the membranes

Level of Cognitive Ability: Analyzing
Client Needs: Physiological Integrity
Clinical Judgment/Cognitive Skills: Recognize Cues
Integrated Process: Nursing Process/Data Collection
Content Area: Maternity: Intrapartum
Health Problem: Maternity: Premature Rupture of the Membranes

Answer: 4
Rationale: Premature rupture of the membranes is usually manifested by a sudden discharge of fluid from the vagina before 37 weeks of gestation. Miscarriage is typically manifested by vaginal bleeding and abdominal pain. Preterm labor is typically manifested by uterine contractions, cramping, and pressure before 37 weeks of gestation. Intrauterine fetal demise is usually manifested by an absence of fetal movements and heartbeat.
Priority Nursing Tip: Infection can cause premature rupture of the membranes, premature labor, and postpartum endometritis.

Test-Taking Strategy: Focus on the **data in the question**, a client who is at 35 weeks of gestation and reports a sudden discharge of fluid from the vagina. Note that all of the conditions noted in the options may occur during this time; therefore, the answer needs to be determined by looking at the clinical manifestations. Recall that amniotic fluid, rather than blood, would be expelled in premature rupture of the membranes; this will assist in eliminating option 1. From the remaining options, it is necessary to know which signs and symptoms are associated with each disorder to answer correctly.

---

96. On data collection of the client diagnosed with stage III Lyme disease, which clinical manifestation would the nurse expect to note?

1 Palpitations
2 A cardiac dysrhythmia
3 A generalized skin rash
4 Enlarged and inflamed joints

Level of Cognitive Ability: Analyzing
Client Needs: Physiological Integrity
Clinical Judgment/Cognitive Skills: Recognize Cues
Integrated Process: Nursing Process/Data Collection
Content Area: Adult Health: Immune
Health Problem: Adult Health: Immune: Lyme Disease

Answer: 4
Rationale: Stage III Lyme disease develops within a month to several months after initial infection. It is characterized by arthritic symptoms such as arthralgia and enlarged or inflamed joints, which can persist for several years after the initial infection. A rash occurs during stage I, and cardiac and neurological dysfunction occur during stage II.
Priority Nursing Tip: The typical ring-shaped rash of Lyme disease does not occur in all clients. Many clients never develop a rash. Additionally, if a rash does occur, it can arise anywhere on the body, not only at the site of the bite.

Test-Taking Strategy: Eliminate options that are **comparable or alike** and are cardiac symptoms. Focusing on the **subject,** signs and symptoms of stage III Lyme disease, will direct you to the correct option.

---

97. A child experienced a basilar skull fracture that resulted in the presence of Battle's sign. Which would the nurse expect to observe in the child?

1 Bruising behind the ear
2 The presence of epistaxis
3 A bruised periorbital area
4 An edematous periorbital area

Answer: 1
Rationale: The most serious type of skull fracture is a basilar skull fracture. Two classic findings associated with this type of skull fracture are Battle's sign and raccoon eyes. Battle's sign is the presence of bruising or ecchymosis behind the ear caused by a leaking of blood into the mastoid sinuses. Raccoon eyes occur as a result of blood leaking into the frontal sinus and causing an edematous and bruised periorbital area.

Level of Cognitive Ability: Analyzing
Client Needs: Physiological Integrity
Clinical Judgment/Cognitive Skills: Recognize Cues
Integrated Process: Nursing Process/Data Collection
Content Area: Pediatrics: Neurological
Health Problem: Pediatric-Specific: Head Injury

Priority Nursing Tip: Leakage of cerebrospinal fluid (CSF) from the ears or nose may accompany basilar skull fracture. CSF can be distinguished from other body fluids because the drainage will separate into bloody and yellow concentric rings on dressing material, called a halo sign. The CSF fluid also tests positive for glucose.

Test-Taking Strategy: Eliminate options 3 and 4, which are **comparable or alike** and relate to the periorbital area. Focusing on the **subject,** the description of Battle's sign, will direct you to option 1.

---

98. When collecting data on a child with meningitis, which finding would indicate the presence of Kernig's sign?
1 Calf pain when the foot is dorsiflexed
2 Pain when the chin is pulled down to the chest
3 The inability of the child to extend the legs fully when lying supine
4 The flexion of the hips when the neck is flexed from a lying position

Level of Cognitive Ability: Analyzing
Client Needs: Physiological Integrity
Clinical Judgment/Cognitive Skills: Recognize Cues
Integrated Process: Nursing Process/Data Collection
Content Area: Health Assessment/Physical Exam: Neurological
Health Problem: Pediatric-Specific: Meningitis

Answer: 3
Rationale: Kernig's sign is the inability of the child to extend the legs fully when lying supine. Brudzinski's sign is flexion of the hips when the neck is flexed from a supine position. Both of these signs are frequently present in clients with bacterial meningitis. Nuchal rigidity is also present with bacterial meningitis, and it occurs when pain prevents the child from touching the chin to the chest. Homans' sign is elicited when pain occurs in the calf region when the foot is dorsiflexed.
Priority Nursing Tip: Meningitis is transmitted by droplet infection. Precautions for this disease include placing the client in a private room or with a cohort client and use of a standard precaution mask.

Test-Taking Strategy: Focus on the **subject,** characteristics of Kernig's sign. It is necessary to know that Kernig's sign is the inability of the child to extend the legs fully when lying supine.

---

99. The nurse collects data on an older client's functional status and ability to perform activities of daily living (ADLs). What is the focus area of the nurse during data collection?
1 Everyday routines
2 Self-care activities
3 Household management
4 Endurance and flexibility

Level of Cognitive Ability: Applying
Client Needs: Health Promotion and Maintenance
Clinical Judgment/Cognitive Skills: Prioritize Hypotheses
Integrated Process: Nursing Process/Data Collection
Content Area: Skills: Activity/Mobility
Health Problem: N/A

Answer: 2
Rationale: To evaluate the client's functional status, the nurse checks the client's ability to perform self-care or ADLs, including bathing, toileting, ambulating, dressing, and feeding. Everyday routines, household management, and physical condition are not components of functional status.
Priority Nursing Tip: For the client having a problem with performing ADLs, an occupational therapist would be consulted. An occupational therapist develops adaptive devices that can help the client perform ADLs.

Test-Taking Strategy: Focus on the **subject,** the ability to perform ADLs. Recalling that ADLs refer to self-care needs will direct you to the correct option.

---

100. The nurse is checking a client diagnosed with Addison's disease for signs of hyperkalemia. Which sign/symptom would the nurse observe with this electrolyte imbalance?

1 Polyuria
2 Cardiac dysrhythmias
3 Dry mucous membranes
4 Prolonged bleeding time

Level of Cognitive Ability: Analyzing
Client Needs: Physiological Integrity
Clinical Judgment/Cognitive Skills: Recognize Cues
Integrated Process: Nursing Process/Data Collection
Content Area: Adult Health: Endocrine
Health Problem: Adult Health: Endocrine: Adrenal Disorders

Answer: 2

Rationale: The inadequate production of aldosterone in clients with Addison's disease causes the inadequate excretion of potassium and results in hyperkalemia. The clinical manifestations of hyperkalemia are the result of altered nerve transmission. The most harmful consequence of hyperkalemia is its effect on cardiac function. Based on this information, none of the remaining options are manifestations that are associated with Addison's disease or hyperkalemia.

Priority Nursing Tip: A low-potassium diet is usually indicated for hyperkalemia, which may be caused by disorders such as impaired renal function, Addison's disease, and potassium-retaining diuretics.

Test-Taking Strategy: Focus on the **subject,** Addison's disease and hyperkalemia. Think about the effects of potassium on the body, and remember that hyperkalemia has a direct effect on cardiac function. This will direct you to the correct option.

---

101. The nurse assists in performing an Allen's test before blood is drawn from the radial artery for an arterial blood gas (ABG) test. This intervention is done to determine the collateral circulatory adequacy of which arterial vessel?

1 Ulnar
2 Carotid
3 Brachial
4 Femoral

Level of Cognitive Ability: Analyzing
Client Needs: Physiological Integrity
Clinical Judgment/Cognitive Skills: Recognize Cues
Integrated Process: Nursing Process/Data Collection
Content Area: Foundations of Care: Acid-Base
Health Problem: N/A

Answer: 1

Rationale: Before radial puncture for obtaining an arterial specimen for ABGs, Allen's test is performed to determine adequate ulnar circulation. Failure to check collateral circulation could result in severe ischemic injury to the hand if damage to the radial artery occurs with arterial puncture. Allen's test does not determine the adequacy of carotid, brachial, or femoral circulation.

Priority Nursing Tip: After obtaining an arterial blood gas specimen, the nurse would ensure that pressure is placed over the area of the puncture for at least 5 or 10 minutes and longer if the client is taking an anticoagulant.

Test-Taking Strategy: Note the words *radial artery* in the question. Focus on the **subject,** arterial blood gas (ABG) specimen drawn from the radial artery, and think about the anatomy of the blood vessels. This will eliminate the incorrect options.

---

102. A pregnant client diagnosed with diabetes mellitus arrives at the primary health care clinic for a follow-up visit. What test would the nurse perform to **best** check insulin function?

1 Urine for specific gravity
2 For the presence of edema
3 Urine for glucose and ketones
4 Blood pressure, pulse, and respirations

Answer: 3

Rationale: In addition to blood glucose testing, the nurse checks the pregnant client with diabetes mellitus for glucose and ketones in the urine at each prenatal visit because the physiological changes of pregnancy can drastically alter insulin requirements. It is important to remember, though, that urine testing for glucose may not be beneficial during pregnancy, because of the lowered renal threshold for glucose; therefore, the degree of glycosuria does not accurately reflect the blood glucose level. Checking the urine for specific gravity, checking for the presence of edema,

Level of Cognitive Ability: Analyzing
Client Needs: Physiological Integrity
Clinical Judgment/Cognitive Skills: Recognize Cues
Integrated Process: Nursing Process/Data Collection
Content Area: Maternity: Antepartum
Health Problem: Maternity: Diabetes

and measuring blood pressure, pulse, and respirations are more related to the client with gestational hypertension.
Priority Nursing Tip: Most oral hypoglycemic agents are not prescribed for use during pregnancy because of their teratogenic effects.

Test-Taking Strategy: Focus on the **subject,** a pregnant client with diabetes mellitus, and on the **strategic word,** *best.* The only option that specifically addresses diabetes mellitus is the correct one.

NURSING PROCESS: PLANNING

103. The nurse is assisting in caring for a client who is receiving total parenteral nutrition through a central venous catheter. Which action would the nurse plan to implement to decrease the risk of infection in this client?

1 Track the client's oral temperature.
2 Administer antibiotics intravenously.
3 Check the differential of the leukocytes.
4 Use of sterile technique for dressing changes.

Level of Cognitive Ability: Applying
Client Needs: Safe and Effective Care Environment
Clinical Judgment/Cognitive Skills: Generate Solutions
Integrated Process: Nursing Process/Planning
Content Area: Skills: Infection Control
Health Problem: N/A

Answer: 4
Rationale: Sterile technique is vital during dressing changes of a central venous catheter (CVC). CVCs are large-bore catheters that can serve as a direct-entry point for microorganisms into the heart and circulatory system. Using aseptic technique helps avoid catheter-related infections by preventing the introduction of potential pathogens to the site. Although the remaining options are reasonable nursing interventions for a client with a CVC, none of them prevents infection. Options 1 and 3 are data collection methods, and option 2 is implemented after the confirmation of an existing infection.
Priority Nursing Tip: Use sterile technique when caring for a client receiving total parenteral nutrition (TPN). Because the TPN solution has a high concentration of glucose, it is a medium for bacterial growth.

Test-Taking Strategy: Focus on the **subject,** preventing infection. Note the relationship between "infection" in the question and "sterile" in the correct option. In addition, the only option that will prevent infection is the correct option.

---

104. The nurse assists with the creation of a plan of care for a client with a spica cast that covers a lower extremity. Which action would the nurse suggest to include in the plan of care to promote bowel elimination?

1 Use a bedside commode.
2 Ambulate to the bathroom.
3 Administer an enema daily.
4 Use a low-profile (fracture) bedpan.

Level of Cognitive Ability: Applying
Client Needs: Physiological Integrity
Clinical Judgment/Cognitive Skills: Generate Solutions
Integrated Process: Nursing Process/Planning
Content Area: Skills: Elimination
Health Problem: Adult Health: Musculoskeletal: Skeletal Injury

Answer: 4
Rationale: A client with a spica cast (body cast) that covers a lower extremity cannot bend at the hips to sit up. A low-profile bedpan or fracture pan is designed for use by clients with body or leg casts and for clients who have difficulty raising the hips to use a standard bedpan; therefore, using a commode or the bathroom is contraindicated. Daily enemas are not a part of routine care.
Priority Nursing Tip: Inform the client and family about keeping the cast clean and dry. The material of a cast can crumble if it becomes wet. This presents a risk of altered skin integrity and subsequent infection.

Test-Taking Strategy: Focus on the **subject,** spica cast care, and the words *covers a lower extremity.* Therefore, choose the measure that promotes elimination for a client who cannot flex the hip.

---

105. The nurse is caring for a postpartum client with thromboembolic disease. Which intervention is **most important** to include when planning care to prevent the complication of pulmonary embolism?

1 Enforce bed rest.
2 Monitor the vital signs frequently.
3 Check the breath sounds frequently.
4 Administer prescribed anticoagulant therapy.

Level of Cognitive Ability: Analyzing
Client Needs: Physiological Integrity
Clinical Judgment/Cognitive Skills: Generate Solutions
Integrated Process: Nursing Process/Planning
Content Area: Maternity: Postpartum
Health Problem: N/A

Answer: 4
Rationale: The purposes of anticoagulant therapy for the treatment of thromboembolic disease are to prevent the formation of a clot and to prevent a clot from moving to another area, thus preventing pulmonary embolism. Although the remaining options may be implemented for a client with thromboembolic disease, the correct option will specifically assist in the prevention of pulmonary embolism.
Priority Nursing Tip: Medications containing aspirin would not be given to clients receiving anticoagulant therapy, because aspirin prolongs the clotting time and increases the risk of bleeding.

Test-Taking Strategy: Note the **strategic words,** *most important.* Focus on the **subject,** preventing the complication of pulmonary embolism. Recall that anticoagulant therapy is prescribed to treat thromboembolic disease.

---

106. The primary health care provider prescribes an isotonic intravenous solution for a client. The nurse plans for the administration of which solution?

1 10% dextrose in water
2 3% sodium chloride
3 5% dextrose in water
4 0.45% sodium chloride

Level of Cognitive Ability: Applying
Client Needs: Physiological Integrity
Clinical Judgment/Cognitive Skills: Generate Solutions
Integrated Process: Nursing Process/Planning
Content Area: Foundations of Care: Fluids & Electrolytes
Health Problem: N/A

Answer: 3
Rationale: Five percent dextrose in water is an isotonic solution, which means that the osmolality of this solution matches normal body fluids. Other examples of isotonic fluids include 0.9% sodium chloride solution (normal saline) and lactated Ringer's solution. Ten percent dextrose in water and 3% sodium chloride solution are hypertonic solutions, and 0.45% sodium chloride solution is hypotonic.
Priority Nursing Tip: Isotonic solutions are isotonic to human cells, and thus very little osmosis occurs.

Test-Taking Strategy: To answer this question accurately, focus on the **subject,** the tonicity of various IV solutions, and note the word "isotonic." It is necessary to recall that 5% dextrose in water is an isotonic solution.

---

107. The nurse is assisting to admit a client who recently underwent a bilateral adrenalectomy. Which intervention is **essential** for the nurse to include in the client's plan of care?

1 Prevent social isolation.
2 Consider occupational therapy.
3 Discuss changes in body image.
4 Avoid stress-producing situations.

Level of Cognitive Ability: Applying
Client Needs: Physiological Integrity

Answer: 4
Rationale: Adrenalectomy can lead to adrenal insufficiency. Adrenal hormones are essential to maintaining homeostasis in response to stressors. None of the remaining options are essential interventions specific to this client's problem.
Priority Nursing Tip: Assist a client to identify the source of stress, and explore methods to reduce stress.

Clinical Judgment/Cognitive Skills: Generate Solutions
Integrated Process: Nursing Process/Planning
Content Area: Adult Health: Endocrine
Health Problem: Adult Health: Endocrine: Adrenal Disorders

Test-Taking Strategy: Note the **strategic word,** *essential.* This indicates the need to prioritize. Remember that, according to **Maslow's Hierarchy of Needs theory,** physiological needs come first. The stress reaction involves physiological processes.

---

108. A perinatal client is admitted to the obstetric unit during an exacerbation of a heart condition. When planning for the client's nutritional requirements, which dietary intervention would the nurse consult the dietitian about?

1 A low-calorie diet to prevent weight gain.
2 A diet low in fluids and fiber to decrease blood volume.
3 A diet adequate in fluids and fiber to prevent constipation.
4 Unlimited sodium intake to increase circulating blood volume.

Level of Cognitive Ability: Applying
Client Needs: Physiological Integrity
Clinical Judgment/Cognitive Skills: Generate Solutions
Integrated Process: Nursing Process/Planning
Content Area: Maternity: Antepartum
Health Problem: Maternity: Cardiac Disease

Answer: 3
Rationale: Constipation can cause the client to use Valsalva's maneuver. This maneuver can cause blood to rush to the heart and overload the cardiac system. A low-calorie diet is not recommended during pregnancy. Diets low in fluid and fiber can cause a decrease in blood volume that can deprive the fetus of nutrients; it can also lead to constipation. Therefore, adequate fluid intake and high-fiber foods are important. Sodium would be restricted to some degree as prescribed by the primary health care provider, because high sodium will cause an overload to the circulating blood volume and contribute to cardiac complications.
Priority Nursing Tip: Encourage adequate nutrition for the pregnant client with a cardiac condition to prevent anemia. Anemia could worsen the cardiac status.

Test-Taking Strategy: Focus on the **subject,** the physiology of the cardiac system, the maternal and fetal needs, and the factors that increase the workload on the heart, to answer the question. Think about what would increase the workload of the heart to direct you to the correct option.

---

109. The nurse is assisting in creating a plan of care for a client prescribed bed rest. Which intervention would the nurse include in the plan to limit renal complications of prolonged immobility?

1 Maintain the client in a supine position.
2 Provide a daily fluid intake of 1000 mL.
3 Limit the intake of milk and milk products.
4 Monitor for signs of a low serum calcium level.

Level of Cognitive Ability: Creating
Client Needs: Physiological Integrity
Clinical Judgment/Cognitive Skills: Generate Solutions
Integrated Process: Nursing Process/Planning
Content Area: Skills: Activity/Mobility
Health Problem: Adult Health: Renal and Urinary: Calculi

Answer: 3
Rationale: The formation of renal and urinary calculi is a complication of immobility. Limiting milk and milk products is the best measure to prevent the formation of calcium stones. A supine position increases urinary stasis; therefore, this position would be limited or avoided. Daily fluid intake would be 2000 mL or more per day. The nurse would monitor for signs and symptoms of hypercalcemia, such as nausea, vomiting, polydipsia, polyuria, and lethargy.
Priority Nursing Tip: The client with calcium oxalate stones may be prescribed to follow a diet decreasing the intake of foods high in calcium and avoiding oxalate food sources. This type of diet will help reduce the urinary oxalate content of urine and stone formation. Oxalate food sources include items such as tea, almonds, cashews, chocolate, cocoa, beans, spinach, and rhubarb.

Test-Taking Strategy: Focus on the **subject,** the complications of prolonged immobility. Eliminate option 1, which refers to maintaining an immobile client in one position. Eliminate option 2 by noting the amount of fluid suggested. From the remaining choices, recalling the effect of the movement of calcium into the blood from the bones will direct you to the correct option.

110. The nurse determines that a tuberculin skin test is positive. Which diagnostic test would the nurse anticipate will be prescribed to confirm a diagnosis of tuberculosis (TB)?

1 Chest x-ray
2 Sputum culture
3 Complete blood cell count
4 Computed tomography scan of the chest

Level of Cognitive Ability: Applying
Client Needs: Physiological Integrity
Clinical Judgment/Cognitive Skills: Generate Solutions
Integrated Process: Nursing Process/Planning
Content Area: Adult Health: Respiratory
Health Problem: Adult Health: Respiratory: Tuberculosis

Answer: 2

Rationale: Although the findings of the chest x-ray examination are important, it is not possible to make a diagnosis of TB solely on the basis of this examination because other diseases can mimic the appearance of TB. The demonstration of tubercle bacilli bacteriologically is essential for establishing a diagnosis. The microscopic examination of sputum for acid-fast bacilli is usually the first bacteriological evidence of the presence of tubercle bacilli. Options 3 and 4 will not diagnose TB.

Priority Nursing Tip: Tuberculosis has an insidious onset, and many clients are unaware that the symptoms are associated with TB until the disease is well advanced.

Test-Taking Strategy: Focus on the **subject**, diagnosing TB. Recalling that the presence of tubercle bacilli indicates TB will direct you to the correct option.

---

111. The nurse is assisting in creating a plan of care for a client diagnosed with Ménière's syndrome. Which nursing intervention would the nurse include to assist the client with controlling vertigo?

1 Instruct the client to cut down on cigarette smoking.
2 Encourage the client to increase the daily fluid intake.
3 Encourage the client to avoid sudden head movements.
4 Instruct the client to increase the amount of sodium in the diet.

Level of Cognitive Ability: Applying
Client Needs: Physiological Integrity
Clinical Judgment/Cognitive Skills: Generate Solutions
Integrated Process: Nursing Process/Planning
Content Area: Adult Health: Ear
Health Problem: Adult Health: Ear: Ménière's Disease

Answer: 3

Rationale: Ménière's syndrome refers to dilation of the endolymphatic system by overproduction or decreased resorption of endolymphatic fluid. The nurse instructs the client to make slow head movements to prevent worsening of the vertigo. Clients are advised to stop smoking because of its vasoconstrictive effects. Dietary changes such as salt and fluid restrictions that reduce the amount of endolymphatic fluid are sometimes prescribed.

Priority Nursing Tip: Instruct the client experiencing an episode of vertigo to avoid watching television because the flickering of lights may exacerbate symptoms.

Test-Taking Strategy: Identify the **subject**, controlling vertigo. Note the relationship between the word *vertigo* and the correct option, which recommends the avoidance of sudden head movements. Noting the words *cut down* in option 1 will assist you with eliminating this option. Recalling that salt and fluid restrictions are sometimes prescribed will also assist you with eliminating options.

---

112. A client is admitted to a mental health unit with a diagnosis of anorexia nervosa. When planning care for this client, which **primary** intervention would health promotion focus on?

1 Providing a supportive environment
2 Examining intrapsychic conflicts and past issues
3 Emphasizing social interaction with clients who are withdrawn
4 Helping the client identify and examine dysfunctional thoughts and beliefs

Level of Cognitive Ability: Applying
Client Needs: Psychosocial Integrity
Clinical Judgment/Cognitive Skills: Prioritize Hypotheses
Integrated Process: Nursing Process/Planning
Content Area: Mental Health
Health Problem: Mental Health: Eating Disorders

Answer: 4

Rationale: Health promotion focuses on helping clients identify and examine dysfunctional thoughts, as well as on identifying and examining the values and beliefs that maintain these thoughts. Providing a supportive environment is important, but it is not as primary as option 4 for this client. Examining intrapsychic conflicts and past issues is not directly related to the client's problem. Emphasizing social interaction is inappropriate at this time.

Priority Nursing Tip: Explain treatments and procedures to a client in a quiet and simple manner. Always allow the client the opportunity to express fears.

Test-Taking Strategy: Note the **strategic word,** *primary.* Focus on the **subject,** health promotion in a client diagnosed with anorexia nervosa. The correct option is the only choice that is specifically client centered.

---

113. The nurse is assisting in preparing discharge plans for a hospitalized client who attempted suicide. Which intervention would the nurse include in the plan as an **immediate** resource?

1 Scheduling weekly follow-up appointments
2 Establishing a contact with a specific crisis resource person
3 Encouraging family and friends to be with the client at all times
4 Providing phone numbers for the primary health care provider and psychiatrist

Level of Cognitive Ability: Applying
Client Needs: Psychosocial Integrity
Clinical Judgment/Cognitive Skills: Generate Solutions
Integrated Process: Nursing Process/Planning
Content Area: Mental Health
Health Problem: Mental Health: Suicide

Answer: 2

Rationale: Crisis times may occur between appointments. Establishing a specific contact with a crisis resource person provides the client with a direct connection for communication and immediate crisis intervention. Providing phone numbers will not ensure available and immediate crisis intervention. Family and friends cannot always be present.

Priority Nursing Tip: Discharge planning and follow-up care are important for the continued well-being of the client with a mental health disorder. Aftercare case managers are used to facilitate the client's adaptation back into the community and to provide early referral if the treatment plan is unsuccessful.

Test-Taking Strategy: Focus on the **subject,** the availability of immediate resources for the client who attempted suicide, and the **strategic word,** *immediate.* Eliminate option 3 first because this is unrealistic. Next, eliminate options 1 and 4 because these will not necessarily provide immediate resources.

114. The nurse is assisting in creating a plan of care for a newborn diagnosed with bilateral club feet. Which information would the nurse plan to include in the parents' education?

1. The regimen of manipulation and casting is effective in all cases of bilateral club feet.
2. Genetic testing is wise for future pregnancies because other children born to this couple may also be affected.
3. If casting is needed, it will begin at birth and continue for 12 weeks, at which time the condition will be reevaluated.
4. Surgery performed immediately after birth has been found to be the most effective for achieving a complete recovery.

Level of Cognitive Ability: Creating
Client Needs: Physiological Integrity
Clinical Judgment/Cognitive Skills: Generate Solutions
Integrated Process: Nursing Process/Planning
Content Area: Pediatrics: Musculoskeletal
Health Problem: Pediatric-Specific: Clubfoot

Answer: 3

Rationale: For the infant with clubfoot, casting would begin at birth and continue for at least 12 weeks or until maximum correction is achieved. At this time, corrective shoes may provide support to maintain alignment, or surgery can be performed. Surgery is usually delayed until the child is 4 to 12 months old. Options 1 and 4 are inaccurate. Option 2 does not specifically address the subject of the question.

Priority Nursing Tip: The nurse needs to monitor the child with a cast or brace for signs of neurovascular impairment. If signs occur, the primary health care provider is notified immediately.

Test-Taking Strategy: Focus on the **subject**, parent instructions for the child with bilateral club feet. Eliminate option 1 because of the **closed-ended word** *all*. Eliminate option 2 because it does not specifically address the subject of the question and relates to the future. Eliminate option 4 because of the word *immediately*.

---

115. Which items would the nurse plan to provide to optimally maintain the integrity of a set of arterial blood gas measurements?

1. A syringe that contains a preservative
2. A heparinized syringe and a bag of ice
3. A heparinized syringe and a preservative
4. A syringe that contains a preservative and a bag of ice

Level of Cognitive Ability: Applying
Client Needs: Physiological Integrity
Clinical Judgment/Cognitive Skills: Generate Solutions
Integrated Process: Nursing Process/Planning
Content Area: Foundations of Care: Acid-Base
Health Problem: N/A

Answer: 2

Rationale: The arterial blood gas sample is obtained using a heparinized syringe. The sample of blood is placed on ice and sent to the laboratory immediately. A preservative is not used.

Priority Nursing Tip: Assist with the specimen draw for an arterial blood gas by preparing a heparinized syringe (if one is not already prepackaged); otherwise, the blood may clot.

Test-Taking Strategy: Focus on the **subject**, arterial blood gas measurements; specific knowledge regarding this procedure is needed to answer this question. Remember that an arterial blood gas sample is obtained using a heparinized syringe, is placed on ice, and is sent to the laboratory immediately.

---

116. A client is experiencing diabetes insipidus as a result of cranial surgery. Which anticipated therapy would the nurse plan to implement?
1 Fluid restriction
2 Administering diuretics
3 Increased sodium intake
4 Intravenous (IV) replacement of fluid losses

Level of Cognitive Ability: Analyzing
Client Needs: Physiological Integrity
Clinical Judgment/Cognitive Skills: Generate Solutions
Integrated Process: Nursing Process/Planning
Content Area: Adult Health: Neurological
Health Problem: N/A

Answer: 4
Rationale: The client with diabetes insipidus excretes large amounts of extremely dilute urine. This usually occurs as a result of decreased synthesis or the release of antidiuretic hormone in clients with conditions such as head injury, surgery near the hypothalamus, or increased intracranial pressure. Corrective measures include allowing ample oral fluid intake, administering IV fluid as needed to replace sensible and insensible losses, and administering vasopressin. Diuretics are not administered. Sodium is not administered because the serum sodium level is usually high, as is the serum osmolality.
Priority Nursing Tip: For the client with diabetes insipidus, monitor electrolyte values, monitor for signs of dehydration, and maintain an adequate intake of fluids.

Test-Taking Strategy: Focus on the **subject,** diabetes insipidus as a result of cranial surgery, and recall that a large fluid loss is the problem in this client. This will assist you with eliminating options 1 and 2. From the remaining choices, recalling that the serum sodium level is already elevated in clients with this disorder or knowing that fluid replacement is the most direct form of therapy for fluid loss will direct you to the correct option.

---

117. The nurse is caring for a client diagnosed with dementia. Which nutritional goal would the nurse plan for with this client?
1 Client will be free of hallucinations.
2 Client will feed self with cueing within 24 hours.
3 Client will be able to prepare simple foods by discharge.
4 Client will identify favorite foods by the time of discharge.

Level of Cognitive Ability: Applying
Client Needs: Physiological Integrity
Clinical Judgment/Cognitive Skills: Generate Solutions
Integrated Process: Nursing Process/Planning
Content Area: Mental Health
Health Problem: Mental Health: Neurocognitive Impairment

Answer: 2
Rationale: The correct option identifies a goal that is directly related to the client's ability to care for self. None of the remaining options are related to the client's self-care needs.
Priority Nursing Tip: In dementia, long-term and short-term memory loss occurs, with impairment in judgment, abstract thinking, problem-solving, and behavior.

Test-Taking Strategy: Focus on the **subject,** needs of a client with dementia. The correct option is the only option that addresses a physiological need. In addition, on the basis of **Maslow's Hierarchy of Needs theory,** physiological needs take precedence. This will direct you to the correct option.

---

118. The nurse is preparing to care for an infant diagnosed with pertussis. Which **priority** problem would the nurse address when planning care?
1 Infection
2 Fluid overload
3 Impaired sleep patterns
4 Inability to expectorate secretions

Level of Cognitive Ability: Analyzing
Client Needs: Physiological Integrity
Clinical Judgment/Cognitive Skills: Prioritize Hypotheses
Integrated Process: Nursing Process/Planning
Content Area: Pediatrics: Throat/Respiratory
Health Problem: Pediatric-Specific: Communicable Diseases

Answer: 4
Rationale: The priority problem for the child with pertussis relates to adequate air exchange. Because of the copious, thick secretions that occur with pertussis and the small airways of an infant, air exchange is critical. Infection is an important consideration, but airway is the priority. A deficient fluid volume is more likely to occur in this infant because of the thick secretions and vomiting. Sleep patterns may be disturbed because of the coughing, but this is not the critical issue.
Priority Nursing Tip: For the client with a respiratory problem, reduce environmental factors that cause coughing spasms, such as dust, smoke, and sudden changes in temperature.

Test-Taking Strategy: Use the **ABCs—airway, breathing, and circulation**—and note the **strategic word,** *priority.* Airway is always the priority. This would direct you to the correct option.

---

119. The nurse is assisting in planning care for an infant who has a diagnosis of hypertrophic pyloric stenosis and is scheduled for surgery. Which intervention would the nurse include to meet the infant's preoperative needs?
1 Administer enemas until returns are clear.
2 Provide the mother privacy to breastfeed every 2 hours.
3 Monitor the intravenous (IV) infusion, intake, output, and weight.
4 Provide small, frequent feedings of glucose, water, and electrolytes.

Level of Cognitive Ability: Analyzing
Client Needs: Physiological Integrity
Clinical Judgment/Cognitive Skills: Generate Solutions
Integrated Process: Nursing Process/Planning
Content Area: Pediatrics: Gastrointestinal
Health Problem: Pediatric-Specific: Developmental GI Defects

Answer: 3
Rationale: Preoperatively, important nursing responsibilities for the child with hypertrophic pyloric stenosis include monitoring the IV infusion, intake, output, and weight and obtaining urine specific gravity measurements. Additionally, weighing the infant's diapers provides information regarding output. Enemas until clear would further compromise the fluid volume status. Preoperatively, the infant receives nothing by mouth unless otherwise prescribed by the primary health care provider.
Priority Nursing Tip: When preparing the infant with hypertrophic pyloric stenosis for surgery, monitor intake and output, the number and character of stools, and patency of the nasogastric tube used for stomach decompression.

Test-Taking Strategy: Focus on the **subject,** preoperative care of a child with pyloric stenosis. Eliminate options 2 and 4 based on the fact that the infant needs to receive nothing by mouth during the preoperative period. Eliminate option 1 knowing that enemas would further compromise the fluid balance status.

---

120. A client who was a victim of a gunshot incident states, "I feel as if I am losing my mind. I keep hearing the gunshots and seeing my friend lying on the ground." Which strategy would the nurse include when **initially** formulating a therapeutic relationship?

1 Teaching the client a variety of relaxation techniques
2 Asking the psychiatrist to prescribe appropriate medication
3 Encouraging the client to talk about the incident and feelings related to it
4 Encouraging the client to think about just how lucky he or she is to still be alive

Level of Cognitive Ability: Analyzing
Client Needs: Psychosocial Integrity
Clinical Judgment/Cognitive Skills: Generate Solutions
Integrated Process: Nursing Process/Planning
Content Area: Mental Health
Health Problem: Mental Health: Violence

Answer: 3
Rationale: When developing a therapeutic relationship, it is important to acknowledge and validate the client's feelings. Although teaching the client relaxation techniques may be helpful at some point, it is unrelated to the subject of the question. Options 2 and 4 are nontherapeutic techniques, and they do not promote a therapeutic relationship.
Priority Nursing Tip: The nurse would always encourage the client to express thoughts and feelings as they address identified areas of concern.

Test-Taking Strategy: Focus on the **subject,** initiating a therapeutic relationship with a gunshot victim, and note the **strategic word,** *initially.* Eliminate options that do not encourage further discussion about the client's feelings. Teaching the client how to relax may be helpful at some point, but not at the beginning of the therapeutic relationship. Remember to address the client's feelings.

---

121. The nurse is caring for a hospitalized child with a diagnosis of rheumatic fever who has developed carditis. The parent asks the nurse to explain the meaning of carditis. On which description of this complication of rheumatic fever would the nurse plan to base a response?

1 Involuntary movements affecting the legs, arms, and face
2 Inflammation of all parts of the heart, primarily the mitral valve
3 Tender, painful joints, especially in the elbows, knees, ankles, and wrists
4 Red skin lesions that start as flat or slightly raised macules, usually over the trunk, and that spread peripherally

Level of Cognitive Ability: Applying
Client Needs: Physiological Integrity
Clinical Judgment/Cognitive Skills: Generate Solutions
Integrated Process: Nursing Process/Planning
Content Area: Pediatrics: Cardiovascular
Health Problem: Pediatric-Specific: Rheumatic Fever

Answer: 2
Rationale: Carditis is the inflammation of all parts of the heart, primarily the mitral valve, and it is a complication of rheumatic fever. Option 1 describes chorea. Option 3 describes polyarthritis. Option 4 describes erythema marginatum.
Priority Nursing Tip: Initiate seizure precautions if a child with rheumatic fever is experiencing chorea.

Test-Taking Strategy: Focus on the **subject,** the complications of rheumatic fever–induced carditis. Note the relationship between the word *carditis* in the question and *heart* in the correct option.

---

122. The nurse assisting to admit a 7-month-old infant with febrile seizures would anticipate the need for which equipment when planning care for this infant?

1 Restraints at the bedside
2 A code cart at the bedside
3 Suction equipment and an airway at the bedside
4 A padded tongue blade taped to the head of the bed

Level of Cognitive Ability: Applying
Client Needs: Physiological Integrity
Clinical Judgment/Cognitive Skills: Generate Solutions
Integrated Process: Nursing Process/Planning
Content Area: Pediatrics: Neurological
Health Problem: Pediatric-Specific: Seizures

Answer: 3

Rationale: Suctioning may be required during a seizure to remove secretions that obstruct the airway. An airway would also be readily available. During a seizure, the infant needs to be placed in a side-lying position, but would not be restrained. It is unnecessary to place a code cart at the bedside, but a cart would be readily available for use after the seizure subsides if needed. A padded tongue blade would never be used; in fact, nothing would be placed in the mouth during a seizure.

Priority Nursing Tip: If a child experiences a seizure, lower the child to the floor and protect the child's head from injury.

Test-Taking Strategy: Use the **ABCs—airway, breathing, and circulation**—to answer the question. Option 3 is the only choice that specifically relates to the airway.

---

123. A 10-month-old infant is hospitalized for respiratory syncytial virus (RSV). On the basis of the developmental stage of the infant, what intervention would the nurse include in the plan of care?

1 Restrain the infant with a total body restraint to prevent any tubes from being dislodged.
2 Follow the home feeding schedule, and allow the infant to be held only when the parents visit.
3 Wash hands, wear a mask when caring for the infant, and keep the infant as quiet as possible.
4 Provide a consistent routine, and touch, rock, and cuddle the infant throughout the hospitalization.

Level of Cognitive Ability: Applying
Client Needs: Physiological Integrity
Clinical Judgment/Cognitive Skills: Generate Solutions
Integrated Process: Nursing Process/Planning
Content Area: Developmental Stages: Infant
Health Problem: Pediatric-Specific: Bronchitis/Bronchiolitis/Respiratory Syncytial Virus

Answer: 4

Rationale: A 10-month-old infant is in the trust versus mistrust stage of psychosocial development, according to Erik Erikson, and the sensorimotor period of cognitive development, according to Jean Piaget. Hospitalization may have an adverse effect. A consistent routine accompanied by touching, rocking, and cuddling will help the child develop trust and provide sensory stimulation. Total body restraint is unnecessary and an incorrect action. Touching and holding the infant only when the parents visit will not provide adequate stimulation and interpersonal contact for the infant. RSV is not airborne (a mask is not required), and it is usually transmitted by the hands.

Priority Nursing Tip: According to Erikson's theory of psychosocial development, each psychosocial crisis must be resolved for the child or adult to progress emotionally. Unsuccessful resolution can leave the person emotionally disabled.

Test-Taking Strategy: Focus on the **subject**, a 10-month-old infant who is hospitalized with RSV and appropriate interventions based on the child's developmental state. Note the age and diagnosis of the infant to answer correctly. Also, eliminate options 1 and 2 because of the **closed-ended words** *total* and *only*, respectively.

---

124. A child with a diagnosis of Reye's syndrome is being admitted to the hospital. The nurse assists in creating a plan of care for the child that includes which **priority** nursing action?

1 Monitoring for hearing loss
2 Monitoring intake and output (I&O)
3 Repositioning the child every 2 hours
4 Providing a quiet environment with dimmed lighting

Level of Cognitive Ability: Creating
Client Needs: Physiological Integrity
Clinical Judgment/Cognitive Skills: Prioritize Hypotheses
Integrated Process: Nursing Process/Planning
Content Area: Pediatrics: Neurological
Health Problem: Pediatric-Specific: Reye's Syndrome

Answer: 4

Rationale: Cerebral edema is a progressive part of the disease process of Reye's syndrome. A priority component of care for a child with Reye's syndrome is to maintain effective cerebral perfusion and control intracranial pressure. Decreasing the stimuli in the environment would decrease the stress on the cerebral tissue, as well as neuron responses. Hearing loss does not occur in clients with this disorder. Although monitoring I&O may be a component of the plan, it is not the priority nursing action. Changing the body position every 2 hours would not affect the cerebral edema and intracranial pressure directly. The child would be in a head-elevated position to decrease the progression of cerebral edema and promote the drainage of cerebrospinal fluid.

Priority Nursing Tip: The nurse needs to check the neurological status of a child with Reye's syndrome. Signs of neurological deterioration need to be reported immediately.

Test-Taking Strategy: Note the **strategic word,** ***priority.*** Recalling that increased intracranial pressure is a concern for the child with Reye's syndrome will direct you to the correct option.

---

125. A nursing student is preparing to assist with the running of a clinical conference regarding cerebral palsy. Which characteristic related to this disorder would the student anticipate being included in the discussion?

1 Cerebral palsy is an infectious disease of the central nervous system.
2 Cerebral palsy is an inflammation of the brain as a result of a viral illness.
3 Cerebral palsy is a chronic disability characterized by difficulty with muscle control.
4 Cerebral palsy is a congenital condition that results in moderate to severe developmental disabilities.

Level of Cognitive Ability: Applying
Client Needs: Physiological Integrity
Clinical Judgment/Cognitive Skills: Generate Solutions
Integrated Process: Nursing Process/Planning
Content Area: Pediatrics: Musculoskeletal
Health Problem: Pediatric-Specific: Cerebral Palsy

Answer: 3

Rationale: Cerebral palsy is a chronic disability that is characterized by difficulty with controlling the muscles because of an abnormality in the extrapyramidal or pyramidal motor system. Meningitis is an infectious process of the central nervous system. Encephalitis is an inflammation of the brain that occurs as a result of viral illness or central nervous system infections. Down syndrome is an example of a congenital condition that results in moderate to severe developmental disabilities.

Priority Nursing Tip: Provide the parents of a child with cerebral palsy with information about the disorder, treatment plan, and support services, including support groups.

Test-Taking Strategy: Eliminate options 1 and 2, which are **comparable or alike** and focus on cause rather than a characteristic of the disorder. Next, note the relationship between *palsy* in the question and *muscle* in the correct option.

---

126. A nursing student is asked to assist with the running of a clinical conference about autism. Which characteristic associated with autism would the student plan to include?

1 Normal social play that ceases by age 5
2 Lack of social interaction and awareness
3 The consistent imitation of others' actions
4 Normal verbal but abnormal nonverbal communication

Level of Cognitive Ability: Applying
Client Needs: Psychosocial Integrity
Clinical Judgment/Cognitive Skills: Generate Solutions
Integrated Process: Nursing Process/Planning
Content Area: Pediatrics: Neurological
Health Problem: Pediatric-Specific: Autism Spectrum Disorders

Answer: 2

Rationale: Autism is a severe developmental disorder that begins in infancy or toddlerhood. A primary characteristic is a lack of social interaction and awareness. Social behaviors in children with autism include a lack of or abnormal imitations of others' actions and a lack of or abnormal social play. Additional characteristics include a lack of or impaired verbal communication and marked abnormal nonverbal communication.

Priority Nursing Tip: For the child with autism, determine the child's routines, habits, and preferences and maintain consistency as much as possible. Provide support to parents.

Test-Taking Strategy: Focus on the **subject**, characteristics of autism. It is necessary to recall that the primary characteristic is a lack of social interaction and awareness.

---

127. Which interventions are appropriate to include in the plan of care for a child after a tonsillectomy? **Select all that apply.**

❒ 1 Offer clear, cool liquids when awake.
❒ 2 Administer pain medication as prescribed.
❒ 3 Monitor for bleeding from the surgical site.
❒ 4 Suction every 15 minutes and as necessary.
❒ 5 Initially eliminate milk or milk products from the diet.

Level of Cognitive Ability: Applying
Client Needs: Physiological Integrity
Clinical Judgment/Cognitive Skills: Generate Solutions
Integrated Process: Nursing Process/Planning
Content Area: Pediatrics: Throat/Respiratory
Health Problem: Pediatric-Specific: Tonsillitis and Adenoiditis

Answer: 1, 2, 3, 5

Rationale: After tonsillectomy, clear, cool liquids are encouraged. Options 2 and 3 are important interventions after any type of surgery. Suction equipment needs to be available, but suctioning is not performed unless there is an airway obstruction. Milk and milk products are avoided initially because they coat the throat; this causes the child to clear the throat, thereby increasing the risk of bleeding.

Priority Nursing Tip: After tonsillectomy, suction equipment would be available, but suctioning is not done unless there is airway obstruction because it will disrupt the integrity of the surgical site and cause bleeding.

Test-Taking Strategy: Focus on the **subject**, post-tonsillectomy interventions. Think about the location and complications of this procedure to answer correctly.

---

128. The school nurse is preparing to assist in performing health screening for scoliosis on children ages 9 through 14. Which instruction would the nurse plan to provide to each child?

1 Lie flat and lift the legs straight up.
2 Lie on the right side and then roll to the left side while the arms are held overhead.
3 Walk 10 feet forward and then 10 feet backward with the arms held overhead at both sides.
4 Stand with weight equally on both feet with the legs straight and the arms hanging loosely at both sides.

Level of Cognitive Ability: Applying
Client Needs: Health Promotion and Maintenance
Clinical Judgment/Cognitive Skills: Generate Solutions
Integrated Process: Nursing Process/Planning
Content Area: Health Assessment/Physical Exam: Musculoskeletal
Health Problem: Pediatric-Specific: Scoliosis

Answer: 4
Rationale: To perform this screening test, the child would be asked to disrobe or wear underpants only so that the chest, back, and hips can be clearly seen. The child is asked to stand with weight equally on both feet with the legs straight and the arms hanging loosely at both sides. The nurse checks the child's posture, spinal column, shoulder height, and leg lengths. Lying-down positions and walking forward and backward are incorrect data collection techniques.
Priority Nursing Tip: A complication after surgical treatment of scoliosis is superior mesenteric artery syndrome. This disorder is caused by mechanical changes in the position of the child's abdominal contents that occur during surgery.

Test-Taking Strategy: Focus on the **subject,** plan of care for scoliosis screening procedure. Recall the anatomical location of this disorder and then visualize the screening procedure and the preparation required to adequately assess for this disorder.

---

129. The nurse is assisting in creating a plan of care for a child diagnosed with leukemia who is beginning chemotherapy. Which intervention would the nurse suggest to include?

1 Monitor rectal temperatures every 4 hours.
2 Monitor the mouth and anus each shift for signs of breakdown.
3 Encourage the child to consume fresh fruits and vegetables to maintain nutritional status.
4 Provide meticulous mouth care several times daily using an alcohol-based mouthwash and a toothbrush.

Level of Cognitive Ability: Creating
Client Needs: Physiological Integrity
Clinical Judgment/Cognitive Skills: Generate Solutions
Integrated Process: Nursing Process/Planning
Content Area: Pediatrics: Oncological
Health Problem: Pediatric-Specific: Cancers

Answer: 2
Rationale: When the child is receiving chemotherapy, the nurse would check the mouth and anus each shift for ulcers, erythema, or breakdown. The nurse needs to avoid taking rectal temperatures. Oral temperatures are also avoided if mouth ulcers are present. Axillary or temporal temperatures would be taken to prevent alterations in skin integrity. Bland, nonirritating foods and liquids would be provided to the child. Fresh fruits and vegetables need to be avoided because they can harbor organisms. Chemotherapy can cause neutropenia, and the child would be maintained on a low-bacteria diet if the white blood cell count is low. Meticulous mouth care needs to be performed, but the nurse would avoid alcohol-based mouthwashes and needs to use a soft-bristled toothbrush.
Priority Nursing Tip: Chemotherapy can cause life-threatening neutropenia and thrombocytopenia.

Test-Taking Strategy: Focus on the **subject,** interventions for the child receiving chemotherapy. Think about the adverse effects that can occur with chemotherapy to assist in answering correctly. Remember that life-threatening neutropenia and thrombocytopenia can occur.

---

130. The nurse is assisting in preparing to admit a client from the postanesthesia care unit who has had microvascular decompression of the trigeminal nerve. Which **essential** equipment would the nurse ensure is at the bedside when the client arrives?

1 Flashlight and pulse oximeter
2 Cardiac monitor and suction equipment
3 Padded bed rails and suction equipment
4 Blood pressure cuff and cardiac monitor

Level of Cognitive Ability: Applying
Client Needs: Physiological Integrity
Clinical Judgment/Cognitive Skills: Generate Solutions
Integrated Process: Nursing Process/Planning
Content Area: Adult Health: Neurological
Health Problem: Adult Health: Neurological: Trigeminal Neuralgia

Answer: 1

Rationale: The postoperative care of the client having microvascular decompression of the trigeminal nerve is the same as for the client undergoing craniotomy. This client requires hourly neurological checks as well as monitoring of the cardiovascular and respiratory statuses. Therefore, a flashlight and pulse oximetry are essential items. Cardiac monitoring and padded bed rails are not required unless there is a special need based on a client history of cardiac disease or seizures, respectively. Suctioning is performed cautiously and only when necessary after craniotomy to avoid increasing the intracranial pressure.

Priority Nursing Tip: After surgery for microvascular decompression of the trigeminal nerve, the client's pain is compared with the preoperative pain level.

Test-Taking Strategy: Note the **strategic word,** *essential.* Focus on the **subject,** the essential equipment for a client who just had microvascular decompression of the trigeminal nerve. The client is not necessarily at risk for seizures postoperatively, so option 3 is eliminated first. Eliminate options 2 and 4 because no data in the question indicate that the client had a history of a cardiac problem. In addition, knowing that the procedure is performed via craniotomy enables you to recall that suctioning is done cautiously and only when necessary and also that neurological checks are needed, so a flashlight would be required to perform neurological assessments.

---

131. The nurse is assisting in receiving a client from the emergency department who has a diagnosis of Guillain-Barré syndrome. The client's chief sign/symptom is an ascending paralysis that has reached the level of the waist. Which items would the nurse plan to have available for emergency use?

1 Nebulizer and pulse oximeter
2 Blood pressure cuff and flashlight
3 Flashlight and incentive spirometer
4 Cardiac monitor and intubation tray

Level of Cognitive Ability: Applying
Client Needs: Physiological Integrity
Clinical Judgment/Cognitive Skills: Generate Solutions
Integrated Process: Nursing Process/Planning
Content Area: Adult Health: Neurological
Health Problem: Adult Health: Neurological: Guillain-Barré Syndrome

Answer: 4

Rationale: The client with Guillain-Barré syndrome is at risk for respiratory failure as a result of ascending paralysis. An intubation tray needs to be available for emergency use. Another complication of this syndrome is cardiac dysrhythmias, which necessitate the need for cardiac monitoring. Although some of the items in the remaining options may be kept at the bedside (e.g., pulse oximeter, blood pressure cuff, flashlight), they are not necessarily needed for emergency use in this situation.

Priority Nursing Tip: Monitor respiratory and cardiac status closely and prepare to initiate respiratory support for the client with Guillain-Barré syndrome.

Test-Taking Strategy: Focus on the **subject,** equipment needed for possible emergency use in a client with Guillain-Barré syndrome who is experiencing ascending paralysis. These words tell you that the correct answer will be an option that contains equipment that is not routinely used to provide care. With this in mind, eliminate options 2 and 3 based on the fact that a flashlight is needed for routine neurological checks. From the remaining choices, recalling the complications of this syndrome will direct you to the correct option.

---

132. The nurse is assisting in admitting a newborn infant whose mother is Rh negative. When planning care for the infant's arrival to the nursery, which action would the nurse take?

1 Obtain the newborn infant's blood type and direct Coombs' results from the laboratory.
2 Obtain the necessary equipment from the blood bank needed for an exchange transfusion.
3 Call the maintenance department and ask for a phototherapy unit to be brought to the nursery.
4 Obtain a vial of vitamin K from the pharmacy and prepare to administer an injection to prevent isoimmunization.

Level of Cognitive Ability: Applying
Client Needs: Physiological Integrity
Clinical Judgment/Cognitive Skills: Generate Solutions
Integrated Process: Nursing Process/Planning
Content Area: Maternity: Newborn
Health Problem: N/A

Answer: 1

Rationale: To further plan for the newborn infant's care, the infant's blood type and direct Coombs' results must be known. Umbilical cord blood is taken at the time of delivery to determine blood type, Rh factor, and antibody titer (direct Coombs' test) of the newborn infant. The nurse would obtain these results from the laboratory. Options 2 and 3 are inappropriate at this time, and additional data are needed to determine whether these actions are needed. Option 4 is incorrect because vitamin K is given to prevent hemorrhagic disease of the newborn infant.

Priority Nursing Tip: For the infant with erythroblastosis fetalis, the newborn's blood is replaced with Rh-negative blood to stop the destruction of the newborn's red blood cells; the Rh-negative blood is replaced with the newborn's own blood gradually.

Test-Taking Strategy: Focus on the **subject,** the mother being Rh negative. Note the relationship between the subject of the question and the correct option. In addition, note that the correct option is the only option that addresses data collection.

---

133. The nurse is preparing to assist in the administration of a chemotherapeutic agent via intraperitoneal (IP) therapy. In which position would the nurse plan to place the client before administering this therapy?

1 Supine
2 Semi-Fowler's
3 Trendelenburg's
4 Dorsal recumbent

Level of Cognitive Ability: Applying
Client Needs: Physiological Integrity
Clinical Judgment/Cognitive Skills: Generate Solutions
Integrated Process: Nursing Process/Planning
Content Area: Adult Health: Oncology
Health Problem: N/A

Answer: 2

Rationale: IP therapy is the administration of chemotherapeutic agents into the peritoneal cavity. This therapy is used for intra-abdominal malignancies such as ovarian and gastrointestinal tumors that have moved into the peritoneum after surgery. The client would be placed in a semi-Fowler's position for this infusion because the client may experience nausea and vomiting caused by increasing pressure on the internal organs. Additionally, this treatment may also place pressure on the diaphragm. The positions indicated in the rest of the options would increase pressure in the peritoneal cavity.

Priority Nursing Tip: Malignancies of the abdomen may be treated with the instillation of chemotherapeutic agents into the peritoneal cavity or with external radiation.

Test-Taking Strategy: Focus on the **subject,** care of the client receiving IP therapy. Recalling that this therapy can increase intra-abdominal pressure and cause nausea and vomiting will assist you in eliminating the incorrect options.

---

134. The nurse plans care for a client with alcohol abuse disorder based on which support system?

1 Fresh Start, an option for families of addicts
2 Families Anonymous, an option for those addicted to nicotine
3 Al-Anon, an option for parents of children who abuse substances
4 Alcoholics Anonymous, a major self-help organization for the treatment of alcohol abuse

Answer: 4

Rationale: Alcoholics Anonymous is a major self-help organization for the treatment of alcoholism. Option 1 is a group for families of alcoholics. Option 2 is for nicotine addicts. Option 3 is for the parents of children who abuse substances.

Priority Nursing Tip: As part of the data collection of a client who abuses alcohol, the nurse would ask about the type of alcohol used, how much is consumed, and for how many years.

Test-Taking Strategy: Focus on the **subject,** resources for a client who is personally dealing with alcohol abuse. Note the relationship between this subject and the correct option.

Level of Cognitive Ability: Applying
Client Needs: Safe and Effective Care Environment
Clinical Judgment/Cognitive Skills: Generate Solutions
Integrated Process: Nursing Process/Planning
Content Area: Mental Health
Health Problem: Mental Health: Addictions

---

135. The primary health care provider has prescribed range-of-motion (ROM) exercises for the right side of a client hospitalized for stroke. Which intervention would the nurse's plan include when planning for the client's ROM exercises?

1 Implements ROM exercises to the point of pain for the client.
2 Considers the use of active, passive, or active-assisted exercises in the home.
3 Encourages dependence on the home care nurse to complete the exercise program.
4 Develops a schedule involving ROM exercises every 3 hours during daylight hours.

Answer: 2

Rationale: The nurse must consider all forms of ROM for the client. Even if the client has right hemiplegia, the client can assist with some of his or her own rehabilitative care. In addition, the goal is for the client to assume as much self-care and independence as possible. The nurse needs to teach so that the client becomes self-reliant. Options 1 and 4 are incorrect from a physiological standpoint.

Priority Nursing Tip: The nurse would assist the client who suffered a stroke in establishing a balanced exercise and rest program.

Test-Taking Strategy: Focus on the **subject,** appropriate implementation of ROM exercise. Eliminate options 1 and 4 because the suggested actions may be harmful to the client. From the remaining choices, recalling that dependency is not in the best interest of a client's sense of health promotion will help you eliminate option 3. In addition, note that the correct option is the umbrella option.

Level of Cognitive Ability: Applying
Client Needs: Physiological Integrity
Clinical Judgment/Cognitive Skills: Generate Solutions
Integrated Process: Nursing Process/Planning
Content Area: Skills: Activity/Mobility
Health Problem: Adult Health: Neurological: Stroke

NURSING PROCESS: IMPLEMENTATION

136. A client diagnosed with heart failure is receiving furosemide and digoxin daily. When the nurse enters the room to administer the morning doses, the client reports anorexia, nausea, and yellow vision. Which intervention would the nurse implement **first**?

1 Contact the cardiologist.
2 Administer the medications.
3 Check the morning serum digoxin level.
4 Check the morning serum potassium level.

Level of Cognitive Ability: Applying
Client Needs: Physiological Integrity
Clinical Judgment/Cognitive Skills: Take Action
Integrated Process: Nursing Process/ Implementation
Content Area: Pharmacology: Cardiovascular: Cardiac Glycosides
Health Problem: Adult Health: Cardiovascular: Heart Failure

Answer: 3
Rationale: The nurse would check the result of the digoxin level that was drawn because the client's symptoms are compatible with digoxin toxicity. A low potassium level may contribute to digoxin toxicity, so checking the serum potassium level may give useful additional information, but the digoxin level would be checked first. The medications need to be withheld until both levels are known. If the digoxin level is elevated or the potassium level is not within the normal range, then the cardiologist would be notified. If the morning digoxin level is within the therapeutic range, then the client's complaints are unrelated to the digoxin.
Priority Nursing Tip: The nurse must count the apical heart rate for 1 full minute in a client who is receiving digoxin. If the rate is less than 60 beats/min, the medication is withheld and further investigation is done, because this finding could indicate digoxin toxicity.

Test-Taking Strategy: Note the **strategic word,** *first.* This will assist you with determining that the nurse's action is to further investigate the cause of the client's complaints. Recalling the manifestations of digoxin toxicity and noting the relationship of the name of the medication to option 3 will direct you to this option.

---

137. The nurse is checking the fundus of a postpartum client and notes that the uterus is soft and spongy. Which nursing action is appropriate **initially**?

1 Notify the obstetrician.
2 Encourage the client to ambulate.
3 Massage the fundus gently until it is firm.
4 Document fundal position, consistency, and height.

Level of Cognitive Ability: Applying
Client Needs: Physiological Integrity
Clinical Judgment/Cognitive Skills: Take Action
Integrated Process: Nursing Process/ Implementation
Content Area: Maternity: Postpartum
Health Problem: Maternity: Postpartum Uterine Problems

Answer: 3
Rationale: If the fundus is boggy (soft), it needs to be massaged gently until it is firm and the client is observed for increased bleeding or clots. Option 2 is an inappropriate action at this time. The nurse would document the fundal position, consistency, and height; the need to perform fundal massage; and the client's response to the intervention. The obstetrician will need to be notified if uterine massage is not helpful.
Priority Nursing Tip: The nurse needs to gently massage the fundus of a client experiencing uterine atony and to take care not to overmassage it.

Test-Taking Strategy: Note the **strategic word,** *initially.* Focus on the **data in the question** and note the relationship of these data (soft and spongy) and the data in the correct option (massage the fundus gently until it is firm).

138. A primipara is being evaluated in the clinic during her second trimester of pregnancy. The nurse checks the fetal heart rate (FHR) and notes that it is 190 beats/min. What is the appropriate **initial** nursing action?

1 Document the finding.
2 Tell the client that the FHR is fast.
3 Report the finding to the obstetrician.
4 Recheck the FHR with the client in the standing position.

Level of Cognitive Ability: Applying
Client Needs: Physiological Integrity
Clinical Judgment/Cognitive Skills: Take Action
Integrated Process: Nursing Process/Implementation
Content Area: Maternity: Antepartum
Health Problem: Maternity: Fetal Distress/Demise

Answer: 3
Rationale: The FHR should be between 120 and 160 beats/min. In this situation, the FHR is elevated from the normal range, and the nurse needs to consult with the obstetrician. The FHR would be documented, but option 3 is the appropriate action. The nurse would not tell the client that the FHR is fast at this point in time. Option 4 is an inappropriate action.
Priority Nursing Tip: The normal FHR is 160 to 170 beats/min in the first trimester, but slows with fetal growth to 110 to 160 beats/min near or at term. The obstetrician needs to be notified if the FHR is outside these parameters.

Test-Taking Strategy: Focus on the **subject**, an FHR of 190 beats/min, as well on the **strategic word,** *initial.* Recalling that the normal FHR is between 110 and 160 beats/min will direct you to the correct option.

---

139. A client complains of very dry and irritated skin to the clinic nurse. Which product would the nurse suggest that the client apply to the dry skin?

1 Myoflex
2 Aspercreme
3 Topical emollient
4 Acetic acid solution

Level of Cognitive Ability: Applying
Client Needs: Health Promotion and Maintenance
Clinical Judgment/Cognitive Skills: Take Action
Integrated Process: Nursing Process/Implementation
Content Area: Adult Health: Integumentary
Health Problem: Adult Health: Integumentary: Inflammations/Infections

Answer: 3
Rationale: A topical emollient is used for dry, cracked, and irritated skin. Aspercreme and Myoflex are used to treat muscular aches. Acetic acid solution is used for irrigating, cleansing, and packing wounds infected with *Pseudomonas aeruginosa.*
Priority Nursing Tip: To sustain the hydrating effect, it is best to apply cream or ointment emollients (moisturizers) after bathing.

Test-Taking Strategy: Focus on the **subject,** treatment for dry and irritated skin. Note the relationship between the subject and the word *emollient* in the correct option.

---

140. A client with a history of hypertension has been prescribed triamterene. The nurse reinforces information to the client about the medication and instructs the client to avoid consuming which fruit?

1 Pears
2 Apples
3 Bananas
4 Cranberries

Level of Cognitive Ability: Applying
Client Needs: Health Promotion and Maintenance
Clinical Judgment/Cognitive Skills: Take Action

Answer: 3
Rationale: Triamterene is a potassium-sparing diuretic, and the client would avoid foods that are high in potassium. Fruits that are naturally higher in potassium include avocados, bananas, oranges, mangoes, cantaloupe, strawberries, nectarines, papayas, and dried prunes.
Priority Nursing Tip: Normal potassium levels range from 3.5 to 5.0 mEq/L. A potassium level outside these parameters needs to be reported.

Integrated Process: Nursing Process/ Implementation
Content Area: Adult Health: Cardiovascular/ Diuretics
Health Problem: Adult Health: Cardiovascular: Hypertension

Test-Taking Strategy: Focus on the subject, the fruit that the client needs to avoid. Note that this is asking you to choose the fruit the client would not eat. Recall that triamterene is a potassium-sparing diuretic and that the intake of potassium presents dietary concerns related to the medication.

---

141. A client in the late active first stage of labor has just reported a gush of vaginal fluid. The nurse observes a fetal monitor pattern of variable decelerations during contractions followed by a brief acceleration. After that, there is a return to baseline until the next contraction, when the pattern is repeated. On the basis of these data, the nurse reports the information to the registered nurse and prepares to assist with which **initial** intervention?

1 Take the client's vital signs.
2 Perform a Leopold's maneuver.
3 Perform a manual sterile vaginal exam.
4 Test the vaginal fluid with a Nitrazine strip.

Level of Cognitive Ability: Synthesizing
Client Needs: Physiological Integrity
Clinical Judgment/Cognitive Skills: Take Action
Integrated Process: Nursing Process/ Implementation
Content Area: Maternity: Intrapartum
Health Problem: Maternity: Fetal Distress/Demise

Answer: 3
Rationale: Variable deceleration with brief acceleration after a gush of amniotic fluid is a common clinical manifestation of cord compression caused by occult or frank prolapse of the umbilical cord. A manual vaginal examination can detect the presence of the cord in the vagina, which confirms the problem. On the basis of the data in the question, none of the remaining options are initial actions.
Priority Nursing Tip: Compression of the cord between the fetal head and the forceps used during delivery can cause a drop in the fetal heart rate (FHR). The FHR and pattern are checked, reported, and recorded before and after forceps are applied.

Test-Taking Strategy: Note the **strategic word,** *initial.* Focusing on the **data in the question** and determining the significance of the data will direct you to the correct option.

---

142. The nurse prepares to administer an enteral feeding to a client through a nasogastric tube (NGT). Which is the **priority** intervention for the nurse to complete before administering the feeding?

1 Determining tube placement
2 Auscultating the bowel sounds
3 Measuring the intake and output
4 Establishing the client's baseline weight

Level of Cognitive Ability: Applying
Client Needs: Physiological Integrity
Clinical Judgment/Cognitive Skills: Take Action
Integrated Process: Nursing Process/ Implementation
Content Area: Skills: Tube Care
Health Problem: N/A

Answer: 1
Rationale: The nurse avoids injecting any substance into a client's NGT before verifying tube placement because NGTs can migrate out of the stomach. If the NGT is not in the correct location, subsequent injections or feedings through the tube can lead to serious complications such as aspiration. None of the remaining options are priorities before administering an enteral feeding.
Priority Nursing Tip: After insertion of an NGT, an abdominal x-ray study would be done to confirm placement of the tube. If the tube is incorrectly placed, the client is at risk for aspiration.

Test-Taking Strategy: Note the **strategic word,** *priority.* Use the **ABCs—airway, breathing, and circulation**—and the **steps of the nursing process** to answer the question. The correct option relates to data collection and the risk of aspiration.

---

143. The nurse is asked to assist another health care team member with providing care for a client. On entering the client's room, the nurse notes that the client is placed in this position. The nurse maintains the client's position, knowing that this client is **most likely** being treated for which condition? **Refer to figure.**

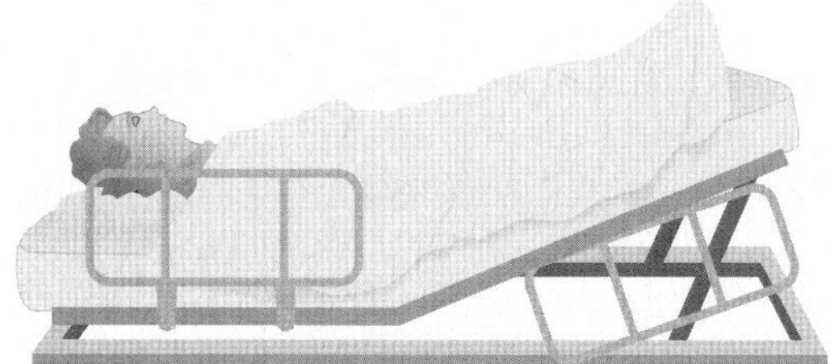

(From Black J, Hawks J: *Medical-surgical nursing: clinical management for positive outcomes,* ed 8, Philadelphia, 2009, Saunders.)

1 Shock
2 A head injury
3 Respiratory insufficiency
4 Increased intracranial pressure

Level of Cognitive Ability: Analyzing
Client Needs: Physiological Integrity
Clinical Judgment/Cognitive Skills: Take Action
Integrated Process: Nursing Process/ Implementation
Content Area: Complex Care: Shock
Health Problem: Adult Health: Cardiovascular: Shock

Answer: 1
Rationale: A client in shock is placed in a modified Trendelenburg's position that includes elevating the legs, leaving the trunk flat, and elevating the head and shoulders slightly. This position promotes increased venous return from the lower extremities without compressing the abdominal organs against the diaphragm. The Trendelenburg's position is no longer recommended for hypotensive clients because the client is predisposed to aspiration and gas exchange is worsened. The remaining options identify conditions in which the head of the client's bed would be elevated.
Priority Nursing Tip: Shock results from the loss of circulatory fluid volume, which is usually caused by hemorrhage. Shock can also be caused by sepsis or hypovolemia (dehydration).

Test-Taking Strategy: Note the **strategic words,** *most likely.* Focus on the **subject,** the position identified in the figure. Eliminate options 2 and 4, which are **comparable or alike** because both relate to a neurological condition. From the remaining choices, eliminate option 3, recalling that the head of the bed is elevated for respiratory conditions.

---

144. The nurse needs to administer 7.5 mg of a medication intramuscularly. The medication label reads "10 mg/mL." How much medication would the nurse prepare to administer? **Fill in the blank.**
Answer:_____ mL

Level of Cognitive Ability: Applying
Client Needs: Physiological Integrity
Clinical Judgment/Cognitive Skills: Take Action
Integrated Process: Nursing Process/ Implementation
Content Area: Skills: Dosage Calculations
Health Problem: N/A

Answer: 0.75
Rationale: Use the following formula to calculate the medication dose:

$$\frac{\text{Desired}}{\text{Available}} \times \text{Volume} = \text{mL per dose}$$

$$\frac{7.5 \text{ mg}}{10 \text{ mg}} \times 1 \text{ mL} = 0.75 \text{ mL}$$

Priority Nursing Tip: After performing a medication calculation problem, ensure that the answer or the amount of medication to be administered makes sense and is not an excessive or extremely small dose.

Test-Taking Strategy: Focus on the **subject,** mL of medication per dose. Use the formula to determine the correct dosage, and use a calculator to verify your answer.

---

145. A client diagnosed with obsessive-compulsive rituals often misses the unit's morning activities because of a bed-making ritual. What nursing action would be therapeutic?

1 Verbalize tactful, mild disapproval of the behavior.
2 Discuss the social implications of the behavior with the client.
3 Help the client make the bed so that the task can be finished quicker.
4 Offer reflective feedback, such as, "I see that you have made your bed several times."

Level of Cognitive Ability: Applying
Client Needs: Psychosocial Integrity
Clinical Judgment/Cognitive Skills: Take Action
Integrated Process: Nursing Process/Implementation
Content Area: Mental Health
Health Problem: Mental Health: Obsessive Compulsive Disorder

Answer: 4
Rationale: Reflective feedback acknowledges the client's behavior. Verbalizing disapproval and discussing social implications would increase the client's anxiety and reinforce the need to perform the ritual. The client is usually aware of the implications of the behavior. Helping with the ritual is nontherapeutic and also reinforces the behavior.
Priority Nursing Tip: If a client is experiencing anxiety, assist the client to perform relaxation techniques.

Test-Taking Strategy: Focus on the **subject,** a client with obsessive-compulsive rituals. Recalling that the purpose of the ritual is to relieve anxiety would assist you with eliminating options 1 and 2, which would increase the client's anxiety. Eliminate option 3 because there is no therapeutic value in participating in the ritual.

---

146. A client who has undergone internal fixation after fracturing a left hip has developed a reddened left heel. What equipment would the nurse use to manage this problem?

1 Trapeze
2 Bed cradle
3 Draw sheet
4 Alternating pressure mattress

Level of Cognitive Ability: Applying
Client Needs: Physiological Integrity
Clinical Judgment/Cognitive Skills: Take Action
Integrated Process: Nursing Process/Implementation
Content Area: Skills: Activity/Mobility
Health Problem: Adult Health: Musculoskeletal: Skeletal Injury

Answer: 4
Rationale: The reddened heel results from the pressure of the foot against the mattress. An alternating pressure mattress is effective at minimizing pressure points. The bed cradle will keep the linens off of the client's lower extremities but will not assist with the management of a reddened heel. A draw sheet and trapeze are of general use for this client, but they are not specific for dealing with the reddened heel.
Priority Nursing Tip: The nurse would perform frequent skin checks on the immobile client.

Test-Taking Strategy: Note the **subject,** a reddened left heel after internal fixation surgery. Think about the item in each option and how it may assist in managing the problem, a reddened heel. The items in options 1, 2, and 3 will have no helpful effect. The correct option addresses the problem stated in the question.

---

147. The nurse is assisting in caring for an infant after a pyloromyotomy is performed to treat hypertrophic pyloric stenosis. In which position would the nurse place the infant after surgery?

1 Flat on the operative side
2 Flat on the nonoperative side
3 Prone with the head of the bed elevated
4 Supine with the head of the bed elevated

Answer: 3
Rationale: After pyloromyotomy, the head of the bed is elevated, and the infant is placed prone to reduce the risk of aspiration. Based on this information, the remaining options are incorrect positions after this type of surgery. The surgeon's prescriptions for positioning need to always be followed.
Priority Nursing Tip: After pyloromyotomy to treat hypertrophic pyloric stenosis, small frequent feedings are introduced as prescribed. This is followed by a gradual increase in the amount and

Level of Cognitive Ability: Applying
Client Needs: Physiological Integrity
Clinical Judgment/Cognitive Skills: Take Action
Integrated Process: Nursing Process/Implementation
Content Area: Pediatrics: Gastrointestinal
Health Problem: Pediatric-Specific: Developmental GI Defects

interval between feedings until a full feeding schedule has been reinstated.

Test-Taking Strategy: Focus on the **subject,** proper positioning after pyloromyotomy. Consider the anatomical location of the surgical procedure and the risks associated with the procedure to answer the question. Visualize each of the positions identified in the options. Keeping in mind that aspiration is a major concern will direct you to the correct option.

---

148. The parent of a child with mumps calls the health care clinic to tell the nurse that the child has been lethargic and vomiting. What instruction would the nurse give to the parent?

1 To continue to monitor the child
2 That lethargy and vomiting are normal manifestations of mumps
3 To bring the child to the clinic to be seen by the primary health care provider
4 That there is nothing to be concerned about as long as there is no fever

Level of Cognitive Ability: Applying
Client Needs: Physiological Integrity
Clinical Judgment/Cognitive Skills: Take Action
Integrated Process: Nursing Process/Implementation
Content Area: Pediatrics: Infectious and Communicable Diseases
Health Problem: Pediatric-Specific: Communicable Diseases

Answer: 3
Rationale: Mumps generally affects the salivary glands, but it can also affect multiple organs. The most common complication is septic meningitis, with the virus being identified in the cerebrospinal fluid. Common signs include nuchal rigidity, lethargy, and vomiting. The child needs to be seen by the primary health care provider.
Priority Nursing Tip: Inform the parents of a child with mumps that bed rest would be encouraged until the parotid swelling subsides.

Test-Taking Strategy: Focus on the **subject,** a child with mumps who has been lethargic and vomiting. Recalling that meningitis is a complication of mumps will direct you to the correct option.

---

149. The nurse is reviewing the prescriptions for a child who was admitted to the hospital with vaso-occlusive pain crisis resulting from sickle cell anemia. Which prescription would the nurse question?

1 Bed rest
2 Intravenous fluids
3 Supplemental oxygen
4 Meperidine hydrochloride

Level of Cognitive Ability: Applying
Client Needs: Safe and Effective Care Environment
Clinical Judgment/Cognitive Skills: Take Action
Integrated Process: Nursing Process/Implementation
Content Area: Pediatrics: Hematological
Health Problem: Pediatric-Specific: Sickle Cell

Answer: 4
Rationale: Meperidine hydrochloride is contraindicated for ongoing pain management because of the increased risk of seizures associated with the use of the medication. The management of vaso-occlusive pain generally includes the use of strong opioid analgesics such as morphine sulfate or hydromorphone. These medications are usually most effective when given as a continuous infusion or at regular intervals around the clock. The remaining options are appropriate prescriptions for treating vaso-occlusive pain crisis.
Priority Nursing Tip: The priority of care for a child with vaso-occlusive pain crisis from sickle cell anemia is to provide hydration and relieve pain.

Test-Taking Strategy: Focus on the **subject,** the prescription to question for treatment of vaso-occlusive pain crisis. Remember that meperidine hydrochloride is associated with an increased risk of seizures.

150. The nurse is caring for an infant diagnosed with laryngomalacia (congenital laryngeal stridor). In which position would the nurse place the infant to decrease the incidence of stridor?

1 Prone
2 Supine
3 Supine with the neck flexed
4 Prone with the neck hyperextended

Level of Cognitive Ability: Applying
Client Needs: Physiological Integrity
Clinical Judgment/Cognitive Skills: Take Action
Integrated Process: Nursing Process/Implementation
Content Area: Pediatrics: Throat/Respiratory
Health Problem: N/A

Answer: 4
Rationale: The prone position with the neck hyperextended improves the child's breathing. Based on that information, none of the remaining options are appropriate positions.
Priority Nursing Tip: A child experiencing respiratory difficulty is never left unattended.

Test-Taking Strategy: Focus on the **subject,** positioning a child diagnosed with laryngomalacia to minimize stridor. Visualize each of the positions identified in the options and the ways in which they may or may not improve breathing to assist with directing you to the correct option.

---

151. The nurse prepares to assist to admit a newborn born with spina bifida, myelomeningocele. Which nursing action is **most important** for the care of this infant?

1 Monitoring the temperature
2 Monitoring the blood pressure
3 Inspecting the anterior fontanel for bulging
4 Monitoring the specific gravity of the urine

Level of Cognitive Ability: Applying
Client Needs: Physiological Integrity
Clinical Judgment/Cognitive Skills: Prioritize Hypotheses
Integrated Process: Nursing Process/Implementation
Content Area: Maternity: Newborn
Health Problem: Pediatric-Specific: Neural Tube Defects

Answer: 3
Rationale: Intracranial pressure is a complication that is associated with spina bifida. A sign of intracranial pressure in the newborn infant with spina bifida is a bulging anterior fontanel. The newborn infant is at risk for infection before the surgical procedure and the closure of the gibbus, and monitoring the temperature is an important intervention; however, checking the anterior fontanel for bulging is most important. A normal saline dressing is placed over the affected site to maintain the moisture of the sac and its contents. This prevents tearing or breakdown of skin integrity at the site. Blood pressure is difficult to check during the newborn period, and it is not the best indicator of infection or a potential complication. Urine concentration is not well developed during the newborn stage of development.
Priority Nursing Tip: In myelomeningocele, the sac (defect) is covered by a thin membrane and is prone to leakage or rupture.

Test-Taking Strategy: Focus on the **strategic words,** *most important.* Eliminate options 2 and 4 because checking blood pressure and specific gravity are common data collection actions, but they are less reliable indications of changes in the status of a newborn than they would be for an older child. From the remaining choices, focusing on the **strategic words** will direct you to the correct option.

---

152. During data collection, the nurse notes that the child's genitals are swollen. The nurse suspects that the child is being sexually abused. Which **priority** action would the nurse take?
1 Document the child's physical findings.
2 Report the case because abuse is suspected.
3 Refer the family to appropriate support groups.
4 Assist the family with identifying resources and support systems.

Level of Cognitive Ability: Applying
Client Needs: Psychosocial Integrity
Clinical Judgment/Cognitive Skills: Take Action
Integrated Process: Nursing Process/Implementation
Content Area: Leadership/Management: Ethical/Legal
Health Problem: Mental Health: Abusive Behaviors

Answer: 2
Rationale: The primary legal responsibility of the nurse when child abuse is suspected is to report the case. All 50 states require health care professionals to report all cases of suspected abuse. Although documenting the findings, assisting the family, and referring the family to appropriate resources and support groups are important, the primary legal responsibility is to report the case. Although the remaining options are appropriate, reporting the findings has priority.
Priority Nursing Tip: The nurse needs to document information related to suspected child abuse in an objective manner.

Test-Taking Strategy: Note the **strategic word,** *priority.* Focus on the **subject,** the possible sexual abuse of a child. Recall that abuse is a crime. Keeping this in mind will direct you to the correct option.

---

153. The nurse is assisting in planning care for an infant with a diagnosis of an encephalocele located in the occipital area. Which item would the nurse use to assist with positioning the child to avoid pressure on the encephalocele?
1 Sandbags
2 Sheepskin
3 Feather pillows
4 Foam half-donut

Level of Cognitive Ability: Applying
Client Needs: Physiological Integrity
Clinical Judgment/Cognitive Skills: Take Action
Integrated Process: Nursing Process/Implementation
Content Area: Pediatrics: Neurological
Health Problem: Pediatric-Specific: Neural Tube Defects

Answer: 4
Rationale: The infant is positioned to avoid pressure on the lesion. If the encephalocele is in the occipital area, a foam half donut may be useful for positioning to prevent this pressure. A sandbag, sheepskin, or feather pillow will not protect the encephalocele from pressure.
Priority Nursing Tip: The nurse needs to monitor the infant with encephalocele closely for signs of neurological deterioration.

Test-Taking Strategy: Eliminate options 1, 2, and 3, which are **comparable or alike** in that they would require the head to remain flat and therefore would not protect the lesion.

---

154. The nurse assisting in caring for a child who has sustained a head injury notes that the neurologist has documented decorticate posturing. During the data collection for the child, the nurse notes the extension of the upper extremities and the internal rotation of the upper arms and wrists. The nurse also notes that the lower extremities are extended, with some internal rotation noted at the knees and feet. On the basis of these findings, what is the **initial** nursing action?

1 Notify the neurologist of the change in posturing.
2 Document that the original positioning is unchanged.
3 Attempt to check the flexibility of the child's lower extremities.
4 Plan to continue to monitor the child for posturing every 2 hours.

Level of Cognitive Ability: Synthesizing
Client Needs: Physiological Integrity
Clinical Judgment/Cognitive Skills: Take Action
Integrated Process: Nursing Process/ Implementation
Content Area: Complex Care: Emergency Situations/Management
Health Problem: Pediatric-Specific: Head Injury

Answer: 1

Rationale: Decorticate (flexion) posturing refers to the flexion of the upper extremities and the extension of the lower extremities. Plantar flexion of the feet may also be observed. Decerebrate (extension) posturing involves the extension of the upper extremities with the internal rotation of the upper arms and wrists. The lower extremities will extend with some internal rotation noted at the knees and feet. The progression from decorticate to decerebrate posturing usually indicates deteriorating neurological function and warrants notification of the neurologist. Although documentation is appropriate, it is not the initial action in this situation. The other options are inappropriate.

Priority Nursing Tip: Decorticate (flexion) posturing is seen with severe dysfunction of the cerebral cortex. Decerebrate (extension) posturing is a sign of dysfunction at the level of the midbrain.

Test-Taking Strategy: Focus on the **subject,** decerebrate and decorticate posturing. Also note the **strategic word,** *initial.* Recalling that progression from decorticate to decerebrate posturing usually indicates deteriorating neurological function will direct you to the correct option.

---

155. The parent of a child with a diagnosis of hepatitis B calls the health care clinic to report that the jaundice seems to be worsening. Which response would the nurse make to the parent?

1 "It sounds as if the hepatitis may be worsening."
2 "It is necessary to isolate the child from others in the home."
3 "The jaundice may appear to get worse before it begins to resolve."
4 "You need to bring the child to the health care clinic to see the primary health care provider."

Level of Cognitive Ability: Applying
Client Needs: Physiological Integrity
Clinical Judgment/Cognitive Skills: Take Action
Integrated Process: Nursing Process/ Implementation
Content Area: Pediatrics: Gastrointestinal
Health Problem: Pediatric-Specific: Hepatitis

Answer: 3

Rationale: The parents would be instructed that jaundice may appear to get worse before it resolves. The parents of a child with hepatitis would also be taught the danger signs that could indicate a worsening of the child's condition, specifically changes in neurological status, bleeding, and fluid retention. Based on this information, the statements in the remaining options are incorrect.

Priority Nursing Tip: Proper hand washing and standard precautions can help prevent the spread of viral hepatitis.

Test-Taking Strategy: Focus on the **subject,** the physiology associated with hepatitis, to answer this question. Remember that jaundice worsens before it resolves. This will direct you to the correct option.

---

156. The nurse is preparing to suction a tracheotomy on an infant. The nurse prepares the equipment for the procedure and would turn the suction to which setting?
1 60 mm Hg
2 90 mm Hg
3 110 mm Hg
4 120 mm Hg

Level of Cognitive Ability: Applying
Client Needs: Physiological Integrity
Clinical Judgment/Cognitive Skills: Take Action
Integrated Process: Nursing Process/ Implementation
Content Area: Skills: Tube Care
Health Problem: N/A

Answer: 2
Rationale: The suctioning procedure for pediatric clients varies from that used for adults. Suctioning in infants and children requires the use of a smaller suction catheter and lower suction settings as compared with those used for adults. Suction settings for a neonate are usually 60 to 80 mm Hg; for an infant, 80 to 100 mm Hg; and for larger children, 100 to 120 mm Hg. The pediatrician prescription and agency procedures are always followed.
Priority Nursing Tip: The nurse would always hyperoxygenate the infant before performing respiratory suctioning.

Test-Taking Strategy: Focus on the **subject**, suctioning of an infant's tracheotomy. Recalling the procedure that is used for an adult will assist with directing you to the correct option.

---

157. A client begins to experience seizure activity while in bed. The nurse would provide which intervention to prevent aspiration?
1 Raise the head of the bed.
2 Loosen restrictive clothing.
3 Remove the pillow and raise the padded side rails.
4 Position the client on the side with the head flexed forward.

Level of Cognitive Ability: Applying
Client Needs: Physiological Integrity
Clinical Judgment/Cognitive Skills: Take Action
Integrated Process: Nursing Process/ Implementation
Content Area: Adult Health: Neurological
Health Problem: Adult Health: Neurological: Seizures

Answer: 4
Rationale: Positioning the client on one side with the head flexed forward allows the tongue to fall forward and facilitates the drainage of secretions, which could help prevent aspiration. The nurse would not raise the head of the client's bed. The nurse would remove restrictive clothing and the pillow and raise the padded side rails, if present, but these actions would not decrease the risk of aspiration; rather, they are general safety measures to use during seizure activity.
Priority Nursing Tip: Never place anything into the mouth of a client experiencing a seizure.

Test-Taking Strategy: Focus on the **subject**, preventing aspiration. Use the **ABCs—airway, breathing, and circulation**—and then visualize the effect that each option would have on airway and aspiration to direct you to the correct option.

---

158. The nurse is assisting in caring for a client who has experienced a stroke and has episodes of coughing while swallowing liquids. The client has developed a temperature of 101 °F (38.3 °C) and an oxygen saturation of 91% (down from 98% previously), is slightly confused, and has noticeable dyspnea. Which action would be taken?
1 Notify the primary health care provider.
2 Administer an acetaminophen suppository.
3 Encourage the client to cough and deep-breathe.

Answer: 1
Rationale: The client is exhibiting clinical signs and symptoms of aspiration, which include fever, dyspnea, decreased arterial oxygen levels, and confusion. Other symptoms that occur with this complication are difficulty with managing saliva, or coughing or choking while eating. Because the client has developed a complication that requires medical intervention, the most appropriate action is to contact the primary health care provider. The remaining options are unrelated to the management of aspiration.
Priority Nursing Tip: During the acute phase of a stroke, monitor the client for signs of increased intracranial pressure because the client is most at risk during the first 72 hours after the stroke.

4 Administer a bronchodilator prescribed on an as-needed basis.

Level of Cognitive Ability: Synthesizing
Client Needs: Physiological Integrity
Clinical Judgment/Cognitive Skills: Take Action
Integrated Process: Nursing Process/Implementation
Content Area: Complex Care: Emergency Situations/Management
Health Problem: Adult Health: Neurological: Stroke

Test-Taking Strategy: Focus on the **subject**, a client who has experienced a stroke and episodes of coughing while swallowing liquids, as well as on the client's specific signs/symptoms. This will indicate that aspiration has most likely occurred. Eliminate options 2, 3, and 4 because they do not assist with alleviating this life-threatening condition.

---

159. Which action would the nurse implement as part of care for a client after a bone biopsy for suspected multiple myeloma?
1 Monitoring the vital signs once a day
2 Keeping the area in a dependent position
3 Administering intramuscular opioid analgesics
4 Monitoring the site for swelling, bleeding, or hematoma formation

Level of Cognitive Ability: Applying
Client Needs: Physiological Integrity
Clinical Judgment/Cognitive Skills: Take Action
Integrated Process: Nursing Process/Implementation
Content Area: Foundations of Care: Diagnostic Tests
Health Problem: N/A

Answer: 4
Rationale: Nursing care after bone biopsy includes monitoring the site for swelling, bleeding, or hematoma formation. The vital signs are monitored every 4 hours for 24 hours. The biopsy site is elevated for 24 hours to reduce edema. A dependent position will increase the risk for bleeding. The client usually requires mild analgesics; more severe pain usually indicates that complications are arising.
Priority Nursing Tip: Inform the client that mild to moderate discomfort is normal after a bone biopsy.

Test-Taking Strategy: Focus on the **subject**, care of the client after bone biopsy. Begin to answer this question by recalling that after this procedure, the client must have periodic assessments. With this in mind, eliminate option 1 because the time frame is too infrequent. Knowing that the procedure is done under local anesthesia helps you eliminate option 3 next. From the remaining choices, recall the principles related to circulation and positioning to direct you to the correct option.

---

160. The nurse is caring for a client with rheumatoid arthritis who is scheduled for an arthrogram involving the use of a contrast medium. Which action by the nurse is the **priority**?
1 Determining the presence of client allergies
2 Asking whether the client has any last-minute questions
3 Telling the client to try to void before leaving the unit
4 Emphasizing to the client the importance of remaining still during the procedure

Answer: 1
Rationale: Because of the risk of allergy to contrast medium, the nurse places the highest priority on checking whether the client has an allergy to iodine or shellfish. The nurse also reinforces information about the test and reminds the client about the need to remain still during the procedure. It is helpful to have the client void before the procedure for comfort.
Priority Nursing Tip: The priority nursing action before any procedure involving the injection of a contrast medium is to ask the client about allergies.

Level of Cognitive Ability: Applying
Client Needs: Physiological Integrity
Clinical Judgment/Cognitive Skills: Take Action
Integrated Process: Nursing Process/ Implementation
Content Area: Foundations of Care: Diagnostic Tests
Health Problem: N/A

Test-Taking Strategy: Note the **strategic word,** *priority.* Recalling the risk associated with the administration of contrast medium will direct you to the correct option.

---

161. The nurse responds to a call bell and finds a client lying on the floor after a fall. The nurse suspects that the client's arm may be broken. Which **immediate** action would the nurse take?

1 Immobilize the arm.
2 Take a set of vital signs.
3 Call the radiology department.
4 Ask the client to describe what happened.

Level of Cognitive Ability: Applying
Client Needs: Physiological Integrity
Clinical Judgment/Cognitive Skills: Take Action
Integrated Process: Nursing Process/ Implementation
Content Area: Adult Health: Musculoskeletal
Health Problem: Adult Health: Musculoskeletal: Skeletal Injury

Answer: 1
Rationale: When a fracture is suspected, it is imperative that the area be splinted before the client is moved. Emergency help would be called for if the client is external to a hospital, and a primary health care provider is called if the client is hospitalized. Vital signs would be taken, but this is not the immediate action. The primary health care provider rather than the nurse prescribes an x-ray examination. The nurse needs to remain with the client and provide realistic reassurance. Although the details of the fall are important, such a discussion is not an immediate need.
Priority Nursing Tip: If a fracture is suspected, immobilize the extremity by splinting, including the joints above and below the fracture site. Monitor circulatory status closely after splinting the extremity.

Test-Taking Strategy: Note the **strategic word,** *immediate.* Eliminate option 3 because the primary health care provider will prescribe radiology films. Option 4 is eliminated next because such a discussion is not a priority. From the remaining choices, noting that a fracture is suspected will direct you to the correct option.

---

162. The nurse is caring for a hospitalized 14-year-old child who is placed in Crutchfield traction. The child is having difficulty adjusting to the length of the hospital confinement. Which nursing action would be appropriate to meet the child's needs?

1 Allow the child to play loud music in the hospital room.
2 Let the child wear his or her own clothing when friends visit.
3 Allow the child to have his or her hair dyed if the parent agrees.
4 Allow the child to keep the shades closed and the room darkened.

Level of Cognitive Ability: Applying
Client Needs: Psychosocial Integrity
Clinical Judgment/Cognitive Skills: Take Action

Answer: 2
Rationale: An adolescent needs to identify with peers and has a strong need to belong to a group. The child would be allowed to wear his or her own clothes to feel a sense of belonging to the group. The adolescent likes to dress like the group and to wear similar hairstyles. Loud music may disturb others in the hospital. Because Crutchfield traction involves the use of skeletal pins, hair dye is inappropriate. The child's request for a darkened room is indicative of a possible problem with depression that may require further evaluation and intervention.
Priority Nursing Tip: Hospitalized adolescents become upset if friends go on with their lives, excluding them. For the hospitalized adolescent, separation from friends is a source of anxiety.

Test-Taking Strategy: Focus on the **subject,** a 14-year-old child having difficulty adjusting to the length of the hospital confinement. Specific knowledge of Crutchfield traction and its limitations, as well as of growth and development concepts, will direct you to the correct option.

Integrated Process: Nursing Process/ Implementation
Content Area: Developmental Stages: Adolescent
Health Problem: Pediatric-Specific: Fractures

---

163. The nurse assists to prepare for a client in leg traction to be admitted to the nursing unit. Which **essential** item will be needed to assist the client to move in bed while in leg traction?
1 A foot board
2 Extra pillows
3 A bed trapeze
4 An electric bed

Level of Cognitive Ability: Applying
Client Needs: Physiological Integrity
Clinical Judgment/Cognitive Skills: Take Action
Integrated Process: Nursing Process/ Implementation
Content Area: Skills: Activity/Mobility
Health Problem: Adult Health: Musculoskeletal: Skeletal Injury

Answer: 3
Rationale: A trapeze is essential to allow the client to lift straight up while being moved so that the amount of pull exerted on the limb in traction is not altered. A foot board and extra pillows do not facilitate moving. Either an electric bed or a manual bed can be used for traction, but this does not specifically assist the client with moving in bed.
Priority Nursing Tip: For the client in traction, ensure that pulleys in the traction device are not obstructed and that ropes in the pulleys move freely.

Test-Taking Strategy: Note the **strategic word,** ***essential.*** Attempt to visualize the items identified in the options, and focus on the **subject,** helping the client in leg traction move in bed. This will direct you to the correct option.

---

164. A pregnant client is receiving rehabilitative services for alcohol abuse. How would the nurse provide supportive care? **Select all that apply.**
❒ 1 Assist the client in identifying supportive strategies.
❒ 2 Initiate the possibility of placing the baby up for adoption.
❒ 3 Stress the need for Alcoholics Anonymous (AA) meetings.
❒ 4 Encourage the client to continue counseling after the birth.
❒ 5 Encourage the client to participate in her rehabilitation care.
❒ 6 Promote communication with co-dependent family members.

Level of Cognitive Ability: Analyzing
Client Needs: Health Promotion and Maintenance
Clinical Judgment/Cognitive Skills: Take Action
Integrated Process: Nursing Process/ Implementation
Content Area: Maternity: Antepartum
Health Problem: Mental Health: Addictions

Answer: 1, 3, 4, 5
Rationale: The nurse provides supportive care by encouraging the client to participate in care and to identify coping strategies. Counseling needs to continue after the infant is born. Communication with family members is important, but not when they are supporting the addiction. It is inappropriate to suggest adoption.
Priority Nursing Tip: Fetal alcohol syndrome is caused by maternal alcohol use during pregnancy.

Test-Taking Strategy: Focus on the **subject,** supportive care to a pregnant client for alcohol abuse. Only the correct options provide the client with an active role in care. The incorrect options create barriers for long-term success in dealing with the problem.

---

165. A client in the second trimester of pregnancy is being assessed at the primary health care clinic. The nurse notes that the fetal heart rate (FHR) is 100 beats/min. Which nursing action would be appropriate **initially**?

1 Document the findings as normal.
2 Notify the obstetrician of the finding.
3 Inform the client that the finding is normal and that everything is fine.
4 Instruct the client to return to the clinic in 8 hours for reevaluation of the FHR.

Level of Cognitive Ability: Applying
Client Needs: Physiological Integrity
Clinical Judgment/Cognitive Skills: Take Action
Integrated Process: Nursing Process/ Implementation
Content Area: Maternity: Antepartum
Health Problem: Maternity: Fetal Distress/ Demise

Answer: 2
Rationale: The FHR should be between 110 and 160 beats/min during pregnancy. An FHR of 100 beats/min would require that the obstetrician be notified and the client be further evaluated. Although the nurse would document the findings, the most appropriate nursing action is to notify the obstetrician. Based on this information, eliminate the options that suggest inaccurate nursing actions.
Priority Nursing Tip: The FHR is usually about twice the maternal heart rate. However, an FHR outside the parameters of 110 to 160 beats/min during pregnancy warrants notification of the obstetrician.

Test-Taking Strategy: Note the **strategic word,** ***initially.*** First, eliminate options 1 and 3, which are **comparable or alike** and inaccurate. From the remaining choices, focus on the **subject,** FHR, recalling that the normal range for the FHR is between 110 and 160 beats/min; this will direct you to the correct option.

---

166. A client admitted to the hospital with a diagnosis of a leaking cerebral aneurysm is scheduled for surgery. Which preoperative intervention would the nurse who is assisting with care plan to implement?

1 Place the client on bed rest.
2 Allow the client to ambulate only in the room.
3 Obtain a bedside commode for the client's use.
4 Encourage the client to be up at least twice a day.

Level of Cognitive Ability: Applying
Client Needs: Physiological Integrity
Clinical Judgment/Cognitive Skills: Take Action
Integrated Process: Nursing Process/ Implementation
Content Area: Adult Health: Neurological
Health Problem: Adult Health: Neurological: Aneurysm

Answer: 1
Rationale: The client is placed on aneurysm precautions, and the client's activity is kept to a minimum to prevent Valsalva's maneuver. Clients often hold their breath and strain while pulling up to get out of bed. This exertion may cause a rise in blood pressure, which increases bleeding. Clients who have bleeding aneurysms in any vessel will have activity curtailed. Therefore, the rest of the options are incorrect actions.
Priority Nursing Tip: The primary concern for a client with a cerebral aneurysm is rupture.

Test-Taking Strategy: Focus on the **subject,** the client's diagnosis of a leaking cerebral aneurysm, and the word *preoperative.* Eliminate options 2, 3, and 4, which are **comparable or alike** in that they all involve out-of-bed activity and are incorrect.

---

167. Which is the **most important** laboratory result for the nurse to present to the primary health care provider on a client who is receiving total parenteral nutrition (TPN)?

1 White blood cell count
2 Serum electrolyte levels
3 Arterial blood gas levels
4 Hemoglobin and hematocrit levels

Level of Cognitive Ability: Analyzing
Client Needs: Physiological Integrity
Clinical Judgment/Cognitive Skills: Prioritize Hypotheses
Integrated Process: Nursing Process/Implementation
Content Area: Skills: Nutrition
Health Problem: N/A

Answer: 2

Rationale: TPN solutions contain amino acids and dextrose in solution with electrolytes, trace elements, and other agents added. The provider uses the electrolyte values (including sodium, potassium, and chloride) and the glucose level to determine the effectiveness of the solution, makes changes to the solution as necessary, and decreases the client's risk of a fluid and electrolyte imbalance. It is important to monitor the serum glucose because parenteral nutrition is usually composed of 10% or more dextrose in water. The remaining options can be suitable tests for a client who is receiving TPN, but these results cover a narrower range of information than serum electrolytes.

Priority Nursing Tip: Check the client who is to receive TPN for a history of glucose intolerance. If the client receives the solution too rapidly, does not receive enough insulin, or contracts an infection, hyperglycemia can occur.

Test-Taking Strategy: Note the **strategic words,** *most important,* to choose the laboratory test that provides better information than the other options. Thinking about the purpose of TPN and its components will direct you to option 2.

NURSING PROCESS: EVALUATION

168. The nurse is evaluating the effects of care for the client with nephrotic syndrome. Which diagnostic result demonstrates the least amount of improvement over 2 days of care?

1 Serum albumin 1.9 g/dL, up to 2.0 g/dL
2 Initial weight 208 pounds, down to 203 pounds
3 Blood pressure 160/90 mm Hg, down to 130/78 mm Hg
4 Daily intake and output record of 2100 mL intake and 1900 mL output and 2000 mL intake and 2900 mL output

Level of Cognitive Ability: Evaluating
Client Needs: Physiological Integrity
Clinical Judgment/Cognitive Skills: Evaluate Outcomes
Integrated Process: Nursing Process/Evaluation
Content Area: Adult Health: Renal and Urinary
Health Problem: Adult Health: Renal and Urinary: Inflammation/Infections

Answer: 1

Rationale: The goal of therapy in nephrotic syndrome is to heal the leaking glomerular membrane. This would then control edema by stopping the loss of protein in the urine. Fluid balance and albumin levels are monitored to determine the effectiveness of therapy. The least amount of improvement is in the serum albumin level because the normal albumin level is 3.5 to 5 g/dL. Option 2 represents a loss of fluid that slightly exceeds 2 L and represents a significant improvement. Option 3 shows improvement because both systolic and diastolic blood pressures are lower. Option 4 represents an increased fluid loss, which indicates improvement.

Priority Nursing Tip: For the client with nephrotic syndrome, bed rest is important if severe edema is present.

Test-Taking Strategy: Focus on the **subject,** the information that identifies the least amount of improvement. Option 2 illustrates the greatest improvement and is eliminated first. Option 4 is also a significant improvement and is eliminated next. From the remaining choices, noting that the blood pressure has decreased significantly will direct you to the correct option.

---

169. A client is being discharged after the application of a plaster leg cast. The nurse determines that the client understands the proper care of the cast when the client states the need to engage in which action?

1 Avoid getting the cast wet.
2 Cover the casted leg with warm blankets.
3 Use the fingertips to lift and move the leg.
4 Use a padded coat hanger end to scratch under the cast.

Level of Cognitive Ability: Evaluating
Client Needs: Physiological Integrity
Clinical Judgment/Cognitive Skills: Evaluate Outcomes
Integrated Process: Nursing Process/Evaluation
Content Area: Adult Health: Musculoskeletal
Health Problem: Adult Health: Musculoskeletal: Skeletal Injury

Answer: 1

Rationale: A plaster cast must remain dry to keep its strength. Air needs to circulate freely around the cast to help it dry. Additionally, the cast also gives off heat as it dries. The cast would be handled using the palms of the hands rather than the fingertips until it is fully dry. The client would never scratch under the cast. A cool hair dryer may be used to relieve an itch.

Priority Nursing Tip: The client with a plaster cast needs to be taught to keep the cast clean and dry.

Test-Taking Strategy: Focus on the **subject,** cast care. Option 4 is dangerous to skin integrity and is eliminated first. Recalling that the cast needs to dry eliminates option 2. Knowing that a wet cast can be dented with the fingertips, causing pressure underneath, helps you eliminate option 3. Remember that plaster casts, when they have dried after application, would not become wet.

---

170. The client recovering from an acute kidney injury demonstrates an understanding of the therapeutic dietary regimen when indicating a need to limit which dietary factor?

1 Fats
2 Vitamins
3 Potassium
4 Carbohydrates

Level of Cognitive Ability: Evaluating
Client Needs: Physiological Integrity
Clinical Judgment/Cognitive Skills: Evaluate Outcomes
Integrated Process: Nursing Process/Evaluation
Content Area: Adult Health: Renal and Urinary
Health Problem: Adult Health: Renal and Urinary: Acute Kidney Injury

Answer: 3

Rationale: Most of the excretion of potassium and the control of potassium balance are normal functions of the kidneys. In the client with renal failure, potassium intake must be restricted as much as possible. The primary mechanism of potassium removal with acute kidney injury is dialysis. None of the remaining options are normally restricted in the client with acute kidney injury unless a secondary health problem warrants the need to do so.

Priority Nursing Tip: Foods that are low in potassium include green beans, applesauce, cabbage, lettuce, peppers, grapes, blueberries, cooked summer squash or turnip greens, pineapple, or raspberries.

Test-Taking Strategy: Focusing on the **subject,** a client recovering from acute kidney injury, will assist you with answering this question. Recalling that potassium balance and excretion are controlled by the kidney will direct you to the correct option.

---

171. The nurse assists a client with a history of anxiety and command hallucinations to harm self or others by reinforcing information about appropriate management techniques. Which client statement indicates that the client understands these techniques?

1. "I shouldn't talk about the voices I hear because it will scare others."
2. "If I take my prescribed medication as I'm supposed to, I won't be so anxious."
3. "I can call my counselor so that I can talk about my feelings and not hurt anyone."
4. "If I get enough sleep and eat well, I will be less likely to get anxious and hear things."

Level of Cognitive Ability: Evaluating
Client Needs: Psychosocial Integrity
Clinical Judgment/Cognitive Skills: Evaluate Outcomes
Integrated Process: Nursing Process/Evaluation
Content Area: Mental Health
Health Problem: Mental Health: Anxiety Disorder

Answer: 3
Rationale: There may be an increased risk for impulsive or aggressive behavior if a client is receiving command hallucinations to harm self or others. The client should call his or her counselor to talk about feelings or command hallucinations. Talking about auditory hallucinations can interfere with the subvocal muscular activity that is associated with a hallucination. The remaining options are general techniques, but they are not specific to anxiety and hallucinations.
Priority Nursing Tip: Monitor the client experiencing command hallucinations for signs of increasing fear, anxiety, or agitation.

Test-Taking Strategy: Focus on the **subject,** anxiety and hallucinations. The incorrect options are all interventions that a client can do to aid general wellness. The correct option is specific to the subject and indicates self-responsible commitment and control over the client's own behavior.

---

172. A perinatal client has been instructed about the prevention of genital tract infections. Which statement by the client indicates an understanding of these preventive measures?

1. "I can douche anytime I want."
2. "I can wear my tight-fitting jeans."
3. "I should avoid the use of condoms."
4. "I need to wear underwear with a cotton panel liner."

Level of Cognitive Ability: Evaluating
Client Needs: Health Promotion and Maintenance
Clinical Judgment/Cognitive Skills: Evaluate Outcomes
Integrated Process: Nursing Process/Evaluation
Content Area: Maternity: Antepartum
Health Problem: Maternity: Infections/Inflammations

Answer: 4
Rationale: Wearing items with a cotton panel liner allows for air movement in and around the genital area. Douching is to be avoided. Wearing tight clothes irritates the genital area and does not allow for air circulation. Condoms would be used to minimize the spread of genital tract infections.
Priority Nursing Tip: Instruct the client with a genital tract infection to avoid the use of perfumed toilet paper, sanitary napkins, and feminine hygiene sprays. These items will irritate the genital area.

Test-Taking Strategy: Focus on the **subject,** the client's understanding of preventing genital tract infections. Options 1, 2, and 3 are incorrect statements regarding prevention of infections.

---

173. Addressing a client with coronary heart disease, the nurse reinforces information about the use of sublingual nitroglycerin tablets prescribed for as-needed use if chest pain occurs. Which client statement helps assure the nurse that the client understands how to self-administer the medication?

1 "I will keep the nitroglycerin in a shirt pocket close to my body."
2 "I won't take the medication until the chest pain actually begins and intensifies."
3 "If I get a headache when I first start taking the nitroglycerin, then I will take an aspirin."
4 "I will discard unused nitroglycerin tablets 3 to 6 months after the bottle is opened and obtain a new prescription."

Level of Cognitive Ability: Evaluating
Client Needs: Physiological Integrity
Clinical Judgment/Cognitive Skills: Evaluate Outcomes
Integrated Process: Nursing Process/Evaluation
Content Area: Pharmacology: Cardiovascular: Vasodilators
Health Problem: Adult Health: Cardiovascular: Coronary Artery Disease

Answer: 4
Rationale: Nitroglycerin may be self-administered sublingually 5 to 10 minutes before an activity that triggers chest pain. Tablets would be discarded 3 to 6 months after opening the bottle (per expiration date), and a new bottle of pills would be obtained from the pharmacy. Nitroglycerin is unstable and is affected by heat and cold, so it would not be kept close to the body (warmth) in a shirt pocket; rather, it needs to be kept in a jacket pocket or a purse. Headache often occurs with early use and diminishes in time. Acetaminophen may be used to treat headache.
Priority Nursing Tip: The nurse needs to teach a client taking nitroglycerin to store the medication in a dark, tightly closed bottle. Additionally, the client needs to be informed that tablets will not relieve chest pain if they have expired.

Test-Taking Strategy: Focus on the **subject**, self-administration of nitroglycerin. Recalling that nitroglycerin loses its potency in 3 to 6 months will direct you to the correct option.

---

174. A client who had a laryngectomy for laryngeal cancer has started oral intake. The nurse determines that the first stage of dietary advancement has been tolerated when the client ingests which type of diet without aspirating or choking?

1 Bland
2 Full liquids
3 Clear liquids
4 Semisolid foods

Level of Cognitive Ability: Evaluating
Client Needs: Physiological Integrity
Clinical Judgment/Cognitive Skills: Evaluate Outcomes
Integrated Process: Nursing Process/Evaluation
Content Area: Foundations of Care: Therapeutic Diets
Health Problem: Adult Health: Cancer: Laryngeal and Lung

Answer: 4
Rationale: Oral intake after laryngectomy is started with semisolid foods. When the client can manage this type of food, liquids may be introduced. A bland diet is inappropriate. The client may be unable to tolerate the texture of some of the solid foods that would be included in a bland diet. Thin liquids are not given until the risk of aspiration is negligible.
Priority Nursing Tip: After laryngectomy (radical neck dissection), place the client in a semi-Fowler's to Fowler's position to maintain a patent airway and minimize edema.

Test-Taking Strategy: Focus on the **subject**, swallowing and aspiration concerns related to a postoperative laryngectomy. Eliminate options 2 and 3 by recalling that a client with swallowing difficulty will not be able to manage liquids. From the remaining choices, recall that a bland diet provides no control over the consistency or texture of the food.

---

175. An older client is a victim of elder abuse. He and his family have been attending counseling sessions for the past month. Which statement, made by the abusive family member, would indicate an understanding of more positive coping skills?

1 "I will be more careful to make sure that my father's needs are 100% met."
2 "I am so sorry and embarrassed that the abusive event occurred. It won't happen again."
3 "I feel better equipped to care for my father now that I know where to turn if I need assistance."
4 "Now that my father is going to move into my home with me, I will have to stop drinking alcohol."

Level of Cognitive Ability: Evaluating
Client Needs: Psychosocial Integrity
Clinical Judgment/Cognitive Skills: Evaluate Outcomes
Integrated Process: Nursing Process/Evaluation
Content Area: Mental Health
Health Problem: Mental Health: Abusive Behaviors

Answer: 3

Rationale: Elder abuse is sometimes caused by family members who are being expected to care for their aging parents. This care can cause the family to become overextended, frustrated, or financially depleted. Knowing where to turn in the community for assistance with caring for an aging family member can bring much-needed relief. Using these alternatives is a positive coping skill for many families. The rest of the options are statements of good faith or promises, which may or may not be kept in the future.

Priority Nursing Tip: When working with caregivers, determine the need for respite care or the need for other support systems.

Test-Taking Strategy: Focus on the **subject,** positive coping skills. The correct option is the only choice that identifies a means of coping with the issues and that outlines a definitive plan for how to handle the pressure associated with the father's care.

---

176. A 24-hour-old term infant had a confirmed episode of hypoglycemia when 1 hour old. Which observation by the nurse would indicate the **need for follow-up**?

1 Weight loss of 4 ounces and dry, peeling skin
2 Breast-feeding for 20 minutes or more, with strong sucking
3 High-pitched cry, drinking 10 to 15 mL of formula per feeding
4 Blood glucose level of 40 mg/dL before the last feeding

Level of Cognitive Ability: Evaluating
Client Needs: Physiological Integrity
Clinical Judgment/Cognitive Skills: Evaluate Outcomes
Integrated Process: Nursing Process/Evaluation
Content Area: Maternity: Newborn
Health Problem: N/A

Answer: 3

Rationale: Hypoglycemia causes central nervous system symptoms (high-pitched cry), and it is also exhibited by a lack of strength for eating enough for growth. At 24 hours old, a term infant would be able to consume at least 1 ounce of formula per feeding. A high-pitched cry is indicative of neurological involvement. Weight loss over the first few days of life and dry, peeling skin are normal findings for term infants. Blood glucose levels are acceptable at 40 mg/dL during the first few days of life. Breast-feeding for 20 minutes with a strong suck is an excellent finding.

Priority Nursing Tip: In the newborn, a low blood glucose level is prevented through early feedings.

Test-Taking Strategy: Note the **strategic words,** *need for follow-up.* These words indicate a **negative event query** and ask you to select an option that is an abnormal finding. Eliminate options 1, 2, and 4, which are **comparable or alike** and are normal findings. The words *high-pitched cry* would direct you to the correct option.

---

177. The nurse assists in collecting data on a child with a diagnosis of celiac disease. Which finding **best** indicates that a gluten-free diet is being maintained and has been **effective?**

1 The child is free of diarrhea.
2 The child is free of bloody stools.
3 The child tolerates dietary wheat and rye.
4 A balanced fluid and electrolyte status is noted on the laboratory results.

Level of Cognitive Ability: Evaluating
Client Needs: Physiological Integrity
Clinical Judgment/Cognitive Skills: Evaluate Outcomes
Integrated Process: Nursing Process/Evaluation
Content Area: Pediatrics: Gastrointestinal
Health Problem: Pediatric-Specific: GI and Rectal Problems

Answer: 1
Rationale: Watery diarrhea is a frequent clinical manifestation of celiac disease. The absence of diarrhea indicates effective treatment. Bloody stools are not associated with this disease. The grains of wheat and rye contain gluten and are not allowed. A balance of fluids and electrolytes does not necessarily demonstrate an improved status of celiac disease.
Priority Nursing Tip: The nurse needs to instruct the parents of a child with celiac disease about lifelong elimination of gluten sources.

Test-Taking Strategy: Note the **strategic words,** *best* and *effective.* Focus on the **subject,** a child with celiac disease. Recalling that watery diarrhea is a manifestation of celiac disease will direct you to the correct option.

---

178. A woman in labor is receiving oxytocin by intravenous infusion. The nurse assisting in monitoring the client knows that which finding indicates an adequate contraction pattern?

1 One contraction per minute, with resultant cervical dilation
2 Four contractions every 5 minutes, with resultant cervical dilation
3 One contraction every 10 minutes, without resultant cervical dilation
4 Three to five contractions in a 10-minute period, with resultant cervical dilation

Level of Cognitive Ability: Evaluating
Client Needs: Physiological Integrity
Clinical Judgment/Cognitive Skills: Evaluate Outcomes
Integrated Process: Nursing Process/Evaluation
Content Area: Pharmacology: Maternity/Newborn: Uterine Stimulants
Health Problem: N/A

Answer: 4
Rationale: The preferred oxytocin dosage is the minimal amount necessary to maintain an adequate contraction pattern, characterized by three to five contractions in a 10-minute period, with resultant cervical dilation. If contractions are more frequent than every 2 minutes, contraction quality may be decreased.
Priority Nursing Tip: A woman in labor who is receiving oxytocin would not be left unattended.

Test-Taking Strategy: Focus on the **subject,** an adequate contraction pattern in a client receiving oxytocin. Recall that an adequate contraction pattern is characterized by three to five contractions in a 10-minute period, with resultant cervical dilation; this will assist you with eliminating the incorrect options.

---

179. A preschooler has a diagnosis of scarlet fever and is on bed rest. What data obtained by the nurse would indicate that the child is coping with the illness and bed rest?

1 The child insists that his parent stay in the room.
2 The child is coloring and drawing pictures in a notebook.

Answer: 2
Rationale: According to Jean Piaget, for the preschooler, play is the best way to understand and adjust to life's experiences. Preschoolers are able to use pencils and crayons, and they can draw stick figures and other rudimentary things. A child with scarlet fever needs quiet play, and drawing will provide that. Based on this information, none of the remaining options address positive coping mechanisms.

3 The parent keeps providing new activities for the child to do.
4 The child sucks his thumb whenever he does not get what he asked for.

Level of Cognitive Ability: Evaluating
Client Needs: Health Promotion and Maintenance
Clinical Judgment/Cognitive Skills: Evaluate Outcomes
Integrated Process: Nursing Process/Evaluation
Content Area: Developmental Stages: Preschool and School Age
Health Problem: Pediatric-Specific: Communicable Diseases

Priority Nursing Tip: Scarlet fever is transmitted via direct contact with an infected person or droplet spread, or indirectly by contact with infected articles, ingestion of contaminated milk, or other foods.

Test-Taking Strategy: Note the **subject**, the coping behavior of a preschooler with scarlet fever. Think about the developmental level of a preschooler. Look at the data obtained by the nurse to determine whether the child is coping with the disease and bed rest. The correct option is a positive coping mechanism for preschoolers. None of the remaining options address positive coping mechanisms.

---

180. A client with gastritis has just taken a dose of trimethobenzamide. The nurse determines that the medication has been **effective** when the client states relief of which sign/symptom?
1 Nausea
2 Heartburn
3 Constipation
4 Abdominal pain

Level of Cognitive Ability: Evaluating
Client Needs: Physiological Integrity
Clinical Judgment/Cognitive Skills: Evaluate Outcomes
Integrated Process: Nursing Process/Evaluation
Content Area: Pharmacology: Gastrointestinal: Antiemetics
Health Problem: N/A

Answer: 1
Rationale: Trimethobenzamide is an antiemetic agent that is used for the treatment of nausea and vomiting. The medication is not used to treat heartburn, constipation, or abdominal pain.
Priority Nursing Tip: Antinausea medications cause drowsiness; therefore, safety is a concern when they are administered.

Test-Taking Strategy: Note the **strategic word,** *effective.* Focus on the **subject,** the intended effect of trimethobenzamide. Recalling that trimethobenzamide is an antiemetic will direct you to option 1.

---

181. The nurse is reinforcing instructions to the client of a child with a diagnosis of strabismus of the left eye. Which statement by the client indicates that the client understands the procedure for patching?
1 "I will place the patch on both eyes."
2 "I will place the patch on the left eye."
3 "I will place the patch on the right eye."
4 "I will alternate the patch from the right eye to the left eye every hour."

Level of Cognitive Ability: Evaluating
Client Needs: Physiological Integrity
Clinical Judgment/Cognitive Skills: Evaluate Outcomes

Answer: 3
Rationale: Patching may be used for the treatment of strabismus to strengthen the weak eye. With this treatment, the good eye is patched; this encourages the child to use the weaker eye. The treatment is most successful when it is performed during the preschool years. The schedule for patching is individualized and prescribed by the ophthalmologist.
Priority Nursing Tip: Strabismus is also known as "squint" or "lazy eye."

Test-Taking Strategy: Focus on the **subject**, patching the eye related to the treatment of strabismus. Remembering that this condition involves a lazy eye will direct you to the correct option. It makes sense to patch the unaffected eye to strengthen the muscles in the affected eye.

Integrated Process: Nursing Process/Evaluation
Content Area: Pediatrics: Eye/Ear
Health Problem: Pediatric-Specific: Eye Focus and Alignment Disorders

---

182. The nurse is collecting data on a client with gestational hypertension who was admitted to the hospital 48 hours ago. Which current data would indicate that the condition has not yet resolved?

1 Urinary output increased
2 Presence of trace urinary protein
3 Client complaints of blurred vision
4 Blood pressure reading at prenatal baseline

Level of Cognitive Ability: Evaluating
Client Needs: Physiological Integrity
Clinical Judgment/Cognitive Skills: Evaluate Outcomes
Integrated Process: Nursing Process/Evaluation
Content Area: Maternity: Antepartum
Health Problem: Maternity: Gestational Hypertension/Preeclampsia and Eclampsia

Answer: 3
Rationale: Client complaints of headache or blurred vision indicate a worsening of the condition and warrant immediate further evaluation. The remaining options are all signs that the gestational hypertension is being resolved.
Priority Nursing Tip: Signs of preeclampsia are hypertension and proteinuria. Note that some primary health care providers do not consider proteinuria a reliable indicator of preeclampsia.

Test-Taking Strategy: Note the words *not yet resolved.* This asks you to select an option that is an abnormal finding. Focus on the **subject**, identifying a symptom of gestational hypertension that still exists. Eliminate options that are normal findings (options 1 and 4). From the remaining choices, note that option 2 contains the word *trace* and is the most normal finding of options 2 and 3.

---

183. A client has begun medication therapy with betaxolol. The nurse determines that the client is experiencing the intended effect of therapy if which observation is noted?

1 Edema present at 3 +
2 Weight loss of 5 pounds within 2 days
3 Pulse rate increased from 58 to 74 beats/min
4 Blood pressure decreased from 142/94 mm Hg to 128/82 mm Hg

Level of Cognitive Ability: Evaluating
Client Needs: Physiological Integrity
Clinical Judgment/Cognitive Skills: Evaluate Outcomes
Integrated Process: Nursing Process/Evaluation
Content Area: Pharmacology: Cardiovascular: Beta-blockers
Health Problem: N/A

Answer: 4
Rationale: Betaxolol is a beta-adrenergic blocking agent used to lower blood pressure, relieve angina, or eliminate dysrhythmias. Side/adverse effects include bradycardia and symptoms of heart failure, such as weight gain and increased edema.
Priority Nursing Tip: Beta-adrenergic blocking agents are used with caution in clients with diabetes mellitus because they may mask the symptoms of hypoglycemia.

Test-Taking Strategy: Focus on the **subject**, the intended effect of the betaxolol. Remember that beta-adrenergic blocking agent medication names end with the suffix *-lol.* Recalling the action of the medication will direct you to the correct option.

---

184. When a client with asthma is prescribed a xanthine bronchodilator, the nurse reinforces information about beverages to avoid with this medication. The nurse determines that the client understands the information if the client chooses which beverage from the dietary menu?

1 Cola
2 Coffee
3 Chocolate milk
4 Cranberry juice

Level of Cognitive Ability: Evaluating
Client Needs: Physiological Integrity
Clinical Judgment/Cognitive Skills: Evaluate Outcomes
Integrated Process: Nursing Process/Evaluation
Content Area: Pharmacology: Respiratory: Medications for Restrictive Airway Disease
Health Problem: Adult Health: Respiratory: Obstructive Pulmonary Disease

Answer: 4
Rationale: Cola, coffee, and chocolate contain xanthine and would be avoided by the client who is taking a xanthine bronchodilator. This could lead to an increased incidence of cardiovascular and central nervous system side effects that can occur with the use of these types of bronchodilators.
Priority Nursing Tip: Theophylline, a bronchodilator, increases the risk of digoxin toxicity and decreases the effects of lithium and phenytoin.

Test-Taking Strategy: Focus on the **subject**, an acceptable beverage to consume. Note that options 1, 2, and 3 are **comparable or alike** in that they all contain some form of stimulant; therefore, these options can be eliminated.

---

185. A client is prescribed glipizide once daily. What intended effect of this medication would the nurse observe for?

1 Weight loss
2 Resolution of infection
3 Decreased blood glucose
4 Decreased blood pressure

Level of Cognitive Ability: Evaluating
Client Needs: Physiological Integrity
Clinical Judgment/Cognitive Skills: Evaluate Outcomes
Integrated Process: Nursing Process/Evaluation
Content Area: Pharmacology: Endocrine: Oral Hypoglycemics
Health Problem: N/A

Answer: 3
Rationale: Glipizide is an oral hypoglycemic agent that is taken in the morning. It is not used to enhance weight loss, treat infection, or decrease blood pressure.
Priority Nursing Tip: Clients prescribed hypoglycemic agents require education regarding the possible side and adverse effects, including signs of hypoglycemia.

Test-Taking Strategy: Focus on the **subject**, the intended effect of glipizide. Recalling that this medication is an oral hypoglycemic will direct you to the correct option.

---

186. A client regularly takes nonsteroidal anti-inflammatory drugs (NSAIDs), and misoprostol has been added to the medication regimen. The nurse would monitor the client for the relief of which sign/symptom?

1 Diarrhea
2 Bleeding
3 Infection
4 Epigastric pain

Level of Cognitive Ability: Evaluating
Client Needs: Physiological Integrity
Clinical Judgment/Cognitive Skills: Evaluate Outcomes

Answer: 4
Rationale: The client who regularly takes NSAIDs is prone to gastric mucosal injury, which gives the client epigastric pain as a symptom. Misoprostol is administered to prevent this occurrence. Diarrhea can be a side effect of the medication, but its relief is not an intended effect. Bleeding and infection are unrelated to the question.
Priority Nursing Tip: NSAIDs are contraindicated in clients with hypersensitivity or liver or renal disease.

Test-Taking Strategy: Focus on the **subject**, the relief of a sign/symptom in a client taking both NSAIDs and misoprostol. This tells you that the misoprostol is being given to treat or prevent the occurrence of a specific sign/symptom. Recalling that NSAIDs can cause gastric mucosal injury will direct you to the correct option.

Integrated Process: Nursing Process/Evaluation
Content Area: Pharmacology: Gastrointestinal: Gastric Protectants
Health Problem: N/A

---

187. A client has received a dose of an as-needed medication loperamide. The nurse evaluates the client after administration to determine whether the client has relief of which sign/symptom?

1 Diarrhea
2 Tarry stools
3 Constipation
4 Abdominal pain

Level of Cognitive Ability: Evaluating
Client Needs: Physiological Integrity
Clinical Judgment/Cognitive Skills: Evaluate Outcomes
Integrated Process: Nursing Process/Evaluation
Content Area: Pharmacology: Gastrointestinal: Antidiarrheals
Health Problem: N/A

Answer: 1
Rationale: Loperamide is an antidiarrheal agent, and it is commonly administered after loose stools. It is used for the management of acute diarrhea and also for chronic diarrhea, such as with inflammatory bowel disease. It can also be used to reduce the volume of drainage from an ileostomy. It is not intended to treat any of the other options.
Priority Nursing Tip: Goals for a client with diarrhea are to identify and treat the underlying cause, treat dehydration, replace fluids and electrolytes, relieve abdominal discomfort and cramping, and reduce the passage of stool.

Test-Taking Strategy: Focus on the **subject,** the intended effect of loperamide. Recalling that this medication is an antidiarrheal agent will direct you to the correct option.

---

188. The nurse has reinforced discharge instructions to the parent of a child who has undergone heart surgery. Which statement by the parent would indicate the **need for further instruction?**

1 "My child can return to school for full days 1 week after discharge."
2 "I should allow my child to play inside but omit outside play at this time."
3 "I should have my child avoid crowds of people for 2 weeks after discharge."
4 "I should call the primary health care provider if my child develops faster or harder breathing than normal."

Level of Cognitive Ability: Evaluating
Client Needs: Safe and Effective Care Environment
Clinical Judgment/Cognitive Skills: Evaluate Outcomes
Integrated Process: Nursing Process/Evaluation
Content Area: Pediatrics: Cardiovascular
Health Problem: Pediatric-Specific: Congenital Cardiac Defects

Answer: 1
Rationale: The child may return to school the third week after hospital discharge, but he or she would go to school for half days for the first week. Outside play needs to be omitted for several weeks, with inside play allowed as tolerated. The child would avoid crowds of people for 2 weeks after discharge, including crowds at day care centers and churches. If any difficulty with breathing occurs, the parent would notify the primary health care provider.
Priority Nursing Tip: After cardiac surgery, the parents would be instructed to keep the child away from crowds for 2 weeks after discharge to decrease the risk of contracting an infection.

Test-Taking Strategy: Note the **strategic words,** *need for further instruction.* This indicates a **negative event query** and asks you to select an option that is an incorrect statement. Recalling the principles related to the prevention of infection and the complications of surgery will direct you to the correct option.

---

189. A client has been taking nadolol for the past month. Which finding would indicate a therapeutic effect of the medication?

1 The client is afebrile.
2 The client has clear breath sounds.
3 The client reports no episodes of headache.
4 The client has a blood pressure of 118/72 mm Hg.

Level of Cognitive Ability: Evaluating
Client Needs: Physiological Integrity
Clinical Judgment/Cognitive Skills: Evaluate Outcomes
Integrated Process: Nursing Process/Evaluation
Content Area: Pharmacology: Cardiovascular: Beta-blockers
Health Problem: N/A

Answer: 4
Rationale: Nadolol is a beta-adrenergic blocking agent that is used to treat hypertension. Therefore, a blood pressure within the normal range would indicate an effective response to the medication. Based on this information, the remaining options are unrelated to the action of this medication.
Priority Nursing Tip: Beta blockers may be prescribed to treat angina, dysrhythmias, hypertension, migraine headaches, and glaucoma and to prevent myocardial infarction.

Test-Taking Strategy: Focus on the **subject,** the therapeutic effect of nadolol. Remember that an evaluation-type question addresses a client's response to a treatment measure. In addition, recalling that medication names that end with *-lol* are beta-blocking agents will direct you to the correct option.

---

190. The nurse is assisting in the care of a client diagnosed with acquired immunodeficiency syndrome (AIDS) who is receiving amphotericin B for a fungal respiratory infection. When evaluating for the effects of the medication, which would indicate an adverse effect?

1 Hypokalemia
2 Hypernatremia
3 Hypochloremia
4 Hypercalcemia

Level of Cognitive Ability: Evaluating
Client Needs: Physiological Integrity
Clinical Judgment/Cognitive Skills: Evaluate Outcomes
Integrated Process: Nursing Process/Evaluation
Content Area: Pharmacology: Immune: Antifungals
Health Problem: Adult Health: Immune: Immunodeficiency Syndrome

Answer: 1
Rationale: Clients receiving amphotericin B may develop hypokalemia, which can be severe and lead to extreme muscle weakness and electrocardiogram changes. Distal renal tubular acidosis commonly occurs, and this contributes to the development of hypokalemia. High potassium levels do not occur. The medication does not cause sodium, chloride, or calcium levels to fluctuate.
Priority Nursing Tip: Amphotericin B is nephrotoxic, and the nurse needs to monitor the client closely for signs of nephrotoxicity such as decreased urine output and elevated blood urea nitrogen levels or creatinine levels.

Test-Taking Strategy: Focus on the **subject,** an adverse effect of amphotericin B, and recall that it is an antifungal medication. It is necessary to recall that hypokalemia is an adverse effect of this medication. This will direct you to the correct option.

---

191. A client is seen in the health care clinic, and a diagnosis of conjunctivitis is made. The nurse provides instructions to the client regarding the care of the disorder while at home. Which statement by the client indicates the **need for further teaching?**

1 "I can use an ophthalmic analgesic ointment at night if I have eye discomfort."

Answer: 2
Rationale: Conjunctivitis is highly contagious. Antibiotic drops are usually administered 4 times a day. Ophthalmic analgesic ointment or drops may be instilled, especially at bedtime because discomfort becomes more noticeable when the eyelids are closed. When purulent discharge is present, saline eye irrigations or applications of warm compresses to the eye may be necessary before instilling the medication.

2 "I do not need to be concerned about spreading this infection to others in my family."
3 "I would apply warm compresses before instilling antibiotic drops if purulent discharge is present in my eye."
4 "I would perform saline eye irrigation before instilling the antibiotic drops into my eye if purulent discharge is present."

Level of Cognitive Ability: Evaluating
Client Needs: Safe and Effective Care Environment
Clinical Judgment/Cognitive Skills: Evaluate Outcomes
Integrated Process: Nursing Process/Evaluation
Content Area: Adult Health: Eye
Health Problem: Adult Health: Eye: Inflammation/Infections

Priority Nursing Tip: Instruct the client with conjunctivitis about the importance of infection control measures such as good hand washing and not sharing towels and washcloths.

Test-Taking Strategy: Note the **strategic words,** *need for further teaching.* This indicates a **negative event query** and asks you to select an incorrect statement. Knowing that this disorder is considered highly contagious will direct you to the correct option.

---

192. The nurse reviews the nursing care plan of a hospitalized preschool child who is immobilized as a result of skeletal traction. The nurse notes concerns related to the child's development because of immobilization and hospitalization. Which evaluative statement indicates a positive outcome for the child?
1 The fracture heals without complications.
2 The caregivers verbalize safe and effective home care.
3 The child maintains normal joint and muscle integrity.
4 The child displays age-appropriate developmental behaviors.

Level of Cognitive Ability: Evaluating
Client Needs: Health Promotion and Maintenance
Clinical Judgment/Cognitive Skills: Evaluate Outcomes
Integrated Process: Nursing Process/Evaluation
Content Area: Developmental Stages: Preschool and School Age
Health Problem: Pediatric-Specific: Fractures

Answer: 4
Rationale: Regression and inappropriate developmental behaviors may be displayed in response to immobilization and hospitalization. With individualized care planning, a positive outcome of age-appropriate behavior can be achieved. The remaining options are appropriate evaluative statements for an immobilized child, but they do not directly address the child's development.
Priority Nursing Tip: For the hospitalized child who is immobilized, focus on the child's ability and needs. Accept regression in the child but encourage independence.

Test-Taking Strategy: Focus on the **subject,** concerns regarding growth and development. Recalling that issues with development involve an individual not performing age-appropriate tasks will direct you to the correct option. All options are evaluative statements, but only the correct option addresses development.

---

193. The nurse has been encouraging the intake of oral fluids for a client in labor to improve hydration. Which indicates a successful outcome of this action?

1 Ketones in the urine
2 A urine specific gravity of 1.020
3 A blood pressure of 150/90 mm Hg
4 The continued leaking of amniotic fluid during labor

Level of Cognitive Ability: Evaluating
Client Needs: Physiological Integrity
Clinical Judgment/Cognitive Skills: Evaluate Outcomes
Integrated Process: Nursing Process/Evaluation
Content Area: Maternity: Intrapartum
Health Problem: N/A

Answer: 2

Rationale: Urine specific gravity measures the concentration of the urine. During the first stage of labor, the renal system has a tendency to concentrate urine. Labor and birth require hydration and caloric intake to replenish energy expenditure and promote efficient uterine function. An elevated blood pressure and ketones in the urine are not expected outcomes related to labor and hydration. After the membranes have ruptured, it is expected that amniotic fluid may continue to leak.

Priority Nursing Tip: The woman in labor is at risk for hypovolemia because of the dehydrating effects of labor. However, if the laboring woman is receiving intravenous fluids, the risk of hypervolemia is present.

Test-Taking Strategy: Focus on the **subject,** a successful outcome related to oral intake. Recalling the relationship of oral intake to urine concentration will direct you to the correct option.

---

194. A goal for a postpartum client states, "The client will remain free of infection during her hospital stay." Which data would support that the goal has been met?

1 Normal appetite
2 Absence of fever
3 Minimal vaginal bleeding
4 Moderate breast tenderness

Level of Cognitive Ability: Evaluating
Client Needs: Physiological Integrity
Clinical Judgment/Cognitive Skills: Evaluate Outcomes
Integrated Process: Nursing Process/Evaluation
Content Area: Maternity: Postpartum
Health Problem: Maternity: Infections/Inflammations

Answer: 2

Rationale: Fever is the first indication of an infection. Therefore, the absence of a fever indicates that an infection is not present. The remaining options are not associated with a postpartum infection.

Priority Nursing Tip: In the postpartum client, a temperature up to 100.4°F (38°C) is normal because of the dehydrating effects of labor.

Test-Taking Strategy: Focus on the **subject,** the physical indications of an infection. The question is asking for a means of evaluating the effectiveness of a goal that relates to infection. Options 1, 3, and 4 are not related to postpartum infection.

---

195. The nurse is monitoring the nutritional status of a client who is receiving enteral nutrition. Which would the nurse monitor as the **best** clinical indicator of the client's nutritional status?

1 Daily weight
2 Calorie count
3 Skinfold measurement
4 Serum prealbumin level

Level of Cognitive Ability: Evaluating
Client Needs: Physiological Integrity

Answer: 4

Rationale: A serum prealbumin level is the most important parameter for determining the effectiveness of a client's nutritional management and nutritional status. Because prealbumin is a major plasma protein with a short half-life, it is sensitive to changes in protein synthesis and catabolism, and it is thus the best clinical indicator of nutritional status. It is a better nutritional index than a daily weight because body weight can be skewed quickly by changes in total body fluid. It is also a better index than anthropomorphic measurements because nutritional status is not necessarily related to skinfold thickness. The calorie count reports the total calories provided to the client without data regarding the client's use of the calories and nutrients.

Clinical Judgment/Cognitive Skills: Evaluate Outcomes
Integrated Process: Nursing Process/Evaluation
Content Area: Skills: Nutrition
Health Problem: N/A

Priority Nursing Tip: Enteral nutrition provides liquefied foods into the gastrointestinal tract via a tube.

Test-Taking Strategy: Note the **strategic word,** *best.* This tells you that the correct option is a better indicator of nutritional status than the remaining options. Remember that the prealbumin is a major plasma protein and is sensitive to changes in protein synthesis and catabolism.

---

196. An adult client with hyperkalemia is prescribed sodium polystyrene sulfonate. Which serum potassium level is a clinical indicator of **effective** therapy?

1 4.9 mEq/L
2 5.4 mEq/L
3 5.8 mEq/L
4 6.2 mEq/L

Level of Cognitive Ability: Evaluating
Client Needs: Physiological Integrity
Clinical Judgment/Cognitive Skills: Evaluate Outcomes
Integrated Process: Nursing Process/Evaluation
Content Area: Pharmacology: Fluid and Electrolyte Balance: Electrolytes
Health Problem: N/A

Answer: 1
Rationale: The normal serum potassium level for an adult is 3.5 to 5.0 mEq/L. Option 1 is the only option that reflects a value within this range. The remaining options identify hyperkalemic levels.
Priority Nursing Tip: Electrocardiographic changes in hyperkalemia include tall-peaked T waves, flat P waves, widened QRS complexes, and prolonged PR intervals.

Test-Taking Strategy: Note the **strategic word,** *effective.* Without knowing the mechanism of action of sodium polystyrene sulfonate, compare each value with normal serum potassium levels. Note that only one value is within normal limits and that effective therapy is very likely to achieve normal results.

---

197. The nurse checks a client after abdominal surgery. The client has a nasogastric (NG) tube in place that is connected to suction. Which observation by the nurse indicates **most** reliably that the tube is functioning properly?

1 The suction gauge reads low intermittent suction.
2 The client indicates that pain is a 3 on a scale of 1 to 10.
3 The distal end of the NG tube is pinned to the client's gown.
4 The client denies nausea and has 250 mL of fluid in the suction collection container.

Level of Cognitive Ability: Evaluating
Client Needs: Physiological Integrity
Clinical Judgment/Cognitive Skills: Evaluate Outcomes
Integrated Process: Nursing Process/Evaluation
Content Area: Skills: Tube Care
Health Problem: N/A

Answer: 4
Rationale: An NG tube connected to suction is used postoperatively to decompress and rest the bowel. The gastrointestinal tract lacks peristaltic activity as a result of manipulation during surgery. The client would not experience symptoms of ileus (nausea and vomiting) if the tube is functioning properly. Although the nurse makes pertinent observations of the tube to ensure that it is secure and properly connected to suction, the client is checked for the effect. A pain indicator of 3 is an expected finding in a postoperative client.
Priority Nursing Tip: To determine the true or actual amount of NG drainage during a nursing shift, subtract the amount of irrigating solution used during the shift from the amount of drainage in the collection device.

Test-Taking Strategy: Note the **strategic word,** *most.* Focus on the **subject,** the proper functioning of the NG tube. Recalling the purpose of an NG tube in a postoperative client will direct you to the correct option.

198. The nurse is assisting in caring for a client who has returned from the postanesthesia care unit after prostatectomy. The client has a three-way Foley catheter with an infusion of continuous bladder irrigation (CBI). Which color description of the urinary drainage would lead the nurse to determine that the flow rate is adequate?

1 Dark cherry
2 Clear as water
3 Pale yellow or slightly pink
4 Concentrated yellow with small clots

Level of Cognitive Ability: Evaluating
Client Needs: Physiological Integrity
Clinical Judgment/Cognitive Skills: Evaluate Outcomes
Integrated Process: Nursing Process/Evaluation
Content Area: Adult Health: Renal and Urinary
Health Problem: Adult Health: Renal and Urinary: Obstructive Problems

Answer: 3
Rationale: The infusion of bladder irrigant is not at a preset rate; rather, it is increased or decreased to maintain urine that is a clear, pale yellow color or that has just a slight pink tinge. The infusion rate would be increased if the drainage is cherry-colored or if clots are seen. Alternatively, the rate can be slowed down slightly if the returns are as clear as water.
Priority Nursing Tip: If the client is receiving an infusion of CBI, use only sterile bladder irrigation solution or the prescribed solution to prevent water intoxication.

Test-Taking Strategy: Note the **subject**, an indication of an adequate flow rate of CBI. With this in mind, eliminate option 4 because clots are not expected. Eliminate options 1 and 2, which reflect inadequate or excessive irrigation flow, respectively.

---

199. The nurse caring for a client with Graves' disease is concerned about the client's caloric intake because of the resulting hypercatabolic state of the disorder. Which situation indicates a successful outcome for this concern?

1 The client verbalizes the need to avoid snacking between meals.
2 The client discusses the relationship between mealtime and the blood glucose level.
3 The client maintains a normal weight or gradually gains weight if it is below normal.
4 The client demonstrates knowledge regarding the need to consume a diet that is high in fat and low in protein.

Level of Cognitive Ability: Evaluating
Client Needs: Physiological Integrity
Clinical Judgment/Cognitive Skills: Evaluate Outcomes
Integrated Process: Nursing Process/Evaluation
Content Area: Adult Health: Endocrine
Health Problem: Adult Health: Endocrine: Thyroid Disorders

Answer: 3
Rationale: Graves' disease causes a state of chronic nutritional and caloric deficiency caused by the metabolic effects of excessive T_3 and T_4. Clinical manifestations are weight loss and increased appetite. Therefore, it is a nutritional goal that the client will not lose additional weight and that he or she will gradually return to the ideal body weight, if necessary. To accomplish this, the client must be encouraged to eat frequent high-calorie, high-protein, and high-carbohydrate meals and snacks.
Priority Nursing Tip: Provide a high-calorie diet to a client with Graves' disease because of the increased metabolic effects that are characteristic of the disorder.

Test-Taking Strategy: Focus on the **subject**, the client's need to manage his or her own hypercatabolic state. Eliminate options 1 and 4 because they would not be beneficial for a client in a hypercatabolic state. Option 2 can be eliminated because discussing the fluctuation in the blood glucose level will not be helpful for a client who is hypercatabolic.

---

200. The nurse is reviewing the results of a client's phenytoin level that was drawn that morning. Which result indicates that the level is therapeutic?

1 3 mcg/mL
2 8 mcg/mL
3 15 mcg/mL
4 24 mcg/mL

Level of Cognitive Ability: Evaluating
Client Needs: Physiological Integrity
Clinical Judgment/Cognitive Skills: Evaluate Outcomes
Integrated Process: Nursing Process/Evaluation
Content Area: Pharmacology: Neurological: Anticonvulsants
Health Problem: Adult Health: Neurological: Seizure Disorder/Epilepsy

Answer: 3
Rationale: The therapeutic range for serum phenytoin levels is 10 to 20 mcg/mL in clients with normal serum albumin levels and renal function. A level below this range indicates that the client is receiving insufficient medication and is at risk for seizure activity. In this case, the medication dose would be adjusted upward. A level above the therapeutic range indicates that the client is entering the toxic range and is at risk for toxic side effects of the medication. In this case, the dose would be adjusted downward.
Priority Nursing Tip: The client prescribed the anticonvulsant phenytoin needs to be informed of the need for monitoring therapeutic serum drug levels to monitor for toxicity.

Test-Taking Strategy: Focus on the **subject,** the therapeutic drug serum level. Recalling that this level for phenytoin is 10 to 20 mcg/mL will direct you to the correct option.

---

201. The nurse reinforces information to a parent regarding the appropriate actions to take when the toddler has a temper tantrum. Which statement by the parent indicates a successful outcome of the teaching?

1 "I will ignore the tantrums as long as there is no physical danger."
2 "I will give frequent reminders that only bad children have tantrums."
3 "I will send my child to a room alone for 10 minutes after every tantrum."
4 "I will reward my child with candy at the end of each day without a tantrum."

Level of Cognitive Ability: Evaluating
Client Needs: Health Promotion and Maintenance
Clinical Judgment/Cognitive Skills: Evaluate Outcomes
Integrated Process: Nursing Process/Evaluation
Content Area: Developmental Stages: Toddler
Health Problem: N/A

Answer: 1
Rationale: Ignoring a negative attention-seeking behavior is considered the best way to extinguish it, provided that the child is safe from injury. Option 2 is untrue and negative. Option 3 gives attention to the tantrum and also exceeds the recommended time of 1 minute per year of age for a time-out. Providing candy for rewards is unhealthy and unlikely to be effective at the end of the day.
Priority Nursing Tip: Anticipate temper tantrums from a toddler. Ensure a safe environment if the toddler displays physical acting-out behaviors.

Test-Taking Strategy: Focus on the **subject,** toddler tantrum management. Recalling that ignoring a tantrum is the best way to extinguish it will direct you to the correct option.

---

202. The nurse is caring for a client who is placed in seclusion because of violent behavior. Which client statement indicates to the nurse that the seclusion is no longer necessary?

1 "I am in control of myself now."
2 "I need to use the restroom right away."
3 "I'd like to go back to my room and be alone for a while."
4 "I can't breathe in here. It feels like the walls are closing in on me."

Level of Cognitive Ability: Evaluating
Client Needs: Psychosocial Integrity
Clinical Judgment/Cognitive Skills: Evaluate Outcomes
Integrated Process: Nursing Process/Evaluation
Content Area: Mental Health
Health Problem: N/A

Answer: 1
Rationale: Option 1 indicates that the client may be safely removed from seclusion. The client in seclusion must be checked at regular intervals (usually every 15 to 30 minutes) for physical needs, safety, and comfort. Option 2 indicates a physical need that could be met with a urinal, bedpan, or commode; it does not indicate that the client has calmed down enough to leave the seclusion room. Option 3 could be an attempt to manipulate the nurse; it gives no indication that the client will control himself or herself when alone in the room. Option 4 could be handled by supportive communication or an as-needed medication, if indicated; it does not necessitate discontinuing seclusion.
Priority Nursing Tip: Within 1 hour of the initiation of restraints or seclusion of a client with a mental health disorder, the psychiatrist must make a face-to-face assessment and evaluation of the client. Agency and state policies and procedures regarding the use of restraints and seclusion are always followed.

Test-Taking Strategy: Focus on the **subject,** removing a client from seclusion. Recalling the purpose and the use of seclusion will direct you to the correct option.

---

203. The nurse has assisted to create a plan of care for a client who is in traction; its interventions focus on the client reassuming self-care. The nurse evaluates the plan of care and determines that which observation indicates a successful outcome?

1 The client denies a need for assistance with care.
2 The client allows the family to perform the care.
3 The client assists in self-care as much as possible.
4 The client allows the nurse to complete the care on a daily basis.

Level of Cognitive Ability: Evaluating
Client Needs: Physiological Integrity
Clinical Judgment/Cognitive Skills: Evaluate Outcomes
Integrated Process: Nursing Process/Evaluation
Content Area: Adult Health: Musculoskeletal
Health Problem: Adult Health: Musculoskeletal: Skeletal Injury

Answer: 3
Rationale: A successful outcome for reassuming self-care is for the client to do as much of the self-care as possible. The nurse would promote independence in the client and allow the client to perform as much self-care as is optimal, considering the client's condition. The nurse would determine that the outcome is unsuccessful if the client denies the need for assistance or allows others to perform the care.
Priority Nursing Tip: To maintain self-esteem and client dignity, the nurse would encourage and maintain client independence in the performance of activities of daily living as much as possible.

Test-Taking Strategy: Focus on the **subject,** reassuming of self-care. Option 1 can be eliminated first because the client is denying a need for assistance. Then eliminate options 2 and 4, which are **comparable or alike** in that they indicate relying on others to perform care.

---

204. The nurse is monitoring a male client with a spinal cord injury who is experiencing spinal shock. Which findings indicate that the spinal shock is resolving? **Select all that apply.**

- ❒ 1 Flaccidity
- ❒ 2 Presence of a gag reflex
- ❒ 3 Positive Babinski's reflex
- ❒ 4 Development of hyperreflexia
- ❒ 5 Return of the bulbocavernosus reflex
- ❒ 6 Return of reflex emptying of the bladder

Level of Cognitive Ability: Evaluating
Client Needs: Physiological Integrity
Clinical Judgment/Cognitive Skills: Evaluate Outcomes
Integrated Process: Nursing Process/Evaluation
Content Area: Complex Care: Trauma
Health Problem: Adult Health: Neurological: Spinal Cord Injury

Answer: 3, 4, 5, 6

Rationale: Spinal shock is associated with acute injury to the spinal cord with temporary suppression of reflexes controlled by segments below the level of injury. It may last for 1 to 6 weeks. Indications that spinal shock is resolving include a return of reflexes, development of hyperreflexia rather than flaccidity, and return of reflex emptying of the bladder. The return of the bulbocavernosus reflex in male clients is also an early indicator of recovery from spinal shock. Babinski's reflex (dorsiflexion of the great toe with fanning of the other toes when the sole of the foot is stroked) is an early returning reflex. The gag reflex is not lost in spinal shock; therefore, its presence is not an indication of resolving spinal shock.

Priority Nursing Tip: For clients with spinal cord injuries above the level of T6, autonomic dysreflexia may occur as a result of autonomic nervous system overstimulation. The clinical manifestations include severe hypertension, throbbing headaches, diaphoresis, nasal stuffiness, flushing above the level of the injury, and bradycardia.

Test-Taking Strategy: Focus on the **subject,** indications that spinal shock is resolving. As you read each option, recall that spinal shock is associated with acute injury to the spinal cord with temporary suppression of reflexes controlled by segments below the level of injury. This will assist in eliminating flaccidity and the presence of a gag reflex as signs that spinal shock is resolving.

---

205. The nurse is assisting in the monitoring of a client with acute respiratory failure on mechanical ventilation via an oral endotracheal tube. Which of the following would be indicative of possible causes of the high-pressure alarm sounding? **Select all that apply.**

- ❒ 1 A kink in the tube
- ❒ 2 The client fighting the ventilator
- ❒ 3 Increased secretions in the airway
- ❒ 4 A cuff leak in the endotracheal tube
- ❒ 5 The client biting on the endotracheal tube
- ❒ 6 The ventilator tubing disconnecting from the endotracheal tube

Level of Cognitive Ability: Evaluating
Client Needs: Physiological Integrity
Clinical Judgment/Cognitive Skills: Analyze Cues
Integrated Process: Nursing Process/Evaluation
Content Area: Complex Care: Acute Respiratory Failure
Health Problem: Adult Health: Respiratory: Acute Respiratory Distress Syndrome/Failure

Answer: 1, 2, 3, 5

Rationale: The high-pressure alarm sounds when the peak inspiratory pressure reaches the set alarm limit. Causes include obstruction of the endotracheal tube because of the client lying on the tube, or water or a kink in the tubing; the client being anxious or fighting the ventilator; an increased amount of secretions in the airway or a mucus plug; the client coughing, gagging, or biting on the oral endotracheal tube; decreased airway size related to wheezing or bronchospasm; pneumothorax; and displacement of the artificial airway and the endotracheal tube slipping into the right main stem bronchus. The low-pressure alarm sounds when there is a leak or disconnection in the ventilator circuit or a leak in the client's artificial airway cuff.

Priority Nursing Tip: The nurse never shuts the alarms on a ventilator to the off position.

Test-Taking Strategy: Focus on the **subject,** the triggers of the high-pressure alarm. Recalling that the high-pressure alarm sounds when the peak inspiratory pressure reaches the set alarm limit assists in eliminating options 4 and 6. In addition, remember that "L" in "low" can be associated with "L" in "leak" for low-pressure alarms.

---

206. The nurse is assisting the clinic nurse in observing a student perform a physical assessment on a client. During the observed assessment, the nurse determines that the student is performing which physical assessment correctly? **Refer to figure.**

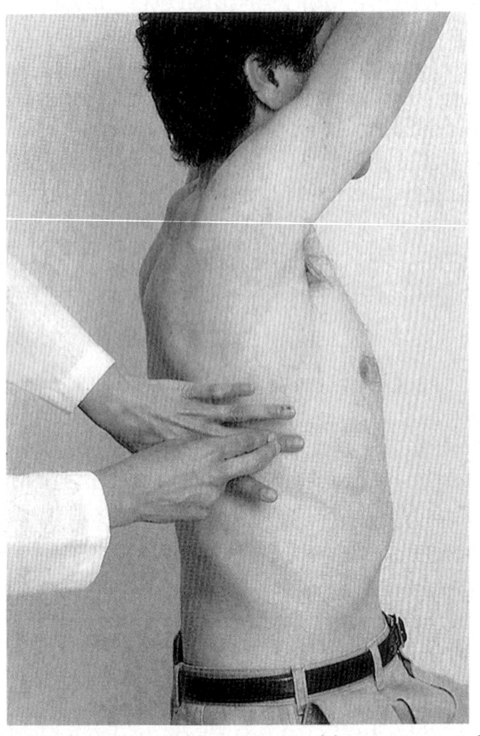

(From Wilson SF, Giddens JF: *Health assessment for nursing practice*, ed 5, St. Louis, 2013, Mosby.)

1 Palpation
2 Inspection
3 Percussion
4 Auscultation

Level of Cognitive Ability: Evaluating
Client Needs: Health Promotion and Maintenance
Clinical Judgment/Cognitive Skills: Evaluate Outcomes
Integrated Process: Nursing Process/Evaluation
Content Area: Health Assessment/Physical Exam: Thorax and Lungs
Health Problem: N/A

Answer: 3
Rationale: To perform percussion, the nurse places the middle finger of the nondominant hand against the body's surface. The tip of the middle finger of the dominant hand strikes the top of the middle finger of the nondominant hand. Palpation is performed using the sense of touch. Inspection is the process of observation. Auscultation involves listening to the sounds produced by the body.
Priority Nursing Tip: When auscultating breath sounds, instruct the client to breathe through the mouth. Monitor the client for dizziness, and provide a rest period if dizziness occurs.

Test-Taking Strategy: Focus on the **subject**, identifying data collection techniques. Recalling the definition of each technique listed in the options will direct you to the correct option. Remember that inspection is observing, palpation uses the sense of touch, and auscultation is listening.